SCIENTIFIC BASIS FOR AYURVEDIC THERAPIES

SCIENTIFIC BASIS FOR AYURVEDIC THERAPIES

EDITED BY
LAKSHMI CHANDRA MISHRA

CRC PRESS

Boca Raton London New York Washington, D.C.

Library of Congress Cataloging-in-Publication Data

Scientific basis for Ayurvedic therapies / edited by Lakshmi C. Mishra.
p. cm.
Includes bibliographical references and index.
ISBN 0-8493-1366-X (alk. paper)
1. Medicine, Ayurvedic. I. Mishra, Lakshmi C. (Lakshmi Chandra)
[DNLM: 1. Medicine, Ayurvedic. WB 50.1 S416 2003]
R605.S376 2003
615.5′3—dc21 2003055156

Direct all inquiries to CRC Press LLC, 2000 N.W. Corporate Blvd., Boca Raton, Florida 33431.

International Standard Book Number 0-8493-1366-X
Library of Congress Card Number 2003055156
Printed in the United States of America 1 2 3 4 5 6 7 8 9 0
Printed on acid-free paper

Preface

There has been increasing public interest in complementary alternative medicine during the past decade in the U.S. that led to the establishment of the Center for Alternative and Complementary Medicine at the National Institutes of Health (NIH), Bethesda, MD, by the U.S. Congress to conduct scientific evaluation of these therapies. The Ayurvedic system of medicine (traditional medical system of India) is recognized by NIH as a complementary and alternative medicine (CAM). Ayurveda has been practiced in India for over 5000 years and is recognized as a complete medical system comparable with allopathic medicine by the government of India. In India, Ayurveda has a complete infrastructure, medical colleges, hospitals integrated with allopathic medicine, research institutes, and scientific journals devoted to Ayurveda. In addition, India's Ayurvedic pharmaceutical industry is governed by the same food and drug laws that regulate conventional drugs. Research in pharmacology, biochemistry, phytochemistry, and clinical trials of Ayurvedic therapies currently constitutes a substantial portion of the total research conducted in government institutes and medical colleges in India.

There has been considerable scientific research effort in Ayurvedic therapies during the past 50 years. This research has not been adequately disseminated to Ayurvedic students and physicians. In order to accomplish the assimilation of this research into practice, three major goals were set for this book: (1) to provide information on pharmacological, biochemical, and clinical investigations on Ayurvedic therapies; (2) to explore the scientific basis of Ayurvedic concepts of diseases, diagnosis, and treatments; and (3) to develop new interpretation of Ayurvedic concepts of therapies based on modern knowledge where possible.

As editor of the book, I used my combination of medical education in Ayurveda and research experience in conventional medicinal pharmacy and pharmacology in developing this text. Disease topics were carefully selected based on the scientific studies available and the prevalence of a disease. Knowledgeable physicians and scientists in these fields were selected based on their scientific contributions in the field to review and evaluate the worldwide literature. In addition, I, along with one Ayurvedic physician, one biochemist, and one overall expert with knowledge in conventional and CAM research methods, read each chapter.

General topics such as Ayurvedic disease management, *panchakarma*, Ayurvedic *bhasmas*, the current status of Ayurveda in India, and clinical research design and evaluation of typical clinical trials of certain diseases were written by experts in their fields.

It is my hope that the book will prove useful to all Ayurvedic and conventional medicine physicians, students and scientists, and the general public. In addition, the book is expected to bring awareness to the community of health-care providers that Ayurveda is significantly more than a few home remedies, yoga, and meditation. It is a fully established system of medicine, has a considerable scientific base, and has therapies that can be used alone or as an adjuvant with conventional health care as practiced in India.

Lakshmi Chandra Mishra
Editor

Acknowledgments

I gratefully thank first and foremost Dr. Betsy B. Singh, professor and dean of the Research Division, Southern California University of Health Sciences (SCUHS), for the encouragement and sincere help given to me in preparing this book. Dr. Singh took great interest in reviewing all the chapters and provided valuable comments in the area of science and clinical research methods. I am thankful to Dr. Sivarama Prasad Vinjamury, associate professor; Dinesha Ninjegowda, Research Division, SCUHS; and Vijay Singh for help in reviewing the chapters. Finally, I thank Neil Shepard and Raheleh Khorsan of the Research Division and Dr. Tarek Adra and Dyba Kalyani, SCUHS students, for the technical support provided.

I sincerely acknowledge the effort of all contributors, particularly those who contributed more than one chapter and made all the required changes requested by reviewers and editors on time. These contributors worked hard to secure the information required for the chapters, to take a scientific approach to the presentation of both the Ayurvedic and conventional medicine data on a particular topic.

Finally, I thank my children, Aparna Rani, Gyan Sagar, Anita Rani, and Dhyan Sagar, for their encouragement during the preparation of this book.

Lakshmi Chandra Mishra
Editor

Editor

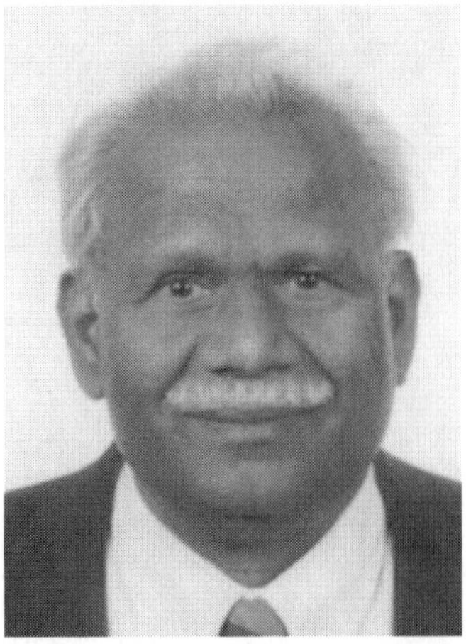

Lakshmi Chandra Mishra, Ph.D., is a professor in the Research Division of Southern California University of Health Sciences and an Ayurvedic medicine practitioner at the University Health Center, Southern California University, Whittier. He has been conducting research on Ayurvedic therapies for musculoskeletal disorders at the university, and stroke in collaboration with faculty at the University of Southern California, School of Pharmacy.

Dr. Mishra received his Bachelor of Indian Medicine and Surgery degree from Bundelkand Ayurvedic College, Jhansi, UP, India, in 1954 and practiced Ayurvedic medicine for several years thereafter. He received his bachelor's and master's degrees in pharmacy from Banaras Hindu University, Varanasi, UP, India, in 1958 and 1959, respectively. He conducted phytochemical and pharmacognostical studies on an Ayurvedic herb for his master's degree thesis. After getting his pharmacy degrees, he worked as a pharmaceutical chemist at the Hindustan Antibiotics Ltd., Pimpari Poona, for 1 year and then as an assistant professor of pharmacology at Maulana Azad Medical College, New Delhi.

After coming to the U.S. in 1963, Dr. Mishra received his Ph.D. in biochemical pharmacology from the State University of New York at Buffalo in 1967. Dr. Mishra worked on cancer chemotherapy research at Roswell Park Memorial Institute in Buffalo for 1 year before joining Microbiological Associates, Bethesda, MD, where he conducted research on anticancer agents that was sponsored by the National Cancer Institute, National Institutes of Health (NIH), Bethesda, MD. He later worked for several federal regulatory government agencies as a pharmacologtist, toxicologist, and branch chief. Dr. Mishra has served on many scientific committees in government and industry. He was an ex-officio member of the National Cancer Advisory Board of the National Cancer Institute, NIH, for 18 years.

Dr. Mishra has extensive background and experience both as a clinician in the traditional and modern practice of Ayurveda and as a bench scientist. His research expertise includes pharmacology, toxicology, pharmaceutical chemistry, pharmacognosy, and phytochemistry. He has authored more than 100 scientific papers, documents, and reports in the fields of Ayurvedic medicine, pharmacology, toxicology, cancer chemotherapy, and health risk assessment, particularly cancer and neurotoxicity risk for exposure to environmental pollutants.

Contributors

Tarek Adra, D. Pharm. Southern California University of Allied Health Sciences, La Habra, California, U.S.A.

Mohammed Abdulkadar Akbarsha, Ph.D. Department of Animal Science, School of Life Sciences, Bharathidasan University, Tiruchirappalli, India

Premalatha Balachandran, M.Sc., Ph.D. National Center for Natural Products Research, Department of Pharmacognosy, School of Pharmacy, University of Mississippi, University, Mississippi, U.S.A.

Sailaja Vani Batchu, B.A.M.S., M.D. (Ayu) Institute of Medical Sciences, Banaras Hindu University, Varanasi, India

Heena A. Bhatt, B.A.M.S., D.H.M.M. Department of Clinical Pharmacology, Seth GS Medical College and KEM Hospital, Bombay, Maharashtra, India

Nandkishore J. Chikhale, M.Sc., Ph.D. Department of Biotechnology, Amravati University, Amravati, Maharashtra, India

Manjusha J. Choukhande, B.A.M.S., M.D., Ph.D. Health Clinic, Amravati University, Amravati, Maharashtra, India

Sudeshna S. Dalvi, M.D. Department of Clinical Pharmacology, Seth GS Medical College and KEM Hospital, Bombay, Maharashtra, India

Milind N. Dudhane, M.Sc., Ph.D. Punjab Rao Deskmukh Medical College, Amravati, Maharashtra, India

Karunakaran Gauthaman, M.Pharm., Ph.D. Department of Biochemistry and Molecular Biology, University of Madras, Guindy Campus Chennai, India

Nithya J. Gogtay, M.D., D.N.B. Department of Clinical Pharmacology, Seth GS Medical College and KEM Hospital, Bombay, Maharashtra, India

Rajgopal Govindarajan, M.V.Sc., Ph.D. Department of Biochemistry and Molecular Biology, University of Nebraska Medical Center, Omaha, Nebraska, U.S.A.

Bharati A. Joshi, B.A.M.S. Bhavan's Swami Prakashananda Ayurveda Research Centre, Juhu, Mumbai, India

Sushil K. Kabra, M.D. Department of Pediatrics, All India Institute of Medical Sciences, Ansari Nagar, New Delhi, India

Anand Kar, Ph.D. Thyroid Research Unit, School of Life Sciences, Devi Ahilya University, Indore, India

Satwinderjeet Kaur, M.Sc., Ph.D. Department of Botanical and Environmental Sciences, Guru Nanak Dev University, Amritsar, Panjab, India

Nilima A. Kshirsagar, M.D., Ph.D. Department of Clinical Pharmacology, Seth GS Medical College and KEM Hospital, Bombay, Maharashtra, India

P.N.V. Kurup, Vaidya Shastry, Vaidya Kalanidhi, H.P.A. (Jamnagar), D. Litt (Jamnagar), Mahamahopadhyaya Office of the Vice Chancellor, Gujarat Ayurved University, Chanakya Bhavan, Jamnagar, Gujarat, India

I. Rajya Lakshmi, M.D. Varun Herbals Pvt. Ltd., Hyderabad, India

Rakesh Lodha, M.D. Department of Pediatrics, All India Institute of Medical Sciences, Ansari Nagar, New Delhi, India

Viswanatha Menon Madhavachandran, B.A.M.S. Experimental Pharmacology Unit, Nagarjuna Herbal Concentrates Ltd., Thodupuzha, Kerala, India

Lakshmi Chandra Mishra, M.Pharm., Ph.D., B.I.M.S. Research Division, Southern California University, Whittier, California, U.S.A.

Shankar K. Mitra, M.D. (Ayu) Research and Technical Services, The Himalaya Drug Company, Makali, Bangalore, India

Ashish A. Mungantiwar, B.Pharm., Ph.D. Macleods Pharmaceutical Ltd., Mumbai, India

Nutan S. Nabar, M.D. (Ayu) CSIR-NMITLI-DM, Bhavan's Swami Prakashananda Ayurveda Research Centre, Juhu, Mumbai, India

Natesh Nagashayana, M.D. (Ayu) Central Government Health Scheme, Basavanagudi, Bangalore, India

Sunanda Panda, M.D. Thyroid Research Unit, School of Life Sciences, Devi Ahilya University, Indore, India

Aashish S. Phadke, M.D. (Ayu), M.I.I.M. (Gold Medal), M.I.O.A., D.Opt. Center for Ayurveda & Panchakarma Therapy, Eye Care Clinic, Vashi; Department of Dravyaguna and Faculty of Department of Shalakyatantra (Ayurvedic Ophthalmology), Y.M.T. Ayurvedic Medical College, Navi Mumbai, Maharashtra, India

Mahendra K. Rai, M.Sc., Ph.D. Department of Biotechnology, Amravati University, Amravati, Maharashtra, India

Sheikh Raisuddin, Ph.D. Department of Medical Elementology and Toxicology, Jamia, Hamdard University, New Delhi, India

Paramesh R. Rangesh, M.D. (Ayu) Research and Development Center, The Himalaya Drug Company, Makali, Banglore, India

I. Sanjeeva Rao, B.A.M.S., M.D. (Ayu), M.D. (Unani) Hyderabad, India

Manoranjan Sahu, M.D. (Ayu), Ph.D. Department of Shalya Shalakya, Institute of Medical Sciences, Banaras Hindu University,Varanasi, India

Krishnamurthy Sairam, M.Pharm., Ph.D. Department of Pharmacology, College of Pharmacy, Kancheepuram, Tamil Nadu, India; University of Kentucky, Lexington, Kentucky, U.S.A.

Ajay Kumar Sharma, M.D. (Ayu), Ph.D. Department of P.G. and Kaya Chikitsa, National Institute of Ayurveda, Jawahr, Jaipur, India

Betsy B. Singh, Ph.D. Research Division, Southern California University of Health Sciences, South Whittier, California, U.S.A.

R.H. Singh, M.D. (Ayu) Faculty of Ayurveda, Institute of Medical Sciences, Banaras Hindu University, Varanasi, India

Subhash Singh, M.D. (Ayu) Central Research Institute, Patiala, Punjab, India

Vijay John Singh, B.S. Argosy University, Irvine, and Southern California University–RD, South Whitter, California, U.S.A.

Venigalla Sridevi, M.D. (Ayu) Arvind Remedies Ltd., Chennai, India

Appian Subramoniam, Ph.D. Ethnopharmacology Unit, Tropical Botanical Garden and Research Institute, Thiruvananthapuram, Kerala, India

Ashok D.B. Vaidya, M.D., Ph.D., F.A.I.M. Bhavan's Swami Prakashananda Ayurveda Research Centre, Juhu, Mumbai, India

Rama A. Vaidya, M.D., Ph.D., D.G.O., D.F.P. Bhavan's Swami Prakashananda Ayurveda Research Centre, Juhu, Mumbai, India

Manjusha Vinjamury, M.D. (Ayu) Center for Ayurvedic Research and Enlightenment, Irvine, California, U.S.A.

Sivarama P. Vinjamury, M.D. (Ayu), M.A.O.M. Southern California University of Health Sciences, South Whittier, California, U.S.A.

Divya Shangari Vohora, M.Pharm., Ph.D. Department of Pharmacology, Hamdard University, New Delhi, India

Introduction

The objective of this book is to explore a scientific basis for Ayurvedic medicine and create a better understanding of Ayurveda among health-care providers and consumers. Books published in the West on Ayurveda generally discuss only a few aspects of Ayurveda such as dietary and lifestyle changes, yoga, breathing exercises, meditation practices, and aroma, gem-stones, color, music therapy, herbs, and other therapies. In fact, these areas cover only a small fraction of the body of classical Ayurveda. These areas offer little or no information about current biochemical, pharmacological, and clinical investigations. During the past 100 years, several hundred Ayurvedic herbs have been investigated with respect to plant chemistry, active chemical constituents, pharmacological effects, safety, and efficacy. However, the basic research on Ayurvedic therapeutic agents has not been adequately integrated into disease management protocols available to most consumers in the West.

The origin of Ayurveda is traced back to four books of knowledge called *vedas*: *Rigveda, Samveda, Yjurveda*, and *Atharveda* (4500 to 1600 B.C.). The information on health care was subsequently developed by many Ayurvedic practitioners and finally compiled into three important books known in Ayurveda as the senior triad (*vriddha traya*): *Charak Samhita, Sushrut Samhita,* and *Ashtang Hridaya Samhita.* The subsequent three books that are commentaries on the senior triads are known as the junior triad (*laghu traya*): *Madhava-nidana, Sarangdhar Samhita,* and *Bhavaprakash Nighantu.* These books contain basic concepts of health and disease, disease management, anatomy and physiology, hygiene, materia medica, pharmacology and therapeutics, herbal formulations, pharmacy, and synthesis of herbo-mineral formulas. Diseases are classified according to organ systems and functions. Specialties such as internal medicine, surgery, pediatrics, gynecology, obstetrics, eye, ear, nose, and throat diseases, geriatrics, eugenics and aphrodisiacs, psychiatry, pharmacology, toxicology, and pharmacy are clearly delineated and discussed in detail in Ayurveda.[1]

Although there is no record of pharmacological testing during the time period when Ayurvedic texts were written, 50 distinct pharmacological categories of medicinal plants were described. The categories include anti-inflammatory, analgesic, antiallergic, antihistaminic, antidiuretic, diuretic, antiemetic, emetic, purgative, astringent, antiasthmatic, antipyretic, and others.[2] Similar to conventional medicine, Ayurvedic medicine has also benefited from advances in science and technology. These advances facilitated the understanding of diseases, the development of better pharmaceutical products, and the implementation of diagnostic techniques. Scientific studies in laboratory animals have now confirmed the pharmacological properties of many Ayurvedic herbs. The old concept of accepting the last word of an Ayurvedic teacher without questioning the scientific underpinning has begun to disappear. A large number of medical schools and medical research institutions, both private and governmental, are currently involved in Ayurvedic research. The government of India has established an agency, the Central Council for Research in Ayurveda and Siddha (CCRAS) under the Ministry of Health and Family Welfare, to sponsor and conduct research in Ayurveda. The agency has been conducting and sponsoring Ayurvedic research all over India for more than 30 years in 70 regional Ayurvedic research institutions. The agency is conducting clinical trials to investigate the effectiveness of Ayurvedic products as well as basic research. Some of the clinical trials conducted by the agency are discussed in Chapter 3, "Clinical Research Design: Limited Systematic Review on Five Diagnosis Categories." The basic research includes pharmacology, biochemistry, plant chemistry, product development, the cultivation of medicinal plants, and manufacturing practices for safe and effective Ayurvedic products.

Basic Concept

Whereas conventional medicine is primarily oriented toward the treatment of disease, Ayurvedic medicine is oriented toward prevention, health maintenance, and treatment. In conventional medicine, drugs are developed based on the concept that the elimination of specific causes of a disease, such as microorganisms, will cure a disease. On the other hand, the belief in Ayurvedic medicine is that a disease is the product of an imbalance in the body and mental elements that reduce the body's resistance to diseases. If the imbalance is corrected and the body's defense mechanisms are strengthened by herbal formulas, lifestyle changes, and diet, then the body will resist a disease with a goal of eliminating it. Herbal and herbomineral products regularly used in Ayurveda are believed to strengthen the body's defenses. Scientific evidence is gradually developing in support of the Ayurvedic concept.[3]

Ayurvedic Physician

Scientific, technical, and engineering advances in the 20th century have been extraordinary. They created an explosion of new information and understanding in molecular biology, biochemistry, physiology, antibiotics, vaccines, genetics, mapping of genome, and the identification of genes responsible for inherited diseases. Ayurvedic physicians have also benefited from these new medical advances. Scientifically based information is the core of the preclinical, clinical, residency, and continuing medical education phases of training.

An Ayurvedic physician must be able to understand and appreciate new scientific knowledge in order to maximize the benefits of Ayurvedic therapies. In order to do so, an Ayurvedic physician must be aware of the current information on the disease processes, inter- and intracellular message transmission, membrane transport, protein interactions, chemical and microbial toxins, autoimmunity, cellular and humoral immunity, and dynamics of neurotransmitters. A physician needs to know about genetics, congenital inborn metabolic problems, pharmacological and biochemical research, and the use of various clinical chemistry data in diagnosis and monitoring disease processes in order to interpret the clinical data. He must understand the basic principles of toxicology and how the knowledge can be used in developing protocols for clinical studies. He must also know how to apply basic science to the Ayurvedic concept of disease management and the use of modern diagnostic methods involving urine and blood chemistry, enzyme assays, histology, pathology, radiology, etc. Finally, the Ayurvedic physician must understand the interaction of spiritual and psychological elements of patients as described in Ayurveda and be able to earn the patient's trust through compassionate and holistic care.

Educational Standards

An Internet search revealed a dozen Ayurvedic colleges in the U.S. offering weekend courses ranging from 1 to 3 years. The curriculums are designed to familiarize students with Ayurvedic therapies, but are inadequate for actual clinical practice. Because Ayurveda is currently unregulated in the U.S., there are no standards to meet or pass any state examination. Because herbs or herbominerals are included under the U.S. Dietary Supplement Health and Education Act (U.S. DSHEA, 1994), Ayurvedic practitioners in the U.S. recommend herbal formulas as dietary supplements along with dietary changes, yoga, and breathing exercises to help remedy certain health problems.

Ayurveda has been recognized as an independent medical system by the government of India for a long time. The Central Council of Indian Medicine (CCIM), Ministry of Health (Regulations 1986, Minimum Education in Indian Medicine) regulates Ayurvedic education and training in India.[4] The curriculum includes 2820 hours of theory and 780 hours of practical and laboratory work over a period of 54 months; this is followed by 1 year of residency leading to a Bachelor of Ayurvedic Medicine and Surgery,[5] formerly Bachelor of Indian Medicine and Surgery. This is an integrated program that teaches Ayurvedic and alopathic courses so that therapeutic options for patients may be maximized.

Reasons for the Current Interest in Ayurveda

The great therapeutic success of synthetic antibiotics, hormones, and vaccines has created an expectation that conventional medicine will be able to discover a cure for every ailment. This expectation has been only minimally met for many diseases (e.g., cancer, arthritis, autoimmune diseases, and AIDS) even after spending hundreds of billions of dollars in research worldwide over the past 30 years. In addition, the synthetic antibiotics and steroids sometimes result in serious adverse effects, such as immunosuppression, gastrointestinal bleeding, and ulcers, after prolonged administration. Ayurvedic therapies generally provide relief without such adverse effects even after prolonged administration. Some formulas known as *rasayanas* are believed to improve the body's defense mechanisms. For example, in one short study for 90 days with *chyawanprash*, a *rasayana*, the following improvements were observed: increased stress tolerance; improved endocrine functions (adrenal and testicular); positive nitrogen balance as indicated by increased serum protein level; and a decrease in urinary levels of nitrogen, creatinine, mucopolysaccharide, and hydroxyproline. The general well-being of the volunteers improved and none of them complained of any physical disorder.[3]

Ayurvedic herbs and formulas often have a wide spectrum of therapeutic activity. For example, *guggul* is recommended in Ayurveda for 25 or more ailments (e.g., inflammatory diseases, a variety of infections, muscle spasm, cough, bronchitis, anemia, endometritis, neurological diseases, skin diseases, urinary system disorders, obesity, osteoarthritis, and rheumatoid arthritis). The reason for this wide spectrum of activity is that *guggul* has anti-inflammatory, anticoagulant, hypolipidemic, and antibacterial activity; it can be beneficial in many health ailments associated with inflammation, infection, obesity, or blood clotting. Additionally, pharmacological activities of herbs may not be confined to one specific chemical constituent. *Guggul* was found to have anti-inflammatory activity in both polar and nonpolar solvents, indicating that several chemical constituents present in it may have anti-inflammatory activity.[5] Similarly, herbs showing neuropharmacological activity *in vitro* did not have the activity concentrated in any one solvent extract. This indicates that several constituents with different chemical physical properties may have the same neuropharmacological activity.[6]

Ayurvedic therapies are known to be relatively economic. For example, a 1-month dose of an Ayurvedic formula for arthritis may be obtained at this time for about $20, which is often the co-payment for brand name prescription drugs for many health insurance and health maintenance organizations. Other alternative nondrug complementary therapies may be even more expensive.

The relative safety of Ayurvedic medicine is another reason for its popularity. Ayurvedic formulas are time tested for safety. These formulas contain vitamins; minerals; biologically active steroids, alkaloids, glycosides, and tannins; and a variety of antioxidants in a natural state. A single herb extract or a pure active chemical constituent may cause some adverse effects under certain conditions and dose levels. For example, *guggul* extract has been shown to produce some anticoagulant effect under certain conditions.[7,8] Ayurvedic text formulas containing *guggul* may be safer than the *guggul* extract; the formulas that have *guggul* in relatively small amounts, along with many other herbs, act as synergists and possibly counteract some of the side effects.

Quality of Ayurvedic Formulas

In order to assure quality of Ayurvedic formulas, the government of India, Ministry of Health, amended the Drugs and Cosmetic Act of 1940 in 1964 to include Ayurvedic drugs (Ayurvedic herbs and herbal formulas). The Act requires the raw materials to be genuine and adequately identified; the formulas must contain ingredients listed on the label and manufacturing must be conducted under prescribed good manufacturing practices conditions. CCRAS developed a formulary of Ayurvedic text formulas called *The Ayurvedic Formulary of India* published in 1978. CCRAS conducted research to establish enforceable standards for Ayurvedic formulas similar to allopathic drugs and promulgated the standards. The book *Pharamcopoeial Standards of Ayurvedic Formulations* was first published in 1976 and subsequently revised in 1987. This effort was followed by the development of *The Ayurvedic Pharmacopoeia of India* in 1989. The pharmacopoeia contains the popular names; macroscopic and microscopic description of herbs; and limits for foreign matter, total ash, acid-insoluble ash, alcohol-soluble extractive, water-soluble extractive, and heavy metals in the same way as prescribed in allopathic pharmacopoeias. It also gives the levels of known chemical constituents, therapeutic uses, and doses.

Organization of the Book

Only a few diseases are selected based on the scientific data available on Ayurvedic therapies. Specialists in treating each disease searched the worldwide literature, critically reviewed the information on the basis of their expertise, and summarized the information in an understandable and easily usable form. Ayurvedic description and therapy of a disease are first described followed by a discussion using current knowledge. Available pharmacological, biochemical, and chemical studies on herbs used in the management of the disease are evaluated to determine if there is an adequate scientific basis for their use. Finally, the overall management strategy of the disease, commonly used therapies, and scientific data are presented.

An attempt is made to first use the English translation or meaning of the Ayurvedic word, followed by the Ayurvedic word in parentheses as often as possible to make the chapters easy to read and understand. In addition, a list of Ayurvedic words is provided in Appendix 1. Other lists provided are botanical and Ayurvedic names of herbs, names and addresses of the manufacturers of Ayurvedic formulas, and a list of journals publishing articles on Ayurvedic therapies. The words *Ayurvedic texts* or *Ayurveda* refer to the senior and junior triads in all chapters.

The book is organized to give a global picture of Ayurveda and to show that these therapies are relatively safe, effective, and have supporting scientific data. It is intended to provide better understanding of Ayurvedic medicine so that wherever appropriate, the integration of these therapies by the health-care providers may become possible.

References

1. Mishra, L., Singh, B.B., and Dagenais, S., Ayurveda: a historical perspective and principles of the traditional healthcare system in India, *Altern. Ther. Health Med.*, 7(2), 36–42, 2001a.
2. Mishra, L., Singh, B.B., and Dagenais, S., Healthcare and disease management in Ayurveda, *Altern. Ther. Health Med.*, 7(2), 44–50, 2001b.
3. Udupa, K.N. and Singh, R.H., *Clinical & Experimental Studies on Rasayana Drugs and Panchkarma Therapy* (monograph), Central Council for Research in Ayurveda and Siddha, New Delhi, India, 1993.
4. Central Council of Indian Medicine (Minimum Standards of Education in Indian Medicine) Regulations, 1986, New Delhi-110055, 13 July, 1989, in *Abstracts of the Gazette of India*, Part III, Section 4, August 5, 1989.
5. Gujral, M.L., Sareen, K., Tangri, K.K., Amma, M.K.P., and Roy, A.K., Anti-arthritic and anti-inflammatory activity of gum (balsamodendrone mukul hook), *Indian J. Physiol. Pharmacol.*, 4, 267–273, 1960.
6. Misra, R., Modern drug development from traditional medicinal plants using radioligand receptor-binding assays, *Med. Res. Rev.*, 18(6), 383–402, 1998.
7. Bordia, A. and Chuttani, S.K., Effect of gum guggulu on fibrolysis and platelet adhesiveness in coronary heart disease, *Indian J. Med. Res.*, 70, 992-996, 1979.
8. Mester, L., Mester, M., and Nityanand, S., Inhibition of platelet aggregation by "guggulu" steroids, *Planta Med.*, 37, 367–369, 1979.

Table of Contents

1

Ayurveda — A Potential Global Medical System

P.N.V. Kurup

CONTENTS

1.1 Introduction

It is a universally accepted fact that good health plays an important role in human development. According to the concepts of Ayurveda, good health is based on the equilibrium of *dosha* (humor), *agni* (digestive fire), *dhatu* (seven body tissues: lymph, blood, muscle, adipose tissue, bone, bone marrow, semen), and *mala* (feces, urine, and other waste products). Furthermore, in Ayurveda there is clear-cut emphasis on maintaining physical, mental, and spiritual well-being as part of good health.[1] The World Health Organization (WHO) defines good health as a state of complete physical, mental, and social well-being and not merely an absence of disease or infirmity,[2] which is in close approximity to the definition of good health mentioned in Ayurvedic classics. Creation of the infrastructure, generation of requisite human resources, and framing of appropriate policies required to meet the health-care needs of its citizens are accepted as some of the main and fundamental responsibilities of a modern state. Every country in the global fraternity aspires to meet the health-care needs of its people through an appropriate and cost-effective approach.

0-8493-1366-X/04/$0.00+$1.50

The contributions of Traditional Systems of Medicine (TSM) for global health care in the past and their importance for the health-care needs of the present and the future are well recognized. The traditional systems of India, which are now called Indian Systems of Medicine (ISM), have a very strong conceptual base and have been practiced uninterruptedly for a very long time; hence they are considered as independent medical systems. Ayurveda, Siddha, and Unani are the three important traditional systems practiced in India. Ayurveda is the oldest and the most widely practiced system among the three. It takes into consideration all aspects of health including mental, physical, and social components.

Considering the comprehensive manner in which all matters related to health are addressed in Ayurveda, it has potential to become a global medical system. However, to achieve this status, some of the shortfalls that are perceived to hinder its progress must be rectified. In the following pages the present status in different subsectors of Ayurveda are reviewed and some of the steps required for further development in the future are suggested.

The matters that require consideration are national policy for the development of Ayurveda in India; role of Ayurveda in the country's health-care delivery; regulatory mechanism to control and regulate manufacturing and utilization of the drugs manufactured in this sector; and facilities available for the generation of trained manpower, including clinical and paramedical personnel, research and development aspects, and globalization of the system.

1.2 National Policy on ISM in India

One of the most important requirements for any system to play a meaningful role in the health care of a country is for that system to receive due recognition from the government. In India, the highest policymaking body regarding the matters concerned with health and family welfare is the Central Council for Health and Family Welfare, set up under Article 226 of the constitution of India. It consists of central health ministers, state health ministers, eminent health experts, nongovernmental organizations with an interest in the health sector, and officials of the central and state governments. It strongly advocates systematic use of the ISM in the primary and secondary infrastructure. In its last meeting, the Council recommended that at least one physician from the ISM and Homeopathy (ISM & H) should be available in every primary health center. Further, it was also resolved to introduce special treatment centers for ISM & H in rural hospitals and to create a wing for these systems in the existing state and district level government hospitals.

The government of India has taken up the matter quite seriously and drafted a national policy on traditional systems practiced in India (www.indianmedicine.nic.in).[3] The policy provides comprehensive coverage of different sectors. Feedback and suggestions have been collected from concerned organizations. This will form the basic material to frame the National Policy after completing the process of consulting different state governments and different ministries of government of India. Some highlights of the draft policy are as follows:

- It addresses the system in the areas of current relevance while at the same time delineating the immense opportunities that lay ahead.

- It plans to build upon the positive features of ISM & H, which are their modest cost, low level of technological input, and growing popularity. There is a possibility of expansion of activity in a wide range of related fields. To maximize utilization of this opportunity a range of strategies has been recommended.
- It seeks to revamp the curriculum of the educational institutes to reorient the approach of the practitioners of these systems to increase their relevance, credibility, and professionalism.
- It strongly advocates enforcement of good manufacturing practices (GMP) by placing acceptable levels of regulation and enforcement covering manufacture and certification of drugs.
- Several measures have been mentioned for the scientific and sustainable utilization of the medicinal plant-based resources of the country. It advocates adoption of a collaborative approach. Emphasis has been placed on utilizing the experience and scientific base available in the research councils of the country; for example, the Central Council for Scientific and Industrial Research (CSIR), the Indian Council for Agriculture Research (ICAR), and institutes under the Department of Science and Technology.
- To protect the intellectual property rights (IPR) of the resources of this sector, creation of an extensive database and a traditional knowledge digital library (TKDL) has been advocated.
- It also highlights the importance of utilization of local health traditions in the national health-care programs. It seeks to provide support of the operational research studies and efficacy trials for this purpose.
- The policy encourages propagation of Ayurveda and other ISM throughout the world, especially in areas where there is special interest in these systems, through Indian missions abroad. This policy will promote creation of a larger constituency for the practitioners of these systems. Promoting ISM as part of health tourism is being planned. Other approaches include international collaboration and academic exchange between interested groups.
- It has been strongly recommended that there should be an increase in the share of ISM in the national health budget.
- The policy also seeks to involve and promote the importance of ISM physicians in various national health programs.
- It seeks to establish and build the credibility of the ISM sector by encouraging certification and establishment of quality marking of products to allay the concern expressed in some quarters about the quality, safety, and efficacy of the products used.
- It recommends effecting policy changes to cover nutraceuticals and food supplements. The Drugs and Cosmetic Act would be amended to cover intermediates and partially processed plant-based products. The enactment of the ISM Product Information Promotion and Regulation Act is under consideration.
- There will be policy support and taxation incentives to promote high standards of manufacture.
- It seeks to support evidence-based research to determine the efficacy of ISM drugs and therapies, generation of data on safety and efficacy, along with standardization.
- There will be strong encouragement for undertaking research on basic principles of Ayurveda and the medico-historical approach.

TABLE 1.1

Summary of Medical Care, Medical Manpower, and Facilities Available under ISM as of 1 April 1999

Facilities	Ayurveda	Unani	Siddha	Yoga	Naturopathy	Homeopathy	Total
Hospitals	2,258	196	224	8	21	297	3,004
Beds	40,313	4,872	1,811	101	733	12,836	60,666
Dispensaries	14,416	970	363	42	56	7,155	23,028
Registered practitioners	367,528	41,221	12,915	—	388	189,361	611,413

Source: www.indianmedicine.nac.in-; Annual Report 2000–2001.

There is a feeling that formulation of a national policy has been delayed inordinately; however, the fact that a comprehensive draft has been prepared and is being circulated among all the agencies involved in its implementation indicates that the matter has been taken seriously and there will be a discernible change in the Ayurvedic sector for the better in the future. The fact that such a detailed draft policy has been prepared and the government of India has initiated steps to enforce GMP in the ISM drug-manufacturing sector clearly indicates that it is earnest in its desire to develop and ensure mainstreaming of the ISM sector and its practitioners. The expenditure in this sector has gradually and significantly increased from Rs. 21683.60 million (US $433.66 million) in 1996–1997 to Rs. 40792.60 million (US $815.95 million) in 2000–2001.

1.3 Role of Ayurveda in India's Health Care

Ayurveda is quite popular, being practiced throughout the country including tribal and remote areas where other modes of therapies are not readily available. Though it does not have as an elaborate organized structure as its modern counterpart, it plays a major role in meeting the health-care needs of a large section of India. There are separate directorates of the ISM & H in 18 states. Though Ayurveda is popular in all these states, this system is more prevalent in the states of Kerala, Himachal Pradesh, Gujarat, Karnataka, Madhya Pradesh, Rajasthan, Uttar Pradesh, and Orissa. In the state of Tamilnadu the Siddha system is prevalent.

At present there are 611,413 practitioners of TSM, 26,032 hospitals/dispensaries, and approximately 8,500 Ayurvedic drug manufacturers in the country. There are more than 190 Ayurvedic colleges turning out more than 7,000 Ayurvedic graduates and around 700 postgraduates every year (Tables 1.1 and 1.2). The government of India is well aware of the resources and is taking steps to integrate ISM in primary health care and national health programs. This growing attitude change is demonstrated by the drafted national policy mentioned above.

1.4 Academic Role of Ayurveda in Future Health Care

The concepts of proper lifestyles, dietary habits, and daily and seasonal routines followed in Ayurveda can be adopted with suitable modification to different countries in different

TABLE 1.2

Number of Undergraduate and Postgraduate Colleges and Institutions In India (1 April 1999)

Facilities	Ayurveda	Unani	Siddha	Total
Undergraduate colleges	196	40	2	238
Admission capacity	7070	1280	150	8500
Postgraduate colleges	49	3	2	54
Admission capacity	645	35	70	750

Source: www.indianmedicine.nac.in-; Annual Report 2000–2001.

parts of the globe after giving due consideration to the cultural milieu existing in each country and also the constitutional profile of each population. Attempts can also be made to utilize the medicinal plant resources of these countries for meeting the health-care needs of their people after categorization of the plants according to Ayurvedic concepts. Drugs used in ISM can be used as adjuvant to the main drugs used in conventional medicine. Therapeutic approaches such as *Panchakarma, Ksarasutra,* etc. can certainly be integrated into other health systems, broadening the choices available to physicians and patients.

1.5 Education and Training

At present, more than 190 undergraduate Ayurvedic colleges in India offer a curriculum for a Bachelor of Ayurvedic Medicine and Surgery (BAMS) degree. This program takes 5½ years to complete and runs according to the standards of the Central Council of Indian Medicine (CCIM), which is a statutory body that regulates the ISM education in the country. During the 5½ years of education, the student must go through internship for a period of 1 year. The 10 + 2 (10 years of school education followed by 2 years of predegree study) students with Science Group are eligible to take admissions in the degree course. This is similar to the requirement for the admission to the MBBS (allopathy) degree program. In fact, in many states there is a common entrance test to admit candidates to these courses. BAMS contains many modern subjects in its course material; however, nothing is taught in MBBS colleges about Ayurveda or any other ISM. This is a paradox, as many modern medicine graduates prescribe Ayurvedic drugs — especially in difficult-to-cure diseases like hepatitis — without any training in Ayurveda. The Department of ISM, being perceptive of this situation, has prepared course material containing basic concepts and fundamentals of ISM & H for incorporation in MBBS curricula. This has been forwarded to the Medical Council of India for appropriate action. In most states, e.g., Uttar Pradesh, Rajasthan, and Gujarat, Ayurvedic colleges are state supported.

Because it is necessary that Ayurvedic graduates understand modern advances in medical diagnostic methods, medical technology, and drug treatment, the present curriculum contains about 50% conventional medicine, and clinical and preclinical subjects. The CCIM, which is the apex body in matters related to the education and practice of Ayurveda in the country, is initiating steps to revise the curriculum to suit the present-day requirement by placing emphasis on practical-oriented teaching. Furthermore, at present there is no facility to impart training in some of the important disciplines, like *Vriksha* Ayurveda (a subdivision of Ayurveda that deals with matters related to cultivation of plants) and *Pasu* Ayurveda (Ayurvedic veterinary science), at the undergraduate level. Steps have to be initiated to include them as subjects for study at the undergraduate level.

1.5.1 Postgraduate Education

Postgraduate education is available in over 30 research institutes and offers specialization in 16 clinical and preclinical Ayurvedic specialty areas such as medicine, surgery, pediatrics, pharmacology, pathology, pharmacy, and *Rasa Vigyan*. Besides the mainstream institutes, the National Academy of Ayurveda, run by the government of India, was established to impart intensive training in different specialties for graduates and postgraduates of Ayurveda under the guidance of eminent scholars (similar to the traditional custom of *Guru Shishya* Parampara; interested readers can obtain more information from the Web site of the Department of ISM as well as a CD released by the department[3–5]).

At the present time, Gujarat Ayurvedic University is the only university exclusively devoted to Ayurveda and allied sciences in India. Its constituent institutes include the (1) Institute for Postgraduate Training and Research in Ayurveda financed by the government of India, (2) Shri Gulabkunverba Mahavidyalaya funded by the Gujarat State, (3) Institute of Ayurvedic Pharmaceutical Sciences, (4) Institute of Ayurvedic Medicinal Plant Sciences, (5) International Center for Ayurvedic Studies, and (6) Mahrishi Pananjali Institute for Yoga and Naturopathy Education and Research. The last three institutes are self-financed. The Gujarat Ayurvedic University has signed the Memorandum of Understanding (MOU) with nine Ayurvedic institutions functioning in Japan, Australia, the Netherlands, Italy, Argentina, and Germany to coordinate and facilitate the globalization of Ayurveda through academic collaboration. Earlier, Medical (Ayu) Institute of Russia had signed the MOU with the government of India, in which the Gujarat Ayurvedic University is also one of the implementing authorities.

The Ayurveda Faculty of the Institute of Medical Sciences, Banaras Hindu University, Varanasi, Uttar Pradesh, which is under the Central Government administration, also has similar programs. It has excellent facilities for imparting postgraduate training in different disciplines of Ayurveda. It is collaborating in international research programs and attracting graduates for training and research in Ayurveda, conducting basic research and publishing in international journals. It has an advantage of sharing the research facilities and clinical research with the medical institute's research program. National Institute of Ayurveda, Jaipur, Rajasthan also has an excellent research facility and similar training programs and collaborations. The other postgraduate research centers also have very good facilities and are involved in various important research collaborations.

1.5.2 Para Ayurvedic Staff

At present there is only one institute attached to Gujarat Ayurved University that conducts courses in Ayurvedic pharmacy. There is an urgent need to establish many such institutes to generate requisite manpower for the Ayurvedic drug manufacturing and dispensing sector. This can be facilitated by formulating a national policy making it compulsory after an initial grace period to appoint only qualified persons in the Ayurvedic manufacturing, dispensing, and drug regulatory sectors. There is also a dearth of institutions to impart training in Ayurvedic nursing. There is a need to open many such institutes and the present practice of recruiting nurses trained in modern medicine has to be phased out. If such persons are recruited, they should be made to undergo orientation training in Ayurveda. Many special therapeutic approaches like Panchakarma, Ksarasutra, and Marmavidhya are of great importance in Ayurveda.

1.6 Research and Development

There are research councils and institutes functioning throughout the country on different aspects of Ayurveda. In 1971, the government of India established a research council, the Central Council for Research in Indian Medicine, Homoeopathy & Yoga (CCRIMH), which was subsequently developed into four independent councils in 1978. The Central Council for Research in Ayurveda and Siddha (CCRAS) is an apex body for the formation, coordination, development, and promotion of research on scientific lines in Ayurveda and the Siddha System of Medicine. The council has 89 field units under it, and they have been reorganized into 30 institutes and units including the Headquarters Office (List 2 in this chapter). The research activities in various fields can be broadly categorized as follows:

- *Clinical research*, encompassing clinical studies and programs in survey and surveillance, community health, and tribal health.
- *Drug research*, encompassing medico-botanical surveys, cultivation of medicinal plants, pharmacognostical studies, and phytochemical profiling of plants used in Ayurveda, plant tissue culture, pharmacological and toxicological studies, and drug standardization. It also has a breeding program for musk deer, which is the source of the well-known drug *Kasturi*.
- *Literary research*, encompassing publication of rare and classical manuscripts of Ayurveda and Siddha, monographs on the basis of the studies undertaken by the council, scientific journals and bulletins, newsletters featuring activities of the council, and pamphlets on research findings; and preparation of video films on various research achievements.
- *Family welfare research*, including studies on family welfare such as antifertility.

Complete details of the activities and research of CCRAS can be found on its Web site: www.ccras.com.

Besides CCRAS, research activities are carried out in other postgraduate institutes as part of an M.D. dissertation and Ph.D. thesis. Research studies on Ayurvedic drugs and therapies are carried out throughout the country in many conventional medical colleges and research institutes, giving MBBS degrees — though not from an Ayurvedic perspective but as part of conventional drug research. However, some institutes have done important research work on Ayurvedic herbs. The major institutes conducting research on medicinal plants are Seth GS Medical College (Mumbai), Central Drug Research Institute (CDRI, Lucknow), Regional Research Laboratory (Jammu), National Institute for Pharmaceutical Education and Research (NIPER, Mohali), Tropical Botanical Garden and Research Institute (TBGRI, Trivandrum), Central Institute of Medicinal and Aromatic Plants (CIMAP, Lucknow), National Botanical Research Institute (NBRI, Lucknow), pharmacology departments attached to the Institute of Medical Sciences, Banaras Hindu University (Varanasi), KG Medical College (Lucknow), SPARC (Mumbai), University Department of Pharmaceutical Sciences, Punjab University, etc. In-house research activity is undertaken by some of the large Ayurvedic drug manufacturers like Himalaya Drug Company, Dabur Research Center, Zandu Research Foundation, etc. (Lists 1 and 2 in this chapter).

The present research approach, especially in the area of drug development and therapeutics, needs to consider single plant as well as Ayurvedic concepts and text formulas. Research protocols are often prepared without giving due consideration to the Ayurvedic conceptual base that underlies employing a drug in a particular disease or clinical condition. The tendency is to treat medicinal plants used in Ayurvedic therapeutics as a source material for drug prospecting for a single herb or chemical constituent and not for a drug formulation. Ayurveda has a very well-developed discipline of Ayurvedic pharmacy and drug formulation called *Bhaisajya Kalpana*, which deals in great detail with different methods of drug preparations, use of adjuvant, maintaining ideal conditions, collecting and processing drugs in a particular season at a particular stage and site, and others. There is urgent need to study the impact of changes made in drug formulation and manufacturing processes on the expression of biological activity and therapeutic efficacy.

Existence of the "therapeutic gap" in modern medicine is well known.[6] Though tremendous progress has been made in the treatment of many dreaded diseases, remedies are yet to be found for treating diseases like tuberculosis, cancer, rheumatoid arthritis, AIDS, etc. In these areas TSM drugs and procedures may have beneficial effects. Similarly, TSM drugs could be beneficial in the treatment of iatrogenic disorders like parkinsonism and to attenuate drug-induced toxicity when administered as adjuvant. Intensive research efforts are required to explore these possibilities.

1.7 Medicinal Plant Resources

The drugs used in the ISM are mainly plant based, in addition to a few materials of mineral and animal origin. Thus the therapeutic efficacy of the drugs used in these systems is greatly dependent on the use of pure and genuine raw materials in their preparation. According to the estimation of the Department of ISM,[3] about 1100 medicinal plants are estimated to find use in ISM & H drug preparation, and 500 of these are more commonly used.

There are many problems in ensuring a constant supply of drugs; avoiding overexploitation of medicinal plant resources; and also ensuring the quality of raw drugs and the conservation, cultivation, and preservation of medicinal plants. To look into these matters, the government of India has set up a Medicinal Plant Board, which has been given the responsibility of coordinating all matters related to medicinal plants. The Planning Commission set up a task force under Dr. D.N. Tewari, to *inter alia* provide policy directives on (1) conservation and sustainable use of medicinal plants, (2) growth of domestic and foreign trade, (3) development of an equitable market system, (4) regulation of this sector to maintain quality control, and (5) protection of IPR of medicinal plants.

1.8 Ayurvedic Herbs and Herbal Formula Manufacturing

Ayurvedic medicines are marketed in various forms. They are available in the classical forms like *gutikas* (tablets), *churnas* (powder), *asavas* and *aristas* (fermented products), *ghritas* (medicated ghee), and *kashayams* (decoctions). For topical use, drops, creams, lotions, liniments, and ointments are available. Dried plant extracts in capsule form are also in use. In addition, many patent drugs are sold in other modern drug presentation forms like syrups, granules, creams, lotions, etc., which constitute around 65% of the market share. There are more than 8500 manufacturers of Ayurvedic drugs in the country, of which the annual return of 10 firms is more than Rs. 50 crores (approximately US $5 million — $1.00 is roughly equal to Rs. 48 crores), of 25 firms is between Rs. 5 and 50 crores, of 965 firms is between Rs. 1 and 5 crores, and the remaining is very small with an annual turnover of less than Rs. 1 crore. The market share of Ayurvedic drugs is around Rs. 3500 crores and that of Siddha drugs is around Rs. 5 crores.[3]

Ayurveda is covered by the Drugs and Cosmetic Act (1940) and Rules (1945) of the country, and the manufacturer is expected to comply with the rules delineated under this act. In 1960, Chapter IV and other related chapters were added. Chapter IV deals with the manufacture, sale, and distribution of drugs and cosmetics; Chapter IV-A, which was subsequently added, deals with provisions related to Ayurvedic, Siddha, and Unani drugs. In this chapter, 19 sections dealing with different aspects have been described. All the drug manufacturing and dispensing activity in the country is covered under this act. According to Clause 3(a) of this act, the definition of Ayurvedic drugs includes all medicines intended for internal and external use for or in the diagnosis, treatment, mitigation, or prevention of disease or disorder in human beings or animals and manufactured exclusively in accordance with the formulae prescribed in the authoritative texts of Ayurveda (which have been specified in the First Schedule of the act). Clause 3(h) describes patent and proprietary medicines. This refers to formulations prepared utilizing the drugs listed in the formulae mentioned in the authoritative texts and mentioned under Schedule I but excludes drugs administered by parenteral route and formulations mentioned in the books in the First Schedule.[7] Schedule E_1 of the act contains a list of poisonous substances under the Ayurvedic and Unani system. In addition to the above, other acts that are relevant to the manufacturing of Ayurvedic drugs are the (1) Medicine and Toiletry Preparation Act, (2) Magic Remedies and Objectionable Advertisement Act, (3) Poisons Act, (4) Weights and Measurement Act, (5) Shops and Establishment Act, (6) Dangerous Drugs (Psychotropic and Narcotic Substances) Act, (7) Patents Act, and, in the future, the (8) Biodiversity Act (which is in the offing).

Three types of agencies are involved in the administration of the acts and rules mentioned above: the Drug Technical Advisory Board and Drug Consultative Committee, which act as advisory bodies;[8] drug testing laboratories, which provide support by shouldering the analytical responsibilities; and licensing and controlling authorities, which function as the executive wing. The Technical Advisory Board and the Drug Consultative Committee have been set up to advise the government on matters relating to ISM drugs. The Drug Technical Advisory Board (Ayurveda, Siddha, and Unani Technical Advisory Board) has been functioning regularly. The Drug Controller General of India is in charge of licensing and enforcing the above acts and rules. At the state level are drug controllers or Food and Drug Administration Commissioners who shoulder this responsibility. The drugs manufactured in the Ayurvedic sector are also under their controlling authority. In some states, like Kerala, there are officers trained in Ayurveda who provide technical assistance to the enforcing authorities.

Manufacturing of Ayurvedic drugs, except in accordance with the prescribed standards, is prohibited. It is essential to obtain a license from the licensing authority to manufacture Ayurvedic drugs. Separate licensing is required for each of the manufacturing premises maintained by the manufacturer. Manufacturing activity can also be undertaken through a loan license. For drug manufacturing, it is necessary to maintain a certain level of hygiene and optimum manufacturing conditions. These conditions are specified in Schedule T of the act (mentioned under the schedule to the rules). On 23rd June 2000 an amendment was made in the above act to specify GMP for Ayurveda, Siddha, and Unani drugs. Notice was made to ensure that (1) raw materials used in the manufacture of drugs are authentic, of prescribed quality, and are free from contamination; (2) drugs are manufactured according to standard conditions; (3) adequate quality control measures are adopted; and (4) the manufactured preparations released to the marketplace are of acceptable quality.

The ISM drug-manufacturing industry is in the process of technical upgrading to comply with GMP norms prescribed by the government of India. To achieve the objectives listed above, each licensee is expected to evolve methodology and procedures for following the prescribed process of manufacture of drugs, which should be documented as a manual and kept for reference and inspection. However, teaching institutions and registered, qualified *Vaidyas*, *Siddhas*, and *Hakeems* who prepare medicines on their own to dispense to their patients and not to sell such drugs in the market are exempt from the purview of this practice. Part I of two parts contains specification regarding the maintenance of factory premises; Part II contains the list of machinery, equipment, and minimum manufacturing premises required.

For the implementation of drug testing provisions under the Drugs and Cosmetics Act (1940) and Rules (1945), it is necessary to evolve pharmacopoeial standards. At present, pharmacopoeial standards are available for 258 drugs, and 654 formulations have been published in the *Ayurvedic Formulary of India*. The Department of ISM is developing pharmacopoeial standards through pharmacopoeial committees. Three volumes of Part I of the pharmacopoeia, called *Ayurvedic Pharmacopoeia*, have been published containing 258 monographs. The target is to cover 600 single drugs.

At present, there are more than 8000 licensed pharmacies in the country manufacturing Ayurvedic drugs. There is the Mumbai-based Ayurvedic Drug Manufacturer's Association which can be contacted for further details about issues related to Ayurvedic drug manufacturing.

A drug-control cell in the Department of ISM deals with various issues pertaining to quality control, import, export, classification of drugs under the Drugs and Cosmetics Act, patents, and the establishment of a TKDL. It monitors and coordinates implementation of legislation relating to drugs of ISM & H. The agency may be a good source for information on matters related to regulations.

1.9 Globalization of Ayurveda

Globalization of Ayurveda has gained momentum. Many active groups have been formed in many parts of the world, including developed countries, to spread the concept and practice of Ayurveda. This is due primarily to the following three reasons: (1) the holistic approach advocated by Ayurveda in therapeutic practice, (2) it has one of the most extensive and profound conceptual bases among the TMSs of the world, and (3) its survival for more than 2 millennium as a vibrant medical system. It is believed that Ayurveda has the potential to develop into a global health-care system.

The first requirement is to undertake globalization of Ayurvedic education to generate high-quality, competent manpower with the requisite communication skills to teach the principles and practice of the system. There is a requirement to start introductory, short and long-term courses as per the local requirement and situation in different parts of the world. It is also necessary to start similar types of courses in the premier Ayurvedic institutes in India. Some universities have already taken a step in this direction by starting short- and long-term courses under its International Center for Ayurvedic Studies. Another important requirement is to translate important Ayurvedic literature to major international languages.

The second requirement is to globalize Ayurvedic practice and marketing of Ayurvedic drugs. There are many obstacles to achieve this, especially in the developed countries. The laws regulating these aspects are quite rigid and a lot of time, effort, and finance will be required to comply with them. They do not take into consideration the conceptual uniqueness of Ayurveda. A two-pronged strategy is required to overcome this problem. The first one is to undertake multicenter collaborative studies on internationally acceptable guidelines to prove therapeutic utility and safety of Ayurvedic drugs and practices. The second one is to establish Ayurvedic clinics and hospitals in countries where there is no such barrier. Standardization of Ayurvedic drugs and formulations should be given top priority — without this it would not be possible to promote the utilization of Ayurvedic drugs at the global level. Another aspect needs to be taken into consideration is the possibility of existence of constitutional differences among different races and communities as per the concepts of Ayurveda. Also, it would be necessary to explore the possibility of utilization and integration of locally available flora into Ayurvedic practice of the particular country or region.

Facilities have been established in many countries to impart short- and long-term training in Ayurveda. Such facilities are available in the U.S., Argentina, Australia, Brazil, New Zealand, South Africa, Czech Republic, Greece, Italy, Hungary, the Netherlands, Russia, U.K., Israel, Japan, Nepal, and Sri Lanka.

1.10 Research at the International Level

At present, there are no international collaborative studies to validate the therapeutic claims of Ayurvedic preparations except for some studies carried out on medicinal plants used in Ayurveda. A recent review[9] points out that more than 13,000 plants have been investigated during the past 5 years. A number of medicinal plants have been shown to possess important pharmacological activities in preclinical testing; however, the generated leads have not been adequately followed up with double-blind, placebo-controlled clinical trails. The following drugs are identified for such studies based on existing biological and clinical data: *Curcuma longa, Boswellia serrata, Picrorhiza kurroa, Terminalia chebula, Emblica officinalis, Bacopa monnieri, Boerhaavia diffusa, Phyllanthus niruri, Celastrus paniculatus, Ocimum sanctum, Gymnema sylvestre, Momordica charantia, Commiphora mukul, Withania somnifera, Pterocarpus marsupium, Tinospora cordifolia, Trichopus zeylanicum,* and *Terminalia arjuna.* One of the main lacunae that becomes apparent for any reviewer of this sector is that most of the studies are undertaken on an individual pharmacologic-effect basis. These studies need to be organized and reviewed. Such a review of these studies is likely to provide scientific basis to the traditional usage of Ayurvedic therapies. It is also of utmost importance that sufficient attention be paid to the conceptual basis that underlies selection of a drug or group of drugs to treat a particular disease condition. Furthermore, many more studies are required to be undertaken on multicomponent formulations and assessment of possible drug interactions when a person who is already on modern drugs takes herbal preparations. If the recent trends are any indications, interest in medicinal plant-based preparations and traditional medical systems is bound to increase.

List 1: Postgraduate Study Centers

1. Central Drug Research Institute, Chattar Manzil Palace, Lucknow 226 001

2. Dabur Research Foundation, 22, Site IV, Sahibabad, Ghaziabad 201 010
3. Himalaya Drug Company, Research and Development Centre, Makali, Bangalore 563 123
4. Institute of Medical Sciences, Faculty of Ayurveda, Banaras Hindu University, Varanasi 226 004
5. Institute of Postgraduate Teaching and Research in Ayurveda, Gujarat Ayurved University, Post Box no. 4, Jamnagar 361 008
6. National Institute of Ayurveda, Madhav Vilas Palace, Ajmer Road, Jaipur 302 002
7. National Institute of Pharmaceutical Education and Research (NIPER), Sector 67, SAS Nagar, Mohali, Punjab
8. National Botanical Research Institute (NBRI, Lucknow), Rana Pratap Marg Lucknow 226 001
9. R.A. Podar Medical College, Dr. Annie, Bessant Road, Worli, Mumbai 400 018
10. Regional Research Laboratory, Canal Road, Jammu, Jammu and Kashmir 181 001
11. State Ayurvedic College, Tulsidas Marg, Turia Ganj, Lucknow 226 004
12. Swami Prakashananda Ayurveda Research Centre (SPARC), 13th N A S Road, Mittal Nagar, JBPD-Scheme, Juhu, Mumbai 400 049
13. Tropical Botanical Garden and Research Institute (TBGRI), Pacha, Palode Trivandrum 695 562
14. Zandu Research Foundation attached to Zandu Pharmaceutical Works Ltd., 70, Gokhale Road South (Dadar), Mumbai 400 025

List 2: Regional Research Institutes (RRIs)

RRIs under Central Council for Research in Ayurveda and Siddha (CCRAS), 61-65, Institutional Area, Opp. D-Block, New Delhi 110058, Ph: 011-5528748/5536520/5624457 (O), 5614971 (R).

Addresses

1. Road No. 66, Punjabi Bagh, New Delhi 110026, Ph: 011-5919128/5411059, Fax: 5464546
2. R.A. Podar College, Worli, Mumbai 400 018, Ph: 022-4947822, Fax: 4947833 (O) 0250-462991 (R)
3. 4, CN Block, Sector V, Bidhan Nagar, Calcutta 700 091, Ph/Fax: 033-3673808
4. RCRI, AA Govt. Hospital Campus, Arumbakkam, Chennai 600 106, Ph: 044-6214809(O), 6214925 (G), 6265857 (R)
5. Cheruthuruthy, Via. Shoranur, Trichur, Kerala 679 531, Ph/Fax: 0488-462366, 462543 (O), 462544 (H), 622175 (R)
6. No. 1, Bhubaneswar 751 009, Ph/Fax: 0674-530125, 531941 (H), 570650/570705 (R)
7. Moti Bagh Road, Patiala 147 001, Ph/Fax: 0175-212393, 228361(H), 212348 (R)

8. Govt. Ayurvedic Hospital, Amhho, Gwalior 474 009, Ph/Fax: 0751-323307, 430317 (Fax), 327959 (R).
9. 474/6, Sitapur Road, Lucknow 206 020, Ph/Fax: 0522-369156, 362341/732238(R)
10. Indira Colony, Jhotwara, Bani Park, Jaipur 320 016, Ph/Fax: 0141-200812/206063, 392174/399646 (R)
11. 1044 Jagnada Chowk, KDK College Rd., Nandanwan, Nagpur 440 009, Ph/Fax: 0712-714230, 242310 (R)
12. Govt. Central Pharmacy Annexe, Ashoka Pillar, Jayanagar, Bangalore 560 011, Ph/Fax: 080-6562030, 2272208 (R)
13. Poojapura, Trivandrum 695 012, Ph/Fax: 0471-340628, 342070 (R)
14. Indira Gandhi Municipal Stadium Complex A, First Floor, North Wing, Vijayawada 520 010, Ph/Fax: 0866-472535, 481512 (R)
15. Govt. Pharmacy (Upstairs), Indira Nagar, Gorimedu, Pondicherry 605 5006, Ph: 0413-272420 (O), 202097 (R)
16. D Block, Rajindra Memorial Res. Institute Bldg., Agam Kuan, Patna – 800 007, Ph/fax: 0612-631678, 345775 (R).
17. Borsojai (Bhetapara), Beltola, Guwahati 781 028, Assam, Ph: 0361-303714
18. Tadung, Gangtok, Sikkim 737 102, Ph/Fax: 03592-31494, 81649/81662 (R)
19. New Itanagar 791 111 (Arunachal Pradesh), Ph/Fax: 0361-212284, 211498 (O), 212520 (R)
20. 20, Rewari Chowk, Jammu 180 005, Ph/Fax: 0191-546475
21. Gandhi Bhawan, Mandi 175 001 (HP), Ph/Fax: 01905-35236
22. Tarikhet 263 663 (Uttaranchal), Ph/Fax: 05966-64227, 64222(R)
23. Gwalior Road, Jhansi 284 003 (UP), Ph/Fax: 05174-442132
24. Tajmanzil, Sardar Bagh, Junagadh 362 001, Ph/Fax: 0285-631631
25. Nehru Garden, Kothrud, Pune 411 029, Ph: 020-5383138, Fax: 5386715, 5442338 (R)
26. Indian Institute of History of Medicine, Osmania Medical College Buildings, Putlibowli, Hyderabad 500 095, Ph/Fax: 040-4657388, 3511259 (R)
27. CSMDRIA, A.A. Govt. Hospital Campus, Arumbakkam, Chennai 600 106, Ph: 044-6214823/6207566 (O), 6282487 (R)
28. Dr. A. Laksmipati Research Centre for Ayurveda, VHS Medical Centre, Adyar, Chennai 600 113, Ph: 044-2541537
29. Regional Research Institute (Ay), Hastinapur 250 404, Ph/Fax: 95123380176, 95123380338 (R)
30. CCRAS Main Office, #61-65, Institutional Area, Opp. D. Block, New Delhi 110 058, Ph: 5528748/5624457

Further details can be obtained from the Council's headquarters:
Address: Jawahar Lal Nehru Bhartiya Chikitsa Avum Homeopathy Anusandhan Bhavan, No. 61-65, Institutional Area, Opp. D Block, Janakpuri, New Delhi 110 058 (India)
Ph: 91-011-5614970/71/72, Fax: 91-011-5528748
E-mail: ccras@ndf.vsnl.net.in or ccras@del6.vsnl.net.in

References

1. Shastri Ambika Dutta, *Sushrut Samhita*, 8th ed., Chowkhembha Sanskrit Samsthan, Varanasi, 1982, 64 (or Chap. 15, Verse 48).
2. Park, G.E., *Textbook of Preventive and Social Medicine*, 9th ed., M.F. Banarasi Das Bhanot, Jabalpur, India, 1983, p. 12.
3. Web site: www.indianmedicine.nac.in.
4. Anon., South-East Asia Progress Towards Health for All 1977–2000, World Health Organization, New Delhi, 2000.
5. CD: Information Gateway on Ayurveda, prepared by ISM & H, Government of India.
6. Satyavati, G.V., An overview of pharmacological studies in India on medicinal plants and natural products (1975–1982), A sequel to the chapter Pharmacology of medicinal plants and natural products, in *Current Research in Pharmacology in India (1975–1982)*, Indian National Science Academy, New Delhi, 1984.
7. Narayana, D.B.A., Forensic Ayurveda and GMPs, in *Proceedings National Workshop on Internationally Acceptable Standards for Ayurvedic Formulations*, Ravishankar, B., Ed., July 20–21, Institute of PG Teaching and Research in Ayurveda, Gujarat Ayurved University, Jamnagar, India, 2000, p. 36.
8. Jain, N.K., *A Textbook of Forensic Pharmacy*, Vallabh Prakashan, Delhi, 2001.
9. Dahanukar, S.A., Kulkarni, R.A., and Rege, N.N., Pharmacology of medicinal plants and natural products, *Indian J. Pharmacol.*, 32, S81, 2000.

2

Health Care and Disease Management

Lakshmi Chandra Mishra

CONTENTS

2.1 Introduction

In Ayurveda, health is defined as the state where physical body, senses, and psyche are in original or natural state with respect to body and function. Although the genetic makeup of an individual determines the basic body constitution with respect to *dosas* (biomaterials) and psychological factors, total health is determined by physical and psychological environment. It is currently believed that the expression of genes largely depends on environmental factors. Consistent with this belief, Ayurveda emphasizes the role of environmental factors, daily routine, seasonal changes, lifestyle, diet, regular exercise, and body tonics (*rasayana*) in maintaining health. It also emphasizes that all needs of the body and senses must be in balance in order to avoid illness and maintain good health — a scientifically valid concept.[1]

0-8493-1366-X/04/$0.00+$1.50

The founding fathers of Ayurveda believed that the world is made up of five elements called *Panch-mahabhuta*. Their criterion was that an element must not be "divisible into" a new material. They determined that earth, water, fire, air, and space are indivisible and therefore designated them as the five basic elements (*Panchmahabhuta*). The human body in Ayurveda was also believed to be made up of these five elements. In order to understand the whole body physiology, Ayurveda postulates three main factors called *tridosa*, which are also called biomaterials, biofactors, or bioenergies. These *tridosas* or biomaterials are *vata*, *pitta*, and *kapha*. The primary dominant elements in *vata*, *pitta*, and *kapha* are air, fire, and earth, respectively. According to the *tridosa* theory the total human body consists of an intensive interplay of a solid material substrate referred to as *kapha*, chemical activity (biofire) referred as *pitta*, and an energy pool of motion and movement referred to as *vata*. These three *dosas* coexist in a predetermined proportion and function in a complementary manner to overall function of the total organism in spite of their opposite properties and functions. The existence of the *dosas* can be understood at both the macromolecular and micromolecular levels. A balance in the activity of these *dosas* is necessary for health.

The human body according to Ayurveda is made up of somatic *dosas* (*vata*, *pitta*, and *kapha*) and psychic components (*dosas*), body tissues (*dhatus*), and waste products (*malas*). The three psychological components are *satogun*, *rajogun*, and *tamogun*. A close interdependence among the somatic and psychological components exists; if one component is out of balance, the others are also out of balance. The imbalance or vitiation of *vata*, *pitta*, or *kapha* is considered the major factor in the causation of a disease.[1]

Ayurveda has a concept of *agni* (fire) for all digestive and metabolic activities. Use of the word "fire" can be rationalized based on the fact that fire generates carbon dioxide as a result of burning carbon-based materials, and metabolism of carbon-based nutrients in the body also generates carbon dioxide. Digestion and absorption processes are called digestive fire (*pakwagni*) and the enzymic action causing transformation of nutrients into various tissue materials is called tissue fire (*dhatwagni*). Food must not only be digested and absorbed from the intestine and circulate in the blood plasma, but also must be absorbed by the tissue cells in order to be assimilated by the body. There are seven primary supportive tissues (*dhatus*) in the body: (1) plasma, (2) blood, (3) muscular tissue, (4) osseous tissue, (5) adipose tissue, (6) marrow and myeloid tissue, and (7) reproductive tissue. All tissues are made up of cells with different structures and functions connected with other cells through minute channels or pores (*suksma srotas*) to receive and distribute nutrients and excrete metabolic waste products. This description of cellular communication in Ayurveda is consistent with the modern understanding of intercellular uptake and release of substrates and metabolites. All tissues have a material called activator, essence, or hormone (*ojas*) which has specific properties and functions that are perceived to produce a healthy essence. The properties and balance of excretory products (stool and urine) and breakdown products of tissues (nitrogenous products) are also important factors in determining health and disease.[1]

2.2 *Tridosas*[1]

2.2.1 *Vata*

Vata literally means "air." The description of *vata* in Ayurveda includes the following: dry, cold, light, penetrating, mobile, transparent, and rough-like air and responsible for all

TABLE 2.1

Classification of *Vata*

Vata	Location	Function
Prana	Central nervous system and some vital centers of the brain	Controls the action of other *vatas*
Apana	Lumbo-sacral, gluteal, genito-urinary, inguinal, and visceral regions	Regulates discharge of seminal fluid, menstrual fluid, feces, urine, and aids in childbirth
Vyana	The heart (the fluid pumping system), nonconscious reflexes produced along the spinal cord (corresponds to autonomic nervous system)	Controls contraction and relaxation of muscles, blood circulation, lymph circulation, sweating, and other secretions of the body through the stimulation of nerves
Udana	The chest, umbilical area, nasal and pharyngeal passages	Controls speech, respiration, energy, body luster, and consciousness and also influences the respective centers in the brain
Samana	The entire abdomen	Controls digestion and assimilation of food, as well as excretion of waste products

Signs and symptoms of deranged vata are indicative of neurological problems

Causes of Deranged *Vata*	Symptoms of Deranged *Vata*
Overworking, grief, worry, lack of sleep, intentional retention of bodily waste, excess exercise or sexual indulgence, and ingestion of bitter, pungent, astringent, or dry foods	Irregular movement of the limbs, tearing pain, throbbing suppression of secretions, contraction of muscles (spasms), roughness of the skin, formation of bone cavities, suspension of bowel movements, and an astringent taste in the mouth

kinds of movements in the body, speed, impulse, and odor. *Vata* is a part of every cell; however, the major sites of *vata* are believed to be the colon, lower back, calf muscle, ear, bones, and joints. Some organs of the body also have a higher level of *vata* biofactor than other organs, such as the brain, spinal cord, autonomic nervous systems, and motor and sensory systems. *Vata* biofactor is responsible for functions of the central, autonomic, and peripheral nervous systems. *Vata* controls the respiratory, blood, lymphatic, excretory, and reproductive systems, as well as all types of movements. It is also responsible for the cognitive and neocognitive function of the brain, and secretion of various chemical neurotransmitters and hormones. This description of *vata* resembles the functions of central, peripheral, and autonomic nervous systems. The following six main *chakras* (extrasensory channels) of *vata* correspond to modern autonomic nervous system plexuses, further substantiating that *vata*, in fact, resembles the nervous system:

1. *Agya chakra* – nasociliary extension of the cavernous plexus of the sympathetic nervous system
2. *Vishuddha chakra* – pharyngeal plexus of the sympathetic nervous system
3. *Anahat chakra* – cardiac plexus of the sympathetic nervous system
4. *Manipur chakra* – plexus of the cholinergic
5. *Swadhistan chakra* – hypogastric plexus
6. *Muladhar chakra* – pelvic plexus

Among *tridosas*, *vata* is more critical because it controls p*itta* and *kapha* in order to accomplish various physiological functions. *Vata* is classified into five types based on the organ site and function as shown in Table 2.1.

TABLE 2.2
Classification of *Pitta*

Pitta	Location	Function
Pachak	Stomach and small intestine	Controls bile and pancreatic juices
Ranjaka	Stomach, duodenum, liver, spleen, and pancreas	Enzymes responsible for digestion and metabolism; provide nutrients, blood constituents, and the formation of the blood cells in the spleen
Sadhak	Heart	Responsible for life span, complexion, energy, body temperature, body luster
Bhrajak	Eye	Responsible for vision
Alochak	Skin	Responsible for the heat, moisture, and health of the skin, as well as the vasomotor mechanism and adaptation to the surrounding environment

Signs and symptoms of deranged pitta are indicative of digestive, metabolic, and enzymatic problems

Causes of Deranged *Pitta*	Symptoms of Deranged *Pitta*
Pitta may be deranged by ingestion of salty, hot, irritating, or sharp-tasting foods, as well as by anger	Burning sensation in the stomach, redness, digestive system disturbances, excessive sweating, fainting, symptoms of intoxication, pungent and sour taste, and inability to see white and dark red color

2.2.2 *Pitta*

The second *dosa* is *pitta*, which indicates *agni* (fire, heat energy), and the description in Ayurvedic texts includes heat, sharpness, sourness, and moisture. It is responsible for appetite, thirst, digestion, metabolism, body heat, normal eyesight, softness of the body, luster, mental calmness, and intelligence. This description of *pitta* resembles that of digestion, metabolism, oxidation, conjugation, reduction, phosphorylation, enzymes, and hormones. Although *pitta* is present in every cell in the body, it is classified based on five major anatomical locations shown in Table 2.2. Although *pitta*, like *vata*, exists in every cell of the body, the major sites of *pitta* are believed to be the stomach, duodenum, liver, spleen, pancreas, heart, eyes, and skin.

2.2.3 *Kapha*

The third *dosa* is *kapha*, which is described in Ayurveda as moist, steady, cool, heavy, soft, and slimy materials. *Kapha* is responsible for the normal body moisture, stability of the joints, firmness of the body, a proportionate bulk, weight, strength, endurance, and courage. The description of *kapha* resembles those of the lymphatic system, immune system, body fat, and mucous and mucoid systems. *Kapha* balances *pitta* in functions by providing basic materials for conversion into body tissues by enzymes, a kind of biochemical feedback mechanism. *Pitta* generates heat from the enzymatic activities, while *kapha* provides ways to eliminate the heat through the skin, lungs, urine, and feces via fat and moisture.

Although *kapha* is basically the same in all cells of the body, it is classified into five types based on location and functions as shown in Table 2.3. Again, like *vata* and *pitta*, *kapha* is present in every cell of the body and its major sites are believed to be the chest, stomach, brain, tongue, and synovial membrane of bone joints.

TABLE 2.3

Classification of *Kapha*

Kapha	Location	Function
Avalambak	Chest	Enables other *dosas* to perform their function by supplying humidity and body water, blood, fluid
Kledak	Stomach	It is liquid, mucoid, sweet, cooling in nature, and moistens the bolus
Bodhak	Tongue	Controls saliva and other juices that moisten the mouth, helps the bolus descend, and creates taste
Tarpak	Brain	Controls vision, hearing, smell, taste, and touch
Shleshaka	Synovial areas of bone joints	Provides lubrication

Signs and symptoms of deranged kapha are indicative of lipid metabolism and mucus-secreting system

Causes of Deranged *Kapha*	Symptoms of Deranged *Kapha*
Overexposure to cold weather; excessive sleep; day sleeping; excessive, sweet, fatty, and oily food; low level of physical activity	Excess of moisture, hardness of tissues, itching, feeling cold or heavy, low secretary activity, mucous membranes heavily coated with mucous, reduced activity of limbs, swelling, weak digestive power, sleepiness, pale skin, salty taste, and slow recovery after an illness

2.3 Body Constitution (*Prakriti*)[1]

Although all biomaterials are natural elements of the body, people may have the predominance of one or a combination of two of the biomaterials that determine general physical and psychological characteristics and the tendency (susceptibility) to develop certain diseases. Table 2.4 shows the characteristics of body constitutions according to predominance of biomaterials and tendency to develop certain diseases.

2.4 Mental Components (*Mano Guna*)

Charak describes attributes of mental components as desire for pleasure, aversion to pain or misery, intelligence, mind, will power, logical faculty (*vicarna*), memory, knowledge gained from experience (*vijnana*), ability, and perception. Based on these attributes, mental components are divided into three classes: godly (*satogun*), kingly (*rajogun*), and evil (*tamogun*). Manifestations of these classes of mental components and characteristic constitutions are shown in Tables 2.5 and 2.6, respectively.[1]

2.5 Health Care

Health care in Ayurveda is essentially aimed at balancing the *dosas* and *gunas*, bringing them into equilibrium. With this goal in mind, management of a disease is designed to

TABLE 2.4
Characteristics of Dosha Constitutions

***Vata* Constitution**	***Pitta* Constitution**	***Kapha* Constitution**
Characteristics		
Low body weight, light bone structure, fast to act, forgetful, artistic, loves esoteric material, is shy and sensitive, enthusiastic	Healthy body, well-developed muscles, well-functioning metabolism, an urge for physical activities, an interest in science and technical subjects, good speaking ability, aggressiveness, hostile tendency, impatience, tendency to baldness, good mental ability, excellent memory, loves intellectual activities	Heavy body weight, solid body structure, strength, endurance, secure feeling, self-confident, not easily rattled, somewhat lethargic, patient, polite, generous, materialistic tendency, greedy, passive, tendency to sleep too much
Diseases Prone To		
Rheumatism, nervous disorders, sciatica, insomnia, dry skin, constipation, receding gums, weak bones, infertility, impotence, colic, flatulence, stuttering, ringing in the ears, irregular menstruation with cramps, varicose veins, paralysis, blood clotting, anorexia, shivering fits, poor blood circulation	Stress-related diseases; high blood pressure; coronary diseases; thrombosis; ulcers; cancer of the stomach, intestine, and skin; psoriasis; inflammation of the lymph system; infectious diseases; inflammation of the spleen; hepatitis, urinary tract infection; heartburn	Nausea, colds, bronchitis, asthma, kidney stones, swollen lymph nodes, benign tumors, dropsy, goiter, lung and breast cancer, fungal infections, digestive system problems, obesity

TABLE 2.5
Characteristics of Mental Components

Godly (*Satogun*)	**Kingly (*Rajogun*)**	**Evil (*Tamogun*)**
Compassion, self-control, forbearance, devotion to truth, proper conduct, faith in god, knowledge gained from self-realization (*Jnana*), intelligence, resolution, comprehension, nonattachment	Sensitivity to pain, restlessness of mind, lack of true understanding, egoism, lack of honesty, lack of compassion, false pride, overconfidence, buoyancy of spirit, strong desires, anger	Despondency, agnosticism and atheism, tendency to evil conduct (*adharma*), dull intellect, lack of knowledge and insight, perverted mind, physical and mental inertia, somnolence

TABLE 2.6
Characteristics of Mental Constitutions (*Manasik Prakriti*)

Godly (*Satvik*)	**Kingly (*Rajsik*)**	**Evil (*Tamsik*)**
Pure-minded, compassionate, loving, and righteous person who is capable of enduring all degrees of hardship and pain through willpower	Egotistic, ambitious, proud, competitive, controlling, and power-hungry person who may be made to submit to pain and unpleasant medical treatment through persuasion and logic	Lazy, sleepy, depressed, greedy, irritable, irresponsible, and selfish person with a large appetite who is horrified at the prospect of bodily pain

TABLE 2.7
Eight-Point Diagnosis

Examination	*Vata*	*Pitta*	*Kapha*
1. Pulse	Thread-like, feeble, snake-like motion	Moderately heavy, and jumps like a frog	Heavy, slow, flows like swan
2. Urine	Black–brown color	Dark brown color	Cloudy appearance
Drop of sesame oil spreads on the surface of urine gives:	Wave-like movement	Multiple colors, like rainbow	Pearl-like droplets
3. Stool	Uniform, dark color	Yellowish color	Bulky foul smell
4. Tongue	Black to brown, dry, coarse, furred, pigmented	Red, yellow, or green, soft, sharp, moist	Whitish color, pale coated, big, soft, flabby
5. Eye	Small, conjunctiva, muddy, iris is dark gray or brown	Moderate size, sharp, more sensitive to light	Large, moist, oily, conjunctiva is white
6. Skin	Dry, coarse, wrinkled, dusky	Wheat color, copper-like color, shiny, moist	Soft, off-white, smooth, moist
7. Speech and voice	Coarse and dry	Sharp	Heavy
8. General appearance	Mental disorders, anxiety, distress, pain, weakness, and strength are important factors in diagnosis		

diagnose which biomaterials and components are in excess or not and how they can be brought into balance.[2]

2.5.1 Diagnosis

Diagnosis of a disease in Ayurveda is essentially done by inspection, palpation, and interrogation. The specific examination includes the standard eight-point examination: (1) pulse, (2) urine, (3) stool, (4) tongue, (5) eye, (6) skin, (7) speech and voice, and (8) general appearance (Table 2.7). Additional examinations are made to assess digestive capacity, personal habits, body appearance, and patient's resilience. The other elements of diagnosis are the most recent reason for the illness, warning symptoms, clear symptoms, various diagnostic tests, and pathogenesis.

Management of an illness considers elimination of causes of the imbalance of *dosas*, administration of various herbal formulas, dietary and lifestyle interventions to bring *dosas* back into balance, elimination of *chinta* (serious worry), and nurturing the soul to regain spiritual health (*Samana*).

2.5.2 Disease Management

Charak Samhita describes four components of a disease management scheme: (1) the physician, (2) the drug, (3) the patient, and (4) the attendant. A physician must have proper training, knowledge, and experience. A remedy must be abundantly available, effective, and relatively safe. A patient must provide all information to the physician about the disorder and be compliant. An attendant (a nurse) must have the knowledge of patient care, dexterity, loyalty, and cleanliness.

Management of illness primarily consists of four procedures: (1) cleansing (*samsodhan*), (2) palliation (*samsaman*), (3) rejuvenation (*kaya kalp*), and (4) mental and spiritual healing (*sattvavajaya*, or psychotherapy). The management of an illness starts with cleansing and

TABLE 2.8

Group of Herbs Used To Mitigate *Vata*[3]

Medicinal Plant	Botanical Name	Medicinal Plant	Botanical Name
Bhadradaru		*Vrsciva*	*Boerhavia diffusa*
Nata	*Caesalpinia bonduc* (L.)	*Devahvaya*	*Cedrus deodru*
Kustha	*Saussurea lappa* cob	*Two Salpaparni*	
Dashmula		*Kandukari*	*Mueuna pruriens*
Two Bala	*Sida cordifolia* Linn.	*Abhiru*	*Asparagus racemoses*
Vellantara	*Vativera zizanoides*	*Vira*	*Roscoea procera*
Aranika	*Premna integrefolia* Linn.	*Jivanti*	*Leptadenia reticulata*
Buka	*Osmanthus fragrans*	*Rsbhaka*	*Microstullus wallachi* Lindl
Vrsa	*Addhatoda vasica* Nees	*Brihatee*	*Solanum anguivi* Lam.
Asmabheda	*Bergenia ligulala* wall	*Kantakaree*	*Solanum surattense* Burm. F.
Gokantaka	*Tribulus teriatris*	*Saliparni*	*Desmodium gangeticum*
Itkata	*Sesbania bispinosa*	*Prasniparni*	*Uraria picta*
Sahacara	*Baeleria prionitis* Linn.	*Goksuraka*	*Tribulus terristris*
Bana	*Bareleria stringosa*	*Hansapadi-Adiantum Lunilatum-Burm*	*Podophyllum hexandrum royle*
Gundra	*Typha elephantia* Roxb	*Kasa*	*Saccharum spontaneum* Linn
Bhalluka	*Oroxylum indicum* Vent.	*Vrksadani*	*Loranthus longifolius*
Karambha	*Pergularia extensa*	*Nala*	*Arundo donax* Linn
Partha	*Gynandropsis pentaphylla*	*Two Kusa*	*Desmostachya bipinnata*
Vrscikali	*Pergularia extensa*	*Guntha*	*Typha angustata*

includes five procedures called *panchakarma*, all of which are not necessarily done at the same time or to all patients. This topic is described in detail in Chapter 4.

Panchakarma is a major therapeutic procedure in Ayurveda known to be useful for all diseases of all the body organs and functions because the elimination of toxic products, endogenous or exogenous, can contribute to overall management of an ailment. It is understandable that if the body organs are not eliminating toxic products from the body, toxic symptoms will develop over a period of time. The major cause of body ailments is the toxic products produced by body metabolism, microorganisms, synthetic chemicals, xenobiotics, or drugs. *Panchakarma* is discussed in detail in Chapter 4.

Palliation essentially consists of compound preparations of herbs and minerals for diet and lifestyle interventions. Ayurvedic texts describe seven types of palliation: (1) digestive power enhancement, (2) toxic waste (*ama*) elimination, (3) fasting, (4) observing thirst, (5) yoga exercise, (6) lying in the sunlight or sunbathing, and (7) breathing exercise and meditation. A variety of formulas are used to improve digestion, eliminate *ama*, and balance *dosas*. Examples of herbs used to subdue deranged or vitiated *dosas* are shown in Tables 2.8 through 2.10. Fasting also helps in acute indigestion, dysentery, diarrhea, and acute fever.

2.5.2.1 An Example of Ayurvedic Case Management

To illustrate a typical Ayurvedic therapy, the management of *Ama-vata* (rheumatoid arthritis) is given below. It includes biopurification and detoxification by dietary interventions and necessary *panchakarma* procedures and administration of herbal formulas. The first step is elimination of *ama* (the incompletely digested food material in the intestine, collagen materials, allergens, mucus, mucoid materials, crystals like uric acid) by reducing the diet to near or total fasting if possible. The diet consists of very small quantities of double-boiled rice and watery *mung dal* (lentils) for the first 5 days, with the addition of small amounts of vegetables for the next 5 days, and then one piece of bread (*roti*) for an

TABLE 2.9

Herbs Used To Mitigate *Pitta*[3]

Herb	Botanical Name	Herb	Botanical Name
Durva	*Cynodon dactylon*	*Abhiru*	*Asparagus racemoses*
Ananta	*Alhagi camelorum*	*Sitapaki*	*Abrus precatorius*
Nimba	*Azadirachta indica* A.	*Priyangu*	*Setaria italica* Beauv
Vasa	*Litesa glutinosa*	*Two Sthira*	*Desmodium gangeticum*
Atmagupta	*Mueuna pruriens*	*Padmak*	*Prunus cerasoides*
Gundra	*Typha elephantine* Roxb	*Vanya*	*Cyperus rotundus* Linn.
Nyagrodhadi group			
Nyagrodha	*Ficus vengakensis* Linn.	*Two Meda* (fat)	*Litsea monpetala*
Tuga	*Bamboo mann*	*Mudgaparni*	*Vigna trilobata*
Rddhi	*Sphaeranthus inducus*	*Mashaparni*	*Teramnus labialis*
Shringee	*Pistacia chinensis* Bunge	*Rsabhaka*	*Microstullus wallachi*
Amrita	*Tinospora cordifolia*	*Jivaka*	*Microstyllus wallachi* Lindl
Jivanti	*Leptadenia reticulata*	*Madhuka*	*Sapotaceae*
Two Kakoli	*Roscoea procera*		
Sarivadi group (used to treat burning sensation, bleeding disease, thirst, and fever)			
Pippala	*Piper longum* Linn.	*Usira*	*Vativeria zizanoides*
Sadaphala	*Ficus glomerata*	*Kasmarda*	*Cassia sophera*
Two Rodhra	*Symplocos racemosa* Roxb	*Yashti-madhu*	*Glycyrrhiza glabra*
Arjun	*Terminalia arjuna*	*Kadamba*	*Anthocephalus chinensis*
Kapitana	*Thespesia populnea*	*Virala*	*Diospyros tomentosa*
Somavalka	*Acacia suma* Kurz	*Madhuka*	*Sapotaceae*
Plaksha	*Ficus lucescens* Blume		
Amaara	*Vitex nigundo* Linn.		
Padmakadi group (increase breast milk to subjugate *vata* and *pitta*)			
Padmaka	*Prunus cerasoides*		

additional 5 days. This treatment is generally given for a minimum of 1 month. During this period, hot fomentations are applied and no ghee (dehydrated milk fat), vegetable oil, meat, or animal fat is given. It is believed that this treatment increases the metabolic power of the body, resulting in breakdown and excretion of the disease-producing vitiated materials (*ama*), collagen, uric acid, sugar, urea, fat, etc. To augment the process of cleansing, ginger juice or dry ginger is given daily in the early morning on an empty stomach. *Chirata* or *Swertia chirayita*, a bitter herb, is also given to improve digestion.

After 1 month of this treatment, ghee (dehydrated butter) may be given to help in removing fat-soluble materials from the body. A medicated enema (*basti*) containing sesame (*til*) oil may be started and continued for 1 month for this purpose. At this point the treatment is stopped for 4 to 8 weeks and the reduced diet treatment is resumed. Once the acute phase has subsided, the patient is asked to exercise, first with passive movements and then with active movements (yoga exercises using various body positions). Yoga instructions are recommended to help the patients do these exercises correctly.

This treatment is often accompanied by an oral administration of Ayurvedic herbal formulas two to three times per day. The formulas often used are *Yograj-guggul* or *Mahayograj-guggul* (formulas from Ayurvedic text) with gold *bhasma* (gold formula made by oxidizing gold with heat using herbs). A physician must carefully examine the patient for other illnesses and organ disorders to determine a suitable antiarthritis formula, depending on accompanying health conditions.

TABLE 2.10

Group of Herbs To Mitigate *Kapha*[3]

Aragvadhadi Group (used to treat vomiting, leprosy, fevers, mitigate kapha, itching, diabetes, and clean bad wounds)

Medicinal Plant	Botanical Name
Aragvadha	*Cassia fistula*
Indrajava	*Holerrhina antidysenterica* wall
Patali	*Stereospermum colais*
Kakatitka	*Abrus precatorius* Linn.
Nimba	*Azadirachta indica* A.
Amrata	*Tinospora cordifolia* Miers
Madhurasa	*Marsedenia tenacissima*
Sruvavrksa	*Flacourtia indica*
Patha	*Steohania japonica* Miers
Bhunimba	*Andrographis paniculata*
Sairyaka	*Barleria prionitis* Linn.
Patala	*Cydonia oblonga*
Two *Karanja*	*Pongamia pinnata*
Saptacchada	*Alstonia scholaris* R.
Agni	*Plymbago zeylanica* Linn.
Susavi	*Momoridca chirantia* Linn.
Phalsa	*Grewia subinaequalis* DC
Bana	*Barleria stringosa*
Ghonta	*Acaia catechu* Willd *badari* (Hem), *Zyziphus jujuba* Lam.
Arka	*Calotropis gigantea* (L.)
Alarka	*Calotropis procera*
Nagadanti	*Croton oblongifolius*
Visalya	*Gloriosa superba* Linn.
Bharangi	*Clerodendrum indicum*
Rasna	*Acampe papikkosa*
Vrscikali	*Pergularia extensa*
Prakirya	*Cesalpinia bonducella* Fleming
Pratyakpuspi	*Achyranthes aspera* Linn.
Pitataila	*Abrus precatorius* Linn.
Udakirya	*Pongamia glabra* Vent.

2.5.3 Dietary Management and Lifestyle Changes

Dietary and lifestyle interventions are initiated according to the disturbed *dosas* and the physical and mental constitution of a person; these interventions are accompanied by spiritual nurturing, removing serious worry, exercise, and yoga practice. If *vata* were disturbed, the diet would include oils, butter, and sweet food. If *kapha* were disturbed, the diet would include bitter, sour, vinegary, spicy, dry food. If *pitta* were disturbed, the diet would include mild tasting food, grains, lentils, and moderate amounts of sweets and oils. Patients are given a restricted diet of small quantities of *mung dal* (a type of lentil) or yogurt and rice. Depriving the patient of drinking water helps in ascites, edema, and certain kidney diseases where large amounts of water are retained in the body.

TABLE 2.11

Ayurvedic Herbs Known To Have Confirmed Therapeutic Effects

Disease/Symptoms	Herb	Popular Name
Edema	*Achyranthes aspera* Linn.	*Apamarga*
Mental distress	*Acorus calamus* Linn.	*Vacha*
Bronchiolar constriction	*Adhatoda zeylanica* Medic.	*Vasa*
Intestinal worms	*Butea monosperma* Lam	*Palasha*
Arthritis, inflammation, and high cholesterol	*Commiphora mukul* Wightii	*Guggul*
Bone fracture	*Cissus quadrangularis* Linn.	*Vajravalli*
Malaria	*Alstonia scholaris* R. Br.	*Saptaparna*
Liver disorders	*Andrographis paniculata* Nees	*Bhunimba*
Cardiac disorders	*Artemisia vulgaris* Linn.	*Nimba*
	Terminalia arjuna	*Arjuna*
Bacterial or virus	*Azadirachta Indica* A. Juss	*Nimba*
Memory problem	*Bacopa monnieri* (Linn.) Pennell	*Brahmi*
Inflammation and diuretic need	*Boerhaavia diffusa*	*Punarnava*
Severe constipation	*Cassia angustifolia* Vahl.	*Rechani*
Muscle spasm	*Cedrus deodara* (Roxb.)	*Devadaaru*
Memory problem	*Celastrus paniculatus* Willd.	*Jyotishmati*
Nerve weakness	*Centella asiatica* (Linn.) Urban.	*Mandukaparni*
Malaria and fevers	*Caesalpinia crista* Linn.	*Natakaranja*
Inflammation	*Curcuma longa* Linn.	*Haridraa*
Diabetes	*Eugenia jambolana* Lam.	*Jamboo*
Dysentry	*Holarrhena antidysenterica* Wall.	*Kutaja*
Convulsions	*Masilea minuta* Linn.	*Sunisannak*
Liver toxicity	*Picrorhiza kurroa* Royle.	*Kutuka*
Mild constipation	*Plantago ovata* Forsk	*Ishadgola*
Skin white spot	*Psoralea corylifolia* Linn.	*Bakuchi*
Low breast milk	*Pueraria tuberosa* DC.	*Vidarikanda*
Low muscle mass	*Sida rhombifolia* Linn.	*Mahabala*
Fever	*Swertia chirata* Buch.-Ham.	*Kairata*
Heart weakness	*Terminalia arjuna* W. and A.	*Arjuna*
Mental distress, physical exhaustion, and inflammation	*Withania somnifera* Dunal	*Ashwagandha*

Healthy lifestyle is very important to maximize the effect of palliative treatment. Ayurveda strongly recommends that the patient utilize a regular sleeping schedule, about 8 hours of sleep each night, rising early in the morning; do regular exercise; and eat breakfast and engage in other dietary recommendations according to seasons. In order to maximize the effectiveness of palliative treatment, *Vyayam* (exercise, yoga, stretching), breathing exercises, and sunbathing are necessary. It is important that some appropriate form of exercise be done at a maximum tolerated effect (MTE) level during the treatment period; this may be with the help of a physical fitness trainer. The concept of MTE is similar to a therapeutic dose of pharmacologic agents to get maximum beneficial effect. Exercise is likely to create a need for nutrients inside the cells. It is believed to open up the microchannels (*shrotas*) in the body cell for nutrients and for medicine to enter. It is particularly important in maximizing the effectiveness of therapies in management as well as prevention of chronic musculoskeletal disorders.

2.5.4 *Bhasma*

The oxidized form of metal and mineral preparations, called *bhasma*, is also extensively used in Ayurvedic medicine. *Bhasmas* are metal or mineral powder formulas made by specific Ayurvedic text procedures with several herbs and herbal extracts and subjected to very precise heat treatment. The common metals and minerals used in making *bhasmas* for therapeutic use are gold, silver, copper, mercury, iron, zinc, tin, arsenic, gypsum, lime, alum, borax, silica, diamond, ruby, emerald, saphire, jade, moonstone, sunstone, turquoise, and mica.

Procedures to make *bhasmas* are very complicated and involve dozens of steps and many herbs and herbal extracts. These procedures detoxify toxic metals like mercury. If any of the steps in the procedure are either omitted or not properly carried out, then safety is compromised. The pure metal salts do not account for unique pharmacological properties of their *bhasmas*. For example, pure mercury salts do not account for the antiarthritic activity of mercury *bhasma*. There are several hundred metal *bhasmas* described in texts. The science and art of *bhasmas*, a separate branch of pharmacy known as *Rasa Shastra*, is described in Chapter 6.

2.5.5 *Rasayana*

The word *rasayana* is made up of two Sanskrit words, *rasa* (nutrition) and *ayana* (transportation in the body). Thus, *rasayana* refers to compound preparations containing multiple herbs and minerals that improve transportation of nutritional materials to body tissues. The fundamental underlying theme of *rasayanas* is nutrition. They are part of the overall balanced diet. *Rasayanas* are claimed to improve vitality, rejuvenate body tissues, improve immunity, and prevent aging. *Rasayanas* may act in a variety of ways by improving the nutritional value of the food, digestion and absorption of nutrients, transportation of nutrients to tissues, bioavailability of nutrients, metabolism of nutrients in tissues, immunity, and by cleaning the *srotas* (microcirculatory channels or pores) which improve uptake of micronutrients. Basically, *rasayanas* are classified into three categories: (1) *Ajasrika rasayana* (nutrition, dietary) is taken regularly with food as nutrition; (2) *Kamya rasayana* (normal health promoter) is indicated to improve vigor, vitality, and to make a healthy person feel better; and (3) *Naimittika rasayana* is indicated to promote vitality in a particular disease. *Kamya rasayana* is further classified into three categories: (1) *Pranakamya rasayana* (promoter of life vitality and longevity); (2) *Medhakamya rasayana* (promoter of intellect); and (3) *Srikamya rasayana* (promoter of skin complexion and luster). Ayurvedic physicians should be consulted to determine the appropriate rasayana required depending upon the health needs.

Rasayanas are the Ayurvedic equivalent to modern dietary supplements. It is understandable that vitamins, minerals, and biologically active steroids, alkaloids, glycosides, tannins, and a variety of antioxidants present in *rasayanas* would be a good source in providing necessary nutrients to the body. Sometimes an overdose of pure vitamins in modern dietary supplements can cause serious side effects. There is virtually no possibility of an overdose of any specific vitamin or mineral from a *rasayana*.

2.5.6 Formulas

The drug treatment in Ayurveda primarily consists of herbal formulas, *bhasmas*, *rasas* (mercury is always an ingredient of *rasas*), and medicated oils and ghee (for topical application, nasal drops, and enemas). A single herb is rarely administered to a patient in Ayurveda; generally a formula made up of several herbs is used. They are always given with other foods or herbal items, e.g., honey, ghee, ginger, etc., which help mitigate toxicity and may increase absorption of certain ingredients, thus obtaining the desired therapeutic effect. Herbal formulas are favored in Ayurveda because the founders of Ayurveda recognized the possible synergistic and counterbalancing effects of herbs.

Sometimes none of the herbs in a formula exhibit therapeutic effects individually, but the formula could nevertheless be effective. Recently, a formula (*Trasina*) made up of *Withania somnifera*, *Tinospora cordifolia* (Wild*)* Miers, *Eclipt alba* Hassk, *Ocimum sanctum* Linn, *Picrorrhiza kurroa* Royal ex Benth, and *Shilajit* (rock sweat, collected from rocks) showed beneficial activity in diabetic rats, whereas no such effect was seen with individual herbs.[4] This example illustrates the fact that a rapid screening program to assess biologic activity of single herbs or purified constituents of a herb may not necessarily confirm or disprove a health claim because of possible synergistic effects of the combination of drugs or adjuvant. Ayurvedic formulas are analogous to vegetarian food where an experienced cook makes the difference in taste and benefits. All the chemical constituents of milk consumed individually are not likely to give benefits equal to that of an equivalent amount of whole milk consumed. It is therefore important that Ayurvedic formulas as described in Ayurvedic texts be evaluated for therapeutic benefits along with the individual active herbs.

There are several thousand formulas described in Ayurvedic texts that are recommended for over 200 well-identified diseases. In the 1970s, a panel of Ayurvedic experts was appointed by the government of India to evaluate the formulas in Ayurvedic texts. The panel compiled an "Ayurvedic Formulary of India."[5] It has over 560 evaluated formulas including 22 *bhasmas* and 55 *rasas* and *yogas* (preparations containing mineral drugs as main ingredients). Some formulas have dozens of herbs; for example, *Jirakadi Modaka* has 46 herbs and *Shiva Gutika* has 49 herbs.

Individual plants and plant constituents have been studied for therapeutic activity in recent scientific studies. Therapeutic effects have been confirmed by clinical and biological testing for many of them. A few examples are given in Table 2.11.

2.5.7 Yoga

Yoga is used not only as a therapy, but also to improve general health and vitality. Yoga is defined as the inhibition of fluctuations of consciousness.[6] In effect, it restrains mental activity. Mind in total is composed of three faculties: brain, intellect, and ego. Yoga teaches the means by which the mind is controlled and redirected into constructive channels.

Pantanjali, a famous sage, advocated two methods to control the mind: constant practice and detachment. Although Yoga is conceived today as a combination of physical postures and breathing exercises, Ayurvedic texts actually describe several components of Yoga such as ethical practices, punctuality of daily routine, physical-posture exercises, breathing exercise, sensorial practices, and meditation practices. Today, breathing and physical-posture exercises are collectively known as Yoga. The practice of Yoga alone or in combination with other Ayurvedic therapies has been noted in Ayurvedic texts as beneficial in certain diseases, such as hypertension, bronchial asthma, anxiety, neurosis, gastrointestinal disorders, headache, insomnia, obesity, anxiety, and depression. It is suggested that the autonomic nervous system is improved by Yoga, resulting in a relatively hypometabolic state, thereby lessening the energy demands on the body. The efficiency of the cardiovascular and respiratory systems is also significantly enhanced by Yoga.

2.5.8 Massage

Vital points exist where muscle, cartilage, nerves, and bones join each other. The life energies are believed to be concentrated at these points. There are 22 vital points on the upper extremities, 22 on the lower extremities, 12 in the abdominal areas, 14 in the back, and 37 in the neck and head. Manipulation and massage of these points has been used in Ayurveda to treat diseases and strengthen the body. Ayurvedic massage is the combination of massage with medicinal oils and acupressure. Because lipophilic materials can be easily absorbed through skin, medicated oil massage can be a very effective therapy. Specific medicated oils and types of strokes are chosen based on the disturbed *dosas*, body constitution, injury, and disease condition.

The basic strokes of massage include (1) friction where pressure is applied by thumb and finger tips more on muscular part, and gentle pressure on bony parts; (2) kneading, deep or superficial; (3) rounding; (4) wringing or twisting; (5) chucking; (6) stroking; (7) percussion; (8) vibrations; (9) joint movement; and (10) soft, gentle massage with thumbs and palm. Ayurvedic massage is useful for general weakness, fatigue, arthritis, musculoskeletal disorders, tennis elbow, lumbago, frozen shoulder, backache sprains, and aches. Massage is also found useful for nervous system disorders, psychosis, drug addiction, gynecological disorders, menopausal syndrome, postdelivery recovery, myocardial infarction, ischemic heart disease, functional heart disease, cold hands and feet due to bad circulation, varicose veins, psychological problems, obesity, loss of weight, stamina, and disturbed digestive system.[7] Contraindications for massage therapy are fever, indigestion, and patients undergoing cleansing processes.

Massage is also advised for healthy people to maintain their health and relieve muscular fatigue after a heavy physical activity or exercise.

2.6 Summary

Basically, Ayurvedic health care is based on the principle that body, mind, and soul must be in harmony for health and happiness. Each of these has to be nurtured for an individual to create health. Ayurveda recommends daily activities in detail, e.g., getting up before sunrise, routine physical exercise, meditation, and diet according to the body constitution with seasonal adjustments in lifestyle and sexual activities to maintain an optimum balance of *dosas* to prevent illness. Unhealthy lifestyles, exposure to various physical, chemical, and biological agents, extreme weather conditions, unhealthy diets, and overexertion from physical or mental activities are considered the major causes of imbalance of *dosas*. Cleansing of the body from waste products of the illness is necessary to eradicate an illness and prevent its recurrence. Finally, management of an illness essentially consists of elimination of causes of the imbalance of *dosas*, administration of various Ayurvedic formulas, dietary changes to bring *dosas* back into balance, elimination of serious worry, and nurturing the soul to regain spiritual health.

Research activity on Indian medicinal plants over the past 50 years has been extensive. Data on more than 5000 Indian medicinal plants have been complied in the *Compendium of Indian Medicinal Plants* by Rastogi and Mehrotra.[8] The data include research studies on pharmacological and therapeutic activity, pharmacognosy, plant chemistry, and established chemical structures of chemical constituents. Research on more than 500 popular Indian medicinal plants are similarly described in *The Treatise of Indian Medicinal Plants* by

Chatterjee and Pakarashi.[9] Data on several hundred selected medicinal plants are also compiled in other books.

Ayurveda, the traditional health-care system of India, is a complete and holistic health-care system that contains both preventive and therapeutic aspects. It has a defined diagnostic system covering all physiological functions and organs, as well as specific treatments and management techniques for each disease. Although Ayurveda is thousands of years old, many of its core principles are consistent with modern medicine. Ayurvedic medicine offers a wealth of relatively effective, safe, and economic health-care therapies. Its therapies provide relief for many chronic illnesses such as musculoskeletal disorders, rheumatoid arthritis, osteoarthritis, diabetes, obesity, nervous disorders, etc. Ayurvedic medicine has been successfully integrated with allopathic medicine in India. Certainly, a great potential exists for its integration into the health-care system in the U.S.

References

1. Mishra, L., Singh, B.B., and Dagenais, S., Ayurveda: a historical perspective and principles of the traditional healthcare system in India, *Altern. Ther. Health Med.*, 7(2), 36–42, 2001a.
2. Mishra, L., Singh, B.B., and Dagenais, S., Healthcare and disease management in Ayurveda, *Altern. Ther. Health Med.*, 7(2), 44–50, 2001b.
3. Shikantha Murthy, K.R. (translator), Sodhanadigana Samgraha, in *Vagbhatt's Ashtanghradaya*, Vol.1, Krishnadas Academy, Varanasi, UP, India, 1999, chap. 15.
4. Bhattacharya, S.K., Satyan, K., and Chakrabaarti, A., Effect of Trasina, an Ayurvedic herbal formulation, on pancreatic islet superoxide dismutase activity in hyperglycemic rats, *Indian J. Exp. Biol.*, 35, 297–299, 1997.
5. Ayurvedic Formulary of India, 1st ed., Government of India, Ministry of Health and Family Planning, Department of Health, Government of India Press, Delhi, 1978.
6. Murthy, A.R.Y., Ayurveda and yoga, in *Principles of Ayurvedic Therapeutics*, Vinaya Kumaar, A., Ed., Shri Satguru Publications, New Delhi, India, 1995.
7. Ranade, S. and Rawat, R., *Healing Touch: Ayurvedic Message*, Chaukhambe Sanskrit Pratisthan, Delhi, India, 2000.
8. Rastogi, R.P. and Mehrotra, B.N., *Compendium of Indian Medicinal Plants*, Central Drug Research Institute, Lucknow, and National Institute of Science Communication, New Delhi, printed at Publication and Information Directorate of Council of Scientific and Industrial Research, New Delhi, India, Vol. 1, 1990; Vol. 2, 1991; Vol. 3, 1993; Vol. 4, 1995; Vol. 5, 1998.
9. Chatterjee, A. and Pakrashi, S.C., *The Treatise of Indian Medicinal Plants*, Publication and Information Directorate, New Delhi, National Institute of Science Communication (CSIR), Dr. Krishnan Marg, New Delhi, India, Vol. 1, 1991; Vol. 2, 1992; Vol. 3, 1994; Vol. 4, 1995; Vol. 5, 1997.

3

Clinical Research Design: Limited Systematic Review of Five Diagnostic Categories

Betsy B. Singh, Sivarama P. Vinjamury, and Vijay John Singh

CONTENTS

3.1 Introduction

Ayurveda, the Indian System of Medicine (ISM), may be the least well known of the complete systems of medicine in the West, despite being one of the oldest. According to the definition used by the National Center for Complementary and Alternative Medicine (NCCAM),[1] World Health Organization (WHO), and other organizations, Ayurveda qualifies as a complementary and alternative medicine (CAM).[2]

Certain techniques used as therapies in this system of medicine have been assimilated in the West but not practiced as a whole system. For example, yoga, oil massages, meditation practices, and body cleansing (both internal and external) are used frequently in the West as part of health-promoting behaviors; they are rarely perceived as part of a larger holistic traditional medical practice. Often the practitioners of these techniques have not completed full Ayurvedic medical training and have merely focused on learning

0-8493-1366-X/04/$0.00+$1.50

the technique via the apprenticeship method. The training is limited to studies with practitioners in India, whereas others have merely taken weekend seminars. Some training is now available in the U.S. for those who wish to get a certificate or some other training credential. These programs are not full time and last between 1 and 2 years.[3] No equivalent program of the Ayurvedic medical schools in India, which require 5 ½ years of training before practice is allowed, exists.[4] As a result, there are quite a variety of credentials held by the practitioners of Ayurvedic therapeutic techniques. In addition, because licensing is not required by most states in America, there is not a consistent and focused movement torward establishing the practice. It is also questionable as to whether those programs that teach both professionals and paraprofessionals certain Ayurvedic treatment techniques (e.g., yoga) without the whole context of Ayurvedic theoretical underpinning will do more than produce isolated therapies originally designed to be part of a whole.

This disassociation of the Ayurvedic treatment repertoire will minimize optimization of patient recovery potential as the synergistic advantages will be lost. Because these practices are rarely coordinated by a trained Ayurvedic physician in the West, research into the utilization of Ayurvedic bodywork practices, cleansing, and Ayurvedic herbals used independently or in an integrated medical scenario with allopathic treatment techniques is essential. Research in Ayurveda must be done with rigor and with an expectation of perusal by Western trained physicians who wish to integrate these techniques into their health-care practices. Without research data that will convince the Western trained physician that a patient can benefit or at least will not be harmed, Ayurveda will continue to remain an underutilized therapeutic option for patients.

Research must be done to identify which practices and herbals are both safe for specific conditions, with or without certain co-morbidities, and that are able to produce optimized patient recovery. Because individual practices have begun to be used primarily as a consumer-driven enterprise, research respecting the character and tradition of Ayurvedic medical parameters must be conducted within the context in which the practice is likely to occur.

3.2 Empiricism in Medical Knowledge Development

It is interesting to note that many Western-trained physicians question, for example, the scientific underpinning or rationale for the use of Ayurvedic medicine, homeopathy, and traditional Chinese medicine. However, empirical explanations for use of health treatments, much like the role of empiricism in a biological lab, are often ignored as a source of evidence. Empiricism draws upon close observation and experimentation.[5] So, when past Ayurvedic physicians observed changes in a patient's condition after administering a treatment, it should not have been considered philosophical or traditional knowledge, per se. It is not less valid than observations made and recorded in a laboratory experiment.

When clinical case notes are passed on to colleagues and to the next generation of doctors being trained, it is no less valid than descriptive case studies published today in peer-reviewed medical journals. In balance, it might be helpful to note that if the highest scientific rigor were demanded of allopathic medicine as is being demanded of CAM practices, including Ayurveda, conventional medical practice would not meet the mark either. In 1983 the U.S. Office of Technology stated that only 10 to 20% of all procedures currently used in medical practice had been shown effective by controlled trial.[6] Currently, data indicate that only 20 to 37% of procedures in conventional medicine have been subjected to the same standards as demanded for CAM.[7]

3.3 Ayurveda: An Evidence-Based Medicine

An accurate understanding of what evidence-based medicine (EBM) really means might be helpful in understanding the relative role of science and clinical knowledge. EBM, which has become a buzz word concerning medical decision making, refers to a triangulated set of information that the physician should use to determine the best treatment for a particular patient.[8] Here, Western medicine is coming closer to a holistic treatment approach, closer to the parameters of treatment in Ayurvedic practice. The three factors of EBM are the following:

1. Best available relevant scientific evidence concerning the effectiveness and efficacy of the proposed treatment
2. Physician knowledge based on practice experience
3. Patient's own preferences for treatment modalities if they do not contradict 1 or 2 above

In order to make the best utilization of this triangulation of information, physicians must be familiar with the treatment perspectives described in the scientific literature. If there is a dearth of information or the studies are conducted without scientific rigor, patients are put into jeopardy; either therapies that might help will not be considered, or physicians will be concerned about validity and reliability of data based on quality of data in studies reported.

3.3.1 Overcoming Barriers of Research

There have indeed been barriers to CAM research, in general, which also affected Ayurvedic research. They have included structural barriers in the West where conventional medical institutions received the largest share of funds to investigate therapies for which no one in the institution receiving the funds had any firsthand knowledge. Collaborations were often not equitable, even when CAM therapists were co-investigators. Publication bias has been a problem in the past. With specific journals dedicated to publishing CAM literature, the situation may improve. However, both CAM investigators and journal editors must produce and ensure the quality of data presented. In this way, those persons who are skeptical will learn that CAM researchers can produce good, relevant science.

Expectations for randomized controlled trials (RCTs) can be another barrier. It is appropriate for preclinical studies to be done along with quasi-experimental designs prior to conducting RCTs whenever possible.[9] It is important for the investigators in RCTs to have established factors that will allow for accurate calculation of sample size, to determine possible sources of bias in executing such a trial, the usefulness of outcome measures chosen, and that the dosages (if applicable) and delivery schedule of the therapeutic product or intervention are optimized before moving to an RCT. If these factors, minimally, are not known, then the investigators must do Phase II clinical work to establish this information. It behooves all of us to recognize research at the case study, case series, or outcome study level for the scientific building blocks that they are.[10]

3.4 Research Designs: A Look at a Hierarchy of Design

Several clinical study types can be implemented by those clinicians who do not have the funds or expertise to engage in larger research projects. These clinicians may consider adding to the body of knowledge through executing one of the following designs.

3.4.1 Case Studies

3.4.1.1 Retrospective Case Study

This case-study design can offer information about an unusual case that might help colleagues problem solve if they have a similar case. In this research design, there would be no prior planning to investigate the diagnosis or treatment. The term *retrospective* is used to refer to its structure. Generally, the authors of such a study give detailed information about the demographic, diagnosis profile, and general health parameters of the patient of focus. The therapy utilized and the patient progress are noted in detail. This is a particularly useful tool when the disease presents in an unusual manner, the patient's progress is unanticipated, or a unique therapy has been tried.

A prospective descriptive case study is structured identically to the retrospective model given above except that the clinician plans in advance to conduct the study. Like the retrospective case study described above, the information is for the most part qualitative. It is hoped that the prospective nature of the study will encourage the clinician to take even more detailed SOAP (clinical) notes than would have been the case normally; this creates a rich information source for those clinicians who might find the information useful in the future. Both retrospective case studies and prospective case studies can be case series. This change in name merely means that multiple (generally 5 to 10) patients with a similar diagnosis or similar treatment will be presented.

Probably the most useful study of this design type is the structured or experimental case study and case series. This design involves *a priori* design time. The specific patient diagnostic parameters, type and duration of treatment, outcome measures, number of patients in the sample (n = 1 to 10), and analyses would be planned in advance. This structure allows for quantitative information in addition to the standard qualitative information to be gleaned from the investigation. This type of design is particularly helpful when details of the therapy and consequences are required to determine optimum delivery of a new therapy or new combination of therapies or when there are questions about the effectiveness of a therapy for an esoteric group of sufferers from a particular diagnosis.

3.4.1.2 Outcome Studies

Another design that might be considered is an outcome study. This design is similar in structure to the experimental case study described above. However, it would best be built upon a case study where notions of percentage of improvement are available so that power calculations could be generated. Whenever possible, knowing the number of participants needed to show differences, generally moderate differences, is important. Otherwise, investigators are left using cookbook guesses that may defeat the purpose of the study. Patients serve as their own control, and their improvement is noted through standardized measures from baseline (period just prior to treatment beginning) to various measurement points until the end of treatment. Often 25 to 30 persons are enrolled if prior data are not available to determine sample size needs. Because patients serve as their own control, it is a very useful design to refine the therapy, refine study protocol, and have larger sample size data to inform an RCT design.

Because there is no control group and patients serve as their own control (a better match would be hard to imagine), attention to possible sources of bias in the design is important. If covariants are known, efforts should be made to eliminate them in the design or to collect data on these factors and control them in the analysis. This design does not address issues of potential placebo effect; whenever possible, these studies are followed by homogeneous and heterogeneous RCTs. Many questions that can be answered by this design cannot be answered by RCTs. The scientific question to be asked coupled with the data that already exist in the literature may mean that an RCT is not the best design.

3.4.1.3 Randomized Controlled Trials

RCTs are best done when there is information in the existing literature at a quasi-experimental level (e.g., outcome study) to inform the RCT. It is important to minimally:

1. Have a specific research question that can be answered by a multigroup comparison.
2. Know the optimum effective dose or equivalent for the medical practice before starting.
3. Know the precise number of subjects needed to be able to detect differences among the groups.
4. Know that the placebo or sham arm of the study will not be obvious to the participants (blinding is maintained).
5. Know the approximate number of dropouts expected due to possible rigors of the protocol.
6. Take precautions to control potential biases and not merely rely on random assignment to condition or pure randomization to equally disburse individual differences among the groups in the study.
7. Have a precise analytical plan with the person manipulating the data (biostatistician or methodologist) blinded to group assignment as completely as the persons in contact with the patients.

It is obvious that preliminary data at quasi-experimental levels must be collected before the sophistication of an RCT design is cost effective. Guessing on information required to inform an RCT will result in poor data, which may be considered valid in today's medical culture merely because it uses the word *randomized* in the title. It is far better to contribute to the body of knowledge with a well-done case study or outcome study than to report a flawed RCT.

3.4.1.4 Systematic Reviews and Meta-Analyses

Two additional designs that contribute to a consensus building about a therapy or diagnosis are systematic reviews and meta-analyses. Both designs are secondary analyses of previously done work. Generally, these two designs have utilized RCT data and not included information from quasi-experimental designs with the assumption that RCTs constitute the highest level of data collection for individual trials. Both homogeneous and heterogeneous RCTs are used in both.

A systematic review is a qualitative method of evaluation of a group of RCTs on a specific therapy or diagnosis for the most part. The fewer the RCTs, the smaller the data pool from which conclusions are drawn. Currently, systematic reviews in CAM suffer from too few RCTs on the topic, design flaws of the RCTs (e.g., inadequate sample size), and changing expectations of expected research rigor in CAM during the most recent past. Other levels of data must continue to be relied upon for clues to prescribing and safety parameters.

A meta-analysis is difficult at this point, but some have been attempted. This research strategy is similar to systematic reviews except that the analysis is a quantitative one. The authors of such analyses generally attempt to get raw data from authors of RCTs, normalize the data across the trials they have collected, and use this pooled data attempt to determine the overall safety or efficacy of a particular therapy. This is even a more difficult task than a Systematic Review strategy. These designs are best left to biostatisticians or methodologists at this time. Even they have difficulty getting sufficient information in which to conduct a meta-analysis, as the total information required is rarely reported in full in a published article.

3.5 Southern California University Research Model

The authors of this chapter have pursued a stepwise approach to development of a research track in Ayurveda, just as in other medical treatment modalities. Even though effectiveness and efficacy of certain therapies were established via traditional knowledge and through clinical data used in conventional medicine, this research group has chosen to investigate Ayurvedic therapies holistically and to investigate specific herbals within a reductionistic science-based approach as well. Animal work concerning mechanism of action and safety and toxicity has been conducted with standard models. Additionally, each diagnosis and therapy pursued are first tested in a structured case study design, a case series, and outcome study before moving onward to an RCT. In this way, the team utilizes the traditional knowledge base to develop the research questions and design both basic science and clinical studies. Design structure and outcome measures are then used that will satisfy scientists regardless of the continent on which they live.

Unlike their knowledge of recently formulated conventional drugs, these authors have the advantage of knowing the long history of use of many of the herbal formulas or processes in Ayurveda. However, we still collect adverse event data and report them (lack of them) so that those physicians who read the studies will have as much detail as possible about the potential benefit to their patients. Until there are many fully trained Ayurvedic physicians in the West, access to knowledge about the appropriate use of therapies and formulas may have to come from doctors initially trained in the West. It is best that we become "bilingual": Ayurvedic medical benefits should be presented both in the context of Ayurvedic practice and in a framework that the conventional physician will understand and ultimately feel comfortable using in his or her practice with appropriate patients.

3.6 Review of Quasi-Experimental Data

The clinical trial data in five monographs on epilepsy,[11] asthma,[12] hyperlipidemia,[13] urinary diseases,[14] and liver diseases[15] generated by Central Council for Research in Ayurveda and Siddha, Ministry of Health, India, were reviewed and analyzed in this chapter for effectiveness of the following herbs and herbal formulas:

1. AYUSH 65 in epilepsy
2. *Naradeeya lakshmi vilasa rasa* in bronchial asthma
3. *Shwasa kesari* tablets in bronchial asthma
4. *Guggulu* in hyperlipidemia (short-term study)
5. *Guggulu* in hyperlipidemia/hyperlipoproteinemia (long-term study)
6. *Varuna* in urinary tract infection, benign prostatic hyperplasia (BPH), urolithiasis, and miscellaneous disorders
7. *Kulattha* in urolithiasis
8. *Varuna* and *Kulattha* in urolithiasis
9. *Kulattha* and *Gokshuru* in urolithiasis
10. *Katuki* in hepatocellular jaundice, chronic hepatitis, and cirrhosis
11. *Katukyadi* yoga in hepatocellular jaundice, chronic hepatitis, postinfective hepatitis, obstructive jaundice, chronic cholecystitis, and postcholecystectomy syndrome
12. *Kumariasava* in hepatocellular jaundice, chronic hepatitis, and obstructive jaundice
13. *Kumariasava* in hepatocellular jaundice, chronic hepatitis, and obstructive jaundice
14. *Daruharidra* in hepatocellular jaundice, chonic hepatitis, postinfective hepatitis, and obstructive jaundice

3.6.1 Clinical Data

Table 3.1 shows the rating of the data included in the monographs along two parameters: (1) quality assessment of the data using the Singh Scale for quasi-experimental designs and (2) safety assessment using the Safety Assessment Score for Controlled Clinical Trials© (SAS-CT). The Singh Q-E Quality Assessment Scale© scores 10 factors with 15 possible points. The 10 areas are the following:

1. Background and significance of literature review
2. Adequacy of treatment
3. Power calculation

4. Description of product and procedure
5. Description of sample selected
6. Description of outcome measures
7. Data report
8. Attention to possible bias in experimental design
9. Bias present in design or operationalization of design
10. Comparison of dropouts and competitors

Of the factors listed, 1, 2, 3, 5, and 6 have two points possible due to the specific subfactors listed (see Table 3.1 for more details). The safety score was derived by using the SAS-CT system which queries six global issues with subfactors being scored to produce a possible point score of 100. As the clinical trials reviewed here were not controlled, the scores were modified for the safety assessment. Full scores were given if the scoring category was satisfied for the single group receiving the therapy. Table 3.1 gives both summed scores for each data set reviewed within the monograph for both scales and gives partials across factors for all data sets reviewed.

All authors and three research assistants acknowledged here participated in the systematic review process using both scales. Each article was primarily reviewed by two people with a third person as an arbitrator for reconciliation purposes. This mechanism guaranteed that four to five people reviewed each article in order to produce the scoring offered in the table.

The studies reviewed here with the Singh Q-E Quality Assessment Scale received full points on the factors of the background and significance of study, sample description, clarity of outcome measures utilized, and clarity of tables and data reported. Twelve of thirteen data sets utilized outcome measures with established, known, or reported reliability and validity. Ten of the thirteen articles were believed to be without operationalization flaws and presented the protocol in sufficient detail to allow for replication. Nine of the data sets optimized treatment to patients and seven of the thirteen justified the dosage of herbal treatments or therapies offered. Overall, this is quite a good showing. These results should encourage others to read the literature that is originating in India and other non-Western venues with the attitude that the data presented are going to be consistent with the quality of trials available in the West.

The SAS-CT scores were a bit more mixed. This factor is important, because people in the West are particularly interested in safety information on herbals and procedures that are less well known to them. Of the 13 studies reviewed, the range of scores was from 0 to 100. Four studies got perfect scores for reporting safety issues and five got no points. Other scores were 17, 21, 44.1, 47, and 88. It must be noted that an investigator should address the issues around safety: the occurrence of adverse events, the severity of them should they occur, whether they are likely related to the trial or not, and what the dropout rate is and were these due to adverse events minimally. For example, it is impossible to tell whether five articles did not report adverse events because none occurred, or the information was merely not reported. A simple sentence saying (1) that there were no adverse events and (2) there were no dropouts would go a long way to assist those reading data to assess safety. A reader cannot assume that a product is safe if there is nothing about adverse events mentioned; he or she can only wonder.

Evaluation of Clinical Trials of Typical Ayurvedic Therapies

Quasi-Experimental Designs: Singh's Scale	Factors and Study Codes*													
	EPI	ASTH 1	ASTH 2	LIPID 1	LIPID 2	VARUNA	KULA	V+K	K+G	KATUKI	KYOGA	ASAV	DARU	MEAN
Background and significance or literature review														
Adequate knowledge of disease	1	1	1	1	1	1	1	1	1	1	1	1	1	1
Adequate knowledge of treatment	1	1	1	1	1	1	1	1	1	1	1	1	1	1
Adequacy of treatment														
Optimum dose, duration	1	1	1	1	1	0	0	0	0	1	1	1	1	0.69
Dose justification	1	1	1	0	0	0	0	0	0	1	1	1	1	0.53
Power calculation														
Number needed reported	0	0	0	0	0	0	0	0	0	0	0	0	0	0
Sufficient number recruited	0	0	0	1	1	0	0	0	0	1	1	0	0	0.3
Description of product and procedure														
Sufficient for replication	1	1	1	1	1	1	0	0	0	1	1	1	1	0.76
Description of sample selected														
Demographics	1	1	1	1	1	1	1	1	1	1	1	1	1	1
Diagnosis-related information	1	1	1	1	1	1	1	1	1	1	1	1	1	1
Outcome meaasures														
Clearly stated	1	1	1	1	1	1	1	1	1	1	1	1	1	1
Validity and reliability established	0	1	1	1	1	1	1	1	1	1	1	1	1	0.92
Data reported														
Report consistent with data tables etc.	1	1	1	1	1	1	1	1	1	1	1	1	1	1
Attention to possible biases	0	0	0	1	1	1	0	0	0	0	1	1	1	0.46
No operationalization flaws	1	1	1	1	1	1	1	1	1	0	1	0	0	0.76
Comparison of dropouts vs. completers	0	0	0	1	1	0	0	0	0	0	0	0	0	0.15
Total	**10**	**11**	**11**	**13**	**13**	**10**	**8**	**8**	**8**	**11**	**13**	**11**	**11**	**10.46**

TABLE 3.1 (continued)

Evaluation of Clinical Trials of Typical Ayurvedic Therapies

SAS-CT (Safety Assessment Scores for Controlled Clinical Trials)	Factors and Study Codes*													
	EPI	ASTH 1	ASTH 2	LIPID 1	LIPID 2	VARUNA	KULA	V+K	K+G	KATUKI	KYOGA	ASAV	DARU	MEAN
AEs NR (adverse events not related)	27.0	0.0	27.0	27.0	27.0	0.0	0.0	0.0	0.0	0.0	0.0	27.0	27.0	12.5
ADRs (adverse drug reactions)	27.0	0.0	0.0	27.0	27.0	0.0	0.0	0.0	0.0	17.0	21.0	27.0	27.0	13.3
SAEs NR (serious adverse events not related)	13.5	0.0	0.0	13.5	13.5	0.0	0.0	0.0	0.0	0.0	0.0	13.5	13.5	5.2
SADRs (serious adverse drug reactions)	13.5	0.0	13.0	13.5	13.5	0.0	0.0	0.0	0.0	0.0	0.0	13.5	13.5	6.2
DOs AEs/SAEs NR (dropouts due to AEs and SAEs NR)	3.5	0.0	3.5	9.5	9.5	0.0	0.0	0.0	0.0	0.0	0.0	9.5	9.5	3.5
DOs ADRs/SADRs (dropouts due to ADRs and SADRs)	3.5	0.0	3.5	9.5	9.5	0.0	0.0	0.0	0.0	0.0	0.0	9.5	9.5	3.5
Total	**88.0**	**0.0**	**47.0**	**100.0**	**100.0**	**0.0**	**0.0**	**0.0**	**0.0**	**17.0**	**21.0**	**100.0**	**100.0**	**44.1**

*Study codes:

EPI = Effect of AYUSH 65 in epilepsy.

ASTH 1 = Effectiveness of *Naradeeya Lakshmi vilasa rasa* in bronchial asthma.

ASTH 2 = Effectiveness of *Shwasa kesari* tablets in bronchial asthma.

LIPID 1 = Effectiveness of *Guggulu* in hyperlipidemia (short-term study).

LIPID 2 = Effectiveness of *Guggulu* in hyperlipidemia/hyperlipoproteinemia (long-term study).

VARUNA = Effectiveness of *Varuna* in urinary tract infection, BPH, urolithiasis, and miscellaneous disorders.

KULA = Effectiveness of *Kulattha* in urolithiasis.

V+K = Effectiveness of *Varuna* and *Kulattha* in urolithiasis.

K+G = Effectiveness of *Kulattha* and *Gokshuru* in urolithiasis.

KATUKI = Effectiveness of *Katuki* in hepatocellular jaundice, chronic hepatitis, and cirrhosis.

KYOGA = Effectiveness of *Katukyadi* yoga in hepatocellular jaundice, chronic hepatitis, postinfective hepatitis, obstructive jaundice, chronic cholecystitis, and postcholecystectomy syndrome.

ASAV = Effectiveness of *Kumariasava* in hepatocellular jaundice, chronic hepatitis, and obstructive jaundice.

DARU = Effectiveness of *Daruharidra* in hepatocellular jaundice, chonic hepatitis, postinfective hepatitis, and obstructive jaundice.

Acknowledgments

The following research assistants participated in the systematic review process but did not participate in manuscript preparation: Xiao-Dong Liu, Ph.D., Tarek Adra, Pharm.D., Carol Cho, B.Sc., and Chintan Acharya.

References

1. What is Complementary & Alternative Medicine?, http://www.nccam.nih.gov/health/whatiscam/, accessed July 6, 2002.
2. World Health Organization, The promotion and development of traditional medicine, in *Report of a WHO Meeting, Technical Report Series 622*, Geneva, Switzerland, 1978.
3. Svoboda, R.E. and Bhattacharya, B., Ayurveda, in *Complementary and Alternative Medicine Secrets: Questions & Answers about Integrating CAM Therapies into Clinical Practice*, Kohatsu, W., Ed., Hanley & Belfus, Philadelphia, 2002, p. 65.
4. Hammerly, M., Integrative medicine: who gives a CAM?, *Wellness eJournal*, 2000, accessed July 7, 2002.
5. Smith, R., The ethics of ignorance, *J. Med. Ethics*, 18, 117–118, 1992.
6. White, A. and Ernst, E., The case for uncontrolled clinical trials: a starting point for the evidence base for CAM, *Complement Ther. Med.*, 9(2), 111–116, June 2001.
7. Imrie, R., The evidence for evidence based medicine, *Complement Ther. Med.*, 8, 123–126, 2000.
8. Sackett, D.L., Rosenberg, W.M.C., Gray, J.A.M., et al., Evidence-based medicine: what it is and what it isn't, *Br. Med. J.*, 312, 71–72, 1996.
9. Linde, K. and Jonas, W.B., Evaluating complementary and alternative medicine: the balance of rigor and relevance, in *Essentials of Complementary and Alternative Medicine*, James, W.B. and Levin, J.S., Eds., Lippincott–Williams & Wilkins, Philadelphia, 1999, p. 57.
10. Singh, B.B. and Berman, B.M., Research issues for clinical designs, *Complement Ther. Med.*, 5, 3, 1997.
11. *Ayush-56: An Ayurvedic Anti-Epileptic Drug*, Central Council for Research in Ayurveda and Siddha, Ministry of Health & Family Welfare, Government of India, New Delhi, 1997.
12. Goyal, H.R., Ed., *Tamaka Shwasa (Bronchial Asthma): A Clinical Study New Delhi*, Central Council for Research in Ayurveda and Siddha, Ministry of Health & Family Welfare, Government of India, New Delhi, 1997.
13. Malhotra, S.C., Ed., *Pharmacological & Clinical Studies of Guggulu (Commiphora Wightii) in Hyperlipidaemia/Lipid Metabolism*, Central Council for Research in Ayurveda and Siddha, Ministry of Health & Family Welfare, Government of India, New Delhi, 1992.
14. Singh, L.M., Shukla, J.P., and Deshpande, P.J., *Management of Mutramari (Urinary Calculi) by Three Ayurvedic Drugs: Varuna, Kulattha, and Goksuru*, Central Council for Research in Ayurveda and Siddha, Ministry of Health & Family Welfare, Government of India, New Delhi, 1987.
15. Singh, G. and Chaturvedi, G.N., *Clinical Studies on Kamala (Jaundice) and Yakrt Rogas (Liver Disorders) with Ayurvedic Drugs*, Central Council for Research in Ayurveda and Siddha, Ministry of Health & Family Welfare, Government of India, New Delhi, 1988.

4

Panchakarma Therapy in Ayurvedic Medicine

Ajay Kumar Sharma

CONTENTS

4.1 Introduction

One of the fundamental concepts of Ayurvedic management of diseases is to eliminate toxic materials (vitiated *dosas*) from the body in order to cure a disease. *Panchakarma therapy* (PKT) is designed to eliminate the toxic materials. It is postulated that the toxic materials of the body need to be eliminated radically before a palliative therapy is given. The palliative therapy in the form of drugs and diets may not be effective unless the body channels are properly cleansed and toxic materials are eliminated.

PKT is believed to purify or cleanse all the body tissues and to bring about the harmony of neurohumours (*tridosas*) (i.e., *vata, pitta, kapha,* and *manasa dosas* [i.e., *satva, raja,* and *tama*]) and to obtain long-lasting beneficial effects. PKT is not merely a therapeutic regi-

0-8493-1366-X/04/$0.00+$1.50

men, but it may be considered a management tool when used at certain tissue and body parts. It promotes and preserves the individual's normal health.

PKT[1–3] is an important component of Ayurvedic management of diseases. It is the comprehensive method of internal purification of the body through emesis (*vaman karma*), purgation (*virechana karma*), enema (*vasti karma*), errhines (*nasya karma*), and bloodletting (*raktamokshana*). This chapter will review the ancient classical concepts, traditional practices, and recent advances made in this important field with proper evaluation and rational assessment. Evidence obtained at our hospitals and at other research institutes in treating a variety of diseases with PKT is discussed along with its possible use as an adjunct to allopathic therapies.

PKT is indicated in arthritis, paralysis, neuromuscular diseases and in respiratory, gastrointestinal, ENT, and several blood-related disorders with great benefits. PKT is contraindicated in certain conditions like acute fevers, in various debilitating diseases, and in certain tumors and cancers of different organs; it is also contraindicated in children, the elderly, and pregnant women. PKT is indicated for both the healthy and diseased. The five elimination procedures are usually advised in the sequence of emesis, purgation, enema, errhines, and bloodletting, although it is not mandatory. Either one or all five procedures are advised as per the need and condition of the person undergoing PKT. Based on the health of the individual and stage and type of the disease, only one of the five procedures may be done without following a sequence. However, proper preparation and follow-up treatment are implemented for even one cleansing procedure.

The classical PKT is done in three stages:

1. Preparatory procedures (PREP) (*purva karma*) — These procedures are done to prepare the body to undergo a proper and thorough cleansing. They involve applying as well as ingesting oils and fats, sweating, and also advising which herbs to use to improve the digestion and metabolism in tissues.
2. Main cleansing procedures (MCP) (*pradhana karma*) — These procedures consist of five purification procedures especially designed to eliminate toxic materials from the imbalanced dosas of the body. They are emesis, purgation, enema, errhines, and bloodletting.
3. Postprocedures (*pashchata karma*) — These procedures consist mainly of recuperative measures in the form of diet, lifestyle changes, and rejuvenating herbs.

4.2 *Panchakarma* Therapy Procedures

4.2.1 Preparatory Procedures[4,5]

PREP are used to facilitate PKT effectiveness. They include (1) digestive juice stimulants (*dipana*), (2) digestant (*pachana*), (3) oleation (*snehana*), and (4) sudation (*swedana*). All procedures are discussed below.

4.2.1.1 Digestive Juice Stimulants (Dipana) and Digestants (Pacana)

Digestive juice stimulants are agents that directly stimulate biofire (*agni*) and allow undigested food to be processed without stimulating digestive enzymes. Administration of

TABLE 4.1
List of Commonly Used Digestants and Digestive Stimulant Drugs

No.	Formula Name	Dose	References
1	*Panchakoladi churna*	1–3 g	BR[a] 30/35
2	*Hingvasshtaka churna*	1–3 g	BR 10/59
3	*Lavana bhaskara churna*	1–3 g	BR 10/79–87
4	*Chitrakadi vati*	500 mg to 1 g	BR 8/26,27
5	*Arka vati*	500 mg to 1 g	BR 857
6	*Agnitundi vati*	250–500 mg	BR 10/93,94
7	*Shunthi ghrita*	20–50 g	BR 29/200, 201
8	*Pippalyadi ghrita*	20–50 g	BR 5/1319–1322
9	*Dashmoolarishta*	20–30 ml	BR 74/357–371
10	*Drakshasava*	20–30 ml	BR 8/170–174

[a]BR = Bhaishajaya Ratnavali.

digestants and digestive juice stimulants is an essential prerequisite of PKT; the objective is to improve the digestion both at the cellular and gastrointestinal tract level.

Normal digestion is achieved with the administration of medicated dehydrated butter (*ghee*) mixed with digestants and digestive juice stimulants. Dehydrated butter is a potent biofire stimulant agent. Commonly used digestants and digestive juice stimulants are described in Table 4.1.

Any preparation is usually administered for 3 to 7 days, depending on the age, disease, and condition of the patient. Signs and symptoms of satisfactory stimulation of digestion are (1) feeling of lightness in the body, (2) improved appetite, (3) feeling of thirst, and (4) well-formed stool without any mucus.

4.2.1.2 Oleation Therapy (Snehana Karma)[4,5]

Any procedure or substance that increases the availability of lubricants, which produce lubrication in the body externally or internally, is called oleation therapy (OT). It is often used as an independent therapeutic procedure for disorders of *vata* as well as PREP for PKT. It is essential to administer OT to an individual before subjecting him or her to MCP to mobilize the toxic materials from their respective sites.

OT may be given externally by applying the oily materials on the skin or internally via ingestion, enema, or nasal route. External application consists of massage, application as a thin layer on the skin, application on the scalp, as ear drops, holding the oily material in the mouth for a few minutes, applying on the feet, etc.

4.2.1.2.1 Classification of Oleating Drugs and Agents

OT materials may be of animal or vegetable origin. Examples of animal origin materials include dehydrated butter, animal fat, bone marrow, fish oil, and milk. Vegetable origin materials include sesame oil and mustard oil.

The oleation substance selected for administration to the patient on the basis of a underlying disease is shown in Table 4.2. Some standard preparations used for internal oleation are listed in Table 4.3. These are to be swallowed orally with lukewarm milk or water in the prescribed dose as indicated in Table 4.3.

OT is indicated prior to sudation as PREP, dry skin, *vata* dominance, excessive loss of blood, and eye disorders. It is contraindicated in patients with aggravated *kapha* and all conditions where PKT is contraindicated.

Internally medicated ghee is given for 3 to 7 days at the break of dawn (6 to 7 A.M.), based on the person's constitution and digestive power (*agni* and *kostha*). Usually this is

TABLE 4.2

Selection of Oleating Materials Based on Underlying Diseases

No.	Oleating Drug	Disease Indicated
1	*Tikta ghita, mahatikta ghita,* or *vasa ghita*	Skin and blood disorders
2	*Kalyana ghita, brahmi ghita, mahakalyana ghita*	Mental disorders, epilepsy, insanity, etc.
3	*Maha sneha, pancatikta ghita*	Paraplegia

Note: Adjuvants are recommended along with oleating materials.

No.	Adjuvant	Oleating Material
1	Lukewarm water	In all types until specified; otherwise, dehydrated butter
2	Vegetable soups	Oils
3	Gruel made of rice	Fat, bone marrow

TABLE 4.3

Some Standard Preparations of Internal Oleation

No.	Disease	Oil/Dehydrated Butter	Dose	Reference
1	Bronchial asthma	*Manhanshiladi ghrita*	20–30 ml	CC[a] 17/145
2	Skin disease	*Mahatikta ghrita*	20–30 ml	CC 7/144–150
3	Psychosis	*Mahakalyanaka ghrita*	20–30 ml	CC 9/42–44
4	Epilepsy	*Panchagavya ghrita*	20–30 ml	CC 10/17
5	Cardiovascular accident (stroke)	*Bala taila*	20–30 ml	CC 28/148–156
6	Osteoarthritis, arthritis	*Eranda taila*	20–30 ml	CD[b] 25/6
7	Hepatobiliary disorders	*Draksha ghrita*	20–30 ml	BR[c] 12/135
8	Irritable bowel syndrome	*Shunthi ghrita*	20–30 ml	BR 8/555
9	Gynecological disorders	*Phala ghrita*	20–30 ml	BR 67/74-77
10	Tuberculosis	*Pipali ghrita*	20–30 ml	BR 14/237
11	Hemorrhagic diathesis	*Vasa ghrita*	20–30 ml	CC 4/88
12	Hemorrhoids	*Vyoshadya ghrita*	20–30 ml	BR 8/187
13	Anemia	*Pathya ghrita*	20–30 ml	CC 16/50

[a]CC = *Charak Chikitsa.*
[b]CD = *Chakradatta.*
[c]BR = *Bhaishajaya Ratnavali.*

preceded with easily digestible and compatible food with plenty of fluids a day earlier in order to obtain proper oleation.

4.2.1.2.2 Massage Therapy (External Oleation Therapy)

External OT is achieved through massage and is done all over the body. For massaging the head, cold or lukewarm oil should be used. The rest of the body should be massaged with lukewarm oils. Massaging the body is to be done from 15 to 35 min. The massage should be carried out in seven different postures:

1. Sitting posture with extended legs
2. Lying down in supine posture
3. Lying down in left lateral position
4. Lying down on the front side of the body (over the back region)

5. Lying down in right lateral position
6. Lying down in supine posture
7. Sitting postures with extended legs from 2 to 5 min in each posture, depending upon the underlying disease

The massage should be done in a downward direction (i.e., away from the heart) over larger areas or big organs and in circular form over joints or the lower back.

Proper and regular practice of massage therapy results in the following benefits:

1. Improves eyesight
2. Induces sound sleep
3. Improves the quality of skin by making it tender, delicate, and strong
4. Corrects stiffness, rigidity, and induces elasticity in the body by softening the muscles, ligaments, and tendons
5. Relieves exertion, tiredness, and weakness due to various physical activities
6. Relieves and controls vitiated *vata dosa* in the body
7. Delays the aging process and strengthens the body

Massage therapy produces all these effects by lubricating the microcirculatory channels, displacing the exudates which may relieve tension and pain, and preparing smooth passages (microchannels) for elimination of toxic materials during sudation therapy.

The standard preparations used for massage therapy are described below:

1. Oils used for head massage
   a. *Candanadi taila* (Bhaishajaya Ratnavali [BR] 14/292–295)
   b. *Brahmi taila*
   c. *Jyotismati taila*
2. Oils used for body massage
   a. *Vatika* disorders
      i. *Narayana taila* (Chakradatta [CD] 22/120–130)
      ii. *Bala taila* (BR 26/273–283)
      iii. *Dasmula taila* (BR 65/89)
   b. *Paittika* disorders
      i. *Kshira Bala taila*
      ii. *Candanadi taila*
      iii. *Candan Balalaksadi taila*
   c. *Kaphaja* disorders
      i. *Sahacaradi taila* (BR 61/134–135)
      ii. *Dasmula taila*

Oleating materials given alone without any other carrier substances are also effective in providing oleation. In certain cases, some other substances such as rice, fruit juices, soup, curd, buttermilk, and lentils are added.

The following instructions are given to patients to maintain equilibrium of physiological factors during and after OT:

1. Avoid day sleeping.
2. Avoid a coarse and constipating diet.
3. Drink warm water.
4. Abstain from sexual activities.
5. Suppress normal urges.
6. Avoid speaking loudly.
7. Avoid anger and anxiety.
8. Avoid exposure to heat and cold.
9. Avoid walking in open air.
10. Avoid exercise and hard work.

OT is done to obtain maximum benefit. Either excess or inadequate oleation may cause problems. Features of adequate oleation include improved digestion, lightness of the body, oiliness of the skin, neuraesthenia, lethargy, semisolid stool, and visual fat in the stool. OT is considered inadequate if the patient passes dry and hard stools and presents with features like movement of flatus upward (bumping), weak digestive power, burning sensation in chest, and dryness of skin. Features of excessive oleation are heaviness and stiffness in the body, drowsiness, anorexia, nausea, dyspepsia, excessive salivation, and frequent evacuation of mucoid stools.

The possible complications of OT include indigestion, nausea, anorexia, gastrointestinal tract upsets, drowsiness, stiffness, skin diseases, anemia, edema, and piles. These complications can be easily treated by frequent use of lukewarm water externally and internally, with the administration of herbs like *Piper longum, Terminalia chebula, Termanalia belarica, Emblica officinalis* and *Comiphora mukul,* honey, and symptomatic treatment.

4.2.1.3 Sudation and Fomentation Therapy (Svedana Karma)[4,5]

The therapeutic production and induction of sweat by a variety of methods is termed sudation therapy (ST). It relieves stiffness, heaviness, and coldness of the body and induces sweating. It is administered to liquefy the oleated toxic materials (brought about by OT), which are spread throughout the body, and direct them to the alimentary canal for elimination by any one of the four cleansing procedures.

ST is administered after OT and it precedes emesis therapy in the sequence of PKT. Besides being the principal PREP of PKT, ST may also be a specific treatment for a number of disorders, especially in *vata*-dominant diseases where it may be a main treatment.

4.2.1.3.1 Types of Sudation Therapy

ST may be applied with the use of direct application of heat (e.g., hot bed, affusion, steam kettle, sudatorium, etc.) or indirect application of heat (e.g., exercise, wearing heavy clothes, exposure to sun rays, etc.). It may be used on the basis of properties of drug used, like unctuous or wet ST and dry ST, which are indicated in *vata* and *kapha*-dominant diseases, respectively. ST may be applied either to one part of the body as a localized ST or to the whole body as a generalized ST.

ST is indicated in patients of various types of paralysis, musculoskeletal disorders, coryza, cough, stiffness, and need for undergoing PKT. ST is contraindicated in patients with hemorrhages, diarrhea, eruptive skin diseases, alcoholism, pregnancy, and in patients of *pitta*-dominant constitution or who are emaciated.

4.2.1.3.2 *Procedure of Sudation Therapy*

ST must be performed after proper OT. In localized sudation, steam vapors of decoction of dashamula (or any other drug) are to be used on the affected parts. In generalized ST, medicated vapors are made to pass all over the oleated patient's body. ST should be done for a maximum of 30 to 45 min. Medicated vapors are generated by boiling the herbs in water.

The process of ST should be stopped when sweat appears over the forehead and there is relief from pain, stiffness, and heaviness. ST is considered inadequate if the patient does not produce any sweating and there is no relief from pain or coldness. A burning sensation of the body, fainting, vertigo, and appearance of blisters may occur if ST is done more than advised.

During and after ST, the blood pressure, pulse rate, respiratory rate, and temperature are monitored to make sure they are within normal limits. Direct exposure to cold water or cold air should be avoided at least for 1 h, and a bath in lukewarm water is indicated after ST. Generally, emesis should be given on the second day after ST and purgation after about a 3-day interval.

The standard preparations used for ST (for producing medicated steam) are:

1. *Dashamula kwatha* (decoction) — Sushruta Samhita Sutra Sthana 39/68–69
2. *Rasanasaptaka kwatha* (decoction) — CD Amavata– 8

4.2.1.3.2.1 *Physical Effects of Sudation Therapy* — Various procedures of ST therapeutically induce sweating, which cleanses microchannels, liquefies toxic materials, and expels toxic materials along with sweat. It recovers vascular insufficiency of the joints and muscles and produces relaxation. These factors might be responsible for improving blood circulation and local metabolic processes, causing relaxation of local structures and producing relief of local symptoms, functional recovery, and a slowdown of the disease process being treated. These therapeutic measures are classically *antivata* and relieve all *vata* manifestations and control the disease process. During ST, the body temperature rises to more than 2 to 3°C, which results in increased sweating.

4.2.1.3.3 *Review of Scientific Data on Oleation, Massage, and Sudation Therapies*[6–11]

R.H. Singh and G.N. Chaturvedi at Banaras Hindu University (BHU), Varanasi, studied the effect of internal oleation clinically[7,10] in patients with hyperchlorhydria and peptic ulcer after internal administration of *dadimadya ghrita* as a palliative therapy. They observed significant clinical improvement in these patients, including a decrease in gastric acid secretions and evidence of healing ulcers confirmed on radiological examinations. Other researchers also tried internal oleation with different *ghrita* preparations for peptic ulcers and reported similar observations.[11]

Scientific studies conducted on the role of oleation and sudation on a series of patients of rheumatoid arthritis and other chronic arthropathies by R.H. Singh at BHU, Varanasi, are reproduced here.[8,9] Similar studies have been conducted by this author and his team on rheumatoid arthritis at the National Institute of Ayurveda, Jaipur, and similar observations were recorded.[6]

Another clinical trial tested the role of *Pinda Sweda*, a type of preparatory procedure, as a main therapeutic procedure in rheumatoid arthritis, in which application of oil over the affected part is followed by fomentation with a hot rice paste cloth bundle. At the end of

TABLE 4.4
Herbs Used in PKT as Emetics

Medicinal Plant	Botanical Name
Madanaphala	*Randia dumatorum*
Madhuka	*Sapotaceae*
Kututumbi	*Lageneria vulgaris*
Nimba	*Azadirachta indica* A.
Bimbi	*Coccinia grandis (l.)* Voight
Visala	*Citrullus colocynthis* Schrad
Trapusa	*Cucumis sativus* Linn.
Kutaja	*Holarrhena antidysenterica* Linn.
Murva	*Celosia cristata* Linn.
Devdali	*Luffa echinata*
Vidanga	*Embelia ribes* Burm
Viduli	*Salix caprea* Linn.
Dahana	*Toddalia asiatica* Linn.
Citra	*Ipomea remiformi* Chois
Kosavati	*Luffa aegyptica* Mill-Hock
Karanja	*Pongamia pinnata* Pierre

30 days the researchers observed significant changes in both clinical symptoms, such as stiffness and pain, as well as in laboratory tests such as erythrocyte sedimentation rate and urinary hydroxyproline. Improved vascularity at the joints was also observed when the pre- and postangiograms were compared.

4.2.2 Main Cleansing Procedures (*Pradhana Karma*)

4.2.2.1 Biopurificatory Therapeutic Emesis — Emesis Therapy (Vamana Karma)[12]

Emesis therapy (ET) is a process by which the contents of the stomach including *kapha* and *pitta dosas* are expelled out of body through the mouth. It is one of the MCPs that eliminates toxic materials from upper parts of the body.

Herbs used in PKT as emetics are detailed in Table 4.4.

ET is indicated for patients of asthma, respiratory disorders, sinusitis, rhinitis, anorexia, dyspepsia, peptic ulcers, and skin diseases and in healthy individuals in different states where *kapha dosa* is aggravated within normal limits (e.g., in the spring season for preserving normal health and preventing diseases). It is contraindicated in patients of hematemesis, cardiovascular diseases, and cachexia and in children and the elderly.

4.2.2.1.1 Procedure of Emesis Therapy

ET is usually the first main procedure of PKT done after a proper preparation of the body. After the PREP, OT and ST are done; the out-of-balance *kapha* is further increased in the body by giving oily food, fatty food, animal meat, milk, and curd for the next 24 h before the induction of emesis. On the morning of ET (between 7 and 8 A.M.), a gruel mixed with ghee in large quantities or 2.5 l of milk or decoction of *Glycerrihza glabra* or sugarcane juice is given to the patient. After 10 min, emesis is induced by administering a certain combination of emetic herbs made into a paste mixed with ghee. Milk or decoction of *Glycerrihza glabra* or sugarcane juice is used as a vehicle to push the paste down.

TABLE 4.5

Criterion of Assessment of Purification of the Body by Emesis Therapy

No.	Parameters	Active Purification	Moderate Purification	Mild Purification
1	No. of bouts	8	6	4
2	Total output and input	Output > input	Output > input	Output < Input
3	Contents vomited	Bile and *pitta*	Bile and *pitta*	Bile and *pitta*
4	Signs and symptoms	To be observed for adequate emesis	To be observed for adequate emesis	To be observed for adequate emesis

Items commonly used in standard preparation are:

1. Powder seeds of *Randia dumatorum* (6 to 10 g [4 parts])
2. Powder of *Acorus calamus* (3 to 5 g [2 parts])
3. Rock salt (3 to 5 g [1 part])
4. Honey (20 ml)

Thoroughly mix the preparations and make them into a paste. Mix in 100 ml of warm milk or lukewarm water and ask the patient to swallow. If the patient is getting an urge to vomit, instruct him or her to do so. Start counting the number of bouts of vomiting and observe its contents.

4.2.2.1.2 Criteria for Proper Emesis Therapy

A bout is the number of times the emetic drug is vomited out after its administration to the patient. Adequacy of emesis is assessed in terms of the number of bouts, ratio of total output/input, its contents, and signs and symptoms produced after ET. A proper emesis will have the sequence of expulsion of saliva, drug, *kapha*, *pitta* (yellowish bile), and *vata dosa* as the end point. The criteria of assessment for effective ET are described in Table 4.5.

After completing emesis, the patient is asked to inhale smoke from medicated cigars prepared with specific drugs that expel residual *dosas*, toxic materials, *kapha*, and unctuousness in the throat, mouth, nose, and microchannels. The patient is advised to avoid speaking loudly, overeating, physical exertion, anger, and anxiety during and after the therapy to maintain normal physiology of the body and avoid complications.

The persistent urge to vomit, heaviness in the body, itching, and abdominal pain may occur in the case of an incomplete emesis of gastric contents. Complications such as hematemesis, frothy vomiting, fainting, cardiac pain, clouding of vision, throat pain, and weakness may occur in uncontrolled excessive vomiting. The physician should monitor the subject constantly and stop the whole process at the right time.

4.2.2.1.3 Review of Scientific Data on Emesis Therapy

A clinical trial for assessing the role of ET in 30 patients with bronchial asthma was carried out by this author and his team on various scientific parameters. After the completion of the ET, it was observed that there was significant improvement in clinical symptoms, including marked improvement in breath-holding time, vital capacity, and respiratory rate. Similarly, statistically significant changes ($p > 0.05$) were observed in ESR, total serum proteins, serum electrolytes, lipid profile, and radiological changes.

TABLE 4.6

Herbs Used in PKT as Purgatives

Medicinal Plant	Botanical Name
Kutaki	*Picrorrhiza kurrora*
Eranda	*Ricinus communis*
Triphala (*haritaki, bibhitaka, amalaki*)	3 fruits = *Terminalia chebula, Termanilia belerica, Embelica officenalis*
Gavaksi	*Citrullus colocynthis schrad*
Snuhi	*Euphorbiorbia nerrifolia* Linn.
Trivritta	*Operculina turpenthum*
Nilini	*Indigofera tinctoria* Linn.
Tilvaka	*Locos racemosa* roxb.
Aragvadha	*Cassia fistula* Linn.
Kampillaka	*Mallotus philippinensis*

TABLE 4.7

Dose Schedule for Various Purgatives[a]

No.	Drug of Choice	Soft Bowel	Medium Bowel	Costive Bowel
1	*Ricinus communis* oil	5–20 ml	20–50 ml	50–100 ml
2	*Operculina turpenthum* powder	1–3 g	3–6 g	5–10 g
3	*Vitis vinifera, cassia fistula, terminalia chebula* decoction	10–20 ml	25–50 ml	50–100 ml
4	*Croton tiglium, Euphorbia neerifolia*	60–125 mg	125–250 mg	500–1000 mg
5	*Pluntago ovata*	3 g	3–6 g	6–12 g

[a]Purgatives are based on practical experiences.

All the patients reported relief in heaviness in the chest, expectoration, cough, breathlessness, and a feeling of well-being and lightness in the chest immediately after emesis. The success rate of ET was approximately 75% in cases of bronchial asthma.

4.2.2.2 *Purificatory Purgation — Purgation Therapy (Virecana Karma)*

Purgation therapy (PT) is a specific process for elimination of *pitta dosa*. PT procedure involves elimination of *pitta* dominating *dosas* and toxins of the body through the rectal route.

PT is indicated mainly in patients suffering with hemorrhage from the upper parts of the body, poisoning, chronic jaundice, various gastrointestinal tract disturbances, asthma, skin disorders, epilepsy, insanity, and other *pitta* disorders. PT is contraindicated in patients with anorectal injury, prolapse of the rectum, bleeding from lower parts of the body, diarrhea, emaciating chest diseases, excessive oleation, and after enema. It is also contraindicated in children, the elderly, and patients who are weak, tired, have fasted, pregnent women, or persons desirous of coitus and pregnancy.

4.2.2.2.1 Procedures of Purgation Therapy

Internal oleation is done prior to PT. A diet containing fatty materials, liquid, warm/hot liquid or solid food, and meat soups is given to the patient. General instructions to be followed in ET are also to be followed in PT.

The dose of the drug to be administered for purgation is decided according to both the nature of the purgative drug and the patient, as described in Table 4.7. The purgative recipe is administered at least 2 h after sunrise (between 7 and 8 A.M.). During PT, the

TABLE 4.8

Assessing Success of Therapeutic Purgation on the Basis of Clinical Manifestations

No.	Parameters	Good Purgation	Medium Purgation	Mild Purgation
1	No. of bouts	15–30	10–15	5–10
2	Quantity of feces in liters	1.5–2	1–1.5	0.05–1
3	Order of contents	Mucin/*kapha*	Mucin	Mucin
4	Symptoms	Signs and symptoms as per textual description	Signs and symptoms as per textual description	Signs and symptoms as per textual description

stomach should preferably be empty, in contrast to emesis where the stomach must be full. Depending on their mode of action and degree of purgation produced, purgative drugs may be grouped as mild purgatives (e.g., *Operculina turpenthum* root), moderate purgatives (e.g., *Cassia fistula*), and drastic purgatives (e.g., *Euphorbia nerrifolia* milk). Various herbs and drugs used in PKT as purgatives are described in Table 4.6.

4.2.2.2.2 *Criteria for Proper Purgation Therapy*

The patient should be assessed for proper purgative effect as shown in Table 4.8. A proper purgation induces a feeling of lightness in the body and abdomen with improved appetite. The sequence of expulsion in proper PT is urine, stool, *pitta*, drug, *kapha*, and *vata*. If the patient has dyspepsia, heaviness in the abdomen or body, vomiting, and constipation, this suggests inadequate purgation. Signs and symptoms of excessive purgation include pain in the abdomen, blood-mixed serous discharge through the anus, syncope, weakness, and drowsiness. The physician should constantly monitor the subject and stop the whole process at the right time.

4.2.2.2.3 *Review of Scientific Data on Purgation Therapy*[14–16]

A clinical trial for assessing the role of PT in 30 patients with hepatitis (jaundice) was carried out by this author and his team on various scientific parameters. After the completion of the PT, it was observed that there was significant improvement in clinical symptoms such as anorexia, pruritis, nausea, and abdominal discomforts. There were significant changes in laboratory tests such as ESR, 24-h stercobilinogen, and D-xylose excretion.

All the patients reported relief in the feeling of lightness in the body and abdomen and improved appetite. The success rate of PT was approximately 85% in cases of hepatitis (jaundice).

After purgation, these patients were put on a short course of posttherapy dietetic regimen for 2 to 3 days. Within 7 days after purgation, these patients showed notable symptomatic improvement ($p < 0.05$). The D-xylose excretion test applied on these patients within a week of completion of the total procedure showed a statistically significant ($p < 0.001$) increase in D-xylose excretion rate, indicating improved absorption power, which determines the rate of purification of microchannels in these patients.

4.2.2.3 *Biopurificatory Therapeutic Enema — Enema Therapy (Vasti Karma)*[17]

Enema therapy (ENT) is a procedure in which medicated oils, decoctions, and decoctions with pastes of herbs or oils are introduced into the large intestines through the rectum with the help of an enema apparatus.

TABLE 4.9

Herbs Used in PKT to Make Decoctions for Enema

Medicinal Plant	Botanical Name
Madanaphala	*Randia dumatorum*
Kutaja	*Holarrhena antidysenterica* Linn.
Kustha	*Saussurea costus*
Devadali	*Luffa echinata*
Vaca	*Acorus calamus*
Dasmula (group of ten drugs: *bilva, agnimantha, syonaka, kasmarya, patala, saliparni, prsniparni, brhati, kantakari, goksura*)	*Aegle marmelose, Premna integrifolia, Oroxylum indicum, Gmelina arboria, Stereospermum suaveolens, Desmodium gangeticum, Ureria picta, Solanum indicum, Solanum surrattense, Tribulus terrestris*
Devadaru	*Cedrus deodaru* (Roxb)
Rasna	*Acampe papillosa*
Yava	*Hordeum vulgare*
Methi	*Foeniculum vulgare* Mill
Krtavedhanam	*Luffa acutangula* Roxb
Kulattha	*Dolichos biflorus* Linn.
Saindhava lavan	Rock salt
Madhu (honey)	Honey

TABLE 4.10

Proposed Quantity of Decoction-Based Enema According to Various Age Groups

No.	Age	Maximum Quantity of Decoction-Based Enema
1	1 year	50 ml
2	10 years	400 ml
3	15 years	900 ml
4	18–70 years	1200 ml
5	Above 70 years	1000 ml

Note: The dose of oil-based enema according to age of the patient is recommend. Examples are *Sneha vasti* – 300 ml, *Anuvasana vasti* – 150 ml, and *Matra vasti* – 75 ml.

4.2.2.3.1 *Classification of Enema Therapy*

ENT can be classified in different groups on the basis of drugs that are used in an enema, such as (1) a decoction-based enema in which drugs used for the enema contain decoction in a larger quantity, or (2) an oil-based enema in which oil is the main ingredient. Usually, a combination of decoction and oil enema is given; decoction alone is not indicated at any time. According to therapeutic actions of the drugs, the enema can be an oleation enema that produces oleation of the body, a roborant enema that improves strength and general status of health, a purifying enema that removes toxic materials from the body, or a depleting enema that reduces fat content of the body tissue leading to sound health.

ENT may also be classified according to the number of enemas administered during the full course of therapy:

1. *Karma vasti* — Total of 30 enemas, 12 decoction-based and 18 oil-based enemas administered on alternate days
2. *Kala vasti* — Total of 16 enemas, 6 decoction-based and 10 oil-based

TABLE 4.11

Two Types of Topical Errhines (*Nasya*)

No.	*Pratimarsha Nasya* (Topical)	*Marsha Nasya* (Topical)
1	Never produces complications	May produce complications
2	Dose: 2 drops B.D.	Dose: Maximum – 10 drops Moderate – 8 drops Minimum – 4 drops
3	Indicated in all seasons and all age groups	Needs consideration of seasons and age
4	Least oleus material used	Excess oleus material used
5	Slow acting and less potent	Quick action and highly potent

3. *Yoga vasti* — Total of 8 enemas, 3 decoction-based and 5 oil-based

Various herbs used in PKT to make decoctions for enemas are described in Table 4.10.

ENT is indicated in various gastrointestinal tract disorders, helminthiasis, urogenital disorders, lithiasis, neuromuscular disorders, articular diseases, venereal diseases, convulsions and paralytic disorders, and anorectal disorders. ENT is contraindicated in patients with intestinal obstruction, perforation, ascites, cholera, dysentery, anal inflammation, anemia, and anasarca.

4.2.2.3.2 *Procedure of Enema Therapy*

A decoction-based enema is given on an empty stomach between 5 and 7 P.M. after subjecting the patient to gentle massage and mild fomentation. An oil-based enema is administered 15 to 30 min after having a light diet in the evening. In both types of ENT, the quantity of enema is decided according to the schedule as described in Table 4.11.

Duration of elimination of the enema should be a maximum of 48 min. If expulsion does not occur within the stipulated time, the following complications may occur: tympanitis, distention of abdomen, painful abdomen, renal colic, reverse peristalsis, and pressing pain in the chest region; these complications should be managed accordingly.

Proper release of fecal matter and flatus, a feeling of lightness in the abdomen, suggests proper ENT. It is considered inadequate if the patient has few urges for evacuation, gripping pain, flatulence, and dyspnea.

After resting, the patient may take a bath with warm water. Lukewarm water, milk, gruel made of rice, meat soup, or another light diet is given. Excess of physical and mental exertion is avoided during ENT.

4.2.2.3.3 *Uttara Vasti*

Uttara vasti is the means by which the drugs of enema are made to pass through the penis or vagina or through extra genitalia into the urinary bladder or uterus. A dose of *uttara vasti* is 20 to 40 ml. The remaining description, indications, contraindications, and mode of administration of *uttara vasti* are similar to decoction-based or oil-based enemas.

4.2.2.3.4 *Review of Scientific Data on Enema Therapy*[18,19]

A clinical trial for evaluating the efficacy of ENT was conducted on 30 patients with rheumatoid arthritis with scientific parameters. Patients were subjected to a course of *Vaitarana vasti* (a type of decoction-based enema, *Chakradatta,* Chapter No. 73/32) for 30 days.

TABLE 4.12

Standard Preparations Commonly Used for Errhine Therapy

No.	Drug	Dose (Purification)	Reference
1	*Anu taila*	6 drops in each nostril	CS[a] 5/63–70
2	*Rasnadi taila*	6 drops in each nostril	CC[b] 26/160
3	*Shadbindu taila*	6 drops in each nostril	BR[c] 65/83
4	*Vyaghhri taila*	6 drops in each nostril	BR 63/30
5	*Pathadi taila*	6 drops in each nostril	BR 63/29
6	*Apamarga taila*	6 drops in each nostril	BR 65/113

[a]CS = *Charak Sutra.*
[a]CC = *Charak Chiikitsa.*
[c]BR = *Bhaishajaya Ratnavali.*

Significant changes such as stiffness, pain, and swelling, as well as laboratory tests like ESR, were observed in both clinical symptoms. A decrease in the rate of urinary excretion of hydroxyproline and a trend of restoration of adrenocortical functions, indicating remission of the disease process with control of connective tissue breakdown, were also noted. After the course of the therapy, patients showed statistically significant ($p < 0.001$) increase in D-xylose excretion rate, indicating significant improvement in GIT absorption capacity, clearly indicating the cleansing effect of microchannels after the MCP (i.e., ENT). Scientific study on a current series of patients with rheumatoid arthritis showed relief in symptoms in 70% of the patients.

4.2.2.4 Errhine Therapy (Nasya Karma)

Errhine therapy (ErT) refers to administration of medicines in various forms through the nostrils (i.e., instilling medicated oil in the nose or administering paste, powder, or fumes of errhine drugs in the nostrils). There are two types of ErT: (1) *Pratimarsha nasya* and (2) *Marsha nasya* (Table 4.11). ErT should be administered to patients who are 7 to 80 years old. ErT is indicated in various diseases of the supraclavicular region such as stiff neck and jaw, headache, migraine, graying of hair, baldness, facial palsy, aphonia, stammering or alteration of voice, hoarseness of voice, corrhyza, tonsillitis, sinusitis, rhinitis, and earache. ErT should be avoided in patients who have acute fevers or acute corrhyza or have had purgation or oleus enema, had fasted, and had indigestion. There are five methods of ErT:

1. Inunction (*navana*)
2. Instillation of nasal drops (*avapeedana*)
3. Insufflation (*dhamapana*)
4. Inhalation (*dhuma nasya*)
5. Topical application (*marsha* and *pratimarsha*)

When the oil is being instilled, the head should not be shaken; the patient should not loose his or her temper, speak, sneeze, or laugh. The unctuous material should not be swallowed and should be expectorated properly so that no part of it remains inside. The patient should be instructed to avoid talking, becoming angry, laughing, and swallowing of errhine drugs during the ErT procedure.

Standard preparations commonly used for ErT are listed in Table 4.12, and herbs used in PKT for nasal medication (*nasya*) are described in Table 4.13. The dose of ErT should be determined according to Table 4.14.

TABLE 4.13

Herbs Used in PKT for Nasal Medication (*Nasya*)

Medicinal Plant	Botanical Name
Vidanga	*Embelia ribes* Burm
Apamarga	*Achyranthes aspera* Linn.
Vyosa (3 pungents: *sunthi, pippali, marica*)	*Zinziber officenalis, Piper longum, Piper nigrum*
Darvi	*Beriberis aristata*
Surala	*Vateria indica* Linn.
Bija of sirisa	*Albizia lebbek*
Brihati	*Solanum anguivi* Lam.
Shigru	*Moringa oleifera*
Madhusarkara	*Dolichos biflorus* Linn.
Saindhava lavana	Rock salt

TABLE 4.14

Determination of Dosage in Errhine Therapy

No.	Type of Errhine Therapy	Mild Purification	Moderate Purification	Maximum Purification
1	Snuffing errhine therapy	8 drops in each nostril	16 drops in each nostril	32 drops in each nostril
2	Purificatory errhine therapy	4 drops in each nostril	6 drops in each nostril	8 drops in each nostril
3	Blowing errhine therapy	250 mg	375 mg	500 mg
4	Topical (*marsa nasya*)	6 drops in each nostril	8 drops in each nostril	10 drops in each nostril
5	Topical (*pratimarsh nasya*)	2 drops in each nostril	2 drops in each nostril	2 drops in each nostril
6	Paste (*kalka*)	4 drops in each nostril	6 drops in each nostril	8 drops in each nostril
7	Smoke (*dhumapana*)	1–2 min	2–3 min	Up to 5 min

Adequate ErT produces lightness in the body and head and sensorial happiness. ErT is inadequate if the patient has excessive secretions from the nose, eyes, and mouth and heaviness in the body. Complications such as headache, confusion, and salivation may occur in uncontrolled excessive ErT. The physician should constantly monitor the subject to avoid complications.

After ErT; the patient is given mild sudation over the throat, cheeks, face, and forehead and a soft massage on the feet, palms, and back of the neck; hot water gargling of the mouth and medicated smoking (*dhumapana*) is advised to the patient to clear the mouth and throat of residual *kapha dosa*.

4.2.2.4.1 Review of Scientific Data on Errhine Therapy[20]

Clinical efficacy of ErT was evaluated by the author on 30 patients with chronic sinusitis. At the end of 21 days, after administration of ErT with *Anu Taila*, the researchers noted significant changes such as a growing feeling of well-being, sneezing, nasal secretions, and headache in both clinical symptoms, as well as in laboratory findings such as ESR and radiological findings.

There was a statistically significant ($p < 0.001$) reduction in TLC and ESR. On radiological examinations there was a marked reduction in the haziness of sinuses along with restoration of normal mucosa. Nasal passages and sinuses were thoroughly cleansed after a course of therapy, indicating suppression of the disease process.

In the author's clinic, the success rate of ErT in a current series of patients with chronic sinusitis is about 90%.

4.2.2.5 Bloodletting Therapy (Rakta Mokshana)

Bloodletting therapy (BLT) may be performed with or without the help of metallic instruments. In the latter type, BLT may be administered by application of leech, cow's horn, dried bitter gourd, or coupling glass.

BLT is practiced to remove toxic materials in blood in blood-borne diseases; in *pitta*-predominant diseases; and also in a few *vata* disorders like erysepalis, boils and carbuncles, abscesses, blue and black pigmentation on the face, moles, eczema, leucoderma and vitiligo, scabies, red patches, anorectal inflammation, splenomegaly, jaundice, dyspepsia, anorexia, stomatitis, halitosis (foul-smelling mouth), gingivitis, and gout. It is contraindicated in patients with bleeding disorders, general anasarca, cachexia, anemia, piles, and all conditions where venepuncture is contraindicated.

4.2.2.5.1 Bloodletting Therapy with the Application of Leeches

The patient should be properly screened before leech therapy can be given. Before the BLT is done with a leech, oleation and sudation should be performed the day before. It can be done localized or generalized, depending upon the condition, and the part that is to be leeched should be dried. Then the purified leech is applied to the diseased part. The leech's mouth is covered with a smooth, white, moistened cotton swab. When the leech starts opening its mouth, which is shaped like a horse's hoof, and raising the shoulders, the leech is sucking the blood. If the leech does not start sucking the blood, a drop of milk or blood is placed over the affected part and the leech will start sucking the blood. If at the biting site needling pain and itching occur, then the leech is sucking pure blood. The leech is then removed from the site by pouring rock salt at its mouth. With the removal of vitiated blood after leech therapy, the redness and pain subside immediately.

After the leech is detached, the blood from the sucked area should be allowed to flow for 1 to 3 min and then dressing either with turmeric powder and alum powder or antiseptic solution is applied. Dressing should be kept in place for 6 to 12 h.

4.2.2.5.2 Bloodletting Therapy by the Venesection

Venesection is the process of cutting open a vein under strict aseptic conditions. It is done with sharp instruments and is a more severe form of bloodletting than the application of leeches. When the venesection is done properly, the blood (which is impure) flows automatically. Adequate venesection is considered if the patient feels lightness in the body, a decrease in pain, and a remission of symptoms. Signs of inadequate venesection include swelling, burning sensation, inflammation, pain, itching, and redness at the site of venesection.

4.2.2.5.3 Bloodletting Therapy by Superficial Wounding

Superficial incisions are made over the skin with the help of a scalpel, fine needles, or instruments under strict aseptic conditions. BLT with this method is commonly used in localized blood disorders and in certain skin disorders. It must be done after taking aseptic measures. Antiseptic dressing should be applied over the wound.

BLT improves the collateral circulation of affected parts and cleanses the microcirculatory channels directly by removing toxic materials and exudating from the affected parts. Hirudin, the chemical substance present in the saliva of a leech, has a potent anticoagulant property. It induces bleeding and encourages free flow of blood, removing the virulent substances present at the site of the lesion and helping to restore healthy blood supply. Hirudin checks the inflammatory process especially at specific points where bloodletting is done, which produces rapid symptomatic improvement.

4.3 Beneficial Effects of *Panchakarma* Therapy[21]

The beneficial contribution of PKT is that it removes the toxic materials from the body and provides purification of the body at two levels: (1) the gross level, where various organs and systems of the body are thoroughly cleansed (e.g., cardiovascular system, gastrointestinal tract, chest, etc.); and (2) the cellular level, where purification and cleansing of the body is produced at the level of cells, cell membranes, and molecules. PKT helps bring the whole body to normalcy; starts rejuvenation and revitalization of all body tissues; potentates the pharmacological actions of various drugs and medicines administered after PKT; removes waste products, unwanted materials, various toxins, and stagnant *dosas;* and potentiates physiological functions of all the body systems (e.g., gut absorption improves considerably and metabolism is also corrected). The prognosis of various diseases that are difficult to treat with simple administration of medicines becomes significantly improved (good prognosis) after administration of PKT. PKT not only is a prerequisite for all the therapeutic procedures and medications but also has a full therapeutic role in promoting preventive, curative, and rehabilitative procedures.

If properly performed, PKT does not produce any serious complications. If any minor complications are produced, they are easily manageable. Specialized techniques of PKT are simple to perform and can be carried out at both the outdoor patient and indoor patient (OPD and IPD) levels. There is no need to carry out all PKT practices at one sitting; specific techniques of PKT (any of the MCP) can be recommended to the patient after proper preparation. The toxic materials are eliminated from the body mainly through the alimentary canal.

4.4 Conclusions

Any type of main cleansing procedure of PKT is believed to affect the cleansing of microcirculatory channels by eliminating the toxic metabolites from the body. This helps in the process of curing a disease. Scientific studies indicate that cleansing procedures appear to help in eradicating chronic diseases more effectively.

It was observed by the author in a case study that when PKT was administered as an adjuvant therapy along with the allopathic system of medicines, the results were better than the PKT or allopathic system of medicines given alone.

Acknowledgments

I am thankful to my co-workers, Dr. Uttam Sharma, Dr. Sunil Borkar, Dr. Parshuram Yadav, Dr. Rajesh Gupta, and my son Amit Sharma, for help in writing this chapter. In addition, I am extremely thankful to my revered teacher Prof. R.H. Singh, Dean, Faculty of Ayurveda, Indian System of Medicine, Banaras Hindu University, Varanasi, for extending help and inspiring me to complete this chapter. I am also thankful to my wife, Dr. (Smt.) Praveen Sharma, and daughter, Gauri Sharma, for their help.

References

1. Shri Atri Dev Gupta, *Astanga Hrdya*, Chaukhamba Sanskrit Sansthana,Varanasi, India, 1980.
2. Shri Atri Dev Gupta, *Astanga Sangrah*, Nirnava Sagar Mudranalaya, Bombay, India, 1951.
3. Chaturvedi, G.N. and Shastri, K., *Caraka Samhita*, Chaukhamba Sanskrit Sansthana,Varanasi, India, 1979.
4. Haridasa Shridhara Kasture, *Ayurvediya Pancakarma Vigyana*, Shri Baidya Nath Ayurveda Bhawana Ltd., Allahabad, India, 1999.
5. Singh, R.H., *Panca Karma Therapy*, Chaukhamba Sanskrit Series Office, Varanasi, India, 1992.
6. Singh, D. and Sharma, A.K. (supervisor), A Clinical Study of Snehana, Svedana and Rasnadi Gugulu in the Management of Sandhigata Vata with Special Reference to Osteo Arthritis, M.D. (Ayurveda) Kayacikitsa thesis, National Institute of Ayurveda, Jaipur, India, 2000.
7. Chaturvedi, G.N. and Singh, R.H., Studies on pancha karma therapy. I. Certain physiological and biochemical studies on snehana and different types of vasti therapies, *Nagarguna*, 8(9), 685–691, 1964.
8. Chaturvedi, G.N. and Singh, R.H., Studies on pancha karma therapy. II. Certain experimental studies on the effect of svedana in arthritis, *Nagarjuna*, 8(10), 767–773, 1964.
9. Chaturvedi, G.N. and Singh, R.H., Studies on pancha karma therapy. III. A clinical studies on the treatment of certain neuromuscular and articular disorders with pinda sweda, *Nagarjuna*, 8(11), 29–39, 1964.
10. Herron, R.E. and Fagan, J.B., Lipophil-mediated reduction of toxicants in humans: an evaluation of an ayurvedic detoxification procedure, alternative therapies, 8(5), 40–51, 2002.
11. Singh, R.H. and Chaturvedi, G.N., Studies on pancha karma therapy. VIII. Therapeutic value of snehapana in the management of peptic ulcer syndrome, *Nagurjana*, 11, 572–578, 1967.
12. Warrier, P.K., Bhattathiri, P.P.N., Radha Krishnan, P., and Balachandran, K.P., Evaluation of snehapana in comparison to samana therapy with mahatikta ghrita in parinamasoola (duodenal ulcer), *J. Res. Ayurveda and Siddha*, 8(3–4), 90–105, 1987.
13. Pandey, S.N. and Tripathi, S.N., Studies on Bronchial Asthma and Samsodhana, M.D. (Ayurveda) thesis, Banaras Hindu University, Varanasi, India, 1980.
14. Chaturvedi, G.N. and Singh, R.H., Studies on pancha karma therapy. IV. Role of pancha karma therapy in tamaka swasa vis-à-vis bronchial asthma with particular reference to its pathophysiological basis: a hypothesis, *Nagarjuna*, 8(2), 119–124, 1964.
15. Singh, R.H. and Singh, R.S., Standardisation of vamana and virechana karma, *J. Res. Ayurveda and Siddha*, 13(2), 13–27, 1978.
16. Sharma, A. and Sharma, A.K. (supervisor), Clinical Evaluation of the Role of Samsodhana and Bhargee Sarkara in the Management of Tamaka Sawasa (Bronchial Asthma), Ph.D. Kayacikitsa thesis, National Institute of Ayurveda, Jaipur, India, 2001.
17. Singh, G. and Chaturvedi, G.N., Studies on Virecana with Special Reference to Catheritic Effect of Kutki (Picrorhyza Kurora Royle ex Bigeth), Ph.D. thesis, Banaras Hindu University, Varanasi, U.P., 1975
18. Pandey, V.N., Principles of pancakarma cikitsa, *Nagarjuna*, 13(10), 23–29, 1970.

19. Gupta, A. and Sharma, A.K. (supervisor), Study to Evaluate the Efficacy of Vasti Therapy in Rheumatoid Arthritis (Amavata), M.D. (Ayurveda) Kayacikitsa thesis, National Institute of Ayurveda, Jaipur, India, 1999.
20. Mohite, K. and Sharma, A.K. (supervisor), Clinical Evaluation of Tikta Kshira Vasti in the Management of Sandhigata Vata with Special Reference to Osteo Arthritis, M.D. (Ayurveda) Kayacikitsa thesis, National Institute of Ayurveda, Jaipur, India, 2000.
21. Rai, R. and Sharma, A.K. (supervisor), Clinical Evaluation of Nasya Karma in Pinasa Roga (Pratisayaya), M.D. (Ayurveda) Kayacikitsa thesis, National Institute of Ayurveda, Jaipur, India, 2000.
22. Sharma, A.K., *Panchakarma Treatment of Ayurveda Including Keraliya Panchakarma*, Sat Guru Publications, Delhi, India, 2002.

5

Immunomodulation: Therapeutic Strategy through Ayurveda

Ashish A. Mungantiwar and Aashish S. Phadke

CONTENTS

0-8493-1366-X/04/$0.00+$1.50

5.1 Introduction

Why is it that there is always some lucky soul who does not get sick when the flu is going around the office? Or why is it when the chicken pox is sending all the kids home from school, there are a few who remain untouched? Why do only some in a family develop allergies or bacterial infection? Some attribute this phenomenon to simple luck, whereas others attribute it to strong genes. The answer is a bit more complex.

A large number of diverse disease states threatening mankind, such as chronic and recurrent viral and fungal infections, human immunodeficiency virus (HIV) infection, allergies, and cancer, are believed to have resulted from altered functioning of the immune system. The immune system helps an individual toward establishing an infection-free state. Disturbances in the internal state of order of the host immune system results either in the terms of hyperactivity, hypoactivity, or the inability to distinguish self from nonself that would lead to disease. Such multidimensional response would require proper control through immunomodulation.

It is true that our genes affect our immune system; we call that *influence of natural constitution*. We cannot change our genetic makeup, but we can definitely strengthen our immune system to fight against diseases.

The immune system can be stimulated and suppressed by various physical, chemical, and biological agents. These include steroids, cytotoxic drugs, and various natural products of microbial, animal, and plant origin.[1] Although an antigen-specific immunomodulator is desirable, reliable agents for sustained therapeutic effects are being investigated.

The suppression of the immune system associated with tuberculosis (TB), cancer,[2] surgery,[3] or HIV infection is characterized by a reduction in the number and phagocytic function of neutrophils and macrophages[4] as well as a reduction in the intracellular bactericidal capacity of these cells. This profound suppression of the individual elements of the system allows opportunistic pathogens to overwhelm the host so that secondary infection becomes the most common cause of the mortality in such individuals.[5]

An attempt to overcome this problem has been made by introducing the concept of pro-host therapy.[6] This approach aims at administering drugs to bolster immune defense against infections.[7] Several naturally occurring and synthetic substances like bacillus calmette and guerin (BCG),[8] muramyl dipeptide,[9] interleukin–1 (IL-1),[10] and colony-stimulating factors[11] have been used to enhance resistance against infections. However, these substances share several limitations. One of their major drawbacks is the necessity to administer them parenterally, which often leads to local reactions such as granuloma formation. Another factor is the cost of therapy, which can be prohibitive. Against this background, the potential of Ayurvedic therapy appears to be encouraging.[12]

Ayurveda emphasizes the promotion of health with a concept of strengthening host defense against diseases. The concept of immunostimulation through Ayurveda has been used successfully in the treatment of immunocompromised conditions like acquired immune deficiency syndrome (AIDS), TB, cancer, and hepatic disease.

5.2 Etiology

The cellular components of the immune system, which are essential in controlling infections, include macrophage, T-cell and B-cell subset, natural killer cell, lymphokine

TABLE 5.1

Cytokines Released by CD4 T-cells

Cytokines	Functions	T_H^1-Cells	T_H^2-Cells
IL-2	T-cell proliferation	+	–
IL-3	T- and B-cell proliferation	++	++
IL-4	Activation of T-cell, B-cell, and macrophage	–	++
IL-5	Eosinophil production	–	++
IL-10	Inhibition of T-cell	–	++
IFN-γ	Activation of macrophage	++	–
TNF-α	Stimulation of inflammation	++	–
GM-CSF	Stimulation of macrophage	++	+

activated killer cell, and cytotoxic lymphocyte. Generation of an effective immune response involves two major groups of cells: lymphocytes and antigen-presenting cells. Lymphocytes are one of many types of white blood cells produced in bone marrow that circulate in the blood and lymph system and reside in various lymph organs. The major population of lymphocytes is B-lymphocytes (B-cell) and T-lymphocytes (T-cell). There are two well-defined subpopulations of T-cells: T helper cells (T_H) and T cytotoxic cells (T_C). T_H- and T_C-cells can be distinguished from one another by the presence of either membrane glycoprotein CD4 or CD8 on their surfaces. T-cells displaying CD4 generally function as T_H-cells, whereas those displaying CD8 generally function as T_C-cells. The T_H-cell recognizes and interacts with the specific antigen (microbe). Interaction takes place with the help of major histocompatability complex (MHC) II molecule. Once the interaction takes place, T_H-cell activates and secretes various growth factors known as cytokines. The secreted cytokines play an important role in activating various cells of the immune system, like the B-cell, T_C-cell, and macrophage.[13]

Recently, it has become clear that two distinct subsets of CD4 helper T-cells (T_H^1- and T_H^2-cells) secrete different pattern of cytokines as shown in the Table 5.1. T-cells respond to antigenic stimulation with a transient burst of cytokine production.[14] The key differences are expressions of interferon-gamma (IFN-γ), tissue necrosis factor-alpha (TNF-α), interleukin-2 (IL-2), and granulocyte macrophage colony-stimulating factor (GM-CSF) by T_H^1 clones and interleukin-4 (IL-4) and interleukin-5 (IL-5) by T_H^2 clones. T_H^2-cells stimulate the production of three of the hallmark features of the allergic disease: mast cells, eosinophils, and immunoglobin E (IgE) antibodies. The cytokines responsible for these activities are IL-4 for IgE production[15] and IL-5 for eosionphilia.[16] Cytokines released by T_H^1 lead to a substantial increase in the ability of macrophages to kill a wide variety of intracellular pathogens and to enhance the development of long-term immunity to those organisms.[17]

The understanding of T-cell-mediated immunoregulation suggests a number of potential therapeutic applications in TB, hepatic disorders, HIV infections, etc.

5.2.1 Apoptosis

Apoptosis is a mode of cell death in which single cells are deleted in the living tissue.[18] The term is derived from ancient Greece, meaning the falling of leaves from trees or petals from flowers. It is characterized by structural changes that appear with great fidelity in cells of widely different lineage.

5.2.2 Signal Pathway to Trigger Apoptosis and Its Intervention through Ayurveda

Several pieces of evidence implicate a rise in cellular-free calcium as a critical event for apoptosis. A moderate but sustained increase in intracellular calcium has been demonstrated to produce cell death. However, because calcium is implicated in signaling for a multitude of cellular activities, including proliferation and differentiation, it seems unlikely that a simple influx of calcium from outside the cell activates a specific pathway for apoptotic death. Apart from increased calcium levels, there are signals that contribute toward apoptosis. These are protein kinase A and protein kinase C. Protein kinase C has a negative effect on apoptosis. Therefore, factors that stimulate protein kinase C will inhibit apoptosis. For example, activated macrophage, IL-1, and GM-CSF both activate protein kinase C and inhibit apoptosis.

Inhibition of apoptosis is useful in the treatment in AIDS, making Ayurveda a potential treatment as well. Many ayurvedic medicinal plants have been found to modulate the process of apoptosis. For example, the plants *Boerhaavia diffusa*[19] and *Tinospora cordifolia*[20] have been shown to stimulate macrophage and GM-CSF and inhibit apoptosis.

Other diseases in which apoptosis is implicated are cancer, autoimmune disease, and neurodegenerative disease. The rate at which cancer grows depends on the comparative rates of cell division and cell death. Apoptosis is an efficient way of preventing malignant transformation because it removes genetically malformed cells. Abnormal apoptosis can promote the development of cancer by either allowing the accumulation of normal cells or preventing their removal. AIDS is another condition where the balance between the rate of CD4 death and cell replacement becomes abnormal. It is believed that apoptosis plays an important role in lymphocyte depletion in AIDS.

Neurodegenerative diseases are also becoming the focus of much research as the census of the aging population increases. For example, it is hypothesized that apoptosis may play a role in Alzheimer's disease or motor neurone disease. In addition, anticancer effects produced by several anticancer drugs have been shown to induce apoptosis, thus aiding in removal of cancerous cells. The modulation of apoptosis may assist the manipulation of the aging process. Indian medicinal plants offer prospects for the modulation of the balance between proliferation and apoptosis. The potential of several medicinal plants described in Ayurveda needs to be tapped.

5.3 Immunomodulation and Concept *Rasayana* in Ayurveda

Out of the eight branches of Ayurveda, the *rasayana* and *vajeekarana tantra* branch is the one that is concerned with the immunomodulation. According to Ayurveda, the common cause of all diseases may be due to contact with environmental factors and aging. The latter is inevitable and the other cause can be avoided only by scrupulously puritan patterns of living. Ayurveda claims to be able to slow down the process of aging successfully.

Rasayana is a treatment in which the body constituents are prepared to adapt to a selective tissue endowment program. This concept in modern scientific understanding would mean the enhancement of immune responsiveness of an organism against pathogens by nonspecifically activating the immune system with immunomodulatory agents of plant origin. It is now recognized that immunomodulation could provide an alternative or complement to conventional chemotherapy for a variety of diseased conditions; this is especially the case when host defense mechanisms have to be activated under the conditions of impaired immune responsiveness.

Rasayan drugs are believed to slow down the aging process (*jara*) and provide a defense against diseases (*vyadhi*). *Rasayanas* improve the host resistance of an individual, helping to prevent aging and diseases. Specific diets and lifestyle changes are also advised in *rasayana* therapy.

Rasayana is made up of *rasa* and *ayana*. *Rasa* primarily means essential seven vital tissues: rasa (lymphatics), *rakta* (blood), *mamsa* (muscle), *meda* (adipose tissues), *asthi* (bones), *majja* (bone marrow and nervous tissue), and *shukra* (reproductive element). *Ayana* means the path or channel for the same. So, *rasayanas* are those that bring about proper uptake, growth, and improvement of essential seven vital tissues. *Rasayanas* provide long life, good intellect, the ability to remain young, and general well-being.

5.3.1 Mode of Action of *Rasayanas*

Rasayana drugs act on the immune system. On ingesting the appropriate formulation of the *rasayana* in the appropriate season by a qualified Ayuravedic physician, the beneficial effects of *rasayana* are seen. What, then, are these *rasayana* drugs that have so many vital life-enhancing properties? The ancient writers of Ayurveda have endowed the drugs with multiple properties of delaying aging, improving mental functions, and giving freedom from several diseases including those caused by infections. How can these *rasayanas*, which otherwise seem to be simple herbs having a different number of phytochemicals, influence such a wide variety of body functions? To the scientific mind, it appears impossible to credit one plant with such an apparently disparate variety of effects — almost as though it were a magic potion! It seemed possible only if the drugs were modulating an endogenous system of the body, setting into motion a whole cascade of events that will act on the different organs and produce its myriad actions.

The immune system has connections with a number of other organs and can directly or indirectly influence the actions of many other organs, including the brain. By acting primarily on the immune system like macrophages, the simple chemical of the herbs through the activating cytokine network could produce all the actions that have been attributed to them. This hypothesis was proved scientifically by Dhanukar et al.[24] In one set of experiments, *rasayanas* were given to rats whose macrophages had been overloaded with a fat lipofundin. In this setup, the *rasayanas* were unable to stimulate macrophages further and were thus unable to prevent stress-induced organ damage. *Rasayana* shows myriad actions on other organs by acting on the immune system. The classification of *rasayanas* is presented in Table 5.2.[25]

5.4 Scientific Basis of Ayurvedic Immunomodulation Therapies

Commercially available *rasayana* herbal formulas and supporting clinical and biological studies are listed in Table 5.3. Studies on single *rasayana* herbs are presented here.

5.4.1 *Terminalia Chebula* (*Haritaki*)

Terminalia chebula is an antibacterial, antioxidizing, anti-inflammatory, and immunomodulatory agent. The topical administration of an alcoholic extract of the leaves of *T. chebula* was found to heal much faster as indicated by decreased period of epitheliazation. The tensile strength of the tissue, which was treated with *T. chebula*, was increased by 40%.[26]

TABLE 5.2
Classification of Rasayanas

No.	Classification	Remarks
1	*Kutipraveshika*	Patient has to stay in a very specialized manner in the *kuti* (hut or home) specifically made as per the needs of *rasayana*
2	*Vatatapika rasayana*	Can be given on an out-patient department basis; person can consume it while doing his or her normal duties and staying at his or her own home
3	*Kamya rasayana*	*Rasayana* that are specifically used for benefit of specific system (e.g., for bone marrow *Withania somnifera* and *Asparagus racemosus*)
4	*Naimittika rasayana*	*Rasayana* given only for partial period for certain number of days
5	*Agasrik rasayana*	*Rasayana* commonly used to keep the process of formation of vital tissue (e.g., milk)
6	*Sharira rasayana*	*Rasayana* working on physical levels (e.g., *Emblica officinalis*)
7	*Medhya rasayana*	*Rasayana* working on mind for the improvement of intellect (e.g., *Bacoppa manorial, Centella asiatica*)
8	*Vardhanana rasayana*	Dosage of drug has to be increased slowly and kept at highest level and then once again tapered down (e.g., *Piper longum, Semecarpus anacardium*)
9	*Achara rasayana*	Based on a code of conduct, which keeps oneself to attain good mental and spiritual health; if one follows *Achara rasayana*, one can be keep away from anxiety, stress, and thereby from all diseases that are generated due to stress
10	*Ahar rasayana*	Food is considered as *rasayana* (e.g., milk)
11	*Dravya rasayana*	Drug therapy is considered under this; drug therapy includes single herbal, polyherbal, and herbo-mineral formulation; modern scientific medicine also states that good diet, nutrition, proper lifestyle management, supportive family, good counseling, and stress control help reverse the damage already done to the immune system

Biochemical studies revealed a significant increase in total protein, DNA, and collagen contents in the granulation tissue of the treated wound. Reduced lipid peroxide levels in the treated wounds suggest that *T. chebula* possesses antioxidant activity. The extracts of *T. chebula* were found to significantly suppress yields of cytomegalo virus (CMV) in lungs of mice. Thus, *T. chebula* may be beneficial for the prophylaxis of CMV disease in immunocompromised patients.[27] The extract of *T. chebula* was also found to inhibit human immunodeficiency virus-1 reverse transcriptase with (IC_{50}) ≤ 50 μg/ml.[28]

5.4.2 *Emblica officinalis* (*Amlaki*)

Emblica officinalis is a rich source of vitamin C. The fruits of *E. officinalis* have been used by Ayurveda as potent *rasayana* and also for the treatment of diverse etiology disease. Perhaps there is no other drug in any other system of natural medicine with such a vast range of attributed effects. In an experimental study, it was reported that *E. officinalis* could bring about a significant weight gain in the subjects together with an increase in serum total protein content.[29] It is used as an antioxidizing, antibacterial, and anti-inflammatory agent.[30] The antioxidant activity of *E. officinalis* resides in tannoids. Tannoids have been found to increase superoxide, catalase, and glutathione peroxidase.[31]

TABLE 5.3

Clinical Evidence of Some Compound Formulas

Compound Formula	Clinical and Biological Studies	Ref.
Septilin tablet[a]		
Each tablet contains *Balsamodendron mukul*, Exts. *Maharsnadi*, *Phyllanthu emblica*, *Tinospora cordifolia*, *Rubia cordifolia*, *Moringa pterygosperma*, *Glycyrrhizasperma*	• Septilin possesses immunomodulatory and anti-inflammatory plant principles, which strengthen the nonspecific immune responses of the body; Septilin stimulates the phagocytosis by macrophage activation, increases the polymorphonuclear cells, and helps overcome the infections; Septilin builds up resistance to disease and helps prevent reinfection	
	• Septilin significantly enhanced gain in tensile strength in incision wounds and wound contraction and epithelialization in excision wounds	79
	• One tablet was given to younger patients twice a day, and one tablet was given to elder patients three times a day; doses have been found to be useful for upper respiratory tract infections; 50% of the patients showed excellent results; 30% reported good results with no recurrent attacks upon 6-month follow-up[c]	80
	• Septilin enhances both primary and secondary immune response in mice immunized with sheep red blood cells and counteracts IgG and IgM suppression induced by prednisolone when administered orally with immunosuppressive drug (prednisolone); the mechanism of immune protection by Septilin treatment could probably be due to increased number of activated macrophages by Septilin treatment[d]	81
Mentat Tablet[a]		
Each tablet contains *Hydrocotyl asiatica*, *Withania somnifera*, *Acorus calamus*, *Aspargus racemosus*, *Emblica officinalis*, *Evolvulus alsinoides*, triphala	• Mentat tablets have been used as a general tonic and vitalizer and as a memory enhancer	
	• Clinical studies have shown that it improves memory quotient in normal subjects of different age groups, increases memory span and attenuates fluctuations of attention in normal subjects, and improves learning ability in children[e]	82
Liv 52[a]		
Each tablet contains *Capparis spinosa*, *Cinchorium intybus*, *Solanum nigrum*, *Cassia occidentalis*, *Tamarix gallica*, *Terminalia arjuna*, *Achillca millefolium*, *Mandhura bhasma*	• In a clinical trial of Liv 52 vs. placebo in 60 malnourished children, a dose of one tablet twice a day for 6 months showed significant improvement in body weight, height, total protein, albumin, and globulin levels; appetite also improved remarkably[f]	83
	• Liv 52 significantly improves chronic hepatitis and cirrhosis[g] as observed from clinical trials on 300 patients with hepatitis.	84

TABLE 5.3 (continued)

Clinical Evidence of Some Compound Formulas

Compound Formula	Clinical and Biological Studies	Ref.
Geriforte Tablets[a]		
Each tablet contains *Chyavanprash* concentrate, *Exts. Capparis spinosa, Solanum nigrum, Cassia occidentalis, Terminalia arjuna, Achillea millefolium, Tamarix gallica, Mandhur bhasma*, saffron, amber, makardhwaj, *Asparagus adscendens, Caesalpinia digyna, Asparagus racemosus, Withania somnifera, Glycyrrhiza glabra, Centella asiatica*, shilajeet, *Terminalia chebula, Mucuna pruruiens, Myristica fragrans, Piper longum, Maceeugenia caryophyllata, Elettaria cardomomum, Carum coptieum, Curcuma longa, Exts. Berberis aristata, Adhatoda vasica, Eclipta alba, Celastrus paniculaus, Argyreia apecosia, Abhrak bhasma, loh bhasma, jasa bhasma*	• Geriforte, an indigenous herbo-mineral preparation, claimed to be a useful comprehensive general tonic and restorative	
	• Geriforte prevented stress-induced changes in adrenal, restraint ulcers, liver toxicity, and milk-induced leucocytosis; these properties indicate the presence of antistress (adpatogenic properties) of Geriforte[h]	85
	• A placebo-controlled clinical trial with Geriforte was conducted in 280 postsurgical patients; it was observed that Geriforte therapy promotes cellular regeneration and helps in wound healing by increasing the availability of essential amino acids and elements for primary healing of the operative wounds; a substantial improvement in well-being was observed in 78.57% of patients, and 75% of patients gained weight[i]	86
	• In an open trial in 50 patients, two tablets twice a day for 15 days up to 6 months showed a significant improvement in physical and mental activity and improvement in appetite; weight gain was observed in 80 to 85% of the patients[j]	87
Chyawanprash[b]		
Each supplement contains vitamin C derived from *Emblica officinalis* (*amla*) and several other herbal products	• Ten normal healthy volunteers were given *chyawanprash* for 16 weeks; they received 15 g/day; it was observed that *chyawanprash* reduces postprandial glycemia in the oral glucose tolerance test and reduces blood cholesterol level to a significantly greater extent[l]	88
	• In a controlled clinical study using *chyawanprash awaleha* as an adjuvant in the treatment of pulmonary TB, it was observed that the preparation could augment the recovery process as well as an improved nutritional status of the subjects[m]	58

[a]Himalaya Drug House.

[b]Zandu Pharmaceuticals, Dabur Pharmaceuticals, Baidynath Pharmaceuticals.

5.4.3 *Piper longum* (*Pippali*)

Piper longum is indicated in treatment of chronic dysentery and worm infestations. *Pippali rasayana*, an Ayurvedic herbal medicine prepared from *P. longum* and *Butea monosperma*, is prescribed for the treatment of chronic dysentery and worm infestations. *P. longum* significantly increases macrophage migration inhibition and phagocytic activity.[32] Enhancement of host resistance is the possible mechanism of recovery from giardial infection.

5.4.4 *Glycyrrihza glabra* (*Yashtimadhu* [Parts Used: Roots])

Glycyrrihza glabra is an immunomodulator and antioxidant. Glycyrrhizin, a triterpenoid glycoside obtained from *G. glabra*, is found to inhibit ribonucleic acid (RNA) viruses such as measles; polio vaccine viruses type 1, 2, and 3; and deoxyribonucleic acid (DNA) viruses such as herpes type 1 and 2.[33] Polysaccharide fractions obtained from the root of *G. glabra* induce nitric oxide production from macrophages.[34]

5.4.5 *Allium sativum* (*Lahsuna*)

Allium sativum (garlic) is an antimicrobial, antitumor, hypolipemic, antiarthritic, and hypoglycemic agent. These characteristics have been linked to their influences on immune functions in various ways.[35] The herb has been found to enhance human immune functions by stimulating peripheral blood mononuclear cells. Diallyl sulfide in *A. sativum* is known to exert anticarcinogenic activity.[36] Allicin from garlic has been found to induce programmed cell death and the arrest of proliferation in cancer cells.

5.4.6 *Semecarpus anacardium* (*Bhallatak* [Parts Used: Nuts])

Extract of nut preparation of *Semecarpus anacardium* is effective against a variety of diseases like arthritis, tumors, and infections. An extract of *S. anacardium* at a dose of 150 mg/kg significantly reduced the lysosomal enzyme activity in arthritic animals[37] and displayed significant inhibition of tumor cells with IC_{50} of 1.6 μg/ml.[38]

5.4.7 *Commiphora mukul* (*Guggul*)

Commiphora mukul is used as an anti-inflammatory, antihyperlipidemic, and immunomodulatory agent. A placebo double-blind randomized controlled trial of *C. mukul*, at 50 mg twice daily, was conducted on patients with hypercholesterolemia.[39] *C. mukul* decreased total cholesterol by 11.7%, low-density lipoprotein (LDL) by 12.5%, triglyceride by 12%, and the ratio of total cholesterol/high density lipoprotein (HDL) by 11.1%.

5.4.8 *Tinospora cordifolia* (*Guduchi* [Parts Used: Roots])

Tinospora cordifolia (TC) is used for the treatment of jaundice, skin disease, diabetes, anemia, emaciation, and infections. Plant extracts are known to stimulate macrophages and enhance their phagocytic activity and intracellular killing activity. Immunosuppression associated with deranged hepatic function and sepsis results in poor surgical outcome in obstructive jaundice. *T. cordifolia* was reported to improve surgical outcome by strengthening host defenses.[31] Active principles of *T. cordifolia* were found to possess anticomplementary and immunomodulatory activities. Syringin (TC-4) and cordiol (TC-7) inhibited classical complement pathway. The compound also gave rise to significant increase in immunoglobin G (IgG) antibodies in serum. Both humoral and cell-mediated immunity enhancement were dose-dependent enhanced. *T. cordifolia* has been found to activate the mononuclear cells to release cytokines like GM-CSF and IL-1. Whole aqueous extract of *T. cordifolia* has been evaluated as an adjuvant in clinical conditions like obstructive jaundice, TB, and cancer chemotherapy and has been found to increase the efficiency of conventional therapies. *T. cordifolia* is also shown to specifically stimulate macrophages and enhance their phagocytic activity. In a recent double-blind randomized controlled trial,[40] it also was shown to increase the production of nitric oxide in TB patients, causing increased macrophage stimulations. TB patients who took *T. cordifolia* extract along with conventional anti-TB treatment showed increased radiological recovery and sputum conversion as compared with conventional anti-TB treatment alone.

5.4.9 *Azardicta indica* (*Neem* [Parts Used: Leaves])

Azardicta indica is reported to have several therapeutic effects, including being anti-infective and anxiolytic and having general immunopotentiating ability.[41] It is widely studied for various beneficial properties. The aqueous extracts of neem leaves enhance the phagocytic activity of macrophages. *Neem* is found to enhance the production of IL-2, IFN-γ, and TNF-α. In human volunteers, it stimulated humoral immunity by increasing antibody levels and cell-mediated immunity by increasing total lymphocyte and T-cell count in 21 days. The therapeutic potential of *neem* is mediated through its influence on the immune system, which is in consonance of the Ayurvedic concept of *rasayana*.

5.4.10 *Asparagus racemosus* (*Shatavari* [Parts Used: Whole Plant])

Asparagus racemosus is used as an immunomodulator and antioxidant. The aqueous extract of the whole plant of *A. racemosus* gives protection from biological, physical, and chemical stresses.[42] Treatment with *A. racemosus* significantly inhibited suppression of chemotactic activity and production of IL-1 and TNF-α by murine macrophages induced by 17 weeks of treatment with ochratoxin A.[43] Studies on the mechanisms of action revealed that it produced immunostimulation. Aqueous extracts of *A. racemosus* are also found to suppress the myelosuppressive effects of single and double doses of cyclophosphamide.[44]

5.4.11 *Withania somnifera* (*Ashwagandha* [Parts Used: Roots])

Withania somnifera is one highly acclaimed *rasayana*. *W. somnifera* is an immunomodulatory, anti-inflammatory, and antioxidizing agent. *W. somnifera* effectively inhibits the inflammatory process. It can also bring about a specific reduction in α-2 macroglobulin synthesis, unlike the conventionally used nonsteroidal anti-inflammatory drugs (NSAIDs), and has anti-oxidant activity.[45] The herb is described to act as *rasayana* and *medhya*. In a clinical study on patients of anxiety neurosis, *ashwagandha* was observed to reduce the symptoms of anxiety. One month of treatment with the drug has shown symptomatic relief in mental fatigue, and immediate memory span. In another study, the herb has been shown to be effective in cases of depression. In yet another double-blind placebo-controlled clinical study[46] on the extract of *ashwagandha* involving both normal and depressive volunteers, it was observed that the test extract showed an excellent improvement in mental functions. Experiments with extracts of *Ashwagandha* protected animals against infections in normal and immunosuppressed states induced by hemisplenectomy or surgery. This plant also produced leucocytosis with predominant neutrophilia and prevented leucopenia induced by cyclophosphamide.[47]

5.4.12 *Aloe vera* (*Ghritkumari*)

Aloe vera is a plant exclusively used in skin-care preparation and other health-care products. It is also found to possess anticancer activity. Supplementation of aloe vera gel has been found to suppress the incidence of hepatocarcinogenesis induced by diethylnitrosamine and 2-acetylaminofluorene in male rats.[48] The extract from leaf gel contains glutathione peroxidase activity.[49] The low molecular weight constituent of this extract inhibits the release of reactive oxygen species by human polymorphonuclear leucocytes. The inhibitory effect of these compounds has been shown to be an indirect result of the diminished availability of intracellular free calcium.[50]

5.4.13 *Solanum nigrum* (*Kakamachi*)

Solanum nigrum is an anti-inflammatory and hepatoprotective agent. Steroidal glycosides isolated from *S. nigrum* are found to possess antineoplastic activity against solid tumor cell lines.[51] The hepatoprotective activity of *S. nigrum* may be due to their ability to suppress the oxidative degradation of DNA in the tissue debris.[52]

5.4.14 *Bacopa monnieri* (*Brahmi*)

Bacopa monnieri is used as an antiallergic, antistress, and memory-enhancing agent. In a double-blind randomized controlled clinical trial in 76 subjects,[53] *B. monnieri* showed significant effect on the retention of new information. Follow-up tests showed that the rate of learning was unaffected, suggesting that *B. monnieri* decreases the rate of forgetting newly acquired information.

5.4.15 *Boerhaavia diffusa* (*Punarnava* [Parts Used: Roots])

The plant *Boerhaavia diffusa* (BD) is used as an antiarthritic, immunomodulatory, and antistress agent. Alkaloidal fraction of roots of BD was found to attenuate myelosuppressive effects of cyclophosphamide. BD is known to potentiate macrophage phagocytic activity. It is also shown to increase GM-CSF levels upon oral administration, inhibiting apoptosis.[19]

5.4.16 *Ocimum sanctum* (*Tulasi*)

Ocimum sanctum is used as an antistress, antioxidizing, and immunomodulatory agent. The ethanolic extract of *O. sanctum* revered the changes in plasma levels of corticosterone induced by exposure to acute and chronic stress.[54] Banerjee et al.[55] have studied the modulatory influence of the alcoholic extract of leaves of *O. sanctum* on various enzyme levels in the liver, lung, and stomach of mice. Oral treatment with extract significantly elevated the activities of cytochrome P 450, cytochrome b5, and arylhydrocarbon hydroxylase, all of which are important in the detoxification of carcinogens as well as mutagens. These observations suggest that leaf extract or its active principle may have a potential role in the chemoprevention of chemical carcinogenesis.

5.4.17 *Shilajit* (Asphalt)

Shilajit is an exudate of selected rocks occurring in the Himalaya region. It is a complex mixture of both organic and inorganic matter and is considered to be an effective remedy for many diseases. It was investigated for its effect on memory, learning, and anxiety. It was reported that *Shilajit* enhanced the acquisition of learning and memory in aged rats while exhibiting a marked reduction in anxiety levels. This neurochemical effect of *Shilajit* is attributed to decrease in 5-hydroxytryptamine turnover with an increase in dopaminergic activity.[56] To add the multifaceted activity of *Shilajit*, a study was designed by Oureshi et al.[57] to investigate the cytological and biological effects of *Shilajit* and its response to the changes induced by cyclophoshamide. The study showed that *Shilajit* exhibited cytotoxic effects and inhibited the carcinogenic potential of cyclophosphamide. In experimental studies, it has also been observed that *Shilajit* activates macrophage and enhances cytokine release.[31]

5.4.18 *Chyawanprash Awaleha*: A Polyherbal *Rasayan* Formulation

Chyawanprash awaleha (CA) is a polyherbal Ayurvedic *rasayan* preparation described in Charak Samhita and contains the pulp of *E. officinalis* as the prime ingredient. This preparation is popularly used in India and many other countries as a health supplement.

In a controlled clinical study using CA as an adjuvant in the treatment of pulmonary TB, it was observed that the preparation could augment the recovery process in addition to an improved nutritional status of the subjects.[58]

Recently, the anticarcinogenic property of CA has also been studied. It has been shown to reduce tumor weight in mice. A clinical study was undertaken to estimate the radioprotective effect of CA. The study included patients with head and neck cancers undergoing radiotherapy. It was observed that CA conferred an excellent protection to the tissues from the burning effects of radiation, in comparison with controls.[59] The tumor regression rate was also noted to be higher in the CA-treated group. These results may be suggestive of possible antioxidant effects of *E. officinalis* contained in the preparation.

5.5 Immunomodulation Therapies

5.5.1 Tuberculosis

There is considerable evidence that failure to control or resolve infectious disease often results from an inappropriate rather than insufficient immune response. A good example is TB. In this condition, T-cell immunity is decreased; the T_H-cell is not able to produce sufficient IFN-γ to activate macrophage, which can kill mycobacterium TB. Intervention in this situation could be aimed at expanding protective T_H^1-cells or alternatively enhancing the key protective response macrophage activation by IFN-γ.

Current therapy consists of antibacterial drugs like Rifampicin, Isoniazid, Pyrazinamide, and Ethambutol for a period of 4 to 6 months. Significant success rate is achieved with this regimen. Treatment of TB with *rasayana* has shown significant improvement in treatment period.

Treatment of TB with Ayurveda includes various *rasayana* like *T. cordifolia* and CA. The latter is a wonderful remedy that provides strength and sustenance to the patient. It was mentioned earlier that using CA as an adjuvant in the treatment of pulmonary TB[58] could augment recovery process. It also increases the appetite. The dosage in the beginning should be two teaspoonfuls with milk on an empty stomach twice daily; as the patient gains strength, the dosage should be increased.

A double-blind randomized clinical trial[40] of *T. cordifolia* was conducted in TB patients along with a conventional anti-TB regimen for an initial 2-month intensive period. It was observed that when conventional anti-TB regimen was given along with 500 mg of *T. cordifolia* three times daily, the sputum conversion time was 2 weeks as compared with 4 weeks in the conventional group; there was also hastened radiological recovery as compared with the conventional regimen. This effect was observed due to increased nitric oxide production by *T. cordifolia*, which caused increased macrophage phagocytic activity.

5.5.2 Hepatic Disorder

In recent years, rapid progress has been made in understanding the relationship between various cells of the liver and pathobiology of cellular events responsible for an acute and chronic hepatic damage. Kupffer cells, which are present in the liver, are the most versatile cells. The activity of these cells is a major determinant of outcome of any liver injury.[60] It has been reported that excess activation of Kupffer cells damages the liver,[61–63] whereas hepatic fibrosis is linked with suppressed or subnormal activity of these cells. Thus, modulation of Kupffer[64] cells activity through the immune system would be a weapon against liver disorders.

5.5.2.1 Obstructive Jaundice

In the management of obstructive jaundice, present preoperative therapy aims at decompressing the biliary tract and controlling infection with antibiotics and vitamin K if there is a disturbance in hemostasis. Despite improvement in preoperative care, the surgical outcome of these patients has remained poor.[65,66] Endotoxemia resulting from depressed Kupffer cells is a well-known feature of obstructive jaundice. Based on Ayurvedic literature, it has been observed that *rasayana* like *T. cordifolia* could be a useful therapeutic armamentarium in the treatment of obstructive jaundice. In a clinical trial of *T. cordifolia* as an add-on regimen to conventional therapy, two groups of patients were well matched with respect to clinical features and hepatic and immune functions.[67] The neutrophil activity of these patients was significantly lower as compared with normal healthy donors. After biliary drainage, bactobilia was observed.[67] Therapy with *T. cordifolia* significantly decreased the mortality from 92 to 40%. This was also associated with a decrease in speticemia. *T. cordifolia* was found to potentiate the depressed neutrophil activity.

A randomized double-blind placebo-controlled clinical trial also showed a significant reduction in mortality rates.[20] Moreover, at the cellular level remarkable results were shown; patients suffering from obstructive jaundice taking *T. cordifolia* showed an increase in serum GM-CSF levels. The neutrophils of these patients also showed an increased phagocytic activity, making *T. cordifolia* an effective treatment for patients with obstructive jaundice.[20]

5.5.2.2 Asymptomatic Carriers of Hepatitis B Antigen

In asymptomatic carriers of hepatitis B antigen, elimination of viral antigen is necessary to prevent future hepatic dysfunction and to reduce transmission. Although the role of nonspecific cellular immunity is not clearly defined, defects in monocyte have been reported[68] and immunomodulators like levamisole and interferons have been shown to eliminate antigen.[69] Therapy with *rasayana* such as *T. cordifolia* (16 mg/kg/day) for 2 months led to seroconversion in 37.5% of patients. This rate was three times higher than that observed in the intracellular killing capacity of monocytes.[20]

5.5.2.3 HIV Infection

HIV is a disease starting from the stage of latent infection, progressing into the severe immunodeficiency state of AIDS, and finally ending in death. HIV is a smart bug. Unlike the other lente viruses, which possess only three genes, HIV has six more functional genes. These are responsible for producing numerous drug-resistant mutant variants.

Review of the scenario of the modern highly active antiretroviral therapy (HAART) is depressing. The scenario consists of reverse transcriptase inhibitors and a protease inhibitor. Failure to eliminate the virus from sanctuaries, an increase in the number of resistant variants of the virus, severe toxicity manifestations, a significant increase in risk of TB, very poor improvement in longevity, and prohibitive costs are some of the reasons why HAART cannot be considered as a choice therapy. The practical utility of a vaccine in preventing the disease also holds very little hope.

Under these circumstances, certain studies mentioned in Ayurvedic texts have been examined to find possible solutions. Ayurveda mentions sexually transmitted communicable progressive wasting disorder. Excessive indulgence in sex and abnormal sexual practices are suggested to be the cause of loss of vitality and immunity (*ojakashaya*) leading to a wasting disorder.

According to Ayurveda, the loss of *ojas* is responsible for a progressively wasting disorder. *Ojas* is the creamy by-product of *shukra dhatu*. It is the ultimate strength of the body. Debility, wastage, fear, depression, a feeling of wretchedness, and a loss of coordination in sense and motor organs are all signs of damage to *ojas*. Ayurvedic texts also reveal that *shukra*, the seventh tissue of the body, is of two types. One type is present all over the body and responsible for strength, vitality, and glow (*shukra* is probably related to the steroid hormones of the body). The other type, *beej shukra*, is responsible for gamete production. Ayurveda authoritatively states that the formation of *shukra* begins only after the complete development of bone marrow (*majja dhatu*). The complete formation of *shukra dhatu* occurs in females and males at 16 and 23 years of age, respectively. According to modern endocrinology, adolescent changes occur when red bone marrow in the long bones of a child is transformed into fatty yellow marrow. This produces extra gonadal steroids, which send a positive feedback to the hypothalamus and activate the hypathalmopituitary gonadal axis. This is the beginning of functioning of the gonads. The Ayurvedic hypothesis of the origin of *shukra* from *majja dhatu* appears meaningful.[70]

Cells need oxygen for survival, but the uncoupled single oxygen radical also causes oxidation damage to the cell. It is indeed an oxygen paradox of the cell. In HIV, reactive oxygen species activate nuclear transcription factor, an obligatory factor for HIV replication. It also aids apoptosis of CD4 cells and thus helps disease progression.

With this background of HIV disease pathology, the mind–body holistic concept of Ayurveda should be an interesting option for treating psychological factors and for treating HIV. *Rasayana* that are classified as *achar rasayana*, *ahar rasayana*, and *dravya rasayana* are helpful in reversing the damage already done to the immune system. *Ahaar rasayana* (food as a drug) such as black gram, milk, ghee, and meat are advised. Black grams are well known to be a good source of alpha lipoic acid. Ghee has a special place in increasing the *ojas*.

Some of the plants that have shown anti-HIV activity include *Cichorium intybus*,[70] *Glycyrrhiza glabra*,[71,72] *Grifola frondosa*,[73] *Punica granatum*,[70] curcumin,[70] and aloe vera.[74] In one study, aloe vera juice (20 oz/day) was used in conjunction with essential fatty acids and amino acid supplements to treat 29 patients. There were 15 AIDS, 12 AIDS-related complex (ARC), and two HIV seropositive patients that continued with regular medication, including Azidothymidine (AZT),[74] an antiviral drug used to combat AIDS. After 6 months, all patients showed clinical improvement; 25% of those positive for p24 core antigen converted to nonreactive, anemia induced by AZT showed improvement in all patients, and the patients gained an average of 7% in body weight.

Acemennan, a water-soluble polysaccharide obtained from aloe vera, is found to be responsible for this anti-HIV activity. The anti-HIV activity of acemannan probably results from inhibiting glycosylation of viral glycoproteins. However, the prominent effect is by enhancing the effect of AZT. Researchers believe that use of acemannan may reduce the amount of AZT by as much as 90%.[75] This is quite significant. AZT is extremely expensive and is also associated with side effects such as anemia and a decrease of white blood cell production. Acemannan is commercially available as CARRISYN by Carrington Laboratories in Irving, TX.

In a clinical study in patients in the early stages of AIDS, Acemannan showed some promise. In this study, 14 HIV patients who were prescribed oral Acemannan (800 mg/day) demonstrated significant increases in circulating monocytes and macrophages. In particular, the number of large circulating monocytes increased significantly, indicating improvement in phagocytizing, processing, and presenting cells in blood.[75]

Although Acemannan may be helpful in the beginning stages of AIDS, a recent study[76] indicates that it may be of little value in patients with advanced HIV disease.

Glycyrrhizin, a major constituent of *G. glabra*, is also showing great promise in the treatment of HIV-related disease, including AIDS. In one study, 10 HIV patients without AIDS took 150 to 225 mg of glycyrrhizin daily.[77] After 1 to 2 years, none developed symptoms associated with AIDS or ARC; however, one of the 10 patients in a matched control group developed ARC and two progressed to AIDS and subsequently died. In yet another study, when glycyrrhizin was administered in daily doses of 200 to 800 mg intravenously, after 8 weeks the groups presented increased helper T-cell count, improved helper/suppressor T-cell ratio, and improved liver function.[78]

5.6 Conclusions and Future Prospective

The immune system is a complex system, involving an interwoven network of biochemical mechanism. The concept of rasayana as mentioned is Ayurveda is a holistic approach and constitutes an important approach to handle with subjects of immunity. The objective of research on *rasayana* should focus not only on its immunomodulatory activity, but also on other effects such as antistress, antiaging, antioxidant, adaptogenic, and anti-HIV. The list of herbs in *rasayana* is exhaustive by itself. *Rasayana* formulas provide tremendous potential to be tapped for immunomodulatory activity. It is equally important to arrive at a consensus in regards to the utilization of herbs in a holistic manner in order to deliver their multidimensional benefits to mankind.

References

1. Ziauddin, M. and Phansalkar, N., Studies on the immunomodulatory effects of ashwangandha, *J. Ethnopharmacol.*, 50, 69, 1996.
2. Santos, L.B., Yaranda, F.T., and Scheinberg, M.A., Monocyte and lymphocyte interaction in patients with advanced cancer, evidence for deficient il-1 production, *Cancer*, 56, 1553, 1983.
3. Grzelak, I., Olszewski, W.S., and Engesser, A., Influence of operative trauma on circulating blood mononuclear cells analysis using mononuclear antibodies, *Eur. Surg. Res.*, 16, 15, 1987.
4. Whittaker, J.A., Hughes, A.R., and Khurshid, M., The effect of cytotoxic and anti-inflammatory drugs on the phagocytosis of neutrophils leucocytes, *Br. J. Haematol.*, 29, 273, 1975.
5. Mayer, K.H. and De Torres, O.H., Current guidelines on the use of antibacterial drugs in patients with malignancies, *Drugs*, 29, 262, 1985.
6. Hadden, J.W., Immunomodulators in the immunotherapy of cancer and other diseases, *Trends Pharmacol. Sci.*, 3, 191, 1982.
7. Drews, J., *Immunomodulation in Recent Advances in Infections 2*, Reeves, D.S., Ed., Churchill Livingstone, New York, 1982, p. 89.
8. Hiu, I.J., Water-soluble and lipid free fraction from BCG with adjuvant with anti-tumour activity, *Nature New Biol.*, 238, 241, 1972.
9. Parant, M., Muramyl peptides as enhancers of host resistance to bacterial infections, in *Progress in Leucocyte Biology*, Majde, J.A. and Alan, R., Eds., Alan R. Liss, New York, 1987, p. 235.
10. Dinarello, C.A., Interleukin-1, *Rev. Infect. Dis.*, 51, 1984.
11. Moore, R.N., Hoffield, J.T., Farrar, J.J., and Mergenhagen, S.E., Role of CSF as primary regulators of macrophage functions, *Lymphokines*, 3, 119, 1981.
12. Thatte, U.M. and Dahanukar, S.A., Ayurveda and contemporary scientific thought, *Trends Pharmacol. Sci.*, 7, 247, 1986.
13. Kuby, J., Ed., *Overview of Immune System in Immunology*, W.H. Freeman, New York, 1997, p. 12.
14. Powrie, F. and Coffman, R.L., Cytoregulation of T-cell function: potential for therapeutic intervention, *Trends Pharmacol. Sci.*, 14, 164, 1993.
15. Coffman, R.L. and Carty, J.A., T cell activity that enhances polyclonal IgE production and its inhibition by interferon-γ, *J. Immunol.*, 136, 949, 1986.
16. Sanderson, C.J., O'Garra, A.O., Warren, D.J., and Klans, G.G., Eosinophil differentiation factor also has B cell growth factor: proposed name interleukin-4, *Proc. Natl. Acad. Sci.*, 83, 437, 1986.
17. Murray, H.W., Spitalyny, G.L., and Nathan, C.F., Activation of mouse peritoneal macrophage *in vitro* and *in vivo* by interferon-γ, *J. Immunol.*, 134, 1619, 1985.
18. Wyllie, A.H., Apoptosis (the 1992 Frank Rose Memorial Lecture), *Br. J. Cancer*, 67, 205, 1983.
19. Mungantiwar, A.A., Studies on Immunomodulatory Activity of *Boerhaavia diffusa*, Ph.D. thesis, Bombay University, Bombay, India, 1998.
20. Rege, N.N., *Clinical Prospects of Tinospora Cordifolia: An Immunomodulator Plant in Immunopharmacology Strategies for Immunotherapy*, Upadhyay, S.N., Ed., Narosa Publishing House, Delhi, India, 1999, p. 105.
21. Ranade, S. and Paranjpe, G.R., *Kayachiktsa* (*Marathi*), 3rd ed., Vol. 2, Anmol Publication, Pune, India, 1987, p. 168.
22. Charakacharya, *Charak Samhita*, Commentary by Sashtri, K. and Goraknath, C., 13th ed., Vol. 2, Chaukambha Bharti Academy, Varanasi, India, 1986, p. 5.
23. Sushrutacharya, *Sushrut Samhita* (Sanskrit), Trikamji, J. and Acharya, N.A., Eds., Nirnayansagar Press, Mumbai, India, 1945, p. 2.
24. Thatte, U. and Dahanukar, S., Rasayana concept: clues from immunomodulatory therapy, in *Imuunomodulation*, Upadhyay, S.N., Ed., Narosa Publishing House, Delhi, India, 1995, p. 145.
25. Ranade, S. and Paranjpe, G.R., *Kayachiktsa* (*Marathi*), 3rd ed., Vol. 2, Anmol Publication, Pune, India, 1987, p. 168.
26. Suguna, L. et al., Influence of *Terminalia chebula* on dermal wound healing in rats, *Phytother. Res.*, 16(3), 227, 2002.

27. Shiraki, K., Yukawa, T., Kurokawa, M., and Kageyama, S., Cytomeagolvirus and its possible treatment with herbal medicines, *Nippon Rinsho*, 56(1), 56, 1998.
28. Me Kakkawy, S. et al., Inhibitory effects of Egytian folk medicines on human immunodeficiency virus (HIV) reverse transcriptase, *Chem. Pharm. Bull. (Tokyo)*, 43(4), 641, 1995.
29. Ahmad, I., Mehmood, Z., and Mohammad, F., Screening of some Indian medicinal plants for their anti-microbial properties, *J. Ethnopharmacol.*, 62, 183, 1998.
30. Bhattacharya, A. and Chatterjee, A., Antioxidant activity of active tannoi principles of Emblica officinalis, *Indian J. Exp. Biol.*, 37, 676, 1999.
31. Katiyar, C.K. et al., Immunomodulator products from Ayurveda: current status and future perspectives, in *Immunomodulation*, Upadhaya, S.N., Ed., Narosa Publishing House, New Delhi, India, 1995, p. 163.
32. Agarwal, A.K., Singh, M., and Gupta, N., Management of giardiasis by an immunomodulatory herbal drug Pippali Rasayan, *J. Ethnopharmacol.*, 44, 143, 1994.
33. Badam, L., In vitro studies on the effect of glycyrrhizin from Indian Glycyrrhiza glabra Linn. on some RNA and DNA viruses, *Indian J. Pharmacol.*, 39, 211, 1994.
34. Nose, M., Activation of macrophages by crude fractions obtained from shoots of glycyrrhiza glabra, *Free Radical Biol. Med.*, 23, 302, 1997.
35. Ali, M., Thomson, M., and Afzal, M., Garlic and opions: their effect on eicosonoid metabolism and its clinical relevance, *Prostaglandins Leukot. Essent. Fatty Acids*, 62, 55, 2000.
36. Singh, A. and Shukla, Y., Antitumour activity of diallyl sulfide in two mouse skin models of carcinogenesis, *Biomed. Environ. Sci.*, 11, 258, 1998.
37. Vijayalakshmi, T. and Muthulakshmi, V., Effect of the milk extract of *Semecarpus anacardium* nut on adjuvant arthritis-dose dependent study in Wistar albino rats, *Gen. Pharmacol.*, 27(7), 1223, 1996.
38. Smit, H.F. et al., Ayurvedic herbal drugs with possible cytotoxic activity, *J. Ethnopharmacol.*, 47(2), 75, 1995.
39. Singh, R.B. and Gjosh, S., Hypolipidemic and anti-oxidants effects of *Commiphora mukul* as an adjuvant to dietary in patients with hypercholesterolemia, *Cardiovasc. Drugs Ther.*, 8(4), 659, 1994.
40. Dash, A. et al., Stimulation of nitric oxide synthesis by Tinospora cordifolia in alveolar macrophages and its implications in patients with TB., presented at 33rd Annual Conference of the Indian Pharmacological Society, Gandhinagar, India, December 28–30, 2000.
41. Nirjo, S.M. and Kofi Tsekpo, M.W., Effect of an aqueous extract of Azardicta indica on the immune response in mice, *Onderstepoort J. Vet. Res.*, 66, 59, 1999.
42. Devasagayam, T.P.A. and Sainis, K.B., Immune system and antioxidants, especially those derived from herbal Indian medicinal plants, *Indian J. Exp. Biol.*, 40, 639, 2002.
43. Dhuley, J.N., Effect of some Indian herb on macrophage function in ochratoxin A treated mice, *J. Ethnopharmacol.*, 58, 15, 1997.
44. Thatte, U. and Dahanukar, S.A., Comparative study of Immunomodulatory activity of Indian Medicinal plants, lithium carbonate and glucan, *Methods Find Exp. Clin. Pharmacol.*, 10, 639, 1988.
45. Khafagi, S.H. and Abdul Nabi, M.H., Antigranuloma activity of Iraqui Withania somnifera, *J. Ethnopharmacol.*, 37, 113, 1992.
46. Singh, R.H. and Behere, P.B., Double blind clinical studies on Ashwangandha capsules, unpublished data, 1991.
47. Dahanukar, S.A., Kulkarni, R.A., and Rege, N.N., Pharmacology of medicinal plants and natural products, *Indian J. Pharmacol.*, 32, S81, 2000.
48. Shamaan, N.A. et al., Vitamin C and aloe vera supplementation protects from chemical hepatocarcinogenesis in rats, *Nutrition*, 14, 846, 1998.
49. Sabeh, F., Wright, T., and Norton, S.J., Purification and characterization of a glutathione peroxidase from the Aloe vera plant, *Enzyme Protein*, 47, 92, 1993.
50. t-Hart, L.A. et al., Effects of low molecular weight constituents from aloe vera gel on oxidative metabolism and cytotoxic and bactericidal activities of human neutrophils, *Int. J. Immunopharmacol.*, 12, 427, 1990.

51. Hu, K. et al. Antineoplastic agents. III. Steroidal glycosides from *Solanum nigrum, Planta Medica,* 65, 35, 1999.
52. Sultana, S., Perwaiz, S., Iqbal, M., and Athar, M., Crude extracts of hepatoprotective plants, Solanum nigrum and Cichorium intybus inhibit free radical-mediated DNA damage, *J. Ethnopharmacol.*, 45, 189, 1995.
53. Roodenrys, S. et al., Chronic effects of Brahmi (Bacopa monnieri) on human memory, *Neuropscyhopharmacology,* 27(2), 279, 2002.
54. Sembulingam, K., Semibulingam, P., and Namasivayam, A., Effect of Ocimum sanctum Linn. on noise induced changes in plasma corticosterone level, *Indian J. Physiol. Pharmacol.,* 41, 139, 1997.
55. Banerjee, S., Prashar, R., Kumar, A., and Rao, A.R., Modulatory influence of alcoholic extract of Ocimum leaves on carcinogenic-metabolising enzyme activities and reduced glutathione levels in mouse, *Nutr. Cancer,* 25, 205, 1996.
56. Jaiswal, A.K. and Bhattacharya, S.K., *Indian J. Pharmacol.,* 24, 12, 1992.
57. Oureshi, S. et al. *Fitoterapia,* 65(2), 137, 1994.
58. Katiyar, C.K. et al., Immunomodulator products from Ayurveda: current status and future perspectives, in *Immunomodulation,* Upadhaya, S.N., Ed., Narosa Publishing House, New Delhi, India, 1995, p. 163.
59. Aggarwal, G.N., Radioprotective effect Chyawanprash Awaleha in patients with cancers of head and neck, presented at World Congress on Biotechnological Developments in Medicinal Substances from Plant and Murine Sources, Lucknow, 1995.
60. Lee, W.M., Drug induced hepatotoxicity, *N. Engl. J. Med.,* 333, 1118, 1995.
61. Decker, K., Eicosanoids: signals molecules of liver cells, *Semin. Liver Dis.*, 5, 175, 1985.
62. Shiratori, Y. et al., Modulation of hepatotoxicity by macrophages in the liver, *Hepatology,* 8, 815, 1988.
63. Tsukamoto, H., Gaal, K., and French, S., Insights into the pathogenesis of alcoholic liver necrosis and fibrosis, status report, *Hepatology,* 12, 599, 1990.
64. Toth, C.A. and Thomas, P., Liver endocytosis and Kupffer cells, *Hepatology,* 16, 255, 1992.
65. Dixon, J.M. et al., Factors affecting morbidity and mortality after surgery for obstructive jaundice: a review of 373 patients, *Gut*, 24, 845, 1983.
66. Greig, J.D. et al., Surgical morbidity and mortality in one hundred and twenty nine patients with obstructive jaundice, *Br. J. Surg.*, 75, 216, 1988.
67. Rege, N.N. et al., Immunomotherapy with Tinospora cordifolia: a new lead in the management of obstructive jaundice, *Indian J. Gastroenterol.*, 12, 5, 1993.
68. Dudley, F.J., Fax, R.A., and Sherlock, S., Cellular immunity and hepatitis associated Australia, antigen liver disease, *Lancet*, 1, 723, 1972.
69. Greenberg, H.B. et al., Effect of human leucocyte interferon on hepatitis B virus infection active hepatitis, *N. Engl. J. Med.*, 295, 517, 1976.
70. Palep, H.S., personal communication, 2001.
71. Ito, M. et al., Mechanism of inhibitory effect of glycyrrhizin on replication of human immunodeficiency virus (HIV), *Antiviral Res.*, 10, 289, 1988.
72. Hattori, I. et al., Preliminary evidence for inhibitory effect of glycyrrhizin on HIV replication in patients with AIDS, *Antiviral Res.*, 11, 255, 1989.
73. Nanba, H., Immunostimulant activity in-vivo and anti-HIV activity *in vitro* of 3 branched b-1-6 glucans extracted from maitake mushrooms (Grifola frondosa), presented at 8th Int. Conf. on AIDS, 1992.
74. Pulse, T.L. and Uhlig, E., A significant improvement in a clinical pilot study utilizing nutritional supplements, essential fatty acids and stabilized aloe vera juice in 29 seropositive ARC and AIDS patients, *J. Adv. Med.*, 3, 209, 1990.
75. Anon., Aloe vera may boost AZT, *Med. Tribune*, 8, 4, 1991.
76. Singer, J., A randomized placebo controlled trial of oral acemennan as an adjunctive to antiretroviral therapy in advanced HIV disease, presented in *Int. Conf. AIDS,9*, Abstr. No. B28-2153, 1993.
77. Ikegami, N. et al., Clinical evaluation of glycyrrhizin in HIV infected patients with haemophilia in Japan, presented at 5th Int. Conf. on AIDS, Abstract No. WBP 298, June 1989.

78. Mori, K. et al., The present status in prophylaxis and treatment of glycyrrhizin on HIV infected patients with haemophilia in Japan, *Rinsho Byhori*, 37(11), 1200, 1989.
79. Udupa, A.L. et al., Wound healing profile of septilin, *Indian J. Physiol. Pharmacol.*, 33, 1, 1989.
80. Gaunekar, L. et al., Glinical trial of septilin in recurrent upper respiratory tract infection, *Antiseptic*, 4, 190, 1988.
81. Sharma, S.B. and Ray, S., Effect of herbal preparation on immune response of immunosupressed mice, *Indian J. Physiol. Pharmacol.*, 3, 293, 1997.
82. Kulkarni, S.K., Mentat: multicomponent herbal pschyotropic formulation, *Drugs of the Future*, 21(6), 585, 1996.
83. Patel, R., Malnourished children and Liv-52, *Indian Pract.*, 7, 532, 1993.
84. Patney, N.L., A study of serum glycolytic enzyme and serum B hepatitis in relation to Live 52 therapy, *Med. Surg.*, 26(4), 9, 1986.
85. Singh, N. et al., An experimental evaluation of anti-stress effects of geriforte (an ayurvedic drug), *Q. J. Crude Drug Res.*, 3, 125, 1978.
86. Ghooi, A.M., Post surgical recovery with geriforte following major surgical procedure, *Probe*, 22(2), 103, 1983.
87. Makhani, J.S., Evaluation of geriforte as a general tonic, *Curr. Med. Pract.*, 25(5), 211, 1981.
88. Manjunatha, S. et al., Effect of chyawanprash and vitamin C on glucose tolerance and lipoprotein profile, *Indian J. Physiol. Pharmacol.*, 45, 71, 2001.

6

Ayurvedic Bhasmas

Sheikh Raisuddin

CONTENTS

0-8493-1366-X/04/$0.00+$1.50

6.1 Introduction

Accumulated toxicity data on the hazardous effects of heavy metals have made health scientists afraid of heavy metals. As a result, renewed interest in the beneficial effects of metals and minerals is often viewed with skepticism. However, available literature from all the ancient civilizations indicates that man has used metals in disease treatment since time immemorial. Ayurvedic literature is full of the use of metals. Not only have Ayurveda and other Indian systems of medicine used metals, but their use is also amply described in Chinese and Egyptian civilizations in 2500 B.C.[1] Gold in medicine was also mentioned by Roman physician Pliny and Greek philosopher Dioscrides. Later, Arabic and Persian physicians used gold in various forms in a number of their prescriptions. Besides gold, other metals that are extensively described in Indian and other ancient systems of medicine include silver, arsenic, copper, iron, lead, mercury, and zinc. As far as Ayurveda is concerned, metals have been used mainly as *bhasma* (ash).

Bhasma literally means anything inorganic or organic burnt into its ash. The process of burning in Ayurvedic terminology is known as *marana* (calcination). The process of calcination is also employed for preparation of *bhasmas* of coral, pearl, and shell. The well-known Ayurvedic texts, *Charaka Samhita* and *Susruta Samhita,* which are regarded as the texts scripted by the forefathers of Ayurveda, include ample description of the use of the metals and minerals in the treatment of diseases. It is also reflected in later texts that were attempted to simplify the knowledge of *charaka* and *susruta* (e.g., *Astanga Hridaya, Vagbhata, Mdhahva Nidan, Sharangadhara Samhita,* and *Bhava Prakash*).[2,3] In this chapter, an attempt has been made to describe various medicinal uses of *bhasmas* in general and *swrana bhasma* in particular.

The principles of Ayurvedic treatment are for the most part the same as those of allopathic treatment. They consist of removing the injurious agent, soothing the injured body and mind, and eradicating the cause. The difference lies in the methods adopted by the two systems. In Ayurveda, great importance is given to the study of the various stages of vitiation of the three *dosas* or humours of the body. When an imbalance occurs among three *dosas*, they defile the normal functioning of the body, leading to the manifestation of disease.[4] Consciousness or intelligence (*sattva*), motion or action (*rajas*), and the inertia that resist them (*tamas*) are the three omnipresent nonmaterial qualities (*gunas*) that govern all material forms of basic matter. These material and nonmaterial attributes subsequently dictate the medicinal and healing properties of plants and other healing processes.[5]

Ayurveda uses the concept of purification as a means to eradicate disease rather than to cure as perceived by modern medicine.[5] When treating acute and chronic infections,

Ayurveda does not aim to kill the microbes; restoration of *dosa* balance and host immunity (*rasayna*) ensures elimination of the infectious agent. Numerous Ayurvedic medicinal plants have shown strong chemotherapeutic and immunomodifying effect in experimentally induced infections.[6]

6.2 History of Alchemy in Ayurveda

Ayurvedic literature places great emphasis on the pharmaceutical process known as *samskara*. *Samskara* literally means a process. It is designed to enhance the desirable qualities of the drug being processed. The *samskara* can be classified into two stages: *shodhana* (purification or detoxification of toxic substances) and *bhaishajya kalpana* (formulation of a dosage form). A number of toxic herbal drugs like *Strychnos nuxvomica, Aconitum ferox, Semicarpus anacardium, Commiphora mukul,* and almost all metal and mineral drugs are purified and rendered safe for use, before their use as drugs.

In Ayurveda, *rasayana* is a well-developed concept. Literally, *rasayana* means the augmentation of *rasa,* the vital fluid produced by the digestion of food, which sustains the body through the strengthening of the *dhatus.* It is the *rasa* flowing in the body that sustains life; when it stops flowing, life comes to an end. *Rasayana* is the medium through which the *rasa* is maintained, replenished, and augmented.

In modern terms, the study and practice of *rasayana* such as *rasvidya* is referred to as alchemy. It is generally believed that alchemy appeared in India in the fifth or sixth century A.D. and greatly prospered for the next seven or eight centuries under royal patronage.[7] Hindu *tantriks* developed the mercury-based alchemy in India and related it to the male–female symbolism (*Shiva* and *Parvati*). Mercury was regarded as male principle (*Shiva*) and sulfur as the female principle (*Parvati*).

The laboratory of an Indian alchemist was known as *rasashala,* a place where the alchemists carried out their various operations under the benign influence of the *rasalinga,* a symbol of esoteric potentiality. *Rasalinga* was either a gold amalgam, prepared by triturating gold and mercury, or a compound of mercury and sulfur shaped into a *linga*. The text *Rasaratna Samuchchaya* describes how and where a *rasashala* can be established. It also describes important apparatuses that should be available in a *rasashala*. It is amply clear that knowledge of science of metals and its medicinal usage was well developed in India.

Alchemical or related texts can also be found in other Indian languages like Tamil, Telugu, Kannada, Malayalam, Bengali, Marathi, Oriya, and Gujarati. There are more than 200 works in Tamil on the Siddha system of medicine. Plants occupied an important place in the practices of Indian alchemists. More than 200 names of plants are mentioned in different texts of *Rasashastra*. The Indian alchemists (*rasavadins*) treated the minerals and metals with one medicinal plant or the other to render them the desirable chemical properties. Even mercury considered to be divine was subjected to this process.[7] According to the *Matrakabhedatantram,* "mercury cannot be reduced to bhasma without the help of one or more of medicinal plants."

The plants used were referred to as *divyausadhi* (divine medicinal plants). Mercury is considered to be the king of *rasas* and it is referred to by various names like *parada, rasa, suta, maharasa, rasendra, svarnakaraka, sarvadhatupati,* etc. There are detailed descriptions of a number of compositions with mercury as the chief ingredient. In Indian alchemical texts, the chemical substances have been divided into five main categories: *maharasa, uparasa, dhatu, ratna,* and poisons (*visha*). There are eight *maharasas,* eight *uparasas,* and seven *dhatus,* including three alloys: brass (*pittala*), bell metal (*kamsya*), and a mixture of five metals (*vartka*). The precious gems were placed under the catagory of *ratnas*. Various plant products and minerals having toxic properties are included in the category of poisons.

6.3 Ayurvedic Pharmaceuticals

Ayurvedic medicines are categorized according to whether they promote general health and longevity, enhance sexual vigor, or fight disease. The first category is known as *rasayana*, the second is called *vajikarana*, and the third is *aushadhis*. These categories are not mutually exclusive because some of the *aushadhis* may act as *rasayanas* and vice versa. On the basis of their origin, Ayurvedic medicines are also classified into three groups: (1) *kastha ausadhis* (herbal preparations), (2) *rasa ausadhis* (metallic preparations [e.g., *bhasmas, sindoora*]), and (3) *jangama ausadhis* (animal preparation — prepared from animal products). Depending on their form, method of preparation, ingredients, and pharmacological properties, Ayurvedic medicines are grouped as *Swaras, Kalka, Hima, Phanita, Kashaya, Asavas, Aristas, Awalehas, Churnas, Vati, Gutika, Ghrita, Taila Guggulu, Bhasmas, Pishti, Parpati, Rasayoga, Sindoora, Lepa,* and *Anjana*.[4,8–11]

6.4 Metal and Mineral Drugs of Ayurveda

Metals like gold, silver, copper, lead, tin, and iron, sand (*balu* from river banks), lime and minerals like red arsenic (*manassila*), gems (*manayah*), salts (*lavana*), and red chalk (*gairika*) are indicated as drugs pertaining to earth (*bhauma*). In Indian metallurgy, the term *loha* is often used for metals like gold and silver and minerals containing metals (ores) are called *dhatus*. There are seven *dhatus*: *suvarna* (gold), *rajata* (silver), *tamra* (copper), *trapa* (tin), *tiksna* or *ayas* (iron), *sisa* or *naga* (lead), and *vaikrintaka*.[11] Salts or *lavanas* are mentioned under the *parthive* substances. According to Charaka, there are five salts: *sauvarcala, saindhava, vida, audbhida,* and *samudra*. *Mani* and *ratna*, being synonyms for each other, stand for the modern term "jewel" or "gem."

Mercury is considered eighth metal in *rasa shastra*. It earned the supreme position among the minerals and metals. The learned Acharyas also studied the relation and effects between these metals and planets over the human body and called them *grahanga navaloha*.[11] Metals are grouped as *shuddha, sishra,* and *pooti loha*.[11]

The calcined forms of metals that are termed *bhasmas* in Ayurveda are referred to as *parpams* and *kushta* in Siddha and Unani-tibb, respectively. *Kushta* literally means to kill; in medical terms it is detoxifying the toxic properties of a toxic metal.[12]

Although bhasmas are regarded as chief metal-containing pharmaceuticals of Ayurveda, there are several other preparations prepared from metals. Some of these pharmaceuticals are described below.

6.4.1 *Bhasma*

Animal derivatives such as horns, shells, feathers, and metallic and nonmetallic minerals are normally administered as *bhasmas*. A *bhasma* means an ash obtained though incineration. The starter material undergoes an elaborate process of purification (*shodhana*). This process is followed by the reaction phase, which involves incorporation of some other mineral and herbal extracts. Then the material in pellet form is incinerated in a furnace. The end product is expected to be a nontoxic material. Examples include *swarn bhasma, shankha bhasma,* and *tamra bhasma.*

6.4.2 *Parpati*

These are specialized mercury preparations. The name is derived from the method by which flakes of the compound are obtained. A black sulfide of mercury is obtained by mixing purified mercury and sulfur. Other drugs as per the formula are added to this and mixed well by triturating them in mortar and pestle. A shallow pit is made in fresh cow dung and a banana leaf is placed. The melted compound is poured onto the leaf and is covered with another leaf. Fresh dung is spread on it evenly. When it is cooled the flakes are removed and powdered.

6.4.3 *Rasayoga*

Rasayogas are compound formulations containing mercury and sulfur (in the form of *kajjali*) with other metals or minerals. Most of the ingredients contained in a *rasayoga* are added in the form of *bhasmas*. The final form may be either a pill or powder.

6.4.4 *Sindoora*

Sindoora are prepared by the elaborate process of sublimation. This procedure is termed *kupipakwa vidhi* and the sublimed mineral available on the neck of the sublimation glass flask is called *sindoora. Sindoora* preparations are considered to be more potent than *bhasma* preparations.

6.5 Types of *Bhasma*

Attempts have been made to classify various *bhasmas*. They have been classified on the basis of color and appearance. A more scientific way of classification is on the basis of dominant metal and mineral group.[13] According to this classification, *bhasmas* have been grouped as *rajata* group (silver), *tamra* group (copper), *loha* group (iron), *pravala* group (shells), etc. Often two metals and a metal with mineral are the ingredients of *bhasmas.* For example, *Trivanga Bhasma* contains lead, tin, and zinc. The metals yield three different types of *bhasma* corresponding to the nature of the ingredient used. They appear as best, medium, and inferior quality. Mercury is always used as a basic substance in the process of *marana*.[11]

6.6 Preparation of *Bhasma*: General Procedures

The name *bhasma* is generally applied to all metallic and nonmetallic substances that are subjected to the process of incineration and reduction to ash. Here it is applied to the metals, minerals, and animal products that are, by special processes, calcinated in closed crucibles in pits with cow dung cakes (*puttam*). *Bhasmas* are generally white, pale, or red. The color of the preparation primarily depends on the parent material.[14] The following pharmaceutical steps are used to prepare *bhasmas*.

6.6.1 *Shodhana*

In Ayurveda, purification is called *shodhana*. *Shodhana* is the process through which the external and internal impurities of metals and minerals are removed. Chemical purification is different from medicinal purification. In chemical purification it is only elimination of foreign matters, whereas in medicinal purification the objects are involved in the

1. Elimination of harmful matter from the drug
2. Modification of undesirable physical properties of the drug
3. Conversion of some of the characteristics of the drug to different stages
4. Enhancement of the therapeutic action

There are two kinds of *shodhana*. The first type, *samanya shodhana* (general purification), is applicable to the large number of metals or minerals as heating the thin sheets of metals and immersing them in oil (*taila*), extract (*takra*), cow urine (*gomutra*), and other materials. The second type, *Vishesha shodhana* (special purification), is applicable only to specific metals, minerals, and in certain preparations. *Vishesha shodhana* includes *bhavana, svedana, nirvapana,* and *mardana*.[14]

After *shodhana bhasmas* become soft and malleable for further processing and their metallic property is improved. The main apparatus required includes *dola yantra, khalva yantra,* and *musha yantra*.[11] Various procedures employed for *shodhana* are described below.

When mineral drugs are heated in a furnace in the presence of *dravaka*, substances (liqueficants) like alkali and acid release their *satva*. This is the purest form of any herbal or mineral drug.[11] All the metals except mercury are found in nature in solid state, and they all fuse under high temperature to attain a liquid state. When the temperature lowers they again return to their natural physical form (i.e., in the solid state). But these fused metals in the presence of some liqueficants do not return into their natural solid state even when the temperature lowers (i.e., the metals remain in liquid form). This method of obtaining metals in liquid form is called *dravana* and the obtained liquid metal is called *druti*. *Druti* holds superior character with respect to efficacy, toxicity, and increased shelf life than its native metals and retains its fluidity for a longer time with proper preservation.[11]

Shuddhavarta is a particular stage of heating when the fire becomes strong enough to yield the pure substance (metal, *satva*). At this time the flame becomes golden yellow.[11]

6.6.2 *Marana*

Marana is essentially the burning process or calcination. The purified metal is placed into a mortar and, with a pestle, ground with the juice of specified plants or *kashayas*, mercury (in metallic state), or a compound of mercury such as mercury perchloride (*sauviram*), mercuric subchloride (*ras karpur*), cinnabar (*ingalekam*), or an amalgam of sulfur and mercury (*kajjali*) for a specified period of time. The metal that is intended for *marana* is known as a primary metal (*pradhan dhatu*); the other metal, which is taken in small proportions for the *marana* of the primary metal, is known as secondary metal (*sahaya dhatu*).[14] Small cakes (*chakrikas*) are made with the ground paste of the minerals and dried under the sun. The size and thickness of the cakes depend on the heaviness of the drug and size. The heavier the drug, the thinner the cakes. These cakes are dried well under the shade and placed in one single layer in a mud tray (*sharava*) and closed with another such tray; the clay-smeared cloth keeps both the lid and the container in apposition. The clay-smeared cloth is applied seven times and dried to seal the crucibles properly. A pit is dug in an open space and half the pit is filled with dried cow dung cakes. The crucibles are placed in the half-filled pit and are covered with cow dung cakes up to the brim of the pit. Fire is then ignited on all four sides and in the middle of the pit. When the burning is over, the contents are allowed to cool completely on their own.

Marana differs with the nature of the substance to be calcinated. For example, organic substances such as herbs are burnt in open air, whereas inorganic substances such as metals like *rajata* (silver) are burnt in closed containers. In either case the end product is a *bhasma* of substance taken for *marana*. For example, the end product in the case of silver (*rajata*) is called as *rajata bhasma*. *Marana* of inorganic substances is called *puta* and the process of *marana* of herbs in closed freshly made containers is known as *puta paka*.[13]

Bhasmas obtained by *marana* from primary metals together with herbs (*mulika*) are called *mulika marita bhasma*; the ones where the second metal is taken for the *marana* of primary metal are called *parada* (mercury) *marita*, or *talaka* (arsenic trisulphide) *marita bhasma*, depending upon the second metal used for the purpose. During the process the second metal would finally volatilize itself at the temperature of *marana*, leaving behind the *bhasma* of primary metal.

Very few metals like copper or iron still bear some impurities after the *marana*. In such cases the whole process is repeated until a purified and therapeutically safer product for internal use is obtained. In addition, a process called *amritikarana* is done to make these metals safer.[11] The process consists of heating the product from the *marana* procedure in the presence of some herbal materials to improve safety and therapeutic effect. In this process the required amounts of *triphala* decoction, cow's *ghritika*, and *dhatu bhasma* are placed in an iron pot. Mild heat is applied until the medicinal fluids are completely evaporated. *Bhasma* that remains at the end of this process is safer and possesses higher therapeutic efficacy.

6.6.3 Quality Control of *Bhasma*

Traditionally, the end points of incineration of a metal and its conversion to a *bhasma* state are evaluated based on the following criteria:

1. There should be no *chandrika* or metallic lusture (*nischandrika*).
2. When a *bhasma* is spread between the index finger and thumb, it should be so fine as to get easily into the lines and crevices of the fingers (*rekhapurita*).
3. When a small quantity is spread on cold and still water, it should float on the surface (*varitara*).
4. The *bhasma* should not revert to the original state (*apurnabhava*).[14]

A technique known as the phased spot test has been developed by the investigators of Central Council for Research in Ayurveda and Siddha (CCRAS) of India to identify *bhasmas* and *sindooras*. This technique is very effective and accurate in identifying genuine quality of *bhasmas*. Nearly 30 *bhasmas* and *sinduroos* have been studied based on this technique, and suitable criteria have been established for their identification and quality assessment.[13]

TABLE 6.1

Important *Bhasmas* and Their Main Ingredients

No.	*Bhasma*	Main Ingredient
1	*Abhrak bhasma*	Mica
2	*Hathidanta bhasma*	Charcoal of elephant tusk
3	*Jasad bhasma*	Zinc oxide
4	*Loha bhasma*	Iron oxide
5	*Mandur bhasma*	Iron oxide
6	*Mayurapicha bhasma*	Ashes of peacock feather
7	*Mukta bhasma*	Oxide of pearl
8	*Naga bhasma*	Lead
9	*Parada bhasma*	Mercury compound
10	*Pravala bhasma*	Oxide of coral
11	*Rajata bhasma*	Silver oxide
12	*Sankha bhasma*	Oxide of conch shell
13	*Mukta sukti bhasma*	Oxide of pearl, oyster shell
14	*Talaka bhasma*	Arsenic sulphide
15	*Tamra bhasma*	Cupric oxide
16	*Vanga bhasma*	Tin compounds
17	*Varatika bhasma*	Oxide of cowrie shell

The identification of gold in *makardhwaja,* a powdered mercury preparation, by spot test is simple and spectacular. This effort is one big step toward standardizing Ayurvedic preparations.

6.6.4 Preparation of Gold and Iron *Bhasmas* and Their Chemical Characteristics

Some of the common *bhasmas* and their main ingredients used in Ayuarveda are listed Table 6.1. Methods to prepare two important Ayurvedic *bhasmas* — gold and iron — and their characteristics are presented here as examples.

6.6.4.1 Gold (Swarna) Bhasma

The general preparation of *swarna bhasma* involves the three processes of *shodhana, dravana,* and *marana.* The leaves of gold are heated over fire and dipped in *sesa* (*Sesamum indicum*) oil when they are red hot, and the process is continued seven times separately. The soft leaves are processed in the same manner with buttermilk, cow's urine, and the decoction of *kulatha* (*Dolichos biflorus*), *kanji* (sour gruel processed from rice [*Oryza sativa*]), and radish (*Raphanus sativus*). Finally, the leaves are dried by heat. Care must be taken that the weight of the gold remains unchanged. A measurement of 15 g each of arsenic disulfide, realger (As_2S_2), and red lead (Pb_3O_4) is taken in an earthenware container and mixed thoroughly with 30 ml of latex of *Calotropis gigentea.* The mixture is triturated and the paste thus obtained is dried in sunlight. The process of triturating and drying in sunlight is repeated 7 to 14 times using fresh aliquots of latex, and the final product (~200 g) is obtained. An aliquot of the above product (~10 g) is poured into liquefied metallic gold (10 g) in a closed earthen pot and the mixture is heated above 1000°C. The content is gently stirred and the heating is continued until the mass becomes disintegrated and a homogenous red-brown powder is formed.[15]

All the major Ayurvedic pharmaceutical manufacturers, including Dabur and Zhandu, make *swarna bhasma.* The ingredients of *swarna bhasma* made by Kalptaru Ayurvedic Works, Kolkata, has been reported.[16] The gold content was reported to be 96.76%. It also contained trace quantities of copper and iron. Recently, physicochemical characteristics which resulted in the laboratory following the procedure as per *Rasaratna Samuchchya* of *swarna bhasma* have been reported.[15] An atomic absorption spectrometer (ASS) was employed to study the contents of gold and other metals. The gold content was found to be 20.3%. Some other important metals that were present included iron, magnesium, strontium, copper, arsenic, lead, nickel, zinc, and cobalt.

The organoleptic characteristics of *swarna bhasma* are that it is dark brown, has a faint smell, fine touch, and is tasteless. The standard *swarna bhasma* should contain the following:

1. Free sulfur — no less than 1.43% w/w and no more than 6.39% w/w
2. Sulfur — no more than 3.33% w/w
3. Calcium as Ca — no more than 1.625% w/w
4. Sodium as Na — no more than 0.922% w/w
5. Potassium as K — no more than 0.370% w/w
6. Sulfate — no more than 3.00% w/w
7. Copper — no more than 17.2% w/w
8. Iron oxide (ferric) — no more than 85.0% w/w
9. Iron oxide (ferrous) — no more than 5.7% w/w
10. Iron — no less than 36.0% w/w and not more than 51.96% w/w
11. Phosphate as PO_4 — no more than 1.101% w/w
12. Silica — no more than 3.8% w/w
13. Acid insolubles — no more than 11.93% w/w

Swarna bhasma contains an ash value between 92.10 and no more than 98.20% w/w and an acid-insoluble ash value between 21.20 and 31.18% w/w. The recommended dose is 100 to 250 mg.[14]

6.6.4.2 *Iron (Loha) Bhasma*

Iron *bhasma* preparation uses three basic processes: *shodhana*, *dravana*, and *marana*. Iron is purified by sinking the red-hot leaflet into the fresh *trifala* decoction (*nishechan*) repeatedly nine times. A freshly prepared decoction is used every time. Coarse pieces of sulfur are taken in *khalva yantra* and some amount of *dewadali swaras* are added for *bhavana* (i.e., the sulfur pieces remain in good contact within this medicinal fluid). It is rubbed thoroughly and the process is repeated for at least 7 days. When sulfur powder obtained at the end is sprinkled (*pravap*) over the fused iron, it is kept in liquidity.

Iron *bhasma* should always be prepared with mercury; otherwise, it is not absorbed properly in the intestine. Additional processes are used to obtain the best quality iron *bhasma*. This includes *loha maraka gana, amritkarana*, and *nirutthikarana*. In the *loha maraka*, fresh lemon juice is prepared and a specific amount of *hingula* powder is added. Then these ingredients are mixed thoroughly. Afterward, the process of repeated dipping (*nirvapana*) red-hot iron leaflets in the medicinal fluid is applied to obtain *loha bhasma*. In the *amritkarana* process, equal amounts of *loha bhasma* and *ghrita* are placed in an iron pan and mixed properly under mild heat until the fat disappears. This compound now bears a *yagavahi* character. Finally, the properly prepared *bhasma* and *trifala* decoction (*bhavana drava*) is exposed to heat by the sun (*suryaputa*) or by the process of burning the herbs in closed freshly made mud containers (*putapaka*). At the end of this procedure, *loha bhasma* becomes the end product (*niruttha* and *varttara*) of filtration and separation procedures (*nirutthikarana*).[11]

The organoleptic characteristics of *loha bhasma* are that it is dark brown, has a faint smell, fine touch, and no taste. Iron as Fe_2O_3 is no more than 96.575% w/w, and iron as Fe is no more than 75% w/w present in this *bhasma*. *Loha bhasma* contains an ash value not less than 96.8% w/w and not more than 99.7% w/w. Its acid-insoluble ash is between 0.101 and 2.803% w/w. Its dose is 100 to 250 mg.[14]

6.7 Therapeutic Indications and Scientific Investigations on *Bhasmas*

6.7.1 *Swarna Bhasma*

6.7.1.1 *Indications*

Gold has been used since the Vedic era in India to enhance strength and potency, promote longevity, and combat the aging process in humans. Around the eighth century A.D., gold was used in the form of *bhasma* after proper purification and incineration as described in the *Ayurvedic Pharmacopoeia*. Gold preparations are recommended to promote longevity, combat aging, and treat impotency. They are also used as a tonic, hepatotonic, cardiostimulant, nervine tonic, detoxifier, and an anti-infective drug. *Swarna bhasma* is also used in the treatment of diseases such as anemia, dyspepsia, epilepsy, neurasthenia, loss of memory, bronchitis, asthma, tuberculosis, leucoderma, and rheumatoid arthritis.[9,15] The recommended dose is 100 to 250 mg.[14] In modern medicine, gold is primarily used in rheumatoid arthritis. Some gold compounds used as medicine, in modern medicine are listed in Table 6.2. Of all these gold compounds, auranofin and gold sodium thiomalate (GST) are the most extensively studied.

6.7.1.2 *Animal Studies*

6.7.1.2.1 *Analgesic Activity*

Analgesic activity of *swarna bhasma* was reported in one study involving mice.[17] A Unani calcined gold preparation, *kushta tilan kalan* (KTK), was also used in this study along with the widely used gold drug auranofin. *Swarna bhasma* at 12 to 50 mg/kg body weight by oral route showed analgesic activity against chemical, thermal, electrical, and mechanical stimuli. Whereas the analgesic effect of *swarna bhasma* could be blocked by the treatment of nolaxone, such antagonism was not possible in the case of auranofin. The study suggests involvement of opiodergenic mechanism in the observed analgesic activity of *swarna bhasma*.

6.7.1.2.2 *Immune Response*

Specific and nonspecific immune responses were modified in a positive manner in *swarna bhasma*-treated mice.[18,19] The doses were in the range of 12.5 to 50 mg/kg body weight. *Swarna bhasma* had a stimulatory effect on peritoneal macrophages, which may be helpful to fight against infections. It was suggested that macrophages achieved stimulation possibly due to presentation of the metal to cells in fine emulsified form.

6.7.1.2.3 *Antioxidant Activity*

The antioxidant and restorative effects of *swarna bhasma* in rats have recently been demonstrated.[20] The study was done under ischemia, which was induced by bilateral carotid occlusion under phenobarbitone anesthesia. A number of antioxidant enzymes and lipid

TABLE 6.2

Biologically Active Gold Compounds on the Market

No.	Generic Name	Trade Name	Gold Concentration (%)
1	Gold sodium thiomalate	Myochristin, Myocrisin, Tauredon	50.5
2	Gold thioglucose	Solganal	50.5
3	Gold thioglycoanilid	Lauron	54.2
4	Gold sodium thiosulphate	Sanochrysine, Aurothion, Thiochrysine	402
5	Calcium aurothiothioglycolate	Myoral	64.1
6	Sodium 2-aurothiobenzidazole-4-carboxylalte	Triphal	47.8
7	Sodium auroallylthiourea-*m*-benzoate	Lapion	43.4
8	*S*-triethylphosphine gold 2,3,4,6-teta-*O*-acetyl-1 thio-β-D-glycopyranoside	Auranofin	29.1
9	Chloro (triethylphosphine) gold	SK&F 36914	56.2

Based on information from Lewis, A.J. and Walz, D.T., *Progress in Medicinal Chemistry*, Vol. 19, Elsevier Biomedical Press, New York, 1982, 1–59, and Insel, P.A., *Goodman's and Gilman's: The Pharmacological Basis of Therpaeutics*, 9th ed., McGraw-Hill, New York, 1996, 644.

peroxidation were studied. *Swarna bhasma* (25 mg/kg) had a restorative effect, significantly restoring antioxidant levels in ischemic animals. Biochemical findings supported the histological examination of the brain. The free radical scavenging and antioxidant effects of *swarna bhasma* have also been investigated recently by several groups. Two antioxidant enzymes — superoxide dismutase (SOD) and catalase — were measured after oxidative insult with acetic acid in both *swarna bhasma*-treated mice as well as control serum and liver homogenate of mice.[15] *Swarna bhasma* induced activity of SOD and catalase. Chronic administration of *swarna bhasma* had no toxic effects as assessed by liver function test enzymes and histological investigations.

Biological investigations on *swarna bhasma* are summarized in Table 6.3.

6.7.1.3 Clinical Studies

Gold containing Ayurvedic preparation, *swarna vasanti malti*, was investigated for safety. The *bhasma* was given to 20 male persons at a dose of 100 mg twice a day for 40 days under supervision of Ayurvedic physicians. The total cumulative intake of 160 mg of gold at the rate of 4 mg/day in this form did not have any toxic effect on human body, as evidenced by clinical examination, unaltered body weight, absence of urinary pathology, and by 30 sensitive biochemical and enzymatic tests.[21]

TABLE 6.3

Summary of Scientific Investigations on Swarna Bhasma

No.	Investigation	Model	Ref.
1	Analgesic activity	Mouse, rat	17
2	Immunomodulatory activity: specific immunity	Mouse	18
3	Immunomodulatory activity: nonspecific immunity	Mouse	19
4	Evaluation of safety	Human	22
5	Antioxidant effect	Rat	20
6	Analysis of chemical constituents	—	16
7	Free radical scavenging activity	Mouse	16

6.7.2 *Loha Bhasma*

6.7.2.1 *Indications*

Loha bhasma is a powerful hematinic Ayurvedic drug indicated in anemia. It stimulates the appetite and has a general vitalizing effect. It is readily assimilated in the body.

6.7.2.2 *Animal Studies*

Various *loha bhasmas* made by different manufacturers were screened, and one representative preparation was evaluated for its effect in managing experimentally induced anemia in Charles Foster albino rats. Comparison was made with Fefol®,[22] a widely used standard drug. Anemia was induced by dietary means (agar gel treatment) and by bloodletting (phlebotomy) through the tail vain. Various parameters of hemoglobin estimation, serum ferritin estimation, and total iron and iron binding capacity of serum were studied. *Loha bhasma* was helpful not only in resorting hemoglobin level, but in significantly increasing body weight gain in *bhasma*-treated animals. In some parameters results were better that those observed with Fefol.

No clinical study on iron *bhasma* was found in our literature search.

6.7.3 Copper (*Tamra*) *Bhasma*

6.7.3.1 *Indications*

Tamra bhasma is used as a single drug and also in combination with many medicinal plant extracts. *Tamra bhasma* is used for the management of liver disorder, arthritis, old age disorders, leucoderma, etc.

6.7.3.2 *Animal Studies*

The hepatoprotective effect of *tamra bhasma* has been studied on cumene hydroperoxide-induced peroxidation, reduced glutathione content, and SOD in rat liver homogenate.[23] The drug was orally given for 8 days at different dose levels (0.5, 1.0, and 5.0 mg/100 g body weight). It showed significant reduction in the level of lipid peroxidation. The results suggested that *tamra bhasma* is a strong antioxidant drug and could be used in the management of lipid peroxidation. It showed no acute detectable adverse effects. Levels of SOD were also enhanced by *tamra bhasma*.

The hepatoprotective effects of four Ayurvedic drugs — *kumari asav, kumari kalp, arogyavardhini,* and *tamra bhasma* — against the toxicity of carbon tetrachloride (CCl_4) was established in a series of experiments in rats.[23] The hepatoprotective effect of these drugs was in the following order: *tamra bhasma* < *arogyavardhini* < *kumari kalp* < *kumari asav.* Significant reduction in hepatic necrosis was recorded in all the treated animals.[23,24] Effects of these drugs on acid lipase, alkaline lipase, lipoprotein lipase of the liver and kidney, adipose tissue and hormone-sensitive lipase, acid phosphatase, and beta-glucoridase were also investigated in the animals treated with the above-mentioned drugs.[24–26] Histologically, all the above formulas showed hepatoprotective effects in CCl_4-exposed animals.

6.7.4 *Abhrak Bhasma*

6.7.4.1 *Indications*

Abhrak bhasma is prepared by treating biotite (mica) with the juices of a number of reconstituent plants that make it a powerful cellular regenerator. It is a commonly used Ayurvedic drug against many diseases, including hepatitis. It is also a nervine tonic and is widely used in respiratory tract infections and anemia. It contains iron, magnesium, potassium, calcium, and aluminum in traces. *Abhrak bhasma* is an amorphous powdery drug. Mica mainly contains silicates of iron, magnesium, and aluminum.[27]

6.7.4.2 Animal Studies

The hepatoprotective action of *abhrak bhasma* has been reported in albino rats using a model of hepatitis induced by a single dose of CCl_4 (3 ml/kg body weight). Different doses of *abhrak bhasma* (10, 20, 30, and 40 mg/kg body weight) were used.[27] The centrolobular necrosis induced by a single dose of CCl_4 was reduced significantly by *abhrak bhasma* (10 mg), and liver histology was also protected by a 20-mg dose. Liver acid lipase activity was lowered, whereas alkaline and lipoprotein lipase activity was elevated due to the treatment of CCl_4. *Abhrak bhasma*-treated animals that were exposed to CCl_4 showed marked improvement in enzyme profile.

6.7.5 Mandur Bhasma

6.7.5.1 Indications

Mandur bhasma is prepared by purifying and calcinating iron rust. It is especially useful in anemia, amenorrhea, dysmenorrhea, menorrhagia, chlorosis, and hepatic and splenic disorders. It is also used in diarrhea, chronic bowel complaints, dyspepsia, intestinal worms, nervous system diseases, neuralgia, kidney diseases, and albuminuria. It is a powerful hematinic and tonic and is valuable in the treatment of hemolytic jaundice and microcytic anemia.

6.7.5.2 Animal Studies

The protective effect of *mandur bhasma* (10 mg/kg body weight) has been demonstrated in CCl_4-treated rats.[28] *Bhasmas* were orally administered to animals. Hepatoprotection was established by various enzymatic parameters, lipid peroxidation, and a histological examination of tissues.

6.7.6 Muktashukti Bhasma

Muktashukti bhasma is a compound *bhasma* consisting of pearl (*moti*), *Aloe vera* Linn. (*guar patha*), and vinegar (*kanji*). The *bhasma* is prepared from the outer covering of the shell (pearl-oyster), and is ground and triturated with *A. vera* and vinegar in sufficient quantity to make a homogeneous paste. The recommended proportion of pearl-oyster and *A. vera* is in the ratio of 1:4.

6.7.6.1 Indications

Muktashukti bhasma has been used in the treatment of tuberculosis, cough, chronic fever, conjuctivitis, abdominal discomfort, biliary disturbances, asthma, heart diseases, vomiting, acidity, dyspepsia, dysmenorrhea, general weakness, arthritis, rheumatism, musculoskeletal disorders, etc.

6.7.6.2 Animal Studies

An anti-inflammatory effect of *muktashukti bhasma* has been shown in albino rats by Chauhan et al.[29] The *bhasma* inhibited acute and subacute inflammation in albino rats as induced by subplanter injection of carageenan, histamine, serotonin (5-HT), nystatin, and subcutaneous implants of cotton pellets. In all the test procedures, the anti-inflammatory response of 1000 mg/kg of *muktashukti bhasma* was comparable with the response observed with 300 mg/kg of acetyl salicylic acid, which was used as a standard anti-inflammatory drug. Oral premedication with delayed castor oil-induced diarrhea in rats, indicating its prostaglandin inhibitory activity.[29]

6.7.7 *Sankha Bhasma*

Sankha bhasma is a powder prepared from the calcinated conch shell. It consists mainly of calcium, iron, and magnesium.

6.7.7.1 *Indications*

Sankha bhasma is well known for its antacid and digestive properties. It is useful in hyperchlorhydria, sprue, colic, and hepatosplenomegaly.

6.7.7.2 *Biological Studies*

A mixture of some Ayurvedic medicines that contained *sankha bhasma* and the herbs *Glycrrhiza glabra*, *Terminalia chebula*, and *Piper longum* showed protection against duodenal ulcer in rats.[30] These drugs act on Bruner's gland by improving its secretory status.

6.7.8 Miscellaneous Studies on *Bhasmas*

Yashada bhasma is a specially processed zinc. It is administered in sprue, diabetes, leucorrhea, and hyperhydrosis. The role of the *bhasma* in arresting myopia has been examined in one study.[31]

Contamination of *bhasmas* directly through the herbs used in the preparation and formation of polycyclic aromatic hydrocarbons (PAHs) is expected. Sometimes *bhasmas* may be contaminated with very harmful substances. *Bhasmas* were analyzed and found to contain PAH. The levels of total PAH varied widely (2.32 to 9.55 ppm) among the preparation tested. The benzo[a]pyrene level also varied, the highest concentration being 9.7 ppm.[32]

The studies presented here suggest *bhasmas* may have a hepatoprotective effect. However, efforts should be made to study their beneficial effects on other systems. Especially, evaluation of their immunomodulatory and neuroprotective actions may prove to be rewarding.

A summary of scientific investigations on the above-mentioned *bhasmas* is provided in Table 6.4.

TABLE 6.4

Summary of Scientific Investigations on Other Bhasmas

Bhasma	Investigation	Animal Model	Ref.
Abhrak bhasma	Hepatoprotective activity	Rat	28
Loha bhasma	Antianemic	Rat	23
Mandur bhasma	Hepatoprotective activity	Rat	29
Muktashukti bhsama	Anti-inflammatory activity	Rat	30
Sankha bhasma	Antiulcerogenic activity	Rat	31
Tamra bhasma	Hepatoprotective activity	Rat	24–27

TABLE 6.5

Metal and Mineral Drugs Used in Unani System of Medicine

No.	Metal and Mineral (Unani Name)	Name of Unani Drug (% of Metal and Mineral)
1	Aluminium	*Kushta-e-Zumurrud* (16.55%)
2	Ammonium chloride (*naushadar*)	*Habbe Kabid Naushadri*
3	Antimony (*surma siyah*)	*Kehul-ul-Jawahar*
4	Arsenic (*sankhya*)	*Kushta Sam-ul-far* (18.89%)
5	Borax (*suhaga*)	*Safoof-e-Chutki Atfal*
6	Bromide	*Kushta-e-Sadaf* (2.4458%)
7	Calcium	*Khameera-e-Zaharmohra* (27.16 mg/g)
8	Copper	*Jawarish-e-Jalinoos* (7.82 mg/g ash)
9	Coral (*marjan*)	*Kushta Marjan*
10	Diamond (*almas*)	*Kushta Almas*
11	Gold (*sona*)	*Kushta Tilan Kalan*
12	Iron (*loha*)	*Kushta-e Sadaf* (77 mg%), *Kushta-e-Faulad* (48.75%)
13	Iron rust (*khabsul-hadid*)	*Kushta Khabsul-Hadid*
14	Lead	*Sharbat-e-Khas Khaash* (8.333 mg/g)
15	Magnesium	*Kushta-e-Busud* (44 mg/g)
16	Mercury (*para*)	*Marham Gulabi*
17	Pearl (*moti*)	*Kushta Sadaf*
18	Potassium	*Safoof-e-namak-e-shaikh-ur-raees* (1190 mg%)
19	Shell (*sadaf*)	*Kushta Sankh*
20	Silver	*Kushta-e-Nuqra* (93%)
21	Strontium	*Kushta-e-Kharmohra* (1.32%)
22	Sulphur (*kibreet*)	*Habbe Kibreet*
23	Talc	*Kushta Abhrak*
24	White lead (*safeda kashgiri*)	*Marham Kafoori*

Based on information from Council for Research in Unani Medicine, *Physicochemical Standards of Unani Formulations*, Parts I and II, Central India, New Delhi, India, 1986, and Ali, S.S., *Unani Adviya Mafrada*, Turky Urdu Beaurou, New Delhi, India, 1982, chaps. 3 and 4 (in Urdu).

6.8 Metal and Mineral Preparations of Unani-Tibb

Like Ayurveda, a large number of metal and mineral preparations are used in the Unani system of medicine (Unani-tibb). In Unani-tibb, the procedures of calcination, purification, and trituration are also undertaken to purify and enhance the therapeutic efficacy of drugs. All the important metals (i.e., copper, gold, silver, lead, arsenic, mercury, etc.) are used in this system of medicine. The calcinated drugs of Unani-tibb are termed *kushta*. Drugs derived from shell, oyster, and coral are also used in Unani-tibb. Although there is some similarity between the procedural details of calcination, purification, and trituration, Ayurvedic and Unani-tibb systems of medicine have a number of differences.[5,12] Some of the most widely used drugs prepared from metals and minerals that are used in Unani-tibb are listed in Table 6.5.

6.9 Discussion

Various processes of marana and sodhana involve the incorporation of herbal juices that presumably makes the drugs more efficacious. The drug that is presented in the final form seems to have an enhanced bioavailability, especially through the digestive system. It is also likely that most of the *bhasmas* act as adjuvants and thus may be potentiating the nonspecific immune functions (macrophage activation). They may also activate drug-metabolizing enzymes. Further scientific investigations are warranted. Studies should be undertaken aiming at use of radio-labeled metallic compounds in Ayurvedic medicine and subsequently their distribution and disposition should be tracked down.

Metal and mineral preparations used in Ayurveda, Siddha, and Unani-tibb are often subjected to scientific scrutiny. Analytical laboratories sometimes publish news articles about the existence of heavy metals like arsenic, lead, and mercury in Ayurvedic formulations. This makes the public uneasy to use Ayurvedic and other traditional drugs. However, it is necessary to note that many important metals are essential components of vital molecules of the body; every year the essential nature of some hitherto nonessential elements is established in biological systems.

In Ayurveda, a great emphasis is placed on *shodhana* (purification) and detoxification of metals and other minerals. The process of *shodhana* is followed by the incorporation of various herbal juices to get the final product. This alters the metallic salt forms and the bioavailability. These processes can also convert the metalloids in emulsified form, acting as an adjuvant and eliciting various responses, especially the immune responses. The unabsorbed parts are normally eliminated in the stool after localized activities in the receptor sites of the gut. The activity of any pharmacologically active substance is based on the dose of administration, duration of administration, frequency of administration, and the adjuvant, which may influence bioavailability. In Ayurveda, these principles are the essential parts of therapy. Many of the bhasmas are recommended at very low doses (often in divided doses) and for a specific period of time. Sometimes the dose levels of elements may even normally occur in water sources. Thus, dose is a very important factor in using *bhasmas*.

Metals and minerals in Ayurveda are not essentially the first line of treatment for common diseases. Introduction of metallic preparations is the last resort only when all other methods of treatment have not yielded desired results. One common criticism that is associated with Ayurvedic preparations, particularly those prepared from metals and minerals, is their nephrotoxicity. This may be due to self-medication, which is a common practice because patients do not bother to consult an Ayurvedic physician for proper prescription and, unlike modern medicine, no proper treatment regimen is followed. Another problem relates to drug standardization. The sporadic incidence of environmental contamination may ultimately find its way into plant parts. Due to the use of improper apparatus, contamination may also occur. With the implementation of good manufacturing practices (GMP) in Ayurvedic pharmaceutical industry, these problems will be overcome.

There is also a need to have preclinical and clinical investigations on some selected *bhasmas*. World Health Organization guidelines clearly direct that it is not necessary to carry out detailed toxicological evaluation of the herbs or their compounds originating from traditional systems of medicine. Length of continuity of use is to be taken as testimony of safety.

Acknowledgments

The author wishes to acknowledge contribution of his student, Mehboob Ali, who was immensely helpful in collecting Ayurvedic literature from the library of the Central Council for Research in Ayurveda and Siddha (CCRAS), New Delhi, and other libraries in Delhi.

References

1. Kean, W.F., Hart, L., and Buchanan, W.W., Auranofin, *Brit. J. Rheumatol.*, 82, 560, 1997.
2. Sharma, D.C., India raises standards for traditional drugs, *Lancet*, 356, 231, 2000.
3. Rao, S.K.R., *Encyclopedia of Indian Medicine: Historical Perspective*, Popular Prakashan, Bombay, India, 1985.
4. Zysk, K.G., Traditional Ayurveda, http//:www.hindu.dk.
5. Chopra, A. and Doiphode, V.V., Ayurvedic medicine: core concept, therapeutic principles, and relevance, *Med. Clin. North Am.*, 86, 75, 2002.
6. Frawley, D. and Lad, V., *The Yoga of Herbs*, Motilal Banarsidass Publishers Pvt. Ltd., Delhi, India, 1994.
7. Mahanti, S., History of Science: From Alchemy to Chemistry, Part II, www.vigyanprasar.com.
8. Sharma, P.V., *Dalhana and His Comments on Drugs*, Munshiram Manoharlal Publisher Pvt. Ltd., New Delhi, India, 1982, chap. 1.
9. Dash, B., *Fundamentals of Ayurvedic Medicine*, Bansal & Co., Delhi, India, 1980.
10. Sengupta, K.N., *The Ayurvedic System of Medicine*, 1906 reprint, Logos Press, New Delhi, India, 1984.
11. Pandey, R.S. and Tamrakar, B.P., *Pharmaceutics of Metals in Ayurveda*, Publication Scheme, Jaipur, India, 1988, chap. 1.
12. Said, M., *Hamdard Pharmacopoeia of Eastern Medicine*, Hamdard Foundation, Karachi, India, 1969.
13. Central Council for Research in Ayurveda and Siddha, *Application of Standardised Namburi Phased Spot Test in Identification of Bhasma and Sindura Preparations of Ayurveda*, New Delhi, India, 1991.
14. Raghunathan, K., *Pharmacopoeial Standards for Ayurvedic Formulations*, Central Council for Research in Indian Medicine Homeopathy (CCRIMH), Publ. 15, New Delhi, India, 1976.
15. Mitra, A., Chakraborty, S., Auddy, B., Tripathi, P., Sen, S., Saha, A.V., and Mukherjee, B., Evaluation of chemical constituents and free radical scavenging activity of Swarna bhasma (gold ash), an Ayurvedic drug, *J. Ethnopharmacol.*, 80, 147, 2002.
16. Chopra, R.N., Chopra, I.C., Handa, K.L., and Kapur, L.D., *Chopra's Indigenous Drugs of India*, 2nd ed., Academic Publishers, Calccutta, India, 1982.
17. Bajaj, S. and Vohora, S.B., Analgesic activity of gold preparations used in Ayurveda and Unani-Tibb, *Indian J. Med. Res.*, 108, 104, 1998.
18. Bajaj, S., Ahmad, I., Fatima, M., Raisuddin, S., and Vohora, S.B., Immunomodulatory activity of a Unani gold preparations used in Indian system of medicine, *Immunopharmacol. Immunotoxicol.*, 21, 151, 1999.
19. Bajaj, S., Ahmad, I., Raisuddin, S., and Vohora, S.B., Augmentation of non-specific immunity in mice by gold preparations used in traditional systems of medicine, *Indian J. Med. Res.*, 113, 192, 2001.
20. Shah, Z.A. and Vohora, S.B., Antioxidant/restorative effects calcined gold preparations used in Indian systems of medicine against global and focal models of ischaemia, *Pharmacol. Toxicol.*, 90, 254, 2002.
21. Sharma, D.C., Jha, J., Sharma, P., and Gaur, B.L., Evaluation of safety and efficacy of a gold containing Ayurvedic drug, *Indian J. Exp. Biol.*, 39, 892, 2001.
22. Pandit, S., Biswas, T.K., Debnath, P.K., Saha, A.V., Chowdhury, U., Shaw, B.P., Sen, S., and Mukherjee, B., Chemical and pharmacological evaluation of different Ayurvedic preparations of iron, *J. Ethnopharmacol.*, 65, 149, 1999.
23. Tripathi, Y.B. and Singh, V.P., Role of tamra bhasma an Ayurvedic preparation, in the management of lipid peroxidation in liver of albino rats, *Indian J. Exp. Biol.*, 34, 66, 1996.
24. Patil, S., Kanase, A., and Varute, A.T., Effect of hepatoprotective Ayurvedic drugs on lipase following CCl_4 induced hepatic injury in rats, *Indian J. Exp. Biol.*, 27, 955, 1989.

25. Patil, S., Kanase, A., and Varute, A.T., Effect of hepatoprotective Ayurvedic drugs on lipolytic activities during CCl_4–induced acute hepatic injury in albino rats, *Indian J. Exp. Biol.*, 31, 265, 1993.
26. Kanase, R., Patil, S., and Kanase, A., Effect of hepatoprotective Ayurvedic drugs on lisosomal enzymes during hepatic injury induced by single dose of CCl_4, *Indian J. Exp. Biol.*, 32, 328, 1994.
27. Buwa, S., Patil, S., Kulkarni, P.H., and Kanase, A., Hepatoprotective action of abhrak bhasma, an Ayurvedic drug in albino rats against hepatitis induced by CCl_4, *Indian J. Exp. Biol.*, 39, 1022, 2001.
28. Kanase, A., Patil, S., and Thorat, B., Curative effect of mandur bhasma on liver and kidney of albino rats after induction of acute hepatitis by CCl_4, *Indian J. Exp. Biol.*, 35, 754, 1997.
29. Chauhan, O., Godhwani, J.L., Khanna, N.K., and Pendse, V.K., Antiinflammatory activity of muktashukti bhasma, *Indian J. Exp. Biol.*, 36, 985, 1998.
30. Nadar, T.S. and Pillai, M.M., Effect of Ayurvedic medicines on β-glucuronidase activity of Brunner's glands during recovery from cysteamine induced duodenal ulcers in rats, *Indian J. Exp. Biol.*, 27, 959, 1989.
31. Puri, R.N., Thakur, V., and Nema, H.V., Role of zinc (yashad bhasma) in arrest of myopia, *Indian J. Ophthalmol.*, 31 (Suppl.) 816, 1983.
32. Jani, J.P., Raiyani, C.V., Mistry, J.S., and Kashyap, S.K., Polycyclic aromatic hydrocarbons in traditional medicinal preparations, *Human Exp. Toxicol.*, 10, 347, 1991.

7

Diabetes Mellitus (Madhumeha)

Lakshmi Chandra Mishra and Tarek Adra

CONTENTS

0-8493-1366-X/04/$0.00+$1.50

7.1 Introduction

Diabetes mellitus (DM) is described in Ayurveda as *madhumeha kshaudrameha*, which literally means "excessive urine with sweet taste like honey," or *dhatupak janya vikriti*, which means a disease caused by a defective metabolism leading to derangement in body tissue (seven *dhatus*) transformation process. Historically, Ayurvedic texts have described 20 types of urinary disorders (*pramehas*) based on the predominant dosas (10 *kaphaja*, 6 *pittaja*, and 4 *vataja* urinary disorders) and physical characteristics of the urine (e.g., volume, color, odor, taste, sediments, solid particles, presence of seminal fluid, and mucus). The urine is discharged in excessive quantities and is generally turbid. DM is one of these *pramehas* that may occur in any of the three (*vata, kapha,* or *pitta*) body constitutions.

DM is a very common health problem; almost 3% of the world population or 100 million people suffer from it.[1] It is the fourth most common cause for patient visits to a physician in the U.S. It accounts for nearly 15% of health-care costs in the U.S. DM may result in premature disability, mortality, blindness, end-stage renal disease (ESRD), and nontraumatic limb amputations. DM is also known to increase the risk of heart, cerebral, and vascular diseases by two- to sevenfold. Many of the complications of DM are preventable or can be delayed by appropriate treatment of hyperglycemia and other cardiovascular risk factors.[2] Synthetic drugs like sulphonyl ureas and biguanides may be effective in controlling the blood sugar level for some time, but they may cause side effects like hypoglycemia, nausea, vomiting, cholestatic jaundice, and other health problems. Most type 2 DM patients initially respond to lowering of blood glucose levels (BGLs), but after some time about 20% become resistant and do not benefit from these agents. Patients may also not respond fully to these agents due to the loss of interest in regular diet and exercise, the progression of beta cell failure, drug resistance, and other medical problems.[2] Many patients eventually require insulin treatment.[3]

The Ayurvedic approach to DM management includes life-style dietary interventions, exercise, and a variety of hypoglycemic herbs and herbal formulas depending upon the predominant *dosa*. Cleansing procedures are unique to the Ayurvedic approach to DM. However, the Ayurvedic clinical description of DM, etiology, diagnosis, prognosis, and recommended lifestyle changes are basically similar to those described in Western medicine.

The aim of this chapter is to explore the scientific basis for the Ayurvedic management of DM with single herbs, herbal formulas, and dietary interventions, in addition to understanding the Ayurvedic concept of DM and exploring the underlying science. Available pharmacological, biochemical, and chemical studies on herbs are used to understand the scientific basis of Ayurvedic therapies of DM.

7.2 Clinical Description (*Rog Viakhya*) and Etiology (*Vyadhi Haitu*)

The major signs and symptoms of DM described in classic Ayurvedic texts consist of honeylike sweetness of urine, thirst, polyphagia, lassitude, tiredness, obesity, dysgeusia, constipation, burning sensation in the skin, seizures, insomnia, and numbness of the body. Boils, wounds, and abscesses are often difficult to heal in a diabetic patient and are recognized in Ayurveda. All these symptoms are very similar to those currently described in Western medicine. Ayurvedic physicians also use modern diagnostic chemical analysis of urine and blood for confirmation.

The etiology of DM in Ayurveda is multifactorial. DM may be a familial trait, and overweight (fat — *meda*) patients with this diagnosis may be engaged in a lethargic lifestyle and unhealthy diet (e.g., idle sitting, excessive sleep, overeating sweet and fatty food items, and lack of physical exercise). All these factors are understandable because they all can lead to type 2 DM.[1] Ayurveda divides DM in to two categories: (1) genetic (*sahaja*), occurring in young age from the very beginning of life that has some similarities with the juvenile diabetes or insulin-dependent diabetes; and (2) acquired (*apathyaja*) due to an unhealthy lifestyle that occurs in old age and obese people and has similarities with type 2 DM. In addition, Charak Samhita (100 to 400 A.D.) describes two types of DM: one that occurs in very underweight people (*krsa prameha*) and one that occurs in obese people (*sthula*). The former DM requires restorative (*santarpan*) treatment along the line of insulin treatment and the latter requires fat-reducing (*apatarparna*) treatment. [4]

Type 1 DM is associated with the absence of insulin-secreting capacity of the patient, and this problem accounts for less than 10% of DM patients in the U.S. Type 2 DM patients have some degree of insulin-secreting capacity and account for more than 90% of DM patients in the U.S. Miscellaneous types of DM are very small in number and have various etiological factors (e.g., genetic defect of beta cells, defects in insulin action, diseases of pancreas, endocrinopathies [Cushing's syndrome, hyperthyroidism, and others], and drugs and chemicals [glucocorticosteroids and others]). Other etiological factors are infections (congenital rubella, cytomegalovirus), immune-mediated DM, other genetic syndromes (Down, Klinnefelters, and others), and gestational disorders. Because all types of diabetes may require insulin treatment at some point, the terms "insulin-dependent" and "insulin-nondependent" DM are no longer used.[2]

Recent studies have shown that there is a genetic component in the etiology of type 1 DM. In fact, Kyvik et al.[5] have shown that the cumulative concordance among twins (both twins affected) from birth to age 25 is 70%, which indicates that genetic factors cannot account for 100% of the incidence, but that environmental, immunity, and other factors are contributory. Several genes (HLA-DR3 or HLA-DR4) have been found in 95% of Caucasians with type 1 DM, whereas these genes are found in only 45% of the general DM population.[6] Autoimmunity is suggested to be an important contributory factor because a lymphocyte-rich infiltrate, an indicator of immunological response, was found in pancreatic islets.[7] In addition, 70 to 80% of the patients are found to have islet cell autoantibodies against intracellular islet cell antigens such as glutamic acid decarboxylase islet auto-antigen 2, insulin, and gangliosides.[8] Support for the role of environmental factors came from observations that Finnish children had 60- to 70-fold greater risk of type 1 DM than did Korean children. The incidence of DM in children under 15 in the northeastern U.S. has tripled since the late 1960s, indicating the involvement of environmental factors.[1] Epidemiological studies have shown an association between Coxsackie viruses of group B and pancreatic diseases, including DM, that indicates the possibility of a contributory role of viruses in the etiology of DM.[9] Chemicals such as streptozotocin, alloxan, and pentamidine have also been shown to produce DM by destroying the insulin-producing islet cells.[1]

Type 2 DM has even greater involvement of genetic factors than type 1 DM, but no specific gene has been linked to DM to account for the role. There is no evidence available to show the role of autoimmunity in type 2 DM. The two major problems in type 2 DM are the reduced secretion of insulin from beta cells and development of resistance to insulin in peripheral tissues. Obesity is another major etiological factor, for 80% of type 2 DM patients are obese.[1]

7.3 Pathogenesis (*Samprapti*)

According to classic Ayurvedic texts, DM and all *pramehas* (urinary disorders) start with the derangement of *kapha* that spreads throughout the body and mixes with fat (*meda*) that is similar in physical properties to *kapha* (mucus). *Kapha* mixed with fat passes into the urinary system, thereby interfering with normal urine excertion. Vitiated *pitta, vata,* and other body fluids (*malas*) may also be involved in this blockade. This blockade is believed to be the cause of frequent urination observed in DM. *Pramehas* left untreated may lead to deranged development of the bone marrow, body tissues, nutritional materials (fat, proteins, and carbohydrates), and hormones (*ojas*). The incurable stage of *pramehas* is *madhumeha,* which is insulin-dependent DM. *Madhumeha* may not be described precisely in Ayurveda, but it points in the direction of the current knowledge we have about the disease with respect to neurological damage and insulin (*ojas*) malfunctioning at the production (degeneration of islets of Langerhans in the pancreas) or at the utilization levels. The involvement of tissues (*dushyas*) leading to blood vessels, kidney, eye, and nerve damage is also described in Ayurveda as major complications. DM is described not only as a condition of *madhumeha* (sugar loss in urine), but also as a condition of *ojameha* (immunity and hormone loss) in Ayurveda for the purpose of treatment.

DM is primarily a dysfunction of insulin, a hormone produced by beta cells in the pancreas. Insulin is necessary for cellular uptake of glucose, glycogen formation in the liver and skeletal muscles, conversion of glucose into triglycerides, as well as nucleic acid and protein synthesis. The BGLs are maintained by three factors: (1) the production of glucose by the liver, (2) the uptake and utilization of glucose by the peripheral tissues, and (3) the production and release of insulin by the pancreas. The blood insulin levels are maintained by glucose, which stimulates the synthesis of insulin, and calcium-dependent secretion of insulin by other agents (e.g., amino acids and gastrointestinal hormones). The key feature of DM is impaired glucose tolerance. In a normal person, the BGL returns to normal within an hour after a glucose challenge dose, whereas the level remains high in a diabetic or prediabetic person for many hours.[1]

7.4 Clinical Course and Prognosis (*Sadhyata*)

According to classical Ayurveda, all *pramehas* have the potential to become incurable (*madhumeha*) if left untreated. The *kaphaja* urinary disorders (*pramehas*) are curable because the causative *dosa* and the affected tissues (*dushya*) have the same properties, thus requiring the same type of therapy. Although the *pittaja* urinary disorders are controllable (palliative), the resulting disorder may persist for life because the causative *dosa* is *pitta,* but the tissues and waste products (*dushya*) are different, requiring a different type of therapy. *Vataja* urinary disorders are considered incurable because tissues (*dhatus*) and hormones (*ojas*) undergo deterioration.

Recent studies have observed a relationship between the body constitution and relative amounts of hyperglycemia and insulinemia consistent with the Ayurvedic prognosis.[10–12] *Kapha* constitution patients showed the highest level of insulinemia and the lowest levels of FBS and PPBS. *Vata* patients showed the lowest level of insulinemia and the highest levels of FBS and PPBS. *Pitta* patients were in the middle. Further studies are necessary to confirm these findings.

In Ayurveda the major complications of *kaphaja* urinary disorders are believed to be poor digestion, anorexia, vomiting, drowsiness, coughing, and nasal catarrh. *Pittaja* urinary disorder patients tend to exhibit a pricking pain in the urinary bladder, penis, and scrotum, as well as fever, burning sensations, thirst, sourness of the throat, fainting, and loose bowel movements. *Vata* urinary disorders (diabetes) patients often experience tremors, pain in the cardiac region, abdominal tenderness, insomnia, and dryness of the mouth. The major complications of *vata* DM most commonly include ulcers (eruptions) over joints, muscles, skin, blood vessels, as well as damage to the kidney and the retina.

7.5 Clinical Examination and Diagnosis (*Rog Pariksha* and *Nidan*)

Historically, Ayurveda diagnosis of DM was primarily based on the sweetness of urine that was identified by a swarm of flies and ants over the urine. Ayurvedic physicians currently use urine, blood sugar, and glycohemoglobin (Hb A_{1c}) levels to confirm the diagnosis. The eight-point diagnosis discussed in Chapter 2 is applied to identify the predominant *dosa*. Ancient Ayurvedic texts give the following signs and symptoms of *kaphaja*, *pittaja*, and *vataja pramehas* for diagnosis. Recently, however, Ayurvedic doctors' diagnostic tools evolved to more modern clinical and laboratory methods consistent with those of Western medicine:

1. *Kaphaja pramehas*
   a. *Udaka meha* — The urine is clear; is in large amounts; is white, cold, and odorless; resembles water, sometimes with slight turbidity, and slimy.
   b. *Iksu meha* — The urine is like sugarcane juice and is very sweet.
   c. *Sandra meha* — The urine becomes thick when kept overnight.
   d. *Sura meha* — The urine resembles beer (*sura*) with a clear top and a cloudy bottom portion.
   e. *Pista meha* — The urine is white and thick, similar to a solution of corn flour.
   f. *Sukra meha* — The urine is like semen or mixed with semen.
   g. *Sita meha* — The urine is sweet and very cold.
   h. *Sikata meha* — The urine contains sandlike particles.
   i. *Sanair meha* — The urine is passed very slowly.
   j. *Laala meha* — The urine is slimy and contains threads like that of saliva.
2. *Pittaja pramehas*
   a. *Ksara meha* — The urine is like a solution of alkali in smell, color, and taste.
   b. *Kala meha* — The urine is black.
   c. *Nila meha* — The urine is bluish.
   d. *Haridra meha* — The urine is yellowish, similar to tumeric.
   e. *Manjistha meha* — The urine is foul smelling resembling *manjistha* (*Rubia cordifolia*), a slightly red solution.
   f. *Rakta meha* — The urine is foul smelling, slightly salty, and blood red.
3. *Vataja pramehas*
   a. *Majja meha* — The urine looks like marrow or marrow mixed.

TABLE 7.1

Decoctions to Treat *Kaphaja Pramehas*

Medicinal Plant	Botanical Name	Medicinal Plant	Botanical Name
Decoction #1		Decoction #2	
Katphala	*Myrica esculenta*	*Patha*	*Stephania japonica* Miers
Musta	*Cyperus rotundus*	*Vidanga*	*Embelia ribes*
Lodhra	*Symplocos cocchinchinensis*	*Arjuna*	*Terminalia arjuna*
Haritaki	*Terminalia chebula*		
Decoction #3		Decoction #4	
Haridra	*Curcuma longa*	*Kadamba*	*Anthocephalus chinensis*
Daru haridra	*Berbers aristata*	*Sala*	*Shorea robusta* Geartn.
Tagarai	*Cassia tora* Linn.	*Arjuna*	*Terminalia arjuna*
Vidanga	*Embelia ribes*	*Yavani*	*Carium copticum* Benth Hook
Decoction #5		*Decoction #6*	
Daruharidra	*Berbers aristata*	*Devdaru*	*Polyalthia longifolia*
Vidanga	*Embelia ribes*	*Kushta*	*Saussurea*
Khadira	*Acacia catechu* willd	*Aguru*	*Aqullaria agallocha* roxb.
Dhava	*Anogeissus latifolia*	*Candana*	*Santalum album* Linn.
Candana	*Santalum album* Linn.		
Decoction #7		Decoction #8	
Daruharidra	*Berbers aristata*	*Patha*	*Stephania japonica* Miers
Agnimantha	*Clerodendrum multiflorum*	*Murva*	*Celosia cristata* Linn.
Triphala	*Terminalia chebula, terminalia bellerica,* and *Emblica officinalis* (mixture)	*Gokshura*	*Tribulus lanuginosus*
Patha	*Stephania japonica* Miers		
Decoction #9		Decoction #10	
Yavani	*Carium copticum* Benth	*Cavya*	*Piper chaba* Hunter
Usira	*Vativeria zizanoides* Linn.	*Haritaki*	*Terminalia chebula*
Haritaki	*Terminalia chebula*	*Chitraka*	*Plumbago zeylanica*
Guduci	*Tinospora cordifolia*	*Saptaparna*	*Alstonia scholaris*

b. *Ojas meha* — The urine looks like honey.

c. *Vasa meha* — The urine looks like liquid muscle fat and may be passed frequently.

d. *Hasti meha* — The urine is like that of an elephant in rut, being discharged continuously without force, mixed with lymph and without obstruction.

These urine characteristics may be found in a wide range of pathologies covering all kinds of urinary infections, obstructive uropathies, renal failures, and other health conditions. The *kaphaja iksu meha* and *vataja ojas meha* are the correlate of the modern understanding of DM.

The results of diagnosis are correlated with body constitutions in order to design an individualized therapy.

TABLE 7.2

Decoctions to Treat *Pittaja Pramehas*

Medicinal Plant	Botanical Name	Medicinal Plant	Botanical Name
Decoction #1		Decoction #6	
Usira	*Vativeria zizanoides* Linn.	*Nimba*	*Azadirachta indica* A.
Lodhra	*Symplocos cocchinchinensis*	*Arjuna*	*Terminalia arjuna*
Arjuna	*Terminalia arjuna*	*Guduchi*	*Tinospora cordifolia*
Candana	*Santalum album* Linn.	*Haridra*	*Curcuma longa*
		Utpala	*Nymphaea stellata*
Decoction #2		Decoction #7	
Usira	*Vetiveria zizanoides* Linn.	*Sirisha*	*Albizia lebbek*
Musta	*Cyperus rotundus*	*Sarja*	*Vateria indica* Linn.
Amalata	*Cayratia trifolia*	*Arjuna*	*Terminalia arjuna*
Abhaya	*Terminalia chebula retz*	*Nagakesar*	*Mammea suriga*
Decoction #3		Decoction #8	
Patala	*Cydonia oblonga*	*Priyangu*	*Aglaia elaeagnoidea*
Nimba	*Azadirachta indica* A.	*Kamala*	*Nelumbo nucifera*
Amalaka	*Embilca officinalis* Geartn.	*Utpala*	*Nymphaea stellata*
Gudici	*Tinospora cordifolia* Miers.	*Palasha* flower	*Butea monosperma*
Decoction #4		Decoction #9	
Musta	*Cyperus rotundus*	*Asvattha*	*Ficus religiosa*
Haaritaki	*Terminalia chebula*	*Patha*	*Stephania japonica* Miers
Padmaka	*Prunus cerasoides* D.	*Asana*	*Pterocarpus marsupium*
Kutaja	*Holarrhena antidysenterica* wall.	*Vetasa*	*Salix caprea* Linn.
Decoction #5		Decoction #10	
Lodhra	*Symplocos cocchinchinensis*	*Daruharidra*	*Berbers aristata*
Hribera	*Coleus vettiveroides* Jacob	*Utpala*	*Nymphaea stellata*
Kaliyaka	*Coscinium fenestratum*	*Muskaka*	*Schrebera swietenioides*
Dhataki	*Woodfordia floribunda* Salish		

Note: The decoctions are useful in all types of pramehas. They can be used as impregnated on barley, food, or drinks.

7.6 Therapy (*Chikitsa*)

The principles of Ayurvedic therapy as discussed in Chapter 2 are also applied to treat DM patients. Traditional daily management of DM is carried out with appropriate palliative herbal therapies. These herbs are selected based on their properties, such as *rasa* (taste), *guna* (physicochemical properties), *veerya* (potency), *vipaka* (postdigestive effect), and *prabhava* (unique action), that are necessary to bring about balance in *dosas*. On the basis of this approach, Charak Samhita has prescribed the following palliative treatments specific for *dosa* constitutions: 10 water decoctions for *kapha*, 10 decoctions for *pitta*, and 1 ghee for *vata* in which 17 herbs are collectively cooked.[4,13] These herbs are listed in Tables 7.1 to 7.4.

It is important to note that vigorous exercise is contraindicated in lean and weak patients with severe diabetes. They are advised to perform yoga and breathing exercises (*pranyama*). In fact, certain yoga practices and breathing exercises are believed to stimulate better utilization and production of insulin by stimulating both the pancreas and muscles. Other lifestyle changes recommended are regular walking and reducing the consumption of fat-producing foods such as lard, butter, and oils. The use of bitter gourd, pungent- and astringent-tasting food, asparagus, spinach, turmeric, fenugreek seeds, black pepper, and ginger is encouraged in the diet. Current experience suggests that it is unnecessary to exclude the use of sucrose, provided it is consumed in balance with a normal diet[2] that is consistent with Ayurvedic recommendations. Honey and jaggery are believed to pacify *kapha* and *pitta*, respectively, and may be useful in respective DMs. Patients are also asked to stop smoking tobacco, eliminate alcohol consumption, and restrict sleeping time to about 8 h/day.

Individual herbs are generally not used in Ayurvedic therapies. Because therapies are based on a predominant *dosa* and body constitution, they always include formulas containing many herbs and sometimes various minerals. In Ayurveda, every disease has one or two predominant *dosas* that need to be balanced according to the constitution of the patient; therefore, one therapy may not be applicable to all patients even though the patients share the same disease. Some of the formulations commonly used to treat type 2 DM are listed in Table 7.5. These formulas may also be used concurrently with insulin for the treatment of DM type 1 patients in order to help in decreasing their reliance on this hormone.

Ayurveda recommends that the patient's lifestyle, age, type of work, psychosocial needs, and will power are considered in a management plan. The latter includes the necessary *panchkarmas*, herbal formulas, a healthy meal plan, and blood-sugar monitoring. A physician needs to evaluate the plan at each visit and make necessary modifications.

Ayurvedic physicians currently monitor conventional blood sugar levels in the management of DM. The goal is to keep the premeal glucose level within 80 to 110 mg/day, bedtime glucose level within 100 to 140 mg/day, the low density lipid cholesterol (bad) at <100 mg/day, and the high density lipid cholesterol (good) above 35 mg/dL.[2]

The preventive measures for DM are primarily the adoption of life style and food habits that reduce fat accumulation in the body, because 80% of type 2 DM patients are known to be obese. Regular use of *rasayanas* and hypoglycemic herbal formulas may be useful as a preventive measure, particularly for those who have a family history of type 2 diabetes.

7.7 Scientific Basis

Buanides and sulfonylureas, discovered in the 1920s and 1940s, respectively, are still the most frequently prescribed hypoglycemic agents, although Ciglitazone, Pioglitazone, alpha-glucosidase inhibitors, and others are available.[3] In an 8-year large multicenter clinical trial conducted by the University Group Diabetes Program (UDGP), patients treated with tolbutamide suffered a twofold increase in mortality as compared with insulin-treated patients.[14] The study has not been completely refuted and physicians continue to treat patients with oral hypoglycemic agents, including tolbutamide, because there are few choices available to patients other than insulin where they are resistant to dietary and lifestyle changes.[3] Ayurvedic therapies for DM are effective in controlling blood-sugar levels, either given alone or as an adjunct with other hypoglycemic drugs or insulin. Ayurveda offers alternative

TABLE 7.3

Group of Herbs To Treat *Vataja Pramehas*

Medicinal Plant	Botanical Name
Goksura	*Tribulus terrestris*
Asmantaka	*Mulaka parna (ARU) Ficus cordifolia* Roxb.
Somavalka	*Acacia suma* Kurz
Bhallataka	*Semecarpus anacardium*
Ativisa	*Aconitum heterophyllum*
Lodhra	*Symplocos cocchinchinensis*
Vaca	*Acorus calamus*
Patala	*Stereospermum suaveolens* DC
Arjuna	*Terminalia arjuna*
Nimba	*Azadirachta indica* A.
Musta	*Cyperus rotundus*
Haridra	*Curcuma longa*
Padmak	*Prunus cerasoides*
Yavani	*Carium copticum* Benth
Manjistha	*Rubia cordifolia* Linn.
Aguru	*Aquilaria agalloocha* Roxb.
Candana	*Santalum album* Linn.

Note: Herbs should be collectively cooked in oil for *kapha-vataj* or ghee for *pitta-vataja*.

TABLE 7.4

Herbs to Treat *Kapha-Vataja Pramehas*

Medicinal Plant	Botanical Name
Kampillaka	*Mallotus philippinensis*
Saptacchada	*Alstonia scholaris* R.
Sala	*Shorea robusta* Geratn
Bibhitika	*Terminalia bellirica*
Rohitka	*Aphanamixis polystachya*
Kutaja	*Holarrhena antidysenterica* Linn.
Kapittha	*Limona elephantum*

Note: Herbs can be taken as powder or paste in the dose of 10 g.

choices to control type 2 DM. Our literature search has revealed more than 52 herbs that have been shown to have hypoglycemic activity (Table 7.6). Some of these herbs have been frequently used in Ayurvedic formulas. Studies on six herbs and seven formulas are presented to demonstrate the scientific basis of the Ayurvedic therapies of DM.

7.7.1 *Gymnema sylvestere* R.Br. (Asclepiadacea)

Gymnema sylvestere (GS), a plant popularly known as *gurmara* (meaning sugar destroyer), is derived from a large woody climber that grows in the hills of Behar, Orissa Madhya Pradesh, and the Deccan Peninsula of India. It has been used in Ayurveda to treat DM for 2000 years. The whole plant, seeds, leaves, and roots are taken as a powder or as a decoction in combination with other herbs. The alcohol extract of GS (known as GS4) contains gymnemic acids (a chemically complex mixture of saponins and gurmarin, a polypeptide of 35 amino acids).[15]

TABLE 7.5

Ayurvedic Formulas

Formula	Dose (per day)	Ref.
Kaisora guggul	3 g	AF[a] Section 5:2
Dhanvantra ghrat	12 g	AF Section 6:22
Navayasa churn	1–3 g	AF Section 7:17
Nyagrodhadi churn	1–3 g	AF Section 7:21
Traikantaka ghrat	12 g	AF Section 6:15
Vastyamayantaka ghrat	12 g	AF Section 6:40
Shatavaryadi ghrit	12 g	AP[b] Part II
Agnitundi bati	125 mg twice	Bhasahya Ratnavali
Madhumehar yog	1 tablet twice	Ayurveda Sar Sangraha
Shilajatwadi bati	1 pill twice	Bhasajya Ratnavali
Ayush-82	5 g 3 times	104, 105
Abraga chenodooram	200 mg twice	108
D-400	2 tablets 3 times	109
MA 471	500 mg twice	106
Sandana Podia (*Siddha* formula)	300 mg twice	110
Kadal Azhinjil choornam (*Siddha* formula)	500 mg twice	111
M-93	1 g	112

[a]AF = *Ayurvedic Formulary of India* (Government of India publication).
[b]AP = *The Ayurvedic Pharmacopoeia of India* (Government of India publication).

TABLE 7.6

Scientific Studies on Hypoglycemic Herbs

Plant Name	Ref.	Plant Name	Ref.
Acacia arabica	113	*Momordica charantia*	See text
Achyranthes aspera	114	*Momordica cymbalaria*	162, 163
Aegle marmelos	115, 116	*Mucuna pruriens*	164, 150
Allium cepa	117–119	*Murraya koengii*	165
Allium sativum	120–125	*Musa sapientum*	166–168
Aloe vera	126–130	*Nelumbo nucifera*	169
Andrographis paniculata	131, 132	*Ocimum sanctum*	134, 170–172
Azadirachta indica	133–136	*Phaseolus mungo*	173, 174
Bombax ceiba	137	*Phyllanthus amarus*	175
Caesalpinia bonducella	138	*Phyllanthus urinaria*	176
Calendula officinalis	139	*Picrorrhiza kurroa*	177
Capparis decidua	140	*Polygonatum officinale*	178
Capsicum frutescens	141	*Psidium guajava*	179
Cassia fistula	142	*Pterocarpus marspium*	See text
Catharanthus roseus	134, 143	*Pterocarpus santalinus*	180
Coccina indica	See text	*Punica granatum*	181
Colocassia esculenta	144	*Swertia chirayita*	182–187
Cryptostegia grandiflora	145	*Syzygium alterniffolium*	188
Cyamopsis tetragonoloba	146, 147	*Tecoma stans*	189, 190
Eugenia jambolana	148–152	*Teramus labialis*	191
Ficus bengalonsis	See text	*Tinospora cordofilia*	150, 152 192, 193
Ficus carica	153, 154	*Tinospora crispa*	194–196
Gymnema sylvestre	See text	*Trigonella foenumgraecum*	See text
Hamiltonia suaveolens	155	*Vinca rosea*	197
Hibiscus rosa-sinensis	156–158	*Withania somnifera*	198
Inula racemosa	159		
Mangifera indica	160, 161		

7.7.1.1 Animal Studies

Hypoglycemic activity and mechanism of action of GS have been examined in many animal studies. The following data offer possible mechanisms by which GS might exert its hypoglycemic effect:

1. Increase in the secretion or release of insulin — GS has been shown to stimulate secretion or release of the insulin *in vivo* and *in vitro*.[16–21]
2. Protection of the pancreas from chemical toxins — GS has been shown to have partial protective effect on the pancreas against potent pancreatic toxins like beryllium.[22] It also has been suggested that GS may be promoting the regeneration of islet cells destroyed by streptozotocin in rats.[23,24] Al-DM rats treated with GS lived longer than the untreated diabetic rats, further supporting the regeneration hypothesis.[25]
3. Increased utilization of glucose — GS has been shown to increase the activities of enzymes responsible for the utilization of glucose by insulin-dependent pathways, an increase in phosphorylase activity, and a decrease in gluconeogenic enzymes and sorbitol dehydrogenase.[17]
4. Inhibition of glucose absorption from intestine — GS has been shown to inhibit the absorption of glucose from the intestine.[26]

7.7.1.2 Clinical Studies

Several clinical studies have been done to help authenticate the hypoglycemic effect of GS. These studies are evaluated based on the considerations outlined in Chapter 3.

Our literature search has found two case control studies and two smaller studies. Major drawbacks in these clinical trials are small sample size and inadequate study duration.

1. One group (n = 10) of 4 normal healthy females and 6 males (ages 19 to 25) (nondiabetic) and another group (n = 6) of 2 females and 4 males (ages 35 to 50) (type 2 DM) were studied for the antidiabetic effect of GS.[27] Diabetic patients were given an aqueous decoction of shade-dried GS leaves in a dose of 2 g 3 times/day for 15 days and healthy subjects were given the same dose for 10 days. The fasting blood sugar (FBS) (mg/day) was measured at 30 min postprandial blood sugar (PPBS) and at 2 h PPBS on day 1 before the treatment and on day 10 after daily treatments. Healthy subjects showed mean blood sugar levels of 80, 156, and 76 on day 1 and 69, 132, and 66 on day 10, respectively. Those in the diabetic group showed blood sugar levels of 135, 220, and 152 on day 1 and 110, 180, and 121 on day 10, respectively. Authors concluded that GS treatment demonstrated a blood sugar lowering effect in both normal and diabetic subjects.[27]
2. Eight type 2 DM patients were treated with 10 g of GS leaf powder orally daily for 21 days. The study showed significant reduction ($p < 0.05$) in blood sugar levels, mean fasting BGL, and mean 2-h BGL as compared with baseline.[28]
3. GS4, a water-soluble acid fraction of an alcoholic extract of GS, was supplemented in diet to a group of 22 diabetic type 2 patients.[24] These patients were given oral hypoglycemic therapy plus GS4 (400 mg/day) for 1 to 12 years (mean = 4.6 years). A second group of 25 type 2 DM patients was given only hypoglycemic therapy alone for 1 to 5 years (mean = 2.7 years). Group 1 showed significant improvement ($p < 0.001$) in blood sugar cholesterol and triglycerides levels, whereas group 2 showed fewer effects compared with group 1 ($p < 0.001$). Patients in group 1

developed symptoms of hypoglycemia and the dose of their hypoglycemic agents had to be changed or stopped. The authors suggested that GS supplementation showed an obvious advantage over conventional hypoglycemic therapy alone.[24]

4. Another study[23] done on GS4 reported a synergistic effect of this GS extract on BGLs in 23 type 1 diabetic patients (ages 10 to 31) who continued on insulin therapy plus GS4 as compared with 37 type 1 diabetic patients (ages 8 to 30) who were on insulin therapy alone. The dose of GS4 was 400 mg/day for 6 to 8 months. All patients in the combination therapy developed hypoglycemia and their insulin dose had to be reduced. Insulin doses, fasting glucose, hemoglobin A_{1c}, cholesterol, triglycerides, and free fatty acids were reported for the longest follow-up intervals. Although this study had many design problems, the data derived from it were somewhat encouraging. In fact, the authors concluded that GS4 improved blood glucose homeostasis and showed a better control of hyperlipidemia.[23]

7.7.2 *Momordica charantia* (Cucurbitaceae)

Momordica charantia (MC), a climbing vine, has been widely used in Ayurveda as an antidiabetic, abortificient (whole plant), antirheumatic, and carminative (fruits) agent. It is believed to cure deranged *kapha* and *pitta*.[29] The gourd produced by the plant, known as *karela* in India (bitter gourd), is traditionally eaten as a fried vegetable or as a fresh juice. Pharmacological and clinical studies demonstrating the hypoglycemic activity of MC are summarized here.

7.7.2.1 Animal Studies

The hypoglycemic activity, mechanism of action, and toxicity of MC have been extensively investigated in streptozotocin-induced or alloxan-induced DM (SZ-DM or AL-DM) rat models.[30–44]

Oral feeding of MC at 200 mg/kg/day for 40 days prevented renal hypertrophy as compared with SZ-DM in treated control rats, indicating that MC may have a protective effect against renal toxins.[45] Morevoer, an active hypoglycemic agent, polypeptide-p, with a minimum molecular weight of approximately 11,000 (166 residues), was isolated from fruits, seeds, and tissues of MC. The agent was very effective when administered subcutaneously to gerbils, langurs, and humans in reducing blood sugar levels.[31] MC extracts were also studied in relation to the course of the development of eye cataracts, one of the major side effects of DM. In fact, MC fruit extract given 4 g/kg/day for 20 days to AL-DM rats delayed the cataract formation by 2 months as compared with untreated diabetic rats. Blood sugar level in the diabetic control rats was 307 mg/day compared with 149 mg/day in the diabetic-treated rats. These findings suggest that the protective effect may be dependent upon the maintenance of lower BGLs.[46]

The mechanism of the antidiabetic action of MC has been studied extensively. Fractionation extraction studies using alkaline and acid wash of chloroform extract of MC have shown that the alkaline wash residue produced a hypoglycemic effect 1 h after administration in SZ-DM rats. This same effect was much slower to occur with the residue from the acid wash.[34] On the basis of these results, authors stated that MC may be acting partly via pancreatic and partly via extrapancreatic mechanisms.

7.7.2.1.1 *Increase in Secretion or Release of Insulin*

The increased secretion or release of insulin as a mechanism of the hypoglycemic activity is supported by several studies.[33,35,41] These studies indicate that MC increases (regenerates) or possibly facilitates the recovery of pancreatic beta cells and that viable beta cells in the pancreas that are capable of secreting insulin are still necessary for MC to exert its hypoglycemic effect. Other biochemical effects, such as the reduction in lipid peroxidation reported in SZ-DM rat pancreas and islet cells,[43] may be contributing to MCs hypoglycemic activity.

7.7.2.1.2 *Decreased Synthesis and Increased Utilization of Glucose*

Biochemical studies done on MC have shown that hepatic glucose-6-phosphatase and fructose-1,6-biphosphatase activities are increased and hepatic glucose-6-phosphate dehydrogenase activity is decreased by streptozotocin in SZ-DM rats.[36] MC treatment of SZ-DM rats depressed the phosphatase activities and enhanced the dehydrogenase activity, resulting in depressed synthesis and increased oxidation of glucose, respectively, leading to lowered blood sugar levels. In a comparative study with oral hypoglycemic drugs, MC treatment caused 10 to 15% reduction in BGL, whereas tolbutamide caused 40% reduction in BGL 1 h postadministration.[37] The effect of MC was not accompanied by increased insulin secretion. In SZ-DM rats, MC caused 26% reduction in BGL, whereas metformin, a biguinide, caused 40 to 50% reduction. MC increased the rate of glycogen synthesis in the liver by four- to fivefold as detected by the incorporation of ^{14}C-glucose into glycogen; this suggests that increased glucose utilization in the liver may be a more important mechanism of action of MC.

7.7.2.1.3 *Inhibition of Intestinal Glucose Absorption*

It has been suggested that the inhibition of glucose uptake from the intestine may be an important factor in lowering BGL by MC.[40] Two hypoglycemic chemical constituents were isolated from the plant: (1) the oleanolic acid 3-*O*-monodesmoside, momordin Ic, and (2) oleanolic acid 3-*O*-glucuronide. These chemicals showed a dose–response effect in inhibiting the increase in serum glucose levels in oral glucose-loaded rats, but showed no significant effect on serum glucose levels in normal rats, intraperitoneal glucose-loaded rats, or AL-DM mice. Both chemicals were also found to suppress gastric emptying time in rats, in addition to inhibiting glucose uptake in rat's small intestine in a dose-dependent manner *in vitro*. These results indicate that these chemicals have neither insulin-like activity nor insulin-releasing activity; they apparently inhibit glucose absorption by suppressing the transfer of glucose from the stomach to the small intestine and by inhibiting the glucose transport system at the small intestine brush border. Inhibition of gastric emptying is, at least in part, mediated by capsaicin-sensitive sensory nerves and the central nervous system.[42]

7.7.2.1.4 *Decrease in Insulin Resistance*

A decrease in insulin resistance is also a possible mechanism of action for MC. In fact, a significant increase in the muscle content of facilitative glucose transporter isoform 4 (GLUT4) protein content was found in the plasma membrane of KK-Ay mice, an animal model for type 2 diabetes, after 3 weeks of oral administration of MC. This increase in receptors induced by MC was postulated to be a contributing factor to the lowered insulin resistance in these mice.[39]

7.7.2.1.5 Biochemical Effects of MC

Daily MC fruit extract feeding over a period of 10 weeks was found to reverse the increase of malonedialdehyde, a plasma lipid peroxidation (LPO) product, and LPO in kidney, nonesterified cholesterol, triglycerides, phospholipids, and high density lipoprotein (HDL)-cholesterol in the blood of SZ-DM rats.[44] These biochemical effects may account for the hypolipidemic action of MC.

Other biochemical studies demonstrated the effect of MC on hepatic drug-metabolizing enzymes. One expample is the reversal of a 50 to 100% increase in hepatic anilin hydroxylase (AH) and ethoxyresorufin-*O*-deethylase (EROD) activities in SZ-DM rats after MC feeding. In addition, a decrease (17 to 20%) in aminopyrene *N*-demethylase (ADP) activity and cytosolic glutathionone concentration in SZ-DM rats was brought to normal, and ethoxy-coumarin-*O*-deethylase (ECOD) was even further decreased to 60% of control values by MC. This latter finding was not shown to consistently reverse the effects on drug-metabolizing enzymes in SZ-DM rats. This finding is probably due to the changes in hepatic phase 1 and phase 2 drug-metabolizing enzyme levels in SZ-DM animals and may be associated with the altered gene expression of different citochrome P450 (CYP) and glutathione transferase isozymes.[38] Another theory suggested that the altered metabolism of endogenous substrates and hormonal status in DM may be responsible for changes in the metabolism and oxidative stress in various tissues.[47]

7.7.2.2 Clinical Studies

An insulin-like compound isolated from MC was delivered by injection to 8 male and 1 female patients (ages 16 to 52) and to 5 healthy normal control subjects of the same age range for a period of 3 months to 5 years. The compound produced a consistent hypoglycemic effect in a small number of both type 1 and type 2 patients.[48] In another study, 50 mg/kg of MC powder was administerd twice a day for 7 days to 8 type 2 DM patients (ages 38 to 50). A significant ($p < 0.001$) hypoglycemic effect was also noted in these patients.[49]

Another MC investigation was performed on 9 type 2 DM patients who were allowed to continue on oral hypoglycemic drugs, but were asked to stop the drug 48 h before the glucose tolerance tests. The results showed that the water extract of MC caused a significant reduction in BGLs during the 50-g oral glucose tolerance tests when compared with controls. Insulin levels were statistically higher with MC juice, but no effect on insulin was seen in patients eating fried MC fruits with food.[30] A follow-up to this study by the same authors investigated MC juice and fried MC fruit in 9 type 2 diabetic patients. The patients were treated for 8 to 11 weeks. They took 50 ml of the juice or 230 g of the fried fruit, along their regular oral hypoglycemic agents, but were asked to stop their intake 48 h before the glucose tolerance tests. The authors reported that MC taken as a juice or as fried fruits showed significant hypoglycemic activity.[30]

The fruit juice of MC significantly improved the glucose tolerance of 73% of the patients under investigation in one study;[50] a decoction of MC fruit in 200 ml of boiling water, given 100 ml/day for 3 weeks, produced a significant decrease in hemoglobin A_{1c} from 8.37 to 6.95% in another study.[50] A dose of dry MC fruit powder, 5 g/day for 3 weeks, did not lower blood sugar significantly. Drinking the aqueous suspension of MC fruit pulp also led to a significant ($p < 0.001$) reduction of both FBS and PPBS levels in 86% of the cases studied out of a 100 moderate type 2 DM patients.[52] A significant hypoglycemic activity was observed in 7 type 2 DM patients treated with MC aqueous extract (100 g of the fruit boiled in 200 ml of water, dose of 100 ml) given orally daily for 3 weeks.[51]

As can be deduced from the above data, the results shown in clinical studies are consistent with those obtained from the preclinical studies. This evidence provides a relatively adequate scientific basis for the use of MC in Ayurvedic therapies of DM.

7.7.3 *Trigonella foenum-graecum* Linn. (Leguminose Family)

Trigonella foenum-graecum (TF), known as *methika* in Hindi and Sanskrit and *methi* in Tamil, is an erect aromatic herb, 30 to 50 cm tall.[53] It is widely cultivated in many parts of India. Its seeds are used in cooking as well as treating diabetes, whereas its leaves are eaten as a vegetable. The endosperm of the seed is rich in galactomannan (14 to 15%), young seeds contain carbohydrates and sugar, and mature seeds yield amino acids and fatty acids on hydrolysis. TF seeds also contain carotene, vitamins, and saponins.[53] It is used in Ayurveda as a diuretic, tonic, carminative, astringent, and emoliant. It is also used to treat diabetes, colic, dysentery, diarrhea, coughing, dropsy, rheumatism, rickets, and anemia and to subdue deranged *vata*.[53]

The antidiabetic activity of TF has been confirmed in both animal models[54–64] and type 2 DM patients.[65,66] The hypoglycemic effect of TF has been shown to reside in the defatted seed material. A clear decrease in hyperglycemia and glycosurea and a decreased hyperglycemic effect in an oral glucose tolerance test in TF-treated AL-DM dogs have been shown.[67] The effect was found in the fraction "a" of the defatted portion of the TF seed that contains testa and endosperm and is rich in fibers (79.6%). The fraction "b" that contains the cotyledons and axes and is rich in proteins (52.8%) did not show the effect.

It was also found that saponins isolated from TF seeds enhance food consumption and the motivation to eat and reduce plasma cholesterol levels in rats.[68] It was also postulated that the hypoglycemic activity of TF is not concentrated in any one TF consitituents based on the retention of this activity in all TF parts such as the seed powder, methanol extract, and the residue remaining after the methanol extraction.[58] Chemical analysis of the water extract of the methanol extractive-free residue of the seed powder showed that the major active constituent of the soluble dietary fiber is a galactomannan. Additional hypoglycemic compounds were also present in other fractions. Aqueous extracts of TF leaves given orally and intraperitoneally (i.p.) were also shown to produce a hypoglycemic effect in normoglycemic and AL-DM rats. The oral and i.p. LD_{50} values were shown to be 9 and 1.9 g, respectively, and the main organ affected following i.p. administration was the liver. No major target organ was affected following oral administration.[59]

Several mechanisms of action for TF's hypoglycemic action were proposed. It appears to take effect, at least in part, at the cellular level. In fact, TF antagonized the hyperglycemia caused by alloxan or cadmium in rats. Cadmium has been shown to cause hyperglycemia by increasing the release of epinephrine in intact rats and by decreasing the release of insulin in isolated perfused rat pancreas.[55] A higher level of antioxidants in animals on a TF-supplemented diet as compared with animals on a control diet lead to the assumption that TF seeds used as a supplement in the diet may normalize the disrupted free radical metabolism.[69] Another theory sprung from the fact that TF brought the high glucose-6-phasphatase and fructose 1,6- phosphatase activities in the kidney and liver back to normal levels in diabetic rats. These enzymes are involved in increased production of glucose and fructose.[70] TF powder supplementation also led to the normalization of creatinine kinase's activities in the diabetic rats and restored normoglycemia comparable with insulin and vanadate (an antidiabetic agent).[61] It was also shown that TF seed powder increased the glycolysis and decreased the gluconeogenesis activities back to normal levels in the liver and kidney in diabetic rats.[62]

7.7.3.1 Clinical Studies

Investigation on the hypoglycemic effect of whole TF seeds, extracted TF seed powder, gum isolate from TF seed, cooked TF seed, and cooked TF leaves led to several findings. Gum isolate significantly ($p < 0.05$) reduced BGL and increased insulin levels at 30- and 60-min intervals after administration. The dose was not given. The author repeated the study in 5 diabetic patients given a daily dose of 25 g of defatted TF seeds for 21 days with meals. At the end of the study, the glucose tolerance test showed significant hypoglycemic activity. The dose, number of patients, patients' ages and genders, and diagnostic criteria were not mentioned. The author did conclude that TF was effective following acute as well as chronic administration, its effect was not destroyed by cooking, and it would be a good supplement to a diabetic diet.[71]

A significant hypoglycemic effect of TF was also reported in 10 type 1 diabetic patients in a randomized trial. TF diet significantly ($p < 0.05$) reduced FBS and improved glucose tolerance tests. It also produced 54% reduction in 24-h urinary glucose excretion, a significant reduction ($p < 0.05$) in total cholesterol, and very low density cholesterol and triglycerides.[72]

A crossover randomized trial[66] with a diet enriched with TF seeds was performed on two groups. The first group of 15 type 2 DM patients (ages 32 to 60; 33% females) was randomized and given a TF-enriched diet during the first 10 days or during the second 10 days. The second group of 5 type 2 DM patients (ages 35 to 58) was randomized and given a TF-enriched diet either the first 20 days or the second 20 days of the trial. The authors of this study reported significant hypoglycemic activity ($p < 0.05$) in both groups. However, the participant's gender, demographic data, and data on the use of other hypoglycemic agents were not mentioned.

Another randomized trial[73] was performed on 10 type 2 DM patients (ages 38 to 54) in which 2 groups (5 patients/group) were crossover between placebo and the TF-enriched diet group. Patients were given 25 g of TF seeds incorporated in bread for 15 days. Authors of this study reported significant ($p < 0.05$) hypoglycemic activity of TF and suggested that the use of seeds in the treatment of DM merits further investigation.

A case control study[74] investigated the hypoglycemic effect of TF in 60 type 2 diabetic patients. Patients were kept on a restricted carbohydrate diet and given TF seeds 12.5 g twice a day for 24 weeks. A significant reduction in glycosylated hemoglobin was noted. The authors concluded that TF should be further investigated in the management of DM.

TF (9 g/day in 3 doses for 90 days) in 15 type 2 diabetic patients was found to produce a significant ($p < 0.05$) hypoglycemic effect. It also produced a significant ($p < 0.05$) reduction in serum cholesterol and triglycerides.[75] It was also found to exert a hypoglycemic effect in 20 healthy male volunteers (ages 20 to 30).[65]

The animal studies supported by the clinical experience indicate that TF has a significant hypoglycemic activity and may prove useful in the management of DM. However, studies using various biochemical parameters and endpoints should be carried out to determine efficacy of TF as an adjunct to other hypoglycemic drugs.

7.7.4 *Coccinia indica* Wight (*C. grandis, C. cordifolia* Cogn)

Coccinia indica (CI), known as *Bimbi* or *Kundura* in India, is a climber with branched leaves. CI is found wild in hedges and waste places in different parts of India. Fresh juice from leaves, stem, and roots is used to treat diabetes, glycosuria, enlarged glands, and skin diseases. The leaves and stem are also used as an antispasmodic and expectorant agent in bronchitis.[76]

The hypoglycemic activity of CI has been reported in several animal studies.[77,78] In fact, the oral adminsitration of pectins isolated from CI produced a significant hypoglycemic effect in normal rats.[79] The ethanol extract in glucose-loaded normal rats showed similar results.[80] It was suggested that the hypoglycemic activity of CI is mediated through an insulin secretagogue effect or through an influence on enzymes involved in glucose metabolism.[81] Also, it has been shown that powdered leaf suspension of CI produced a significant hypoglycemic activity in AL-DM dogs but not in normal animals. In a glucose tolerance test, however, the suspension did reduce the blood sugar levels.[78,82] CI root extracts (water or ethanol) have also been shown to have hypoglycemic activity in healthy rabbits.[83–85]

In a clinical double-blind controlled trial,[86] a significant improvement ($p < 0.05$) in the glucose tolerance was seen in 10 of 16 type 2 patients who received CI leaf preparation. In another clinical study,[87] 500 mg/kg dried extract of CI given orally to 30 type 2 diabetic patients for 6 weeks restored the enzymes involved in glucose metabolism back to normal levels.

7.7.5 *Pterocarpus marsupium* (Papilionoidae)

Pterocarpus marsupium (PM), also known as *pitsara, bijasal, pitasal,* or red sandalwood in India, is a moderate to large deciduous tree up to 30 m in height. Cold, aqueous extract of the wood is used to treat diabetes. The paste of the leaves is used to treat abscesses and skin diseases, and the extract of the bark is used as an astringent for gum and is also useful in diarrhea.[88]

The hypoglycemic activity of PM has been reported in several studies.[64,89–94] In fact, an active constituent of PM, epicatechin, was reported to show the hypoglycemic effect in AL-DM rats if given within 24 h after the administration of alloxan; no effect was seen if given after 92 h.[90] This indicates that epicatechin protected the pancreas from the direct toxic effect of alloxan. Three phenolic constituents from PM were isolated and studied for their hypoglycemic activity: marsupin, ptersupin, and pterostilbene. This hypoglycemic effect in diabetic rats was comparable with that of 1,1-dimethylbiguinide.[92]

A significant decrease in BGL in normal rats ($p < 0.001$) 2 h after oral administration of 1 g/kg of aqueous extract of PM was evident in some studies. A significant decrease in BGL in AL-DM rats after the oral dose of PM extract for 21 days was also reported.[64]

In one study,[95] the antidiabetic effect of aqueous, ethanol, and hexane extracts of PM bark in normal and diabetic rats was investigated. The ethanol extract at 0.25 g/kg oral dose showed a more hypoglycemic activity than the aqueous and hexane extracts. The same dose of ethanol extract was also more effective than glibenclamide, an oral hypoglycemic agent.[94] The ethanol extract of PM also exhibited a hypoglycemic effect in healthy normal rats.[95]

These biological studies indicate that PM has substantial hypoglycemic activity and its activity is not concentrated in any one constituent. The studies also show that these active constituents are soluble in water, ethanol, and hexane.

7.7.5.1 Clinical Studies

The Indian Council of Medical Research (ICMR), Collaborating Centers, New Delhi,[93] evaluated the efficacy of PM in newly diagnosed type 2 DM patients. Of 97 patients, 93 completed the daily dose of 2, 3, or 4 g of PM extract treatment for 12 weeks. The fasting and postprandial BGLs in these patients fell significantly ($p < 0.001$) from the initial mean of 151 and 216 mg/day, respectively. No significant change was noted in the mean plasma lipid levels.

The above clinical studies coupled with the previously mentioned biological data provide adequate scientific support for the use of PM in Ayurvedic management of DM.

7.7.6 *Ficus bengalonsis* L. (Moraceae)

Ficus bengalonsis (FB), also known as *Vata, bor, bot,* or Banyan tree, is a large evergreen tree that sends down aerial roots for lateral growth. It is effective in deranged *kapha* and *pitta*. Infusion of the bark is used to treat diabetes. The white milky juice of the plant is helpful when applied on sores, ulcers, and cracked soles of the feet; it is also helpful for inflammation and rheumatism. FB leaves contain quercetin-3-galactoside, rutin, and beta-sitosterol, and its bark contains leucoanthocyanin and two flavonoids.[96]

FB has been shown to have hypoglycemic activity in several animal models. The results of a comparative study of an ethanolic extract of FB bark, a glucoside isolated from the bark, and tolbutamide in normal and AL-DM rabbits showed that the glucoside was more active than the crude extract and half as potent as tolbutamide.[97] Another study also reported that a dimethoxy derivative of leucocyandin 3-*O*-beta-D-galactosyl cellobioside isolated from the bark of FB decreased blood sugar levels very significantly on oral administration in both normal and moderately diabetic rats. It also increased the serum insulin significantly in the diabetic rats at a dose of 250 mg/kg for a 2-h period. In addition, the oral dose of 100 mg/kg of the active principle given to diabetic rats for 1 month produced a significant decrease in blood and urine sugar, certain lipid components in serum and tissues, and glucose-6-phosphatase activity in liver. It further caused a significant increase in body weight and the activities of hexokinase and human menopausal gonadotropin coenzyme A (HMGCoA) reductase in tissues as compared with diabetic control. The authors suggested that the mechanism of action of the principle may be related to its protective and inhibitory action against the insulin-degradative processes.[98]

The extracts of FB bark also showed hypoglycemic activity in SZ-DM rats. In fact, the oral dose caused an enhancement in serum insulin levels in normoglycemic and diabetic rats. Each of these extracts stimulated insulin secretion when incubated *in vitro* with isolated islets of Langerhans from normal as well as from diabetic animals. However, the insulin secretion by beta cells was more apparent in the presence of pelargonidin derivative than in the presence of another leucocyanidin derivative isolated from the bark.[99]

Another study[100] compared the antidiabetic effect of a dimethoxy derivative of perlargonidin 3-*O*-alpha-L rhamnoside isolated from FB bark with glibenclamide (2 mg/kg and 0.5 mg/kg/day for a single dose and chronic dose, respectively). In moderately diabetic rats, 250 mg/kg/day was used in the single-dose study and 100 mg/kg/day of the extract in the chronic-dose study. Fasting blood glucose decreased by 19% and improved glucose tolerance by 29% in the single-dose group. The corresponding effects of glibenclamide were 25 and 66%, respectively, over the control values. In the 1-month treatment group, the FBS levels decreased to almost half of the pretreatment levels in both groups; glucose tolerance improved by 41% in the glibenclamide group and by 15% in the glycoside-treated group. Glycosurea was also decreased in both groups and they appeared healthy.[100]

A glycoside of leucopelargonidin isolated from the bark of FB was compared with a minimal dose of glibenclamide. Significant hypoglycemic, hypolipidemic, and serum insulin-raising effects of the glycoside were demonstrated in moderately diabetic rats. The effect was similar to that of glibenclamide. The main difference was that the former significantly enhanced the fecal excretion of sterols and bile acids, whereas the latter had no such action even though both controlled high blood cholesterol.[101] A very similar isolate, dimethoxy ether of leucopelargonidin-3-*O*-alpha-L-rhamnoside, given orally at 100 mg/kg, produced significant hypoglycemic and serum insulin-raising effects in normal and moderately AL-DM dogs during a 2-h period. The mechanism of action of the glycoside compound seems to be similar to that of drugs that stimulate insulin secretion.

In a toxicity study,[102] a single oral dose (0.2 to 1.8 g/kg) was given to mice. In a different study, daily oral doses (100, 250, and 500 mg/kg) given to rats for a period of 1 month did not show notable toxic effects. The compound was not lethal even at the high dose of 1.8 g/kg in both species. A leucodelphinidin derivative isolated from the bark of FB also showed hypoglycemic activity at a dose of 250 mg/kg in normal and AL-DM rats. The effect was similar to that produced by glibenclamide (2 mg/kg) under the same conditions. However, the plant product was less effective after a glucose load than glibenclamide.[103]

7.8 Clinical Studies on Combination Formulas

7.8.1 Ayush-82

Ayush-82 is a mixture of four herbs: the seeds of *Mangifera indica, Syzygium cuminii,* and *Momordica charantia,* and the leaves of *Gymnema sylvestre.* One hundred type 2 DM patients (ages 40 to 70; 52% male) were given 5 g of Ayush-82 3 times a day for 6 weeks in conjunction with *Shuddha Shilajit.*[104] *Shuddha shilajit* is a mineral preparation of black bitumen purified by *triphala* water. (*Triphala* is a mixture of *Terminalia chebula, terminalia bellerica,* and *Emblica officinalis.*) *Shilajit* was given 500 mg twice a day for 2 weeks. Oral hypoglycemic drugs were withdrawn after 2 weeks of treatment with Ayush-82. All patients were advised to consume a a daily 1200-calorie diet. Although the average blood sugar, FBS, and PPBS levels reduced significantly ($p < 0.001$) in some patients, the control of diabetes was not good because 47% of the patients did not have their diabetes controlled by the end of the study. The study had no comparison arm and the duration of the study was too short.

The duration of treatment was extended to 24 weeks in another clinical trial on 350 type 2 DM patients, and all other parameters were kept the same as in the above study.[105] On the basis of a physician's rating scale, the authors reported that 61% of the patients had a good response, 12.9% had a fair response, and 25.9% had poor response. After the treatment, FBS and PPBS levels were found to be significantly reduced ($p < 0.001$).[105] It is important to note that this clinical trial had no control arm and was not clear about the time and method of withdrawal of the hypoglycemic agent. The results remain encouraging and do support the concept that Ayurvedic formulas, because of their slow duration of action, might yield better results if the treatment duration is extended.

7.8.2 MA-471

MA-471 is a mixture of the following herbs: *Enicostemaa littorale, Phyllanthus niruri, Eugenia jambolana, Melia azadirachta (indica), Terminalia arjuna, Aegle marmelos,* and shilajit. This mixture was found to produce a significant hypoglycemic activity and hypolipidemic activity even in patients resistant to an oral hypoglycemic agent. This activity was demonstrated while studying 69 type 2 DM patients, 6 of whom dropped out due to noncompliance and

3 of whom dropped out due to other illnesses. This study had three arms: (1) patients who never had a hypoglycemic drug and DM was out of control despite dietary intervention and exercise (n = 15), (2) patients who had DM under control through hypoglycemic agents (n = 30), and (3) DM patients who did not respond to maximal dose of oral hypoglycemic agents (n = 15). All patients ingested 500 mg tablets of MA-471 twice a day for an average of 9 months. Arm 3 patients continued to take both M-471 and an oral hypoglycemic agent. The authors observed a significant improvement in other clinical symptoms (e.g., polyurea, fatigue, constipation, moderate improvement in weakness, polydipsia, giddiness, muscle pain, palpitation, and anorexia). The authors deduced from the data that M-471 was beneficial in all groups and that it can be used in conjunction with oral hypoglycemic agents.[106] The results are encouraging and warrant further investigation.

7.8.3 *Abraga Chendooram*

Abraga chendooram (AC) is a mixture of abragum (purified black mica, 80 g), *vengaram* (dehydrated borax, 0.5 g), and *Saranaiver charu* (juice of root of *Trainthema decandra* Linn.); *Adathodaielai charu* (juice from the leaves of *Adhatoda zeylanica* Linn); and *Alam Vizhuthu Kudineer* (root of *Ficus benghalensis* Linn).

Sixty type 2 DM patients (ages 21 to 70) who failed dietary control intervention and showed no evidence of serious complications (e.g., ketoacidosis, nephropathy, neuropathy, or retinopathy) were given 200 mg of AC in capsules twice daily for 45 days while their caloric intake was restricted to 25 calories/kg of ideal body weight. The authors concluded that the study demonstrated hypoglycemic effect and warrants further investigations. The use of other hypoglycemic agents and the actual FBS levels were not shown in this trial.[107]

Another study also investigated AC in 130 type 2 DM patients (57% males). The patients were given 200 mg of the drug in gelatin capsules twice daily for 45 days. The caloric intake was restricted to 25 calories/kg body weight during the treatment. A significant reduction ($p < 0.005$) in FBS and PPBS levels was observed. The authors reported that 57.9% of all patients gave a good response that was defined as FBS and PPBS lower than normal accepted levels and absence of all clinical symptoms; the authors concluded that the treatment could reduce blood sugar levels was combined with dietary controls.[108] Major flaws in the design of this study included its short duration and the lack of defining the use of other hypoglycemic agents. Although these results are encouraging, a long-term study is still necessary to further substantiate the effect of AC.

7.8.4 D-400

D-400 is a mixture of *Eugenia jambolana, Pterocarpus marsupium, Ficus glomerulata, Gymnema sylvestre, Momordica charantia, Ocimum sanctum,* and *shilajit*. This mixture investigated D-400 in 38 diabetic patients (ages 35 to 76). The study had three arms: (1) patients who did not respond to oral hypoglycemic agents (n = 19), (2) patients who did not respond to diet and exercise therapy (n = 8), and (3) patients who were dependent on insulin therapy (n = 6). All patients in all arms were given 2 tablets (weight not known) of the drug 3 times a day for 6 months. The authors concluded that D-400 lowered the blood sugar and cholesterol levels in the groups that failed the oral hypoglycemic therapy and also in arm 2 but was less effective in arm 3 patients.[109] The relative proportion of each ingredient and method of preparation were not cited in the study. Results are encouraging and warrant further investigation.

7.8.5 *Sandan Podia*

Sandana is a mixture of six parts of *Tinospora cordifolia* sugar and one part of each of the following herbs: *Santalum album* (sandalwood) sawdust, *Andropogon citratus* (lemongrass) root, *Vitiveria zizanioides* (vetiver) root, *Syzygium aromaticum* (clove) flower bud, *Anacyclus pyrethrum* (pyrethrum) root, and purified *Shilajit*. The sugar is extracted from *tinospora* by suspending the crushed plant in water overnight, decanting and drying the extract in the sun, and resuspending the material in water overnight. The procedure is repeated three times and the extract is dried and ground into a fine powder. The fine powders are mixed thoroughly and put into 300-mg capsules, which were given to 20 type 2 DM patients (ages 20 to 70) twice a day for 45 days. The FBS and PPBS of the patients decreased significantly ($p < 0.01$) from 164.5 to 114.7 and 281.7 to 171.2 mg/day, respectively. Improvements were also observed in other clinical symptoms, such as polyurea, excessive appetite, weight gain, giddiness, polydipsia, indigestion, vomiting, and abdominal pain.[110] Results are encouraging and warrant a long-term study.

7.8.6 *Kadal Azhinjil Choornam* and *Triphala* Tablets

Kadal, a preparation containing roots and bark of *Salacia chinensis*, and *triphala* were given to 25 type 2 DM patients. *Kadal* was given at 500 mg twice a day and *triphala* was given at 2.5 g three times a day with water for 120 days.[111] Authors reported a hypoglycemic effect, but the results need to be confirmed.

7.8.7 M-93

M-93 is a mixture of four herbs: *Aegle marmelos* (*bilva*), *Azadirachta indica* (neem, *nimba*), *Ocimum sanctum* (*tulsai*), and *Piper longum* (*kalimircha*). Thirty type 2 DM patients (ages 41 to 60) were treated with M-93, 1 g daily for 3 months.[112] Patients with FBS >300 mg/day, chronic renal failure, diabetic neuropathy, and diabetic ketoacidosis were excluded from the study. The authors stated that M-93 showed a positive response after 30 days of therapy and no adverse effect was observed.[112] The results need to be confirmed.

7.9 Summary and Discussion

The review of literature indicates that the Ayurvedic concept of DM, including signs and symptoms, etiology, and strategy of management, is not far from the current knowledge. Herbs used in Ayurvedic therapies and the multi-herbal combination formulas have been found to have a hypoglycemic effect in animal models of DM. Scientific studies done on 52 herbs (Table 7.6) and 7 multiherbal formulas have demonstrated hypoglycemic activity. Considerable information was available about some of the herbs, namely, *gymnema, momordica, trigonella, coccinia, pterocarpus,* and *ficus*, whereas other herbs have not been studied as extensively. This makes Ayurveda a considerable choice as an antidiabetic therapy that is safe, effective, and economic. The mechanism of antidiabetic action of these herbs appears to be multifactorial: increased secretion or release of insulin, efficient use of insulin, increased sensitivity of peripheral tissue to insulin, protective or regenerative effect on pancreas, decreased synthesis, and increased breakdown of glucose. Because these herbs have been used for thousands of years to manage DM patients, biological and mechanistic studies confirming the hypoglycemic effect and clinical trials have not been conducted as rigorously as would have been done for a new synthetic chemical with no human experience.

7.9.1 Future Research Areas

7.9.1.1 Toxicity Studies

Although no serious adverse effects were reported in clinical trials and many of the herbs are traditionally used as vegetables in regular diet, providing some degree of confidence, the following toxicity studies should still be carried out at least on the most frequently used herbs:

1. Single-dose toxicity study to determine LD_{50} dose
2. Subchronic toxicity study (120 days daily dose) in healthy animals and DM animal models to determine the maximum tolerated dose and identify the target toxicity organ
3. Lifetime feeding studies in normal and diabetic animals to determine long-term beneficial effects (increase in survival time), possible protection of pancreas, or toxic effects

7.9.1.2 Biochemical and Pharmacological Studies

There is a need for more biochemical and pharmacological studies. These studies will help determine the optimum therapeutic dose and the major mechanism of the action of herbs, giving the chance to maximize the efficacy by combining different mechanisms of action at their optimum doses.

7.9.1.3 Clinical Studies

Clinical studies necessary to establish management of DM by Ayurvedic therapies are as follows:

1. Definitive clinical studies with a rigorous protocol design; an optimum dose based on toxicological data; Hb A_{1c}, a good marker of DM control; and FBS and PPBS levels
2. Possible relationship between the *dosa* predominance and response to Ayurvedic treatments to validate the Ayurvedic concept of prognosis
3. Potential of Ayurvedic therapies to reduce or eliminate the use of synthetic oral hypoglycemic agents
4. Possible resistance of DM patients to herbs or herbal formulas over a period of time similar to oral hypoglycemic drugs
5. Ayurvedic management and use of herbs in high-risk population of type 2 DM (family history of DM, lifestyle, and obesity) to determine if it can prevent or reduce the incidence of DM
6. Combination of yoga and Ayurvedic therapies to identify any synergistic effects

References

1. Crawford, J.M. and Cotran, R.S., The pancreas, in *Robins Pathological Basis of Disease*, Cotran, R.S., Kumar, V., and Collins, T., Eds., W.B. Saunders, New York, 1999, chap. 20.
2. Sherwin, R.S., Diabetes mellitus, in *Cecil Textbook of Medicine*, Goldman, L. and Bennett, J.C., Eds., W.B. Saunders, New York, 2000, chap. 242.
3. Davis, S.N. and Granner, D.K., Insulin, oral hypoglycemic agents, and the pharmacology of the endocrine pacreas, in *Goodman & Gillman's The Pharamcological Basis of Therapeutics*, Hardman, J.L., Limbird, L.E., Molinoff, P.B., Ruddon, R.W., and Gilman, A.G., Eds., McGraw-Hill, New York, 1995, chap. 60.
4. Sharma, P.V., *Caraka Samhita*, 4th ed., Chaukhambha Orientalia, Varanasi, India, 1998, p. 120.
5. Kyvik, K.O., Green, A., and Beck-Nielsen, H., Concordance rates of insulin dependent diabetes mellitus: a population based study of young Danish twins, *Br. Med. J.*, 312(7026), 913, 1996.
6. Bain, S.C. et al., Genetic factors associated with insulin-dependent diabetes, *Front. Horm. Res.*, 22, 23, 1997.
7. Grewal, I.S. and Flavell, R.A., New insight into insulin dependent diabetes mellitus from studies with transgenic mouse models, *Lab. Invest.*, 76, 3, 1997.
8. Zekzer, D. et al., GAD reactive CD4+Th 1 cells induce diabetes in NOD/SCJD mice, *J. Clin. Invest.*, 101, 68, 1998.
9. Verge, C.F. et al., Number of autoantibodies (against insulin, GAD or ICA512/IA) rather than particular antibody determines risk of type 1 diabetes, *J. Autoimmunol.*, 9, 379, 1996.
10. Bharti, M.S. and Singh, R.H., Constitutional study of patients of diabetes mellitus vis-à-vis Madhumeha, *Ancient Sci. Life*, 15(1), 35, 1995.
11. Chandola, H.M., Tripathi, S.N., and Udupa, K.N., Variations in the progression of maturity onset diabetes according to body constitution, *Ancient Sci. Life*, 13(3–4), 293, 1994.
12. Kar, C.A., Upadhyay, B.N., and Ojha, D., Prognosis of prameha on the basis of insulin level, *Ancient Sci. Life*, 16, 277, 1997.
13. Ashtang Hradayam, translated by Srikantha Murthy K.R., Krishnadas Academy, Varanasi 1, UP. India, 1998.
14. University group diabetes program: a story of the effects of hypoglycemic agents on vascular complications in patients with adult-onset diabetes. II. Motality results, *Diabetes*, 19, 789, 1970.
15. Bone, K., Gymnema sylvester, in *Clinical Applications of Ayurvedic and Chinese Herbs: Monographs for the Western Herbal Practitioner*, Bone, K., Ed., Phytotherapy Press, Warwick Queensland, Australia, 1996.
16. Shanmugasundaram, K.R., Panneerselvam, C., Samudram, P., et al., The insulinotropic activity of *Gymnema sylvestre*, R.Br. and Indian medical herb used in controlling diabetes mellitus, *Pharmcol. Res. Commun.*, 13(5), 475, 1981.
17. Shanmugasundaram, K.R., Panneerselvam, C., Samudram, P., et al., Enzyme changes and glucose utilization in diabetic rabbits: the effect of *Gymnema sylvestre*, R Br., *J. Ethnopharmacol.*, 7(2), 205, 1983.
18. Shanmugasundaram, E.R., Venkatasubrahmanyam, M., Vijendran, N., et al., Effect of an isolate from *Gymnema sylvestre*, R.Br. in control of diabetes mellitus and the associated pathological changes, *Ancient Sci. Life*, 7(3–4), 183, 1988.
19. Shanmugasundaram, E.R., Gopinath, K.L., Radha Shanmugasundaram, K.R., et al., Possible regeneration of the islets of Langerhans in streptozocin-diabetic rats given *Gymnema sylvestre* leaf extracts, *J. Ethnopharmacol.*, 30, 265, 1990.
20. Sugihara, Y., Nojima, H., Matsuda, H., et al., Antihyperglycemic effects of gymnemic acid IV, a compound derived from *Gymnema sylvestre* leaves in streptozotocin-diabetic mice, *Nat. Prod. Res.*, 2(4), 321, 2000.
21. Persaud, S.J., Al-Majed, H., Raman, A., et al., *Gymnema sylvestre* stimulates insulin release in vitro by increased membrane permeability, *J. Endocrinol.*, 163(2), 207, 1999.

22. Prakash, A.O., Mathur, S., and Mathur, R., Effect of feeding Gymnema sylvestre leaves on blood glucose in beryllium nitrate treated rats, *J. Ethnopharmacol.*, 18, 143, 1986.
23. Shanmugasundaram, E.R., Rajeswari, G., Baskaran, K., et al., Use of *Gymnema sylvestre* leaf extract in the control of blood glucose in insulin-dependent diabetes mellitus, *J. Ethnopharmacol.*, 30(3), 281, 1990.
24. Baskaran, K., Kizar Ahamath, B.K., and Radha Shanmugasundaram, K.R., Antidiabetic effect of a lead extract from *Gymnema sylvestre* in non-insulin-dependent diabetes mellitus patients, *J. Ethnopharmacol.*, 30(3), 295, 1990.
25. Srivastava, Y., Venkatakrishna-Bhatt, H., Jhala, C.I., et al., Oral *Gymnema sylvestre* R.Br. leaf extracts inducing protracted longevity and hypoglycemia in alloxan induced rats: review and experimental study, *Int. J. Crude Drug Res.*, 24, 171, 1986.
26. Wang, L.F., Luo, H., Miyoshi, M., et al., Inhibitory effect of gymnemic acid on intestinal absorption of oleic acid in rats, *Can. J. Physiol. Pharmacol.*, 76(10–11), 1017, 1998.
27. Khare, A.K., Tondon, R.N., and Tewari, J.P., Hypoglycemic activity of an indigenous drug (*Gymnema sylvestre*, "Gurmar") in normal and diabetic persons, *Indian J. Physiol. Pharmacol.*, 27(3), 257, 1983.
28. Balasubramaniam, K., Arasaratnam, V., Seevaratnam, S., et al., Hypoglycemic effect if *Gymnema sylvestre* on diabetic patients, *Jaffna Med. J.*, 23, 49, 1988.
29. Chatterjee, A. and Pakrashi, S.C., *The Treatise on Indian Medicinal Plants*, Vol. 5, National Institute of Science and Communication, New Delhi, India, 1997, p. 124.
30. Leatherdale, B.A., Panesar, R.K., Singh, G., et al., Improvement in glucose tolerance due to *Momordica charantia* (karela), *Br. Med. J.*, 282, 1823, 1981.
31. Khanna, P., Jain, S.C., Panagariya, A., et al., Hypoglycemic activity of polypeptide-p from a plant source, *J. Nat. Prod.*, 44(6), 648, 1981.
32. Singh, N., Tyagi, S.D., and Agarwal, S.C., Effects of long term feeding of acetone extract of *Momordica charantia* (whole fruit powder) on alloxan diabetic albino rats, *Indian J. Physiol. Pharmacol.*, 33(2), 97, 1989.
33. Karunanayake, E.H., Jeevathayaparan, S., and Tennekoon, K.H., Effect of *Momordica charantia* fruit juice on streptozotocin-induced diabetes in rats, *J. Ethnopharmacol.*, 30(2), 199, 1990.
34. Day, C., Cartwright, T., Provost, J., et al., Hypoglycemic effect of *Momordica charantia* extracts, *Planta Med.*, 56(5), 426, 1990.
35. Higashino, H., Suzuki, A., Tanaka, Y., et al., Hypoglycemic effects of Siamese *Momordica charantia* and *Phyllanthus urinaria* extracts in streptozotocin-induced diabetic rats (the 1st report), *Nippon Yakurigaku Zasshi*, 100(5), 415, 1992.
36. Shibib, B.A., Khan, L.A., and Rahman, R., Hypoglycemic activity of *Coccina indica* and *Momordica charantia* in diabetic rats: depression of the hepatic gluconeogenic enzymes glucose-6-phosphatase and fructose-1,6-bisphosphatase and elevation of both liver and red-cell shunt enzyme glucose-6-phosphate dehydrogenase, *Biochem. J.*, 292 (Pt 1), 267, 1993.
37. Sarkar, S., Pranava, M., and Marita, R., Demonstration of the hypoglycemic action of *Momordica charantia* in a validated animal model of diabetes, *Pharmacol. Res.*, 33(1), 1, 1996.
38. Raza, H., Ahmed, I., Lakhani, M.S., et al., Effect of bitter melon *(Momordica charantia)* fruit juice on the hepatic cytochrome P450-dependent monooxygenases and glutathione S-transferases in streptozotocin-induced diabetic rats, *Biochem. Pharmacol.*, 52(10), 1639, 1996.
39. Miura, T., Itoh, C., Iwamoto, N., et al., Hypoglycemic activity of the fruit of the *Momordica charantia* in type 2 diabetic mice, *J. Nutr. Sci. Vitaminol.*, 47(5), 340, 2001.
40. Matsuda, H., Murakami, T., Shimada, H., et al., Inhibitory mechanisms of oleanolic acid 3-O-monodesmosides on glucose absorption in rats, *Biol. Pharm. Bull.*, 20(6), 717, 1997.
41. Ahmed, I., Adeghate, E., Sharma, A.K., et al., Effects of *Momordica charantia* fruit juice on islet morphology in the pancreas of the streptozocin-diabetic rat, *Diabetes Res. Clin. Pract.*, 40(3), 145, 1998.
42. Matsuda, H., Li, Y., Yamahara, J., et al., Inhibition of gastric emptying by triterpene saponin, momordin Ic, in mice: roles of blood glucose, capsaicin-sensitive sensory nerves, and central nervous system, *J. Pharmacol. Exp. Ther.*, 289(2), 729, 1999.
43. Sitasawad, S.L., Shewade, Y., and Bhonde, R., Role of bittergourd fruit juice in stz-induced diabetic state *in vivo* and in vitro, *J. Ethnopharmacol.*, 73(1–2), 71, 2000.

44. Ahmed, I., Lakhani, M.S., Gillett, M., et al., Hypotriglyceridemic and hypocholesterolemic effects of anti-diabetic *Momordica charantia* (karela) fruit extract in streptozotocin-induced diabetic rats, *Diabetes Res. Clin. Pract.*, 51(3), 155, 2001.
45. Grover, J.K., Vats, V., Rathi, S.S., et al., Traditional Indian anti-diabetic plants attenuate progression of renal damage in streptozotocin induced diabetic mice, *J. Ethnopharmacol.*, 76(3), 233, 2001.
46. Srivastava, Y., Venkatakrishna-Bhatt, H., and Verma, Y., Effect of *Momordica charantia* Linn. pomous aqueous extract on cataractogenesis in murrin alloxan diabetes, *Pharmacol. Res. Commun.*, 20(3), 201, 1988.
47. Raza, H., Ahmed, I., John, A., et al., Modulation of xenobiotic metabolism and oxidative stress in chronic streptozotocin-induced diabetic rats fed with *Momordica charantia* fruit extract, *J. Biochem. Mol. Toxicol.*, 14(3), 131, 2000.
48. Baldwa, V.S., Bhandari, C.M., Pangaria, A., et al., Clinical trial in patients with diabetes mellitus of an insulin-like compound obtained from plant source, *Ups. J. Med. Sci.*, 82(1), 39, 1977.
49. Akhtar, M.S., Trial of *Momordica charantia* Linn. powder in patients with maturity onset diabetes, *J. Pak. Med. Assoc.*, April, 106, 1982.
50. Welihinda, J., Karunanayake, E.H., and Sheriff, M.H., Effect of *Momordica charantia* on the glucose tolerance in maturity onset diabetes, *J. Ethnopharmacol.*, 17, 277, 1986.
51. Srivastava, Y., Venkatakrishna-Bhatt, H., Verma, Y., et al., Antidiabetic and adaptogenic properties of *Momordica charantia* extract: an experimental and clinic evaluation, *Phytother. Res.*, 7(4), 285, 1993.
52. Ahmad, N., Hassan, M.R., Halder, H., et al., Effect of *Momordica charantia* (Karolla) extracts on fasting and postprandial serum glucose levels in NIDDM patients, *Bangladesh Med. Res. Counc. Bull.*, 25(1), 11, 1999.
53. Chatterjee, A. and Pakrashi, S.C., *The Treatise on Indian Medicinal Plants*, Vol. 2, Publications and Information Directorate, New Delhi, India, 1992, p. 125.
54. Mishkinsky, J.S., Goldschmied, A., Joseph, B., et al., Hypoglycemic effect of *Trigonella Foenum graecum* and *Lupinus termis* (leguminosae) seeds and their major alkaloids in alloxan diabetic and normal rats, *Arch. Int. Pharmacodyn. Ther.*, 210(1), 27, 1974.
55. Ghafghazi, T., Sheriat, H.S., Dastmalchi, T., et al., Antagonism of cadmium and alloxan-induced hyperglycemia in rats by *Trigonella foenum graecum*, *Pahlavi Med. J.*, 8(1), 14, 1977.
56. Ribes, G., Sauvaire, Y., Da Costa, C., et al., Antidiabetic effects of subfractions from fenugreek seeds in diabetic dogs, *Proc. Soc. Exp. Biol. Med.*, 182(2), 159, 1986.
57. Khosla, P., Gupta, D.D., and Nagpal, R.K., Effect of *Trigonella foenum graecum* (Fenugreek) on blood glucose in normal and diabetic rats, *Indian J. Physiol. Pharmacol.*, 39(2), 173, 1995.
58. Ali, L., Azad Khan, A.K., Hassan, Z., et al., Characterization of the hypoglycemic effects of *Trigonella foenum graecum* seed, *Planta Med.*, 61(4), 358, 1995.
59. Abdel-Barry, J.A., Abdel-Hassan, I.A., and Al-Hakiem, M.H., Hypoglycaemic and antihyperglycaemic effects of *Trigonella foenum-graecum* leaf in normal and alloxan induced diabetic rats, *J. Ethnopharmacol.*, 58(3), 149, 1997.
60. Raju, J., Gupta, D., Rao, A.R., et al., Effect of antidiabetic compounds on glyoxalase I activity in experimental diabetic rat liver, *Indian J. Exp. Biol.*, 37(2), 193, 1999.
61. Genet, S., Kale, R.K., and Baquer, N.Z., Effects of vanadate, insulin and fenugreek (*Trigonella foenum graecum*) on creatine kinase levels in tissues of diabetic rat, *Indian J. Exp. Biol.*, 37(2), 200, 1999.
62. Raju, J., Gupta, D., Rao, A.R., et al., *Trigonellafoenum graecum* (fenugreek) seed powder improves glucose homeostasis in alloxan diabetic rat tissues by reversing the altered glycolytic, gluconeogenic and lipogenic enzymes, *Mol. Cell. Biochem.*, 224(1–2), 45, 2001.
63. Zia, T., Hasnain, S.N., and Hasan, S.K., Evaluation of the oral hypoglycaemic effect of *Trigonella foenum-graecum* L. (methi) in normal mice, *J. Ethnopharmacol.*, 75(2–3), 191, 2001.
64. Vats, V., Grover, J.K., and Rathi, S.S., Evaluation of anti-hyperglycemic and hypoglycemic effect of *Trigonella foenum-graecum* Linn, *Ocimum sanctum* Linn and *Pterocarpus marsupium* Linn in normal and alloxanized diabetic rats, *J. Ethnopharmacol.*, 79(1), 95, 2002.

65. Abdel-Barry, J.A., Abdel-Hassan, I.A., Jawad, A.M., et al., Hypoglycaemic effect of aqueous extract of the leaves of *Trigonella foenum-graecum* in healthy volunteers, *East. Mediterr. Health J.*, 6(1), 83, 2000.
66. Sharma, R.D. and Raghuram, T.C., Hypoglycemic effect of fenugreek seed in non-insulin dependent diabetic subjects, *Nutr. Res.*, 10, 731, 1990.
67. Ribes, G., Sauvaire, Y., Da Costa, C., et al., Antidiabetic effects of sub fractions from fenugreek seeds in diabetic dogs, *Proc. Soc. Exp. Biol. Med.*, 182(2), 159, 1986.
68. Petit, P.R., Sauvaire, Y.D., Hillaire-Buys, D.M., et al., Steroid saponins from fenugreek seeds: extraction, purification, and pharmacological investigation on feeding behavior and plasma cholesterol, *Steroids*, 60(10), 674, 1995.
69. Ravikumar, P. and Anuradha, C.V., Effect of fenugreek seeds on blood lipid peroxidation and antioxidants in diabetic rats, *Phytother. Res.*, 13(3), 197, 1999.
70. Gupta, D., Raju, J., and Baquer, N.Z., Modulation of some gluconeogenic enzyme activities in diabetic rat liver and kidney: effect of antidiabetic compounds, *Indian J. Exp. Biol.*, 37(2), 196, 1999.
71. Sharma, R.D., Effect of fenugreek seeds and leaves on blood glucose and serum insulin responses in human subjects, *Nutr. Res.*, 6(12), 1353, 1986.
72. Sharma, R.D., Raghuram, T.C., and Rao, N.S., Effect of fenugreek seeds on blood glucose and serum lipids in type I diabetes, *Eur. J. Clin. Nutr.*, 44, 301, 1990.
73. Raghuram, T.C., Sharma, R.D., Sivajumar, B., et al., Effect of fenugreek seeds on intravenous glucose disposition in non-insulin-dependent diabetic patients, *Phytother. Res.*, 8, 83, 1994.
74. Sharma, R.D., Sarkar, A., Hazra, D.K., et al., Hypolipidaemic effect of fenugreek seeds: a chronic study of non-insulin dependent diabetic patients, *Phytother. Res.*, 10(4), 332, 1996b.
75. Kuppu Rajan, K., Srivatsa, A., Krishnaswami, C.V., et al., Hypoglycemic and hypotriglyceridemic effects of methika Churna (fenugreek), *Antiseptic*, 95(3), 78, 1998.
76. Chatterjee, A. and Pakrashi, S.C., *The Treatise on Indian Medicinal Plants*, Vol. 5, National Institute of Science and Communication, New Delhi, India, 1997, p. 113.
77. Khan, A.K., Akhtar, S., and Mahtab, H., Treatment of diabetes mellitus with *Coccinia indica*, *Br. Med. J.*, 280(6220), 1044, 1980.
78. Singh, N., Singh, S.P., Vrats, S., et al., A study on the anti-diabetic activity of *Coccina indica* in dogs, *Indian J. Med. Sci.*, 39, 27, 1985.
79. Kumar, G.P., Sudheesh, S., and Vijayalakshmi, N.R., Hypoglycemic effect of *Coccinia indica*: mechanism of action, *Planta Med.*, 59(4), 330, 1993.
80. Chandrasekar, B., Mukherjee, B., and Mukherjee, S.K., Blood sugar lowering potentiality of selected Cucurbitaceae plants of Indian origin, *Indian J. Med. Res.*, 90, 300, 1998.
81. Platel, K. and Srinivasan, K., Plant foods in the management of diabetes mellitus: vegetables as potential hypoglycemic agents, *Nahrung*, 41(2), 68, 1997.
82. Ivorra, M.D., Paya, M., and Villar, A., A review of natural products and plants as potential antidiabetic drugs, *J. Ethnopharmacol.*, 27, 243, 1989.
83. Bailey, C.J. and Day, C., Traditional plant medicines as the treatments for diabetes, *Diabetes Care*, 12(8), 553, 1989.
84. Ajgaonkar, S.S., Herbal drugs in the treatment of diabetes: a review, *Int. Diabetes Fed. Bull.*, 24, 10, 1979.
85. Brahmchari, H.D. and Augusti, K.T., Orally effective hypoglycemic principles from *Coccina indica*, *J. Pharm. Pharmacol.*, 15, 411, 1963.
86. Azad Khan, A.K., Akhtar, S., and Mahtab, H., *Coccina indica* in the treatment of patients with diabetes mellitus, *Bangladesh Med. Res. Counc. Bull.*, 5(2), 60, 1079.
87. Kamble, S.M., Kamlakar, P.L., Vaidya, S., et al., Influence of *Coccina indica* on certain enzymes in glycolytic and lipolytic pathway in human diabetes, *Indian J. Med. Sci.*, 52(4), 143, 1998.
88. Chatterjee, A. and Pakrashi, S.C., *The Treatise on Indian Medicinal Plants*, Vol. 2, Publications and Information Directorate, New Delhi, India, 1992, p. 115.
89. Shah, D.S., A preliminary study of the hypoglycemic action of heartwood of *Pterocarpus marsupium* roxb., *Indian J. Med. Res.*, 55(2), 166, 1967.
90. Sheehan, E.W., Zemaitis, M.A., Slatkin, D.J., et al., A constituent of *Pterocarpus marsupium*, (-)-epicatechin, as a potential antidiabetic agent, *J. Nat. Prod.*, 46(2), 232, 1983.

91. Ahmad, F., Khalid, P., Khan, M.M., et al., Hypoglycemic activity of *Pterocarpus marsupium* wood, *J. Ethnopharmacol.*, 35(1), 71, 1991.
92. Manickam, M., Ramanathan, M., Jahromi, M.A., et al., Antihyperglycemic activity of phenolics from *Pterocarpus marsupium*, *J. Nat. Prod.*, 60(6), 609, 1997.
93. Indian Council for Medical Research (ICMR), Collaborating Centers, New Delhi, Flexible dose open trial of Vijayasar in cases of newly-diagnosed non-insulin-dependent diabetes mellitus, *Indian J. Med. Res.*, 108, 24, 1998.
94. Kameswara Rao, B., Giri, R., Kesavulu, M.M., et al., Effect of oral administration of bark extracts of *Pterocarpus santalinus* L. on blood glucose level in experimental animals, *J. Ethnopharmacol.*, 74(1), 69, 2001.
95. Nagaraju, N., Prasad, M., Gopalakrishna, G., et al., Blood sugar lowering effect of *Pterocarpus santalinus* (red sandal) wood extract in different rat models, *Int. J. Pharmacognosy*, 29(2), 141, 1991.
96. Chatterjee, A. and Pakrashi, S.C., *The Treatise on Indian Medicinal Plants*, Publications & Information Directorate, New Delhi, India, 1991, p. 39.
97. Augusti, K.T., Hypoglycemic action of bengalenoside, a glucoside isolated from *Ficus bengalensis* Linn, in normal and alloxan diabetic rats, *Indian J. Physiol. Pharmacol.*, 19(4), 218, 1975.
98. Kumar, R.V. and Augusti, K.T., Antidiabetic effect of leucocyanidin derivative isolated from the bark of *Ficus bengalensis* Linn, *Indian J. Biochem. Biophys.*, 26(6), 400, 1989.
99. Acherkar, S., Kaklij, G.S., Pote, M.S., et al., Hypoglycemic activity of *Eugenia jambolana* and *Ficus bengalensis*: mechanism of action, *In Vivo*, 5(2), 143, 1991.
100. Cherian, S., Kumar, R.V., Augusti, K.T., et al., Antidiabetic effect of a glycoide of pelargonidin isolated from the bark of *Ficus bengalensis* Linn., *Indian J. Biochem. Biophys.*, 29(4), 380, 1992.
101. Cherian, S. and Augusti, K.T., Antidiabetic effects of a glycoside of leucopelargonidin isolated from *Ficus bengalensis* Linn., *Indian J. Exp. Biol.*, 31(1), 26, 1993.
102. Augusti, K.T., Daniel, R.S., Cherian, S., et al., Effect of leucopelargonin derivative from *Ficus bengalensis* Linn. on diabetic dogs, *Indian J. Med. Res.*, 99, 82, 1994.
103. Geetha, B.S., Mathew, B.C., and Augusti, K.T., Hypoglycemic effects of leucodelphinidin derivative isolated from *Ficus bengalensis* (Linn.), *Indian J. Physiol. Pharmacol.*, 38(3), 220, 1994.
104. Chowdhary, D.P. and Dua, M., Hypoglycemic effect of a coded formulation: Aysuh-82, *J. Res. Ayurveda and Siddha*, 19(3–4), 107, 1998.
105. Pandey, V.N., Rajagopalan, S.S., and Chowdhary, D.P., An effective Ayruvedic hypoglycemic formulation, *J. Res. Ayurveda and Siddha*, 16(1–2), 1, 1995.
106. Sircar, A.R., Ahuja, R.C., Natu, S.M., et al., Hypoglycemic, hypolipidemic and general beneficial effects of an herbal mixture MA-471, *Altern. Ther. Clin. Pract.*, 3(5), 26, 1996.
107. Sankar, V.R. and Aggarwal, M.P., Clinical studies of abraga (mica) chendooram in the management of diabetes mellitus (neerazhivu), *J. Res. Ayurveda and Siddha*, 9(1–2), 38, 1988.
108. Shankar, R. and Singhal, R.K., Clinical studies of the effect of abraga (mica) chendooram in the treatment of diabetes mellitus (neerazhivu), *J. Res. Ayurveda and Siddha*, 16(3–4), 108, 1995.
109. Maji, D. and Singh, A.K., Clinical trial of D-400, a herbomineral preparation in diabetes mellitus, *J. Diabetic Assoc. India*, 35(1), 1, 1995.
110. Shankar, R. and Singhal, R.K., Clinical assessement of the effects of sandana (sandal) podi-a in the treatment of diabetes mellitus (neerazhiv), *J. Res. Ayurveda and Siddha*, 15(3–4), 89, 1994.
111. Sivaprakasam, K., Rao, K.K., Yasodha, R., et al., Siddha remedy for diabetes mellitus, *J. Res. Ayurveda and Siddha*, 5(1–4), 25, 1984.
112. Kumar, N. and Kumar, A., A clinical trial of M-93 compound in the management of madhumeha (diabetes mellitus), *J. Res. Ayurveda and Siddha*, 16(3–4), 102, 1995.
113. Wadood, A., Wadood, N., and Shah, S.A., Effects of *Acacia arabica* and *Caralluma edulis* on blood glucose levels of normal and alloxan diabetic rabbits, *J. Pak. Med. Assoc.*, 39(8), 208, 1989.
114. Akhtar, M.S. and Iqbal, J., Evaluation of the hypoglycaemic effect of *Achyranthes aspera* in normal and alloxan-diabetic rabbits, *J. Ethnopharmacol.*, 31(1), 49, 1991.
115. Karunanayake, E.H., Welihinda, J., Sirimanne, S.R., et al., Oral hypoglycaemic activity of some medicinal plants of Sri Lanka, *J. Ethnopharmacol.*, 11(2), 223, 1984.

116. Sachdewa, A., Raina, D., Srivastava, A.K., et al., Effect of *Aegle marmelos* and *Hibiscus rosa sinensis* leaf extract on glucose tolerance in glucose induced hyperglycemic rats (Charles foster), *J. Environ. Biol.*, 22(1), 53, 2001.
117. Mathew, P.T. and Augusti, K.T., Hypoglycaemic effects of onion, *Allium cepa* Linn. on diabetes mellitus — a preliminary report, *Indian J. Physiol. Pharmacol.*, 19(4), 213, 1975.
118. Roman-Ramos, R., Flores-Saenz, J.L., and Alarcon-Aguilar, F.J., Anti-hyperglycemic effect of some edible plants, *J. Ethnopharmacol.*, 48(1), 25, 1995.
119. Babu, P.S. and Srinivasan, K., Influence of dietary capsaicin and onion on the metabolic abnormalities associated with streptozotocin induced diabetes mellitus, *Mol. Cell. Biochem.*, 175(1–2), 49, 1997.
120. Sheela, C.G. and Augusti, K.T., Antidiabetic effects of S-allyl cysteine sulphoxide isolated from garlic *Allium sativum* Linn., *Indian J. Exp. Biol.*, 30(6), 523, 1992.
121. Sheela, C.G., Kumud, K., and Augusti, K.T., Anti-diabetic effects of onion and garlic sulfoxide amino acids in rats, *Planta Med.*, 61(4), 356, 1995.
122. Augusti, K.T. and Sheela, C.G., Antiperoxide effect of S-allyl cysteine sulfoxide, an insulin secretagogue, in diabetic rats, *Experientia*, 52(2), 115, 1996.
123. Kumar, G.R. and Reddy, K.P., Reduced nociceptive responses in mice with alloxan induced hyperglycemia after garlic (Allium sativum Linn.) treatment, *Indian J. Exp. Biol.*, 37(7), 662, 1999.
124. Kasuga, S., Ushijima, M., Morihara, N., et al., Effect of aged garlic extract (AGE) on hyperglycemia induced by immobilization stress in mice, *Nippon Yakurigaku Zasshi*, 114(3), 191, 1999.
125. Patumraj, S., Tewit, S., Amatyakul, S., et al., Comparative effects of garlic and aspirin on diabetic cardiovascular complications, *Drug Delivery*, 7(2), 91, 2000.
126. Ghannam, N., Kingston, M., Al-Meshaal, I.A., et al., The antidiabetic activity of aloes: preliminary clinical and experimental observations, *Horm. Res.*, 24(4), 288, 1986.
127. Al-Awadi, F.M. and Gumaa, K.A., Studies on the activity of individual plants of an antidiabetic plant mixture, *Acta Diabetol. Lat.*, 24(1), 37, 1987.
128. Ajabnoor, M.A., Effect of aloes on blood glucose levels in normal and alloxan diabetic mice, *J. Ethnopharmacol.*, 28(2), 215, 1990.
129. Al-Awadi, F., Fatania, H., and Shamte, U., The effect of a plants mixture extract on liver gluconeogenesis in streptozotocin induced diabetic rats, *Diabetes Res.*, 18(4), 163, 1991.
130. Okyar, A., Can, A., Akev, N., et al., Effect of Aloe vera leaves on blood glucose level in type I and type II diabetic rat models, *Phytother. Res.*, 15(2), 157, 2001.
131. Zhang, X.F. and Tan, B.K., Anti-diabetic property of ethanolic extract of *Andrographis paniculata* in streptozotocin-diabetic rats, *Acta Pharmacol. Sin.*, 21(12), 1157, 2000.
132. Zhang, X.F. and Tan, B.K., Antihyperglycaemic and anti-oxidant properties of *Andrographis paniculata* in normal and diabetic rats, *Clin. Exp. Pharmacol. Physiol.*, 27(5–6), 358, 2000.
133. Sen, P., Mediratta, P.K., and Ray, A., Effects of *Azadirachta indica* A Juss on some biochemical, immunological and visceral parameters in normal and stressed rats, *Indian J. Exp. Biol.*, 30 (12), 1170, 1992.
134. Chattopadhyay, R.R., Possible mechanism of antihyperglycemic effect of *Azadirachta indica* leaf extract. IV, *Gen. Pharmacol.*, 27(3), 431, 1996.
135. Chattopadhyay, R.R., A comparative evaluation of some blood sugar lowering agents of plant origin, *J. Ethnopharmacol.*, 67(3), 367, 1999.
136. Khosla, P., Bhanwra, S., Singh, J., et al., A study of the hypoglycaemic effect of *Azadirachta indica* (Neem) in normal and alloxan diabetic rabbits, *Indian J. Physiol. Pharmacol.*, 44(1), 69, 2000.
137. Saleem, R., Ahmad, M., Hussain, S.A., et al., Hypotensive, hypoglycaemic and toxicological studies on the flavonol C-glycoside shamimin from *Bombax ceiba*, *Planta Med.*, 65(4), 331, 1999.
138. Sharma, S.R., Dwivedi, S.K., and Swarup, D., Hypoglycaemic, antihyperglycaemic and hypolipidemic activities of *Caesalpinia bonducella* seeds in rats, *J. Ethnopharmacol.*, 58(1), 39, 1997.

139. Yoshikawa, M., Murakami, T., Kishi, A., et al., Medicinal flowers. III. Marigold. (1): hypoglycemic, gastric emptying inhibitory, and gastroprotective principles and new oleanane-type triterpene oligoglycosides, calendasaponins A, B, C, and D, from Egyptian *Calendula officinalis*, *Chem. Pharm. Bull.* (Tokyo), 49(7), 863, 2001.
140. Yadav, P., Sarkar, S., and Bhatnagar, D., Action of *Capparis decidua* against alooxan-induced oxidative stress and diabetes in rat tissues, *Pharmacol. Res.*, 36(3), 221, 1997.
141. Tolan, I., Ragoobirsingh, D., and Morrison, E.Y., The effect of capsaicin on blood glucose, plasma insulin levels and insulin binding in dog models, *Phytother. Res.*, 15(5), 391, 2001.
142. Esposito Avella, M., Diaz, A., de Gracia, I., et al., Evaluation of traditional medicine: effects of *Cajanus cajan* L. and of *Cassia fistula* L. on carbohydrate metabolism in mice, *Rev. Med. Panama*, 16(1), 39, 1991.
143. Singh, S.N., Vats, P., Suri, S., et al., Effect of an antidiabetic extract of *Catharanthus roseus* on enzymic activities in streptozotocin induced diabetic rats, *J. Ethnopharmacol.*, 76(3), 269, 2001.
144. Grindley, P.B., Omoruyi, F.O., Asemota, H.N., et al., Effect of yam *(Dioscorea cayenensis)* and dasheen *(Colocassia esculenta)* extracts on the kidney of streptozotocin-induced diabetic rats, *Int. J. Food Sci. Nutr.*, 52(5), 429, 2001.
145. Sharma, A.L., Sapru, H.N., and Chowdhury, N.K., Hypoglycaemic action of *Cryptostegia grandiflora* R.Br.. in rabbits, *Indian J. Med. Res.*, 55(12), 1277, 1967.
146. Srivastava, A., Longia, G.S., Singh, S.P., et al., Hypoglycaemic and hypolipaemic effects of *Cyamopsis tetragonoloba* (guar) in normal and diabetic guinea pigs, *Indian J. Physiol. Pharmacol.*, 31(2), 77, 1987.
147. Frias, A.C. and Sgarbieri, V.C., Guar gum effects on food intake, blood serum lipids and glucose levels of Wistar rats, *Plant Foods Hum. Nutr.*, 53(1), 15, 1998.
148. Teixeira, C.C., Pinto, L.P., Kessler, F.H., et al., The effect of *Syzygium cumini* (L.) skeels on post-prandial blood glucose levels in non-diabetic rats and rats with streptozotocin-induced diabetes mellitus, *J. Ethnopharmacol.*, 56(3), 209, 1997.
149. Achrekar, S., Kaklij, G.S., Pote, M.S., et al., Hypoglycemic activity of *Eugenia jambolana* and *Ficus bengalensis*: mechanism of action, *In Vivo*, 5(2), 143, 1991.
150. Grover, J.K., Vats, V., Rathi, S.S., et al., Traditional Indian anti-diabetic plants attenuate progression of renal damage in streptozotocin induced diabetic mice, *J. Ethnopharmacol.*, 76(3), 233, 2001.
151. Vikrant, V., Grover, J.K., Tandon, N., et al., Treatment with extracts of *Momordica charantia* and *Eugenia jambolana* prevents hyperglycemia and hyperinsulinemia in fructose fed rats, *J. Ethnopharmacol.*, 76(2), 139, 2001.
152. Grover, J.K., Vats, V., and Rathi, S.S., Anti-hyperglycemic effect of *Eugenia jambolana* and *Tinospora cordifolia* in experimental diabetes and their effects on key metabolic enzymes involved in carbohydrate metabolism, *J. Ethnopharmacol.*, 73(3), 461, 2000.
153. Serraclara, A., Hawkins, F., Perez, C., et al., Hypoglycemic action of an oral fig-leaf decoction in type-I diabetic patients, *Diabetes Res. Clin. Pract.*, 39(1), 19, 1998.
154. Canal, J.R., Torres, M.D., Romero, A., et al., A chloroform extract obtained from a decoction of *Ficus carica* leaves improves the cholesterolaemic status of rats with streptozotocin-induced diabetes, *Acta Physiol. Hung.*, 87(1), 71, 2000.
155. Desai, A.C. and Bhide, M.B., Hypoglycaemic activity of *Hamiltonia suaveolen*, *Indian J. Med. Res.*, 81, 86, 1985.
156. Sachdewa, A. and Khemani, L.D., A preliminary investigation of the possible hypoglycemic activity of *Hibiscus rosa-sinensis*, *Biomed. Environ. Sci.*, 12(3), 222, 1999.
157. Sachdewa, A., Raina, D., Srivastava, A.K., et al., Effect of *Aegle marmelos* and *Hibiscus rosa sinensis* leaf extract on glucose tolerance in glucose induced hyperglycemic rats (Charles foster), *J. Environ. Biol.*, 22(1), 53, 2001.
158. Sachdewa, A., Nigam, R., and Khemani, L.D., Hypoglycemic effect of *Hibiscus rosa sinensis* L. leaf extract in glucose and streptozotocin induced hyperglycemic rats, *Indian J. Exp. Biol.*, 39(3), 284, 2001.

159. Tripathi, Y.B. and Chaturvedi, P., Assessment of endocrine response of *Inula racemosa* in relation to glucose homeostasis in rats, *Indian J. Exp. Biol.*, 33(9), 686, 1995.
160. Aderibigbe, A.O., Emudianughe, T.S., and Lawal, B.A., Antihyperglycaemic effect of *Mangifera indica* in rat, *Phytother. Res.*, 13(6), 504, 1999.
161. Aderibigbe, A.O., Emudianughe, T.S., and Lawal, B.A., Evaluation of the antidiabetic action of *Mangifera indica* in mice, *Phytother. Res.*, 15(5), 456, 2001.
162. Rao, B.K., Kesavulu, M.M., and Appa Rao, C., Antidiabetic and hypolipidemic effects of *Momordica cymbalaria* Hook. Fruit powder in alloxan-diabetic rats, *J. Ethnopharmacol.*, 67(1), 103, 1999.
163. Rao, B.K., Kesavulu, M.M., and Apprao, C., Antihyperglycemic activity of *Momordica cymbalaria* in alloxan diabetis rats, *J. Ethnopharmacol.*, 78(1), 67, 2001.
164. Akhtar, M.S., Qureshi, A.Q., and Iqbal, J., Antidiabetic evaluation of *Mucuna pruriens*, Linn seeds, *J. Pak. Med. Assoc.*, 40(7), 147, 1990.
165. Khan, B.A., Abraham, A., and Leelamma, S., Hypoglycemic action of *Murraya koenigii* (curry leaf) and *Brassica juncea* (mustard): mechanism of action, *Indian J. Biochem. Biophys.*, 32(2), 106, 1995.
166. Alarcon-Aguilara, F.J., Roman-Ramos, R., Perez-Gutierrez, S., et al., Study of the anti-hyperglycemic effect of plants used as antidiabetics, *J. Ethnopharmacol.*, 61(2), 101, 1998.
167. Pari, L. and Maheswari, J.U., Hypoglycaemic effect of *Musa sapientum* L. in alloxan-induced diabetic rats, *J. Ethnopharmacol.*, 68(1–3), 321, 1999.
168. Pari, L. and Umamaheswari, J., Antihyperglycaemic activity of *Musa sapientum* flowers: effect on lipidperoxidation in alloxan diabetic rats, *Phytother. Res.*, 14(2), 136, 2000.
169. Mukherjee, P.K., Saha, K., Pal, M., et al., Effect of *Nelumbo nucifera* rhizome extract on blood sugar level in rats, *J. Ethnopharmacol.*, 58(3), 207, 1997.
170. Chattopadhyay, R.R., Hypoglycemic effect of *Ocimum sanctum* leaf extract in normal and streptozotocin diabetic rats, *Indian J. Exp. Biol.*, 31(11), 891, 1993.
171. Agrawal, P., Rai, V., and Singh, R.B., Randomized placebo-controlled, single blind trial of holy basil leaves in patients with noninsulin-dependent diabetes mellitus, *Int. J. Clin. Pharmacol. Ther.*, 34(9), 406, 1996.
172. Rai, V., Iyer, U., and Mani, U.V., Effect of Tulasi *(Ocimum sanctum)* leaf powder supplementation on blood sugar levels, serum lipids and tissue lipids in diabetic rats, *Plant Foods Hum. Nutr.*, 50(1), 9, 1997.
173. Srivastava, A. and Joshi, L.D., Effect of feeding black gram *(Phaseolus mungo)* on serum lipids of normal & diabetic guineapigs, *Indian J. Med. Res.*, 92, 383, 1990.
174. Mani, U.V., Pradhan, S.N., Mehta, N.C., et al., Glycaemic index of conventional carbohydrate meals, *Br. J. Nutr.*, 68(2), 445, 1992.
175. Srividya, N. and Periwal, S., Diuretic, hypotensive and hypoglycaemic effect of *Phyllanthus amarus, Indian J. Exp. Biol.*, 33(11), 861, 1995.
176. Higashino, H., Suzuki, A., Tanaka, Y., et al., Hypoglycemic effects of Siamese Momordica charantia and Phyllanthus urinaria extracts in sterptozocin-induced diabetic rats (the 1st report), *Nippon Yakuraigaku Zasshi*, 100(5), 415, 1992.
177. Joy, K.L. and Kuttan, R., Anti-diabetic activity of Picrorrhiza kurroa extract, *J. Ethnopharmacol.*, 67(2), 143, 1999.
178. Miura, T. and Kato, A., the difference in hypoglycemic action between polygonati rhizoma and polygonati officinalis rhizoma, *Biol. Pharm. Bull.*, 18(11), 1605, 1995.
179. Cheng, J.T. and Yang, R.S., Hypoglycemic effect of guava juice in mice and human subjects, *Am. J. Chin. Med.*, 11(1–4), 74, 1983.
180. Kameswara Rao, B., Giri, R., Kesavulu, M.M., et al., Effect of oral administration of bark extracts of *Pterocarpus santalinus* L. on blood glucose level in experimental animals, *J. Ethnopharmacol.*, 74(1), 69, 2001.
181. Jafri, M.A., Aslam, M., Javed, K., et al., Effect of *Punica granatum* Linn. (flowers) on blood glucose level in normal and alloxan-induced diabetic rats, *J. Ethnopharmacol.*, 70(3), 309, 2000.
182. Sekar, B.C., Mukherjee, B., Chakravarti, R.B., et al., Effect of different fractions of *Swertia chirayita* on the blood sugar level of albino rats, *J. Ethnopharmacol.*, 21(2), 175, 1987.

183. Chandrasekar, B., Bajpai, M.B., and Mukherjee, S.K., Hypoglycemic activity of *Swertia chirayita* (Roxb ex Flem) Karst, *Indian J. Exp. Biol.*, 28(7), 616, 1990.
184. Bajpai, M.B., Asthana, R.K., Sharma, N.K., et al., Hypoglycemic effect of swerchirin from the hexane fraction of *Swertia chirayita, Planta Med.*, 57(2), 102, 1991.
185. Saxena, A.M., Bajpai, M.B., and Mukherjee, S.K., Swerchirin induced blood sugar lowering of streptozotocin treated hyperglycemic rats, *Indian J. Exp. Biol.*, 29(7), 674, 1991.
186. Saxena, A.M., Murthy, P.S., and Mukherjee, S.K., Mode of action of three structurally different hypoglycemic agents: a comparative study, *Indian J. Exp. Biol.*, 34(4), 351, 1996.
187. Saxena, A.M., Bajpai, M.B., Murthy, P.S., et al., Mechanism of blood sugar lowering by a swerchirin-containing hexane fraction (SWI) of *Swertia chirayita, Indian J. Exp. Biol.*, 31(2), 178, 1993.
188. Rao, B.K. and Rao, C.H., Hypoglycemic and antihyperglycemic activity of *Syzygium alternifolium* (Wt.) Walp. seed extracts in normal and diabetic rats, *Phytomedicine,* 8(2), 88, 2001.
189. Lozoya-Meckes, M. and Mellado-Campos, V., Is the *Tecoma stans* infusion an antidiabetic remedy? *J. Ethnopharmacol.*, 14(1), 1, 1985.
190. Roman-Ramos, R., Flores-Saenz, J.L., Partida-Hernandez, G., et al., Experimental study of the hypoglycemic effect of some antidiabetic plants, *Arch. Invest. Med. (Mexico)*, 22(1), 87, 1991.
191. Fort, D.M., Rao, K., Jolad, S.D., et al., Antihyperglycemic activity of *Teramus labialis* (Fabaceae), *Phytomedicine*, 6(6), 465, 2000.
192. Wadood, N., Wadood, A., and Shah, S.A., Effect of *Tinospora cordifolia* on blood glucose and total lipid levels of normal and alloxan-diabetic rabbits, *Planta Med.*, 58(2), 131, 1992.
193. Stanely Mainzen Prince, P. and Menon, V.P., Antioxidant action of *Tinospora cordifolia* root extract in alloxan diabetic rats, *Phytother. Res.*, 15(3), 213, 2001.
194. Noor, H. and Ashcroft, S.J., Antidiabetic effects of *Tinospora crispa* in rats, *J. Ethnopharmacol.*, 27(1–2), 149, 1989.
195. Noor, H., Hammonds, P., Sutton, R., et al., The hypoglycaemic and insulinotropic activity of *Tinospora crispa*: studies with human and rat islets and HIT-T15 B cells, *Diabetologia*, 32(6), 354, 1989.
196. Noor, H. and Ashcroft, S.J., Pharmacological characterisation of the antihyperglycaemic properties of *Tinospora crispa* extract, *J. Ethnopharmacol.*, 62(1), 7, 1998.
197. Chattopadhyay, R.R., Sarkar, S.K., Ganguly, S., et al., Hypoglycemic and antihyperglycemic effect of leaves of *Vinca rosea* linn, *Indian J. Physiol. Pharmacol.*, 35(3), 145, 1991.
198. Andallu, B. and Radhika, B., Hypoglycemic, diuretic and hypocholesterolemic effect of winter cherry (*Withania somnifera,* Dunal) root, *Indian J. Exp. Biol.*, 38(6), 607, 2000.

8

Ayurvedic Therapies for Thyroid Dysfunction

Anand Kar and Sunanda Panda

CONTENTS

0-8493-1366-X/04/$0.00+$1.50

8.1 Introduction

Thyroid problems are among the most common endocrine disorders presently seen worldwide. Patients with thyroid disorders suffer either from hypofunctioning or from hyperfunctioning of the gland. Whereas the former leads to a decrease in the concentrations of circulating thyroid hormones, the latter increases the same. These two dysfunctions are commonly referred as hypothyroidism and hyperthyroidism, respectively.

About 1 to 2% of the adult population is known to suffer from thyroid disorders.[1] According to the 1999 World Health Assembly report, about 1.5 billion persons in more than 110 countries are threatened with thyroid disorders. A World Health Organization (WHO) estimation also indicates that about 200 million people have goiter, although most of the goiters are small and subclinical.

Although small in size, the thyroid is considered to be one of the most important organs of the endocrine system, as it regulates nearly all body functions, including metabolic, respiratory, cardiovascular, digestive, nervous, and reproductive systems either directly or indirectly. Many abnormalities in a person's body can be the result of thyroid dysfunction. In fact, some typical problems directly related to thyroid abnormalities were known since the existence of Ayurveda, the ancient system of medicine in India.

In Ayurveda, the common thyroid-related problem that has been described from time to time is enlarged thyroid gland (*galaganda*),[2] which is now known as the simple goiter, a state of hypothyroidism. Some other diseases that are commonly mentioned in endocrine text,[3,4] such as myxedema, cretinism, Graves' disease, and nodular goiter, have not been well described in Ayurveda symptom-based herbal treatments.

Despite several investigations on the herbal therapies, the use of Ayurvedic medicines in the regulation of thyroid problems continues to require more investigation. The primary aim of this chapter is to review the available literature including the experimental studies conducted to date and then to highlight the scientific basis of Ayurvedic therapies for thyroid dysfunctions. However, before we deal with the treatment of thyroid problems, it is necessary to have a basic understanding of the thyroid gland, its hormone, and functions.

8.2 Basic Understanding of Thyroid Gland: Its Hormones and Functions

The thyroid is a two-lobed gland that lies over the trachea (windpipe) just below the larynx. It synthesizes and secrets two major hormones, thyroxine (T_4) and triiodothyronine

(T_3). Both T_4 and T_3 are iodine-containing chemicals. Because they are the only iodine-containing hormones in the body, an adequate iodine intake is necessary for the optimum functioning of the thyroid gland. Although the entire amount of circulating T_4 is produced in the gland itself, T_3 is mostly generated in liver and kidney by peripheral monodeiodination of T_4 with the help of an enzyme, 5-monodeiodinase (5-D).

Although basically metabolic, thyroid hormones regulate almost all physiological processes directly or indirectly. The hormones are vital to the well-being of a person, and an imbalance in their physiological levels leads to health problems.

8.3 Thyroid Abnormalities: Hypothyroidism and Hyperthyroidism

Hypothyroidism occurs when the thyroid is hypoactive and does not produce enough thyroid hormones. The most common form of hypothyroidic diseases described in Ayurveda is the enlarged thyroid gland (*galaganda*), now known as goiter. In fact, goiter is produced by the inadequate secretion of thyroid hormones, resulting in a positive feedback of a pituitary hormone, thyrotropin (thyrotropin-stimulating hormone [TSH]), on the thyroid gland that ultimately enlarges. This disease process was recognized by early Ayurvedic practitioners.

As thyroid hormones regulate growth and development (both physical and mental) of a person, hypothyroidic children suffer from cretinism (mental retardation). In Ayurveda this is known as a condition of low intelligence *(manda buddhi).*

Hyperthyroidism is the result of excess production and delivery of the thyroid hormones to the peripheral tissues often referred as thyrotoxicosis. In Ayurveda this is believed to be an air or energy disorder (*vata*). Conventional medical text relates it to the production of TSH receptor-stimulating antibodies, leading to enhanced secretion of thyroid hormones, which are responsible for increased metabolism and energy wastage.

At present, diseases such as thyrotoxicosis, exophthalmic goiter or Graves' disease, and thyroid carcinoma and adenoma all come under the category of hyperthyroidism. These diseases can be serious, as the patients may end up with heart ailments and diabetes (*madhumeha*), the two most common modern health problems.[5]

Several symptoms are associated with hypothyroidism and hyperthyroidism. The common symptoms are listed in Table 8.1. A rare symptom, the thickening of the skin over the lower legs (thyroid dermopathy), is also observed in chronic hypothyroid individuals. At the beginning of the thyroid dysfunction, visible symptoms may not be observed.

8.4 Etiology

8.4.1 Hypothyroidism

According to Ayurvedic literature,[2] impairment of air *(vayu)*, mucus or water (*kapha*), and the fat (*meda*) leads to the enlargement of the thyroid gland (galaganda). This is often known as bronchocele. According to common belief, the most common cause of hypothyroidism is iodine deficiency, and this disease is prevalent only in iodine-deficient areas

TABLE 8.1

Common Signs and Symptoms of Hypo- and Hyperthyroidism

Hypothyroidism	Hyperthyroidism
Weight gain	Weight loss
Husky, hoarse voice	Thinning of hair
Tiredness/lethargy	Sweating
Intolerance to cold	Nervousness
Cold hands and feet	Vomiting
Dry skin and hair, brittle nails	Tachycardia
Puffiness of the body	Diarrhea
Periorbital swelling	Tremor
Memory loss	Muscle weakness and fatigue
Constipation	Insomnia
Bradycardia	Angina
Muscle stiffness	Increased appetite
Impotence	Eyelid pain
Anemia	Loss of libido
Depression	Exophthalmos

such as hilly regions or areas with high lime content. In urban areas, iodine deficiency can also be considered a major factor of this disease, as people in these areas are following low sodium diet and using less iodized salt (as a preventive measure for heart problems and high blood pressure). Doctors recommend about 150 μg/day of iodine for normal thyroid function; less than 50 μg/day for a long period may cause goiter.[3] Because of the inadequate iodine in the diet, the thyroid cannot synthesize sufficient amount of T_4 and T_3, resulting in the abnormal increase in circulating TSH, which causes abnormal increase in the size of the thyroid gland (simple goiter).

Other factors causing hypothyroidism are stress, hereditary defects in thyroid iodide transport, thyroglobulin and hormone synthesis, reduction in TSH or thyrotropin-releasing hormone (TRH) (secondary or tertiary hypothyroidism, respectively) and conversion of T_4 to T_3, peripheral resistance to the action of thyroid hormones, excess consumption of adulterated and goitrogenic foods (e.g., cabbage, cauliflower, cassava, peanuts, sweet potatoes, etc.),[4] selenium deficiency, and consumption of heavy metals and pesticides.[6–8] Very often it may be a result of the development of autoimmune antibodies, which destroy the thyroidal tissues by an immunological process.[3]

8.4.2 Hyperthyroidism

According to classic Ayurvedic text, hyperthyroidism is the result of imbalance in air (*vata*) and fire (*pitta*), which govern the neurohormonal system. In the conventional system of medicine, physicians relate constant psychological stress and excess secretion of cortisol with thyrotoxicosis. Apart from genetic susceptibility, an immunological increase in immunoglobin G (IgG) antibodies (sometimes referred as thyroid stimulating antibodies), which act on TSH receptors on the gland to stimulate hormone production, are considered as major factors for hyperthyroidism.[9]

Prevalent data indicate that more young women (ages 20 to 40) suffer from thyroid dysfunctions than do males. This difference may exist because of high-circulating sex steroids, estrogen and progesterone, in females. Thyrotoxicosis may be aggravated during pregnancy, as human chorionic gonadotropin (hCG), a placental hormone, also possesses TSH-like activity.[9] Formation of thyroid carcinoma also increases T_4 and T_3 production.

8.5 Pathogenesis (*Samprapti*)

Although in Ayurveda the pathogenesis of thyroid dysfunctions has not been well described, most available literature relate hypothyroidism with excess of mucus (*kapha*) and fats (*meda*). When the above factors get excited and become out of balance, they produce hormonal (*ojas*) imbalance and then enlargement (a slow process) of the gland, known as *Galaganda*.[2] It may start with loss of appetite and disgust for food or with loss of immunity.

There is limited Ayurvedic literature on hyperthyroidism. However, some physical and behavioral changes do indicate that *vata* and *pitta* lead to insomnia, which may manifest a condition of hyperthyroidism. Excessive sweating, intolerance to heat, and warm soles and palms also indicate the onset of hyperthyroidism.[2]

Conventional medicine describes autoimmunity development as the major pathogenesis process for thyroid dysfunctions. This could be due to genetic predisposition or it could be hormone or virus induced.[10] A characteristic finding in the pathogenesis of hypothyroidism is that there is an accumulation of glycosaminoglycans (mostly hyaluronic acid) in interstitial tissues that generally accounts for the edema. In Graves' disease, sensitized T-lymphocytes stimulate B-lymphocytes to synthesize antibodies that enhance thyroid cell function. Some factors that may also stimulate the immune response of hyperthyroidism are postpartum period of pregnancy, excess iodide or lithium therapy, and glucocorticoid withdrawal.[10]

8.6 Prognosis (*Sadhyata*)

Hypothyroidism always results in a gradual decrease in metabolism with the slowing of mental and physical activity. Patients may experience one or more common symptoms, including sensitivity to cold, dryness of the skin and hair, constipation, anorexia, angina, anemia, and disordered menstrual function. With proper Ayurvedic therapy, these symptoms can be overcome. Goiter in which there is a considerable dyspnea along with emaciation of body, and if there is more than 1 year of standing, may be incurable.[2] According to conventional medical text, untreated myxedema may eventually lead to myxedema coma and death. However, the prognosis has been vastly improved with the use of L-thyroxine with frequent monitoring of the thyroidal status.

With respect to hyperthyroidism, Ayurvedic therapies have been found to provide about 60 to 80% symptomatic relief.[14] With conventional medicine, when patients are treated for 12 to 24 months with antithyroid drugs, prolonged remissions of their illness are generally observed and many patients develop hypothyroidism. With radioactive iodide, 40 to 70% of patients develop hypothyroidism as a side effect within 10 years. Lifetime follow-up is therefore required for all hyperthyroid patients.

8.7 Diagnosis (*Nidan*)

Diagnosis of the thyroid dysfunctions is made on the basis of inspection of the thyroid gland both in Ayurveda and in Western medicine. The size and consistency of the swelling

TABLE 8.2

Commonly Used Ayurvedic Herbal Formulations and Food Supplements for the Treatment of Hypothyroidism

Formulation and Food Supplement	Dose	Major Herbs Used	Manufacturer
Thyro-L#455	2 capsules three times/day	*Laminaria sarassum*	Herbal Doctor Remedies, Monterey Park, CA
B 37 K Para-Thy-Mix	1 tablet/day	Natural iodine from dulse with raw glandular extract	Penn Herb Comp., Philadelphia, PA
Suddha guggulu	2.25 g twice/day	*Commiphora mukul*	Himalya Drug, New Delhi, India
Kanchnar guggulu	500 mg–1.0 g	*Bauhinia variegata, C. mukul*	Dabur Pharmaceuticals, New Delhi, India[a]
Gayatrin	1 to 2 tablets, two to three times/day	*B. variegata, C. mukul*	Arya Aushadhi Pharmaceutical Works, Indore, India
Kelp	1 tablet three times/day (660 mg kelp)	*Fucus vesiculosus*	Herbal Doctor Remedies, Monterey Park, CA

Note: These products are not intended to cure or prevent the disease.

[a]Also from Ayurvedic Formulary of India, Central Council for Research in Ayurveda and Siddha, Ministry of Health and Family Welfare, Government of India, New Delhi.

differ based on the disorder (*dosa*) of *vata, pitta,* or *kapha* involved in causing the dysfunction. Confirmation of diagnosis is done by the estimation of thyroid hormones and thyrotropin by radioimmunoassay (RIA), examination of gland activity by the use of radioiodine, basal metabolic rate (BMR)/oxygen consumption studies, and measurement of autoimmune antibodies.

8.8 Ayurvedic Therapies (*Chikitsa*)

According to the Ayurvedic management of thyroid diseases, the first line of treatment is to clear the blocked channels (*srotas)* in order to balance *vata, pitta,* and *kapha*. Several herbal preparations are also administered to increase the digestive fire at a cellular level and restore metabolism. For the treatment of goiter, some ayurvedic preparations are used to clean *kapha* internally.

Few herbal products are already available for the treatment of thyroid dysfunctions; the popular ones have been mentioned in Tables 8.2 and 8.3. Besides the mentioned drug and food supplements, *Vimbadi* oil (with sesame oil) can be applied four times/day on the goiter.[2] *Yograj guggul* (0.5 to 2.25 g/day) and *Ashwagandha* powder (*churn*) (1 to 6 g/day) are also used in the treatment of hypothyroidism. A study on Liv-52, an Ayurvedic liver tonic, has revealed that it stimulates thyroid hormone secretion, particularly the T_3.[11] In fact, action of the most commonly recommended Ayurvedic drug, *Kanchnar guggul* (prepared from *Bauhinia variegata*), has been found to be similar to that of the allopathic drug Eltroxin.[12]

For the treatment of hyperthyroidism, Charaka has mentioned *Shankapushpi* extract (*rosa*) as a brain tonic (Medhya rasayana, Charaka, Ch.1/30), although this is known to be a very effective supplement. Gupta et al.[14] studied the comparative effects of an allopathic

TABLE 8.3

Common Ayurvedic Herbal Formulations and Food Supplements for the Treatment of Hyperthyroidism

Formulation and Food Supplement	Dose	Major Herbs Used	Manufacturer
Herbal-supra Power (product no. HZ1003)	1 capsule/day	Valerian root, passion flower, hops, skullcap, and wood betony	Viable Herbal Solutions Comp., Morrisville, PA
Biolite	1 capsule/day	Ephedra, kola seed, white willow, kelp, ginger, *Ginkgo biloba*, juniper berries, buchu leaves, *Cascara sagrada*	Bionomics International Inc., Delray Beach, FL
Thyro-H #450	1 capsule three times/day	Oyster shell, nourish yin, scrophularia, *Arnemarrhena fritillaria*	Herbal Doctor Remedies, Monterey Park, CA
Thyrovedic	1 tablet	Garcina, ginger, cambogia	Herbal Doctor Remedies, Monterey Park, CA
Lemon balm	1.5–4.5 g several times/day	*Melissa officinalis*	Herbal Doctor Remedies, Monterey Park, CA
Astrgalagus extract	1 vegicapsule/day	Raw astragalagus powder (250 mg in each capsule)	Suzannes com, Joplin, MO
Shankpuspi syrup	125 mg twice/day	*C. pluricaulis*	Dabur India Ltd., New Delhi, India

TABLE 8.4

Promising Plant Extracts Suggested for the Treatment of Hypothyroidism

Plants	Effective Dose	Tested in	Days Treated	Ref.
Bauhinia variegata	2 g/kg	Animal models	20	12
B. variegata, C. mukul, G. glabra, and C. pluricaulis	100 mg from each plant (Thyrocap)	Humans	15	19
Echhorina crassipes	2 g/kg	Animal models	20	12
Bauhinia purpurea	2.5 mg/kg	Animal models	20	20
Commiphora mukul	0.2 g/kg	Animal models	15	21, 22
Withania somnifera	1.4 g/kg	Animal models	20	23
W. somnifera, C. mukul, B. purpurea	1.4 g, 0.2 g, 2.5 mg/kg	Animal models	30	24
Achyranthes aspera	200 mg/kg	Animal models	7	25
Saussurea lappa	400 mg/kg	Animal models	14	26
Inula racemosa	400 mg/kg	Animal models	21	27

antithyroidic drug, Neomercazole (15 mg three times/day), and the *Shankapushpi* extract (125 mg twice/day) for 9 months. They reported that the plant extract is more effective (as evident by 60 to 80% symptomatic recovery and significant changes in I^{131} uptake and concentration of serum cholesterol ($p < 0.05$ and $p < 0.01$, respectively), with no side effects as compared with the allopathic medicine. Another formulation, *Sutshekhar rasa sada* of Zandu Pharmaceuticals, is sometimes suggested for the amelioration of hyperthyroidism, and the recommended dose is 130 to 250 mg twice/day for 3 to 4 months (as recommended

TABLE 8.5

Promising Plant Extracts Suggested for the Treatment of Hyperthyroidism

Plants	Effective Dose	Tested in	Days Treated	Ref.
Lycopus virginicus	1–2 g	Humans	50	28
Azadirachta indica	100 mg/kg	Animal models	20	29
Momordica charantia	500 mg/kg	Animal models	15	30
Convolvulus plauricaulis	400 mg/kg	Animal models	30	31
Emblica officinalis	30 mg/kg	Animal models	20	32
Ocimum sanctum	0.5 g/kg	Animal models	15	33
Piper betel	0.1 g/kg	Animal models	15	34
Rauwolfia serpentina	2.5 mg/kg	Animal models	30	35
Trigonella foenum-graecum	0.11 g/kg	Animal models	15	36
Moringa oleifera	175 mg/kg	Animal models	10	37
Lithospermum officinale	400 mg/kg	Animal models	1	38
Melissa officinalis, L. verginicus, L. officinale	2 µg, 3 µg, 2 µg	Humans	1	39
Lithospermum ruderale	23 mg/kg	Animal models	5	40

by Zandu). According to some reports, *Potentilla alba* and *Kalanchoe brasiliensis* are also effective for the treatment of thyrotoxicosis.[15,16]

8.9 Conventional Medicine Treatment

Several preparations of L-Thyroxine, including Eltroxin and Synthroid, and thyroid extracts are used for hypothyroidism. Neomarcazole, Methimazole (Tapazole), Carbimazole, and Propyl thiouracil are commonly prescribed for hyperthyroidism. Radioiodine (not in pregnancy) and surgery are suggested in acute cases, but these medicines are not free from side effects[17,18] and are also expensive. A report revealed that 21 patients indicated abnormal T_4 suppression after receiving Carbimazole for 10 to 12 months and the disease relapsed after 1 year of stopping the therapy.[16] With Thyroxine therapy, side effects including bone fracture and sudden increase in heart rate have been observed.[5] As suggested by some other authors,[14] Ayurvedic medicines based on scientific studies appear to be the best choice.

8.10 Scientific Basis

For many years people have been using seaweed, including kelp, as a supplement of iodine, a basic component of thyroid hormones. Several plants have also been screened from time to time and few appear highly promising for the treatment of thyroid dysfunctions. Some important ones have been mentioned in Table 8.4 (for hypothyroidism) and in Table 8.5 (for hyperthyroidism) along with their respective references.[12,19–40] All these scientific studies are presented separately as clinical trials and pharmacological investigations.

8.10.1 Clinical Trials

8.10.1.1 Thyrocap

Thyrocap is a herbal preparation containing solid extracts of *Bauhinia variegata, Commiphora mukul, Glycyrrhiza glabra,* and *Convolvulus plauricaulis* (100 mg of each extract/capsule). This drug was prepared and tried in 50 patients of simple diffuse goiter at a dose of one capsule three times a day for 3 months.[19] After 3 months treatment, a marked improvement was noticed in weakness, fatigability, dyspnea, and reduction in neck swelling. A significant increase in serum T_4 and T_3 concentrations ($p < 0.001$ and < 0.02, respectively) and a decrease in serum cholesterol concentration ($p < 0.02$) confirmed its thyroid-stimulating property.

8.10.1.2 Kanchnara Guggul

Prepared from gum resin of *Commiphora mukul* and bark powder of *Bauhinia variegata, kanchnara guggul* (237 mg three times/day) was given to 899 tribal people of India bearing simple goiter. They were also asked to apply *Kanchnara* ointment simultaneously. Treatment was continued for 10 to 20 months. A 90 to 100% improvement was observed in the swelling of the gland in 163 patients, a 50 to 100% improvement was seen in 148 patients, and up to a 50% improvement was observed in 149 patients.[13] It was also observed that patients over 50 years old exhibited only 40 to 50% improvement.

8.10.1.3 Sankhapushpi Syrup

One hundred sixty thyrotoxicosis patients were divided into three groups. Group 1 (n = 100) received a standard allopathic drug, Neomercazole (15 mg/day), along with Diazepam (tranquilizer; 5 mg/day) B.D.; group 2 (n = 30) received 125 mg of Shakapushpi *(C. pluricaulis)* syrup alone B.D.; and group 3 (n = 30) was treated with equivalent doses of *Shankhapushpi* syrup and Neomercazole. The treatment was continued for 9 months. Maximum improvement (73 to 93%) in clinical features such as tremors, weakness, palpitation, increased appetite, and nervousness was observed in the *Shankhapushpi*-treated group. Thyroidal I^{131} uptake was also minimum in this group. These observations and a significant increase in serum cholesterol ($p < 0.01$) suggested that *Shankhapuspi* is a better thyroid inhibitor as compared with the modern allopathic drug, Neomercazole.[14]

8.10.1.4 Miscellaneous Studies

Some minor investigations have also been made on few plant extracts in relation to the regulation of hyperthyroidism in human beings.

It was discovered that a whole plant extract of *Lycopus verginicus* (bugle weed) at a dose of 1 to 2 g/day for 50 days could decrease serum TSH and T_4 levels in hyperthyroid patients, suggesting that it can ameliorate secondary hyperthyroidism caused by increased TSH.[28] In an *in vitro* study, extracts of *Melissa officinalis* (2 μg), *L. verginicus* (3 μg), *and L. officinalis* (2 μg) were found to decrease the TSH-binding activity in human thyroidal membrane when incubated for 24 h. These results indicate that these plant extracts are effective in secondary hyperthyroidism.[39]

Some scientific investigations have been made on animal models considering different plant extracts to suggest their potential use in further investigation toward the treatment of thyroid dysfunctions. Whereas some have been found to stimulate the production or release of thyroid hormones, others have been found to inhibit the same, indicating their possible use in hypothyroidism and hyperthyroidism, respectively.

8.10.2 Promising Plants for the Treatment of Hypothyroidism (Table 8.4)

8.10.2.1 *Bauhinia variegata*

This plant's water-soluble fraction of total alcoholic extract at a dose of 2 g/kg was fed to Neomercazole (150 mg/kg)-induced hypothyroidic rats (n = 12 in each group) for 20 days. The experiment resulted in enhanced thyroid function as evidenced by increased thyroidal weight ($p < 0.001$), I^{131}uptake and decreased serum cholesterol ($p < 0.05$ for both), and active thyroidal histology.[12] It was found that the action of this plant extract was comparable with Eltroxine.

8.10.2.2 *Echhornia crassipes*

In the same investigation, water-soluble fraction of *E. crassipes* ash at 2 g/kg/day for 20 days was also found to stimulate the thyroid function in the similar manner ($p < 0.001$ in all) as *B. variegata*.[12]

8.10.2.3 *Bauhinia purpurea*

Bark extract of *B. purpurea* at 2.5 mg/kg orally administered to female mice (n = 7 in each group) significantly increased serum T_3 and T_4 concentrations ($p < 0.001$ for both) after 20 days of treatment.[20]

8.10.2.4 *Commiphora mukul*

Commiphora mukul extract at a dose of 200 mg/kg administered for 15 days in mice (n = 10) significantly increased the T_3 concentration ($p < 0.001$) and also the food consumption ($p < 0.001$).[21] A dose of 200 mg of its petroleum ether extract was also earlier reported[22] to enhance thyroidal weight and I^{131} uptake ($p < 0.001$) in melatonin-induced (250 mg/kg) hypothyroid rats (n = 36).

8.10.2.5 *Withania somnifera*

Withania somnifera root extract at 1.4 g/kg, orally administered in albino mice (n = 10 in each group) for 20 days, stimulated both thyroid hormones ($p < 0.001$) without any hepatotoxic effect.[23] In another study, all three extracts (*B. purpurea, C. mukul,* and *W. somnifera*) were administered simultaneously to mice (n = 8) for 30 days at the doses mentioned above. The results showed an increase in both T_3 and T_4 levels ($p < 0.01$ and $p < 0.001$, respectively), suggesting that a combination of the three plant extracts may prove to be an effective treatment for hypothyroidism.[24]

8.10.2.6 *Achyranthes aspera*

Achyranthes aspera leaf extract administered in rats (n = 7) at a dose of 200 mg/kg for 7 days caused an increase of T_3 and T_4 ($p < 0.001$ for both). An increase in blood glucose in this group ($p < 0.05$) further supported the extract's thyroid-stimulating nature.[25]

8.10.2.7 Saussura lapa

Thyroid function stimulation as evidenced by thyroidal histology was reported in rats (n = 7) treated either with 400 mg/kg of *S. lapa* root extract for 14 days[26] or with the equivalent dose of *Inula racemosa* root extract for 20 days.[27]

8.10.3 Promising Plants for the Treatment of Hyperthyroidism (Table 8.5)

T_3 is metabolically the most potent thyroid hormone. Plants that have been found to decrease at least the serum level of this hormone have been suggested to act in the treatment of hyperthyroidism.

8.10.3.1 Azadirachta indica

Two doses (40 and 100 mg/kg) of the leaf extract of *A. indica* was administered in albino mice (n = 7 in each group) for 15 days; the higher dose could decrease the serum concentration of T_3 ($p < 0.05$). It was postulated that the inhibition of T_3 production was mediated through T_4 to T_3 conversion, the principal source of T_3 generation.[29]

8.10.3.2 Momordica charantia

Fruit extract of *M. charantia* (500 mg/kg) orally administered for 15 days decreased serum T_3 and T_4 concentrations ($p < 0.001$ for both) in mice (n = 8 in each group).[30] However, this dose was found to enhance hepatic lipid peroxidation (LPO).

8.10.3.3 Convolvulus pluricaulis

The root extract of *C. pluricaulis* (0.4 mg/kg/day for 30 days) administered to L-thyroxine-induced hyperthyroid mice (n = 7 in each group) decreased serum concentration of T_3 and hepatic 5-D activity. These results indicate that the plant extract-induced inhibition in thyroid function is primarily mediated through T_4 to T_3 conversion.[31]

8.10.3.4 Emblica officinalis

The fruit extract of *E. officinalis* at 30 mg/kg for 20 days decreased both serum T_3 and T_4 concentrations ($p < 0.05$ and < 0.001, respectively) in mice (n = 8 in each group). It was thought to decrease T_3 production particularly by inhibition of peripheral conversion of T_4 to T_3 in extra thyroidal tissues.[32]

8.10.3.5 Ocimum sanctum

The leaf extract (0.5 g/kg) of *O. sanctum* administered to male mice for 15 days (n = 10 in each group) significantly inhibited only T_4 concentration ($p < 0.001$).[33]

8.10.3.6 Piper betel

Administration of the *P. betel* leaf extract (0.1 g/kg) to male mice (n = 7) for 15 days significantly decreased both serum T_3 and T_4 concentrations ($p < 0.01$ for both).[34]

8.10.3.7 *Rauwolfia serpentina*

The *R. serpentina* root extract (2.5 mg/kg) administered to T_4-induced hyperthyroid mice (n = 7 in each group) for 30 days significantly decreased both the serum T_3 and T_4 concentrations ($p < 0.001$ for both).[35]

8.10.3.8 *Trigonella foenum graecum*

T. foenum graecum seed extract treatment (0.11 g/kg for 15 days) given to both mice and rats (n = 7 for both) decreased serum T_3 ($p < 0.01$ in mice and $p < 0.001$ in rats) and increased T_4 concentration ($p < 0.01$ in both mice and rats). The seed extract induced reduction in T_3 level could be the result of inhibition in peripheral conversion of T_4 to T_3 in extra thyroidal tissues.[36]

8.10.3.9 *Moringa oleifera*

M. oleifera leaf extract treatment (175 mg/kg) of female rats for 10 days (n = 14 for each group) decreased serum T_3 concentration ($p < 0.05$) and increased in serum T_4 concentration ($p < 0.05$). This observation suggests the inhibitory activity of the plant extract in the peripheral conversion of T_4 to T_3.[37]

8.10.3.10 *Lithospermum officinale*

An extract from the powdered leaf of *L. officinale*, administered at a dose of 400 mg/kg for 24 h to rats (n = 42), decreased serum T_3 concentration ($p < 0.01$) in TSH-induced hyperthyroidic animals.[38]

8.10.3.11 *Lithospermum ruderale*

The root extract of *L. ruderale* (23 mg/kg/day) administered to TSH-treated guinea pigs (n = 5) for 5 days decreased thyroid weight ($p < 0.01$) and exhibited low active thyroidal histology. The results suggested its antithyroidal nature.[40]

8.10.3.12 *Allium sativum*

A. sativum bulb extract (500 mg/kg) administered to hyperthyroid rats (n = 8) for 15 days showed a decrease in serum T_3 ($p < 0.05$) and cholesterol ($p < 0.05$) concentration.[41]

8.10.3.13 *Nelumbo nucifera*

Rhizome extract of *N. nucifera* (400 mg/kg) administered to rats (n = 8) for 15 days decreased both serum T_3 and T_4 concentrations ($p < 0.01$ and < 0.05, respectively).[42]

8.10.3.14 *Aloe vera*

Diluted parenchyma of *Aloe vera* leaf at 125 mg/kg/day administered for 15 days in mice (n = 7 in each group) has been reported to inhibit both T_4 and T_3 concentrations ($p < 0.05$ and < 0.01, respectively).[43]

8.10.3.15 *Aegle marmelos*

Dried leaf powder extract of *A. marmelos* at a dose of 1 g/kg/day for 15 days significantly ($p < 0.001$) decreased only serum T_3 concentration.[43]

All these findings indicate the plant-specific role in the regulation of thyroid functions. Although some were found to be thyroid stimulatory as evidenced by the increase in serum T_3 and/or T_4 concentrations, the others were inhibitory to either one or both of the thyroid hormones. Although these finding do not claim to cure or treat the thyroid dysfunctions, certainly the plants can be further studied for their potential use in the treatment of hypo- and hyperthyroidism.

8.11 Prevention Strategies

Because thyroid-related problems affect nearly all systems of the body, it is advisable to take some preventive measures, particularly when one or more symptoms of thyroid abnormalities (see Table 8.1) are observed. For the prevention of hypothyroidism, it is important to supply the thyroid gland with adequate quantity of nutrients so that it can manufacture the required amount of thyroid hormones. If hypofunctioning of the gland is suspected, one has to avoid the goitrogenic food such as rapeseed, cabbage, cauliflower, kale, and turnip. One should also ensure the iodine intake of 150 μg/day through food and water supplementation apart from using filtered water with less chloride and fluoride.

Left untreated, hyperthyroidism has a serious consequence and much precaution should be taken for its prevention. Scientists believe that hyperthyroidism has a genetic susceptibility. People who have a family history of thyrotoxicosis should avoid stress, trauma (both physical and mental), and excessive steroid therapy, which are very often considered as causative factors. From a safer point of view, serum T_4, T_3, and TSH should be estimated every year to ascertain the thyroid status and accordingly follow medical advice, if warranted.

8.12 Summary

Considering all the literature available on Ayurvedic therapies in the regulation of thyroid dysfunction, it can be said that the management of the thyroid problems in Ayurveda is nearly similar to the conventional allopathic therapy, because both primarily aim to augment thyroid function (for hypothyroidism) or to reduce it (for hyperthyroidism). However, herbal therapy appears to be safe when compared with the modern allopathic treatment.[14] This is because Ayurvedic preparations include mainly herbs that make the body work more efficiently while supporting many complex functions. Moreover, herbal extracts possess natural antioxidants, which not only help in curing the diseases, but also improve the body's defense system. On the downside, allopathic drugs and chemicals interfere in the body's natural process, resulting in unwanted side effects. Because they offer fewer or no side effects, herbal therapies should be preferred in the treatment of thyroid dysfunctions.

Herbal therapies should be specific, considering the specific type of thyroid diseases and imbalance in the particular type of thyroid or pituitary hormone. In fact, recent researches have revealed a differential role of herbal extracts in relation to the regulation of thyroid function. Although some plant extracts are potent in altering both thyroid hormones, others have been found to be effective in correcting either T_4 or T_3 levels.

8.13 Suggested Future Research

Although some Ayurvedic preparations are already available for the regulation of thyroid dysfunctions, further research is required. Thyroid problems are indirectly related to many other diseases, including diabetes and gastrointestinal, neural, and heart problems. Further investigations on the different aspects of herbal regulation may provide a better understanding on the Ayurvedic management of thyroid dysfunctions. It is suggested that research activities should be undertaken in the following areas:

1. Screening of more plants to find out the highly effective plant extracts for the treatment of thyroid diseases
2. Concentration-dependent studies to identify safe and effective doses
3. Long-term effectiveness studies of the plant extracts to optimize the duration of treatment
4. Comparative studies on the active compounds and crude extracts
5. Target-specific studies on plants acting either at glandular level or at the level of peripheral tissues, including the liver and kidney, which produce maximum amount of T_3 in both human and animal models

Acknowledgments

This chapter is dedicated to the late Shri M.J. Kar (first author's father). We are thankful to Dr. M. Ghollap for his help in literature collection, and Prof. S. Bharti, Prof. K.N. Guruprasad, and Abhishek Kar for their encouragement. Many of our results presented in this chapter are from the investigation made under UGC Research award scheme, sanctioned to A. Kar.

References

1. Pocock, G. and Richards, C.D., The thyroid gland, in *Human Physiology: The Basis of Medicine*, Oxford University Press, New York, 1999, p. 212.
2. Sengupta, N.N., *The Ayurvedic System of Medicine*, Logos Press, New Delhi, India, 1999, p. 268.
3. Ganong, W.F., The thyroid gland, in *Review of Medical physiology*, 7th ed., Appleton and Lange, Norwalk, CT, 1995, p. 295.
4. Turner, C.D. and Bagnara, J.T., The thyroid gland, in *General Endocrinology*, 6th ed., W.B. Saunders, Philadelphia, 1976, p. 178.
5. Williams, J.B., Adverse effects of thyroid hormones, *Drugs and Aging*, 11, 460, 1997.
6. Aaseth, J. et al., Selenium concentrations in the human thyroid gland, *Biol. Trace Elem. Res.*, 24, 147, 1990.
7. Chaurasia, S.S. et al., Free radical mediated membrane perturbation and inhibition of type-I iodothyronine 5′-monodeiodinase activity by lead and cadmium in rat liver homogenate, *Biochem. Mol. Biol. Int.*, 39, 765, 1996.

8. Maiti, P.K. et al., Loss of membrane integrity and inhibition of type-1 iodothyronine monodeiodinase enzyme activity by Fenvalerate in female mice, *Biochem. Biophys. Res. Comm.*, 214, 905, 1995.
9. Hershman, J.M., Hyperthyroidism caused by chronic gonadotropin, in Werner and Ingbar's *The Thyroid: A Fundamental and Clinical Text*, Braverman, L.E. and Utiger, R.D., Eds., Lippincott–Williams & Wilkins, New York, 2000, chap. 32.
10. Greenspan, F.S., The thyroid gland, in *Basic and Clinical Endocrinology*, 4th ed., Greenspan, F.S. and Baxter, J.D., Eds., Appleton and Lange, Norwalk, CT, 1994, p. 160.
11. Dhawan, D. and Goel, A. Hepatoprotective effects of Liv-52 and its indirect influence on the regulation of thyroid hormones in rat liver toxicity induced by carbon tetrachloride, *Res. Exp. Med.*, 194, 203, 1994.
12. Veena, K. et al., Effect of indigenous drugs on experimentally produced goiter, *J. Res. Ind. Med.*, 10, 19, 1975.
13. Ghallop, M., Ghenga roga chikitsa me Ayurveda ek bardan (in Hindi), *Bulletin of Adimzati and Vikash Pradhikaran*, Indore, India, 19, 1991.
14. Gupta, R.C. et al., Probable mode of action of shankpuspi in the management of thyrotoxicosis, *Ancient Sci. Life*, 1, 46, 1981.
15. Prikhod'ko, E.I., Treatment of thyrotoxicosis with the herb *Potentilla alba, V. Del.*, 87, 1976.
16. Ferreira, A.C., Rosenthal, D., and Carvalho, D.P., Thyroid peroxidase inhibition by *Kalanchoe brasiliensis* aqueous extract, *Food Chem. Toxicol.*, 38, 417, 2000.
17. Vitug, A.C. and Goldman, J.M., Hepatotoxicity from antithyroid, *Drugs Horm. Res.*, 21, 229, 1985.
18. Goswami, R. et al., Remission with Carbimazole therapy and associated T_4 suppression acts as an index of relapse on patients with Grave's disease in India, *Indian J. Med. Res.*, 103, 272, 1996.
19. Pandit, R.K., Gupta, R.C., and Prasad, G.C., Effect of an herbal compound: thyrocap in the patients of simple diffuse goiter, *J. Res. Edu. Ind. Med.*, 13, 16, 1992.
20. Panda, S. and Kar, A., *Withania somnifera* and *Bauhinia purpurea* in the regulation of circulating thyroid hormone concentrations in female mice, *J. Ethnopharmacology*, 67, 233, 1999.
21. Panda, S. and Kar, A., Guggulu (*Commiphora mukul*) induces triiodothyronine production: possible involvement of lipid peroxidation, *Life Sci.*, 65, 137, 1999.
22. Singh, A.K., Tripathi, S.N., and Prasad, G.C., Response of *Commiphora mukul* (guggulu) on Melatonin induced hypothyroidism, *Ancient Sci. Life*, 3, 85, 1983.
23. Panda, S. and Kar, A., Changes in thyroid hormone concentrations after administration of Ashwagandha root extract in adult male mice, *J. Pharm. Pharmacol.*, 50, 1065, 1998.
24. Panda, S. and Kar, A., Combined effects of ashwagandha, guggulu and bauhinia extracts in the regulation of thyroid function and on lipid peroxidation in mice, *J. Pharm. Pharmacol.*, 6, 141, 2000.
25. Tahiliani, P. and Kar, A., *Achyranthes aspera* elevates thyroid hormone levels and decreases hepatic lipid peroxidation in male rats, *J. Ethnopharmacol.*, 71, 527, 2000.
26. Chaturvedi, P. et al., Effect of *Saussurea lappa* alcoholic extract on different endocrine glands in relation to glucose metabolism in the rat, *Phytother. Res.*, 7, 205, 1993.
27. Tripathi, Y.B. and Chaturvedi, P., Assessment of endocrine response of *Inula racemosa* in relation to glucose homeostasis in rats, *Ind. J. Exp. Biol.*, 33, 686, 1995.
28. Blumenthal, M., The complete commission: E monographs, in *Therapeutic Guide to Herbal Medicines*, Integrative Medicine Communications, Boston, 1998, p. 98.
29. Panda, S. and Kar, A., How safe is neem extract with respect to thyroid function in male mice?, *Pharmacol. Res.*, 41, 419, 2000.
30. Panda, S. and Kar, A., Excess use of *Momordica charantia* extract may not be safe with respect to thyroid function and lipid peroxidation, *Curr. Sci.*, 79, 222, 2000.
31. Panda, S. and Kar, A., Inhibition of T_3 production in levothyroxine-treated female mice by the root extract of *Convolvulus pluricaulis, Horm. Metab. Res.*, 33, 16, 2001.
32. Panda, S., Bharti, S., and Kar, A., *Emblica officinalis* and *Bauhinia purpurea* in the regulation of thyroid function and lipid peroxidation in male mice, *J. Herbs Spices Med.*, 10, 1, 2002.

33. Panda, S. and Kar, A., *Ocimum sanctum* in the regulation of thyroid function in male mouse, *Pharmacol. Res.*, 38, 107, 1998.
34. Panda, S. and Kar, A., Betel leaf can be both peroxidative and antiperoxidative in nature, *Curr.* Sci., 74, 284, 1998.
35. Panda, S. and Kar, A., Regulation of hyperthyroidism by *Rauwolfia serpentina* root extract in mice, *Pharm. Pharmacol. Commun.*, 6, 517, 2000.
36. Panda, S., Tahiliani, P., and Kar, A., Inhibition of triiodothyronine production by fenugreek seed extract in mice and rats, *Pharmacol. Res.*, 40, 405, 1999.
37. Tahiliani, P. and Kar, A., Role of *Moringa oleifera* leaf extract in the regulation of thyroid hormone status in adult male and female rats, *Pharmacol. Res.*, 41, 319, 2000.
38. Winterhoff, H., Sourgens, H., and Kemper, F.H., Antihormonal effect of plant extracts — pharmacodynamic effects of *Lithospermum officinale* on the thyroid gland of rats: comparison with the effects of iodide, *Horm. Metab. Res.*, 15, 503, 1983.
39. Auf'mkolk, M. et al., Inhibition by certain plant extracts on binding and adenylate cyclase stimulatory effect of bovine thyrotropin in human thyroid membranes, *J. Endocrinol.*, 115, 527, 1984.
40. Noble, R.L., Plunkett, E.R., and Gragham, R.C.B., Direct hormone inactivation by extracts of *Lithospermum ruderale*, *J. Endocrinol.*, 10, 212, 1954.
41. Tahiliani, P. and Kar, A., Mitigation of thyroxine induced hyperglycaemia by two plant extracts, *Phytother. Res.*, 13, 11, 2003.
42. Tahiliani, P. and Kar, A., Relative roles of some plant extracts in the regulation of serum thyroid hormones and glucose concentrations in female rats, *J. Med. Aromatic Plant. Sci.*, 23, 64, 2001.
43. Kar, A., Panda, S., and Bharti, S., Relative efficacy of three medicinal plant extracts in the alteration of thyroid hormone concentrations in male mice, *J. Ethnopharmacol.*, 81, 281, 2002.

9

Obesity (Medoroga) in Ayurveda

Ashok D.B. Vaidya, Rama A. Vaidya, Bharati A. Joshi, and Nutan S. Nabar

CONTENTS

9.1 Introduction

Several centuries ago before foreign rule, India was one of the world's most affluent nations, and the affluence and sedentary habits at that time were known to be the leading cause of obesity.[1,2] This was due to a deadly imbalance of high energy input through rich foods and low energy expenditure due to lack of physical exercise. Daily and seasonal health regimens

0-8493-1366-X/04/$0.00+$1.50

(*swasthavritta* and *ritucharya*) and other modalities, such as detailed instructions on a proper balanced diet and appropriate levels of exercise as per the constitution (*prakriti*) of the person, have been laid out clearly in Ayurvedic texts.[3] It is interesting to note that the world is now again focusing on a healthy lifestyle as key to avoiding risk factors like obesity.[4]

The pioneers of Ayurveda, 2 millennia ago, have described the unhealthy consequences of obesity. Charaka, who may be called as the Indian Hippocrates, described obesity as a disease of the fat tissue (*medoroga*) leading to hugeness (*sthoulyam*).[5] The Sanskrit word *sthoulya* is derived from *sthool*, meaning gross or material.[6] Nondrug and drug modalities to prevent and reduce obesity were elaborated and regularly utilized. Even now there are millions of Indians who do avail themselves of some of these interventions in their daily lives. The prevalence of obesity is higher in urban areas than in rural populations of India, due to a steady erosion of the Ayurveda way of life in the cities as well as the sedentary and overeating habit factor.

Being a holistic system of health care, Ayurveda has emphasized the psychospiritual dimensions in its philosophy; mere drugging without holistic healing is not advocated. The hierarchy of the spiritual, psychological, and physical levels of human health and disease is given due importance.

The disease management approaches in Ayurveda have two basic principles: repletion of the body tissues (*brimhan*) or the depletion (*karshan*) of them, as required. For this process, the groups of modalities used are spiritual and the karmic interventions (*daivavyapashraya*), astral and psychological measures (*satwavajaya*), and nondrug and drug modalities (*yuktivyapashraya*). The holistic base of Ayurveda provides a different kind of evidence than the current reliance on randomized controlled trials.[7] The clinical effects are evident in the field.

This chapter may embolden the open-minded physicians of the world to learn from Ayurveda — a live and growing system of health that is more than 5000 years old.[8] There are leads which can be followed-up proactively for research, too.[9] The current understanding of adipose tissue as an endocrine organ coupled with the successful leads from Ayurveda may form a scientific basis for the management of obesity.[10] Already, *Commiphora wightii* (*guggulu*) is emerging as a drug of global potential for obesity and hyperlipidemia.[11]

9.2 *Agni* and *Srotas* with Reference to Obesity

As per Ayurveda, *agni* is the cosmic fire — the principle of transformations of materials. It is the energy or capacity of the body to convert complex food materials to their constitutents and then to build the body tissues (*dhatus*).[12] The first and foremost level of *Agni* is digestive fire (*jatharagni*).[13] It digests all types of food in the stomach and the small intestine. The digested and absorbed essence of the food material is called *ahar rasa*, which circulates, providing the substrates for tissues. For each of the seven tissues, there is a special energy or digestive power (*dhatwagni*)[14] assimilating the digested substrates. The lipid precursors are acted upon by fat-specific energy (*medodhatwagni*) for its conversion into adipose tissue (*medadhatu*). The channels and the loci where these conversions take place are called *srotas* or *dhatuvahasrotas*. The quality of all the specific energies depends on the quality of the digestive fire, which is protected and maintained carefully. The impairement of the digestive fire and the specific tissue energies lead to poor availability of the constitutents and depletion of tissues (*dhatukshaya*).

With the substrates and energies in balance, all the metabolic activities occur properly in the channels. Defects in the sources with undigested matter block tissue channels. A healthy person is one in whom the activites of humor (*dosa*), tissue (*dhatu*), wastes (*mala*), fire, mind (*manas*), soul (*atma*), and senses are harmonious and in balance.[15]

9.3 Adipose Tissue (*Medodhatu*) and Dynamics

Any disequilibrium in *kapha* humor, fat-specific energy, and waste products of adipose tissues (*kleda*) leads to a dysfunction of adipose tissue — obesity. Adipose channels have two origins: the kidneys, adrenals, and fat around them *(vrukkas)* and the visceral and omental fat (*vapavahan*).[16] These channels draw the nutritive parts (*medoposhakansh*), including lipid, from the antedecent flesh (*mansa dhatwagni*) and the transient lipids (*asthayi*) and then they are converted into a stored form (*sthayi*) of lipid.

Adipose-tissue dynamics is a crucial link for the tissue metabolism. Low adipose energy, despite a normal food intake, could lead to a steady accumulation of fat (*apachith*) and obesity. Excessive consumption of fat and oils, lack of exercise, and overindulgence of wine and sleeping during daytime can disturb the fat channels, as mentioned in Charaka.[17]

9.4 Measurement of Obesity

To determine the normal physique of a person, Charaka gave a standard termed as proportionate body (*samasanhanan nara*), with appropriate measurements and compactness.[18] Gangadhar, a later author, has given the measurements of various parts of body for a normal physic. According to Charaka, fat gets deposited mainly in the abdomen (*udara*), so the measurement of the abdomen size was considered to determine obesity.[19] The exact dimensions given in the text are not relevant today.

9.5 Obesity, Health Risks, and Life Span

Recent importance of obesity control and its adverse impact on health was presaged 1000 years ago by Bhavamishra and Madhavakar. Today, with a better understanding of the reference to the importance of the visceral and abdominal obesity as a cardiovascular risk factor, the reference in ancient texts seems a valuable insight of the seers.[19] We have yet to understand what they have foreseen in the reference about fat accumulation around the kidneys. The management of morbid obesity was considered difficult and the prognosis grave if other risk factors were also present. Decreased life span (*ayu-kshaya*) is stated to be an important consequence of obesity. Even today, early diagnosis and timely management of obesity is mostly neglected because few people realize that obesity is associated with increased mortality.[20] Charaka emphasized that serious diseases (*darun vikar*) arise when fat blocks channels. Sushruta describes several complications of obesity such as tumors and space-occupying lesions like tumorous growth, diabetes mellitus (DM), and

TABLE 9.1

Features of Obesity

Symptom	Charak	Sushrut	Vagbhat	Bhavmishra	Madhavkar
Visceral obesity (*udarvrudhi*)	+	+	+	+	+
Flaccidity (*angashaithilya*)	+	–	–	+	+
Pendulous abdomen (*chalodara*)	+	–	+	+	+
Pendulous breasts (*chala-stana*)	+	–	+	-	+
Pendulous buttocks (*chala-sphik*)	+	–	+	+	+
Heaviness in body (*gourav*)	+	–	–	–	–
Weakness (*dourbalya*)	+	–	–	–	–
Poor self-care (*swakriya-asamarthata*)	+	+	–	–	–
Less coitus (*krichha-vyavaya*)	+	+	–	+	+
Oversleeping (*nidradhikya*)	+	+	+	+	+
Lethargy (*utsaha-nash*)	+	+	+	–	–
Breathlessness (*kshudra-shwasa*)	+	+	–	+	+
Oversweating (*swedati-pravruti*)	+	+	+	+	+
Bad body odor (*dourgandhya*)	+	+	+	+	+
Excessive thirst (*trishnadhikya*)	+	+	+	+	+
Polyphagia (*kshudhadikya*)	+	+	+	+	+
Delicate and tender (*sukumarata*)	+	+	–	–	–
Short life (*ayushyarrhasa*)	+	+	–	+	+

excessive perspiration. Thirty to fifty percent postmenopausal women in the U.S. are said to be overweight.[21]

9.6 Symptoms and Signs

The three major and three minor Ayurvedic treatises (i.e., Charak, Sushruta, and Vagbhat and Madhavnidhan, Bhavaprakasha, and Sharangdhar, respectively) give detailed descriptions of obese individuals and their afflications. Table 9.1 summarizes these descriptions as given by the first five treatises.[15,19,22–24] Bhavamishra describes additional features of obesity such as difficulty in breathing and the emergence of a snoring sound from the throat while breathing. Snoring and daytime sleepiness are important markers of obesity that were well recognized in Ayurveda.[19] In extreme forms of obesity, obesity-hypoventilation (OHV), or Pickwickian syndrome, and obstructive sleep apnea (OSA) are severe as reported in conventional medical literature.[25] They lead to pulmonary hypertension and often to a degree of cardiac failure. There is a spectrum of sleep-related disordered breathing in obesity that varies from simple snoring to OHV. Recognition of the association of OSA, obesity, and daytime sleepiness in conventional medicine is quite recent. Daytime sleeping contributes to obesity. OSA is associated with increased rates of hypertension, stroke, ischemic heart disease, and mortality.[26]

9.7 Obesity and Affect Disorders

Obese people are depressed and often experience sadness as per one of the Ayurvedic texts (*Bhavamishra*).[19] As physicians, we must recognize that obesity, a heterogenous disorder, does have psychopathology as a cause in an individual with a possible familial, environmental,

TABLE 9.2

Etiology of Obesity as per Ayurveda

Ayurvedic Factors	Allopathic Correlates
No exercise (*avyayama*)	Lack of exercise
Dense food (*sleshmal ahara*)	Fattening diet and foods
Daytime sleeping (*diva swapna*)	Obesity sleep apnea
No sexual intercourse (*avyavaya*)	Difficulty in intercourse
No anxiety (*achinta*)	Affect disorders
Genetic (*beeja-dosa*)	Genetic basis
Prodromal signs (*prameha-poorvarupa*)	Hyperinsulinemia
Loss of appetite (*agnimandya*)	Low energy expenditure
Lipotoxicity (*medavrittavayu*)	Defective satiety cascade
Lack of restraint (*ahara-asamyama*)	Environmental food clues
Tissue indigestion (*apathya-dhatwagni*)	Stress and hormones

or hereditary basis. According to modern medicine, specific organic causes may rarely be present. Metabolic and psychological (e.g., depression) pathologies often present together and are associated with dysregulation of the hypothalamo-pituitary adrenal axis.[27] Affect disorders are also reported among obese binge eaters (OBEs). Sixty percent of OBE had one or more psychiatric disorders. Some of the OBEs also had a lifetime prevalence of affective disorders as well as more frequent mood fluctuations and panic attacks.

9.8 Obesity and Diabetes Type 2-NIDDM (*Madhumeha*)

Sushruta, though classifying disorders according to their causes, has stated obesity and DM as the disorders of adipose tissue.[28] Charaka attributes the voracious appetite of obese people to increase in humor (*vata*) and digestive fire, which together rapidly consume ingested food. This leads to increased frequency and amount of food intake. This further increases the fat accumulation, particularly in the abdomen, breasts, and buttocks. The extent of fat accumulation, in these parts is so great that they become pendulous. Clogged fat channels in Ayurveda, as described earlier, then cause preclinical symptoms of urinary disorders (*prameha*) such as perspiration, bad body odor, flaccidity of the body, a desire sleep or sit, thickening of layers on teeth, accumulation of waste in eyes, nose, ears, mouth, etc., sweet taste in mouth, burning sensation of palms and soles, and dryness of the throat and palate.[29]

9.9 Etiological Factors for Obesity (*Karana-Hetu*)

"The central causes of all disease are the vitiated *Malas*, induced by harmful diet and lifestyles."[30] According to Ayurveda, the central cause of almost all diseases is the vitiation of wastes (*malas* — the end products of *dhatus*) and vitation of humor (*dosa* provocation). This is due to harmful regimens of foods and beverages, rest and exercise, restraint and indulgence, etc. (see Table. 9.2). Both Ayurveda and conventional medicine have considered obesity as multifactorial.

TABLE 9.3
Body Mass Index (BMI) and Obesity

Classification	BMI (kg/m^2)
Normal	18.5–24.9
Overweight or pre-obese	25.0–29.9
Obese Class 1	30.0–34.9
Obese Class 2	35.0–39.9
Obese Class 3	>40

9.10 Diagnosis and Markers of Overweight and Obesity

Differences in overweight *(pushta)*, obesity, and morbid obesity *(ati sthoulya)* were recognized in Ayurveda. The measures of normality of the body structure have been described as follows. Charaka described the assessment of obesity by the patient's own fingers (*angulapramana*), breadth, and length (midcarpal–middle finger level) to be borders defined on the abdomen. This may be investigated through the waist–hip ratio (WHR), waist circumference (WC), and body–fat ratio analysis.

According to conventional medicine, the body mass index (BMI) is a simple method of estimating adiposity. It is calculated as weight in kilograms divided by the square of the height in meters (kg/m^2). The World Health Organization (WHO) has classified individuals as per BMI (Table 9.3). Class 3 obese is considered morbidly obese.

It is now well recognized that central or visceral obesity is more important as a risk factor for cardiovascular diseases (CVDs) and noninsulin-dependent DM (NIDDM), independent of general obesity.[31] Accurate assessment for the central and visceral obesity is paramount in evaluation of obesity. WHR and WC correlate better with degree of CVD risks. High accumulation of the upper body fat (abdominal) is associated with high plasma triglyceride levels. A high WHR is shown to be associated with dyslipidemia.

For clinical services and epidemiological studies, the measurements of height, weight, BMI, WHR, or WC are important and suffice. For research purposes, more sophisticated methods like electrical impedence, dual absorptiometry (DEXA), and other imaging techniques such as computered-aided tomography scan (CAT-scan) and magnetic resonance imaging (MRI) may be required. Other markers of obesity are hypertension, hyperpigmentation (*Acanthosis nigricans*), skin tags, hirsuitism, menstrual dysfunctions, and female infertility. Hyperinsulinemia, hyperglycemia (type II DM), and hyperlipidemia are given associated biochemical features.

In a series of 90 cases of polycystic ovarian syndrome (PCOS) with hirsutism at our clinic, only 23% had normal weight. The rest were either overweight or obese. Sixty percent of these women were in their teens.[32] Infertility and menstrual dysfunctions due to anovulation, abortions, and increased fetal wastage, and gestational diabetes are common among women with PCOS.

9.11 Clinical Course and Prognosis of Obesity

The long-term adverse impact on health has been well described in Ayurveda, including diminished life span (*vide supra*). Obesity-related increase in complications like NIDDM and CVDs (including hypertension and arthritis) are well known. However, obesity-related cryptogenic cirrhosis of the liver and hepatocellular carcinoma has recently been recognized. In spite of the rising incidence of obesity and NIDDM, obese individuals are often not screened for nonalcoholic fatty infiltration of the liver and nonalcoholic steatohepatitis (NASH). Early diagnosis and treatment of NASH in overweight and obese patients may prevent hepatocellular carcinoma in cryptogenic cirrhosis of the liver. The incidence of the hepatocellular carcinoma among these patients is reported to be 27%. This rate is similar to that found among hepatitis C virus-related cirrhosis (21%). Early and persistent long-term interventions can certainly alter the progressive course and complications of obesity. Even a 5 to 10% loss in body weight can reduce the risk caused by obesity. Diet, exercise, and stress management can also reduce insulin resistance (IR) in a patient. Ayurvedic way of life is the need for altering the course of obesity.

Weight gains during adolescence in boys and girls, enormous weight gains during and after pregnancy, and peri-post menopausal obesity are noted frequently in clinics that are dedicated to management of obesity. These transitional physiological phases are known to be associated with changes in insulin resistance (IR) and physiological hyperinsulinemia. An antiobesity preventive measure for such physiological phases for smooth transitions may save many individuals, particularly women, a lifetime burden of obesity and its health consequences.

9.12 Prevention of Obesity

The knowledge of the etiological factors and their lifelong avoidance, besides the countermeasures, constitute the foundation of prevention of obesity in Ayurveda and other systems of medicine.[33]

Ayurveda has much to offer for prevention in terms of daily and seasonal regimens, healthy foods, yoga exercise, *panchakarma,* and medicines. The daily routine in Ayurveda involves the following:

1. Going to bed early and waking up early
2. Proper eliminations, tongue cleaning, washing, etc.
3. Meditation
4. Massage
5. Sun-yoga-*asana* (*surya-namaskar*)
6. Proper clothing
7. Suitable, balanced, and measured dietary intake
8. Adequate fluid intake
9. Family, friends, and community relationships
10. Avoidance of undue stress or exertion
11. Pleasant, healthy, and socially permissible sex life
12. Continuing self-education etc.[3]

Similarly, as per the seasons and climate and age of the person, certain regimens are to be followed to maintain health and prevent diseases. *Chyavanprash* in the winter, *gulkand* in the summer, and ginger candy in the monsoon are taken still by millions of Indians as seasonal foods. Bitter and astringent items are also included in the diet.

Education in daily healthy lifestyle should begin very early. Functional information on health, diet, proper exercise, and stress management, given in an incremental manner at the school level, would prove beneficial for prevention of adult obesity. The predictors of weight gain — genetic, metabolic, and demographic — can be identified early and appropriate steps can be taken. Overweight parents have overweight children. In twin studies, heritability estimates are 30 to 50%. Early genetic diagnosis would help identify need for prevention strategies with the advances in genomics. This would assist early Ayurvedic and modern preventive interventions in highly obesity-prone persons.

Breathing yoga practices (*pranayama*) under guidance of a proper expert are advisable for all persons prone to obesity, besides other measures. Meditation and yoga physical and breathing practices (*asanas* and *pranayama*) diminish the sympathetic overdrive, which has a role in inducing IR and obesity. Only massive public health education and values of restraint despite affluence can help prevent the rising prevalence of obesity globally. Ayurveda and modern medical measures have to be individualized for their synergy by practicing doctors and health educators.

9.13 Management of Obesity (*Chikitsa*)

9.13.1 Purification Modalities

The five modes of eliminating Nature's waste by *panchakarma* to reestablish the harmony of *dosas* is a unique gift of Ayurveda.[34] These modes are often preceded by the preparatory oil-therapy (*snehan*) and induced sweating (*swedana*) (see Chapter 4). Oil therapy is not indicated for those who do not exercise or are very obese or very thin.[35] It is also not given to those who have voracious appetites or anorexia. Before oil therapy is carried out in the obese, the vitiated digestive fire will have to undergo drying through controlled dieting and then careful oleation will produce benefit. The oil dose frequency can be individualized as necessary.

Induced sweating usually after oil therapy is indicated to transport the vitiated *dosas* to the trunk (*koshtha*). As per Ayurveda, dry heat, hot poultice, slow hot shower and sauna-bath, and hot-water bottles are used to induce sweating.[36] Sweating can be induced for patients with *kapha* diseases without preceding oil therapy. The parts of the body to be warmed have been described and are followed carefully by the experts. Very obese people are contraindicated for sweating therapy before reducing their weight to a reasonable level with other measures like diet, exercise, and medicine.

Induced therapeutic vomiting is indicated in *kapha*-dominant diseases. The procedures, contraindications, and cautions of this procedure are well described elsewhere in this textbook.[37] Besides preparations for *panchakarma*, follow-up (*paschatkarma*) is equally vital. *Only qualified and experienced vaidyas should engage in panchakarma therapy.*

Of the five purification procedures, the enema (*basti*) is the major component, as it controls the *vata*, which is responsible for the disease. In addition, enemas also cause cleaning of bowels (*malashooddhi*), which reestablish proper balanced metabolism within the tissue elements. Enema decoction of roots of ten medicinal plants (*dashasmool*) and fruits of three medicinal plants (*triphala*) are indicated for their *vataghna* and *tridoshhar* properties frequently used in obesity.[39] To prevent aggravation of *vata*, an oil enema

TABLE 9.4

Preparations To Be Taken after Panchakarma Therapy

Preparation	Frequency of Intake after Elimination Therapy
Gruel (*peya*)	3 times/day
Rice gruel (*vilepi*)	3 times/day
Incomplete soup (*akruta yusha*)	3 times/day
Complete soup (*kruta yusha*)	3 times/day
Incomplete meat soup (*akruta mansarasa*)	3 times/day
Complete meat soup (*kruta mansarasa*)	3 times/day

(*anuwasan basti*) is then given in succession initially. The decoction and oil enemas are given alternately until 8 or 15 days, depending upon symptomatic response. *Shirobasti* of oil is also advisable to counter stress element.

9.13.2 Palliative Therapy

For obese patients, according to the symptoms of *ama*, digestive (*dhatwagni deepan*) and carminative (*pachan*) medications are given. Ayurvedic formulation of a *guggulu kalpa* decoction (e.g., *triphala guggulu, medohara guggulu, arogyavardhini, chandraprabhavati, shilajitvati, loharasayan vati, dashamoolarishta, manjisthadi*) are also advised with appropriate doses (as per age, sex, severity of obesity) with water or decoction of *triphala*.

Gentle oil massage is followed by massage with powders of medicinal plants (turmeric, sandalwood, rosepowder, *manjistha* powder, chickpea flour) along the antidirection of the lanugo hairs, reducing perspiration and its smell.

A diet known as *sansarjankrama* is advised as per the quality results obtained after elimination therapy and the state of digestive fire.[40] It includes rice preparations (*manda, peya, vilepi*) and soups of meat in successive days. Some of the preparations are mentioned in Table 9.4.

The current common treatment of obesity in Ayurveda involves the following:

1. Nondrug modalities of reasonable fasting with dieting, exercise, and yoga and lifestyle changes and counseling to stress, sleep, sex, etc.
2. Diverse formulations and sometimes single plants with appropriate individualized dosage needs

The weight loss is expected to be gradual, long term, and lasting due to integral care rather than drastic weight loss advocated by crash dieting.[38] Individual *prakruti*, aptitude, tastes, profession, peer support, motivation, relationships, and stage of obesity are carefully looked into for a successful outcome of the therapeutic program.

9.13.3 Baseline Acceptance of the Patient's State

Hidden within every obese person, a thin person with a proportionate body is struggling to emerge. Similarly, in every adult there is a hidden child who may regress to oral phase of development under stress.

A physician's nonjudgmental attitude about the patient's body image earns the patient's trust and builds the foundation for a long-term, warm, and effective patient–physician relationship; it is also essential for a sustained motivation, continued long-term compliance management. The repressed sexuality has to be rekindled by subtle and persistent professional counseling, as lack of sexual intercourse is one of the causative factors in obesity in Ayurveda. The aforesaid have to be complemented by lifestyle changes in exercise, sleep, and stress management. The patient's friend, spouse, or family member, as well as the team, has to be firm and supportive for long-term care and compliance (*chatushpada*).

9.13.4 Dietary and Nutrient Diet

The diet for treating obesity has to be individualized as per the level of the caloric needs, energy expenditure, tastes, lifestyle, weight-loss goals, medicines, and other measures used. No formula diets or regimens are usually followed in Ayurveda. In reducing the bulk of a person, food that is heavy but falls in the category of a low-fat diet (*apatarpan*) is beneficial. Roasted pulses (*bharjit dhanya*) such as green beans (*mudga*), dolichos (*kulatha*), and barley (*yava*) are beneficial.

9.13.5 Energy Expenditure and Hormonal Stress

As per Charaka, occasional staying awake at night, sexual intercourse, physical exercise, and mental exertion should also be gradually indulged in to reduce fat. The patients are advised to walk at least 1 h in the morning or evening with regularity and consistency. Adolescent and young adults are advised to engage in vigorous sports and exercise. Movements of shoulder girdle and pelvic girdle are advised to prevent sarcopenia *(mansadaurbalya*). Yoga, particularly physical asanas (*hathayoga*) with mind control (*rajayoga*), is to be integrated in daily routine. Yoga in everyday life (i.e., sun salutations [*suryanamaskar*]) is an excellent dawn practice that has been and continues to be an integral part of Indian life.

9.14 Scientific Basis: Clinical Studies

At hundreds of Ayurvedic hospitals and clinics in India, obesity is being treated with diverse modes. It is desirable to analyze carefully maintained records of many obese patients by pharmacoepidemiological methods. At our Bhavan's Swami Prakashananda and Ayurveda Research Centre (SPARC), we have ambulant care of patients with obesity by Ayurvedic and modern experts. Table 9.5 shows in brief the basal and final body weights and the drug treatment given in female patients with their usual unmodified diet and exercise.

In one study at our clinic, patients were given standard doses of the formulations. It is interesting to note that only two women showed no change, despite the fact that one was given the formulations for 4 months. A weight loss of 1 to 3 kg was observed in four patients within 1 to 2.5 months. There were seven patients who showed a 4- to 6.5-kg weight loss and received the formulations for 3.5 to 6 months. Significant weight loss (4 to 5 kg) occurred in two patients within a month and surprisingly within 1 week in a single subject. Besides *arogyawardhini* there is a widespread use of *medohar-guggulu* (MHG), a formulation based on *Commiphora wightii*, in India. The experiential data suggest the need to increase the dose, as per the individual needs of the patient, and concurrently

TABLE 9.5

Response in Ambulant Obese Patients to Ayurvedic Therapy

Initials	Sex	Age (Years)	Body Weight (kg) Initial	During	End	Treatment Given[a]	Duration (Months)	Change (Δ kg)
AJ	F	40	79	76	75	MHG, AW, SV	6	–4
AS	F	34	64	63	59	AV, TG	1	–5
AG	F	52	75	72	70	MHG, AW, SV	3.5	–5
SS	F	38	95	93	90	MHG, AW	8	–5
MB	F	39	75	—	71	MHG, AW, SV	1	–4
AS	F	33	90	—	86	MHG, AW, SV	1	–4
JP	F	44	60	55.5	53.5	MHG, AW	4.5	–6.5
PM	F	45	98	—	95	MHG, AW, SV	2	–3
LD	F	43	64	63	62	MHG, AW, SV	2	–2
EJ	F	35	63	62	63	MHG, AW, SV	4	0
BS	F	32	64	64	64	MHG, AW, SV	1.5	0
SM	F	54	91	91	90	AW, SV	1.5	–1
MT	F	53	79	78	77	MHG, AW, TG	2.5	–2

Source: Bhavan's Swami Prakashananda Ayurveda Research Centre (SPARC).

[a]MHG = Medoharaguggulu; AW = Arogyawardhini; SV = Shankhvati; TG = Triphalaguggulu.

advise essential diet and exercise measures. Then the magnitude and the rate of weight loss is expected to be more. Our studies with *guggulu* preparations in arthritis have highlighted the need to use larger doses than usually, and hesitantly, prescribed.[41] *Panchakarma,* too, should be judiciously combined for integral therapy. However, some patients who are given higher doses of *guggulu* may complain of gastrointestinal irritation and burning.

At Bhavan's SPARC, the experiential data on the larger doses of different *guggulu* preparations and with a compliance for moderate diet and exercise, as well as steam and massage, showed interesting confirmation of the aforesaid statement of titrating the dose. Thirty-two of 36 patients with an average weight of 81 kg had lost an average of 3.6 kg in 4 weeks with a weight-loss range of 2 to 20 kg; 7 of them had lost more than 10 kg. *Guggulu* has been considered lipolytic (*medohara*) since ancient times. Hypolipidemic effects have been well demonstrated both experimentally and clinically.

In a placebo-controlled trial of 70 obese subjects, Patwardhan et al.[42] showed significant weight loss, decrease in body measurements, and a decline in serum cholesterol and triglycerides with Ayurvedic formulations (i.e., *guggulu* preparations used were *triphala guggul, gokshuradhi guggul,* and *sinhnad guggul*). The placebo group did not show any change in body weight or other variables mentioned above.

9.15 Ayurvedic Drugs and Medicinal Plants for Obesity

For obesity, many plants and formulations have been described in the Ayurvedic texts and are also currently used by Ayurvedic physicians. The herbs are chosen based on Ayurvedic pharmacology, which relies on taste and other physical-chemical properties for its action. Medicinal plants having bitter (*tikta*), pungent (*katu*), astringent (*kashay*) tastes, and light (*laghu*), dry (*ruksha*), rough (*khara*), subtle (*sukshma*), sharp (*tikshna guna*), hot (*ushna veerya*), and pungent *(katu vipak)* properties are used to treat obesity. Substances having sweet (*madhur*), sour (*amla*), and salty (*lavan*) tastes increase fat, whereas bitter, pungent, and astringent tastes have a reverse effect.

Bitter tastes are dry, cold, and light (*ruksha*, *sheeta*, and *laghu*); they stabilize skin and flesh in the body and absorb subtle liquid waste products (*kleda*), excessive fat, excessive mucus, pus, sweat, urine, stool, and humor (*agni* and *apa*)[43] (e.g., neem [*Azadirachta indica* Linn.] and *kutaki* [*Picrorrhiza kurroa*]).

Pungent tastes have similar properties like bitter, light, and dry tastes but are unlike hot tastes. They act on the fat tissue through scraping (*lekhan*) and channels its excretion through sweat, urine, stool, etc. They also destroy coughing (e.g., ginger [*Zingiber officinalis* Roscoe] and *pipali* [*Piper longum*]). Astringent tastes are dry, cool, and heavy; they basically suppress *pitta* but also act on *kapha*.

The property of a substance, called *guna*, is equally important when selecting it as a medicine. In obesity, substances having light, dry, and rough properties are used. It also should have minute and sharp properties. Substances that are light and easy to digest relieve *kapha* and increase *vata* and digestive power (*agni*). They also cause depletion of tissues in the body, scrape out (*lekhan*) excessive fat, and clear the channels of the body for waste. Together, this brings lightness in the body.[44]

Dry substances absorb water and create hardness and dryness. They aggravate *vata* and reduce *kapha*.[45] The rough property of substances increases *vata*, depletes the constitutents of the body, and absorbs water. Substances having these three *gunas* will reduce *kapha* and increase *vatta* in obese patients; combined action of these properties on fat will be through scraping (lekhan), drying, and depleting through various channels in the form of waste. Sharp *(tikshna)* substances act as sharp-edged weapons and cause depletion of tissues and thereby emaciation of the body — this process is called *lekhana*.[46] The hot quality and bitter taste of a substance has light, dry, and sharp and subtle (*sukshma*) properties that act on obesity as described above.

9.16 Formulations Used and Cited (*Aushadhi-Yogas*)

Various formulations containing three to eight medicinal plants in the form of a decoction (*quath*), powder (*churna*), and tablet (*vati*) are widely used based on its description in the ancient text and are given in Table 9.6.[47–55]

9.16.1 Single Plants Used for Obesity

Although Ayurveda commonly uses multiple plants in the formulations, with varying ingredients and concentrations, single plants have also been mentioned in the text. Table 9.7 lists many plants and their parts used either individually or in combination or with a follow-through vehicle (*anupan*). Many of these *tikta/katu* in *rasa* are light, dry, and rapidly acting (*tikshna*) in *guna*, hot in *veerya*, and usually pungent in *vipaka*. Most of these are antiobesity (*medohara*) and pacifying *vata* and *kapha dosas*. The groups of scraping, digestive (*pachaniya*), and appetite stimulating (*deepaniya*) dominate.

TABLE 9.6

Formulations Used for Obesity

Formulations	Plants	Botanical Name	Parts Used
Triphaladiquath	*Haritaki*	*Terminalia chebula* Retz.	Fruits
	Bibhitaki	*Terminalia belerica* Roxb.	Fruits
	Amla	*Emblica officinalis* Gaertn.	Fruits
Bilvadhiquath	*Bilva*	*Aegle marmelos* Corr.	Roots
	Adulsa/Vasa	*Adhatoda vasica* Nees.	Roots
	Kashmiri	*Gmelina arboria* Linn.	Roots
	Patala	*Stereospermum suaveolens*	Roots
Trayushanadya-churna	*Pippali*	*Piper longum* Linn.	Fruits
	Shunthhi	*Zingiber officinale* Roscoe	Rhizome
	Marich	*Piper nigram* Linn.	Seeds
Vidangadi-churna	*Vidanga*	*Embelia ribesburm* Brum. F.	Seeds
	Shunthhi	*Zingiber officinale* Roscoe	Rhizome
	Yavamal/Yavakshar	*Alhaji mourorum*	Seed
	Kantloh Bhasma	Iron formulation	—
	Amla	*Emblica officinalis* Gaertn.	Fruits
Amrutadiguggulu	*Guduchi*	*Tinospora cordifolia*	Stem
	Chota Eliachi	*Elettaria cardmomum*	Seeds
	Vidanga	*Embelia ribes* Burm.	Seeds
	Indrajav	*Holarrhena antidysentrica*	Roots
	Harali		Fruits
	Behada	*Terminalia belerica*	Fruits
	Amala	*Emblica officinalis* Gaertn.	Fruits
	Guggulu	*Commiphora wightii*	Gum

9.17 The Future of Ayurvedic Modalities for Obesity

Certain Ayurvedic modalities bear close resemblance to several nondrug approaches of modern medicines. These modalities can be judiciously combined for individualizing prevention and therapy of obesity and are listed below:

1. Ayurvedic modes of fasting and dietary regulations over long-term period[56]
2. Yoga, *suryanamaskara*, and exercise integrated in daily activities[57]
3. *Shodhana* complementary to obesity programs by *vaidya* experts for induced vomiting, laxation, etc., as per Ayurvedic fundamental principles[58]
4. Advocating frequent sexual intercourse, keeping awake, experiencing anxiety and concern for dear ones and social issues[59]
5. Adopting an inner mind-set change for a new body image

Commonly used drugs and herbs can be adopted by non-Ayurvedic family doctors and obesity specialists who are willing to learn from transcultural healing traditions. These would include the following:

TABLE 9.7

Medicinal Plants in Ayurveda for Obesity

Name	Parts	Dosage per Day	Anupan (With)	Unique Activity	Major Formulation	Ref.
Commiphora wighti (guggulu)	Gum	2–4 g three times/day	Hot water	Rejuvinative	Medohar-guggulu	47, 48
Terminalia chelula (haritaki)	Fruits	1–2 g two times/day	Honey	Memory enhancer	Triphala	49, 50
Tereminalia belerica (bibhitaka)	Fruits	0.75–1.5 g two times/day	Warm water	Sedative	Triphala	51
Emblica officinalis (amalaki)	Fruits	3–6 g three times/day	Cow's milk	Antiaging	Chyavanprash	52
Picrorrhiza kurroa (kutki)	Roots	0.5–1 g two times/day	Honey	Hydrocholeretic	Arogyawardhini	53
Curcuma longa (haridra)	Rhizome	2–4 g three times/day	Warm water	Hypolipidemic	Churna	54
Plantago ovata (isabgol)	Husk	5–10 g one time/day	Cow's milk	Antithirst	Sat-Isabgol	55

1. *Trikatu* — *Piper nigrum*, *Piper longum*, and *Zingiber officinale* with meals[60]
2. *Triphala* — Powder of the fruits of *Terminalia chibula*, *Terminlia berberica*, and *Emblica officinale*[61]
3. Common widely used Indian guggulu (*Commiphora wightii*) preparations in an initial large dose and as subsequent maintenance doses offer 10 to 20% deductions in body weight[62]

In the near future, other single plants and formulations can be investigated by fast-track reverse pharmacology — experiential, exploratory, and experimental research by global collaborative herbal research efforts.

Acknowledgments

The authors acknowledge the substantial help of Chhaya Godse for her assistance in literature search. Sapna Shetty and Anupama Bhaskaran are also thanked for their tireless efforts for typing and retyping the manuscript.

We are indebted to Dr. Lakshmi Chandra Mishra, the editor of this book, for his valuable suggestions on the first and second drafts. We also thank Dr. R. Venkataraman, the president of Bharatiya Vidya Bhavan, for the facilities and inspiration for the review.

Note: For correspondence with Dr. Ashok D.B. Vaidya, e-mail to bhaspa@bom5.vsnl.net.in

References

1. Munshi, V.D. (translator), *Ashtang Hridaya,* Sastum Sahityavardhak Mudranalaya, Ahmedabad, India, 1952, p. 135.
2. Nehru, J.L., *Discovery of India,* J.N. Memorial Fund, Eds., Oxford University Press, New York, 1989.
3. Svoboda, R.E., *Prakriti – Your Ayurvedic Constitution,* 1st ed., Motilal Banarasidas, New Delhi, 1989–1999.
4. Dossey, L., *Meaning and Medicine,* 1st ed., Bantam Books, New York, 1991, p. 66.
5. Shashtri, P.K. (translator), *Charak Sanhita,* 2nd ed., Chaukhambha Sanskrit Sansthan, Varanasi, India, 1983, p. 279.
6. Bhagwat, B.K.. Triphala-guggul in *Sthoulya in Ayurveda Research Papers III,* Kulkarni, P.H., Ed., Ayurved Rasashala, Pune, India, 1995, p. 215
7. Vaidya, A.B., Vaidya, R.A., and Nagral, S.I., Ayurveda and a different kind of evidence: from Lord Macaulay to Lord Walton (1835 to 2001 AD), *J. Assn. Physicians India,* 49, 534, 2001.
8. Vaidya, A.B., We can still learn from Indian medicine, *CIBA-GEIGY J.,* 4, 17, 1979.
9. Bhatt, A.D. et al., Conceptual and methodologic challenges of assessing the short-term efficacy of Guggulu (*Commiphora mukul*) in obesity: data emergent from a naturalistic trial, *J. Postgrad. Med.,* 41, 5–7, 1995.
10. Vaidya, R.A. et al., Clinical endocrine and metabolic studies in the kindred of familial partial lipodystrophy — a syndrome of insulin resistance, *J. Assn. Physicians India,* 50, 773, 2002.
11. Satyavati, G.V., Dwarakanath, C., and Tripathi, S.N., Experimental studies on the hypocholesterolemic effect of *Commiphora mukul* (Guggulu), *Indian J. Med. Res.,* 57, 1950, 1969.
12. Munshi,V.D. (translator), *Ashtang Hriday,* Sastum Sahityavardhak Mudranalaya, Ahamdabad, India, 1952, p. 101.
13. Munshi, V.D. (translator), *Ashtang Hriday,* Sastum Sahityavardhak Mudranalaya, Ahmedabad, India, 1952, p. 111.
14. Shastri, P.K. (translator), *Charak Sanhita,* Part II, 2nd ed., Chaukhambha Sanskrit Sanathan, Varansi, India, 1983, p. 380.
15. Acharya, J.T. (translator), *Sushrut Sanhita of Sushrut,* Nirnay Sagar Press, Mumbai, India, 1915, p. 65.
16. Shastri, P.K. (translator), *Charak Sanhita,* Part I, 2nd ed., Chaukhambha Sanskrit Sanathan, Varansi, India, 1983, p. 593.
17. Shastri, P.K. (translator), *Charak Sanhita,* Part I, 2nd ed., Chaukhambha Sanskrit Sanathan, Varansi, India, 1983, p. 595.
18. Shastri, P.K. (translator), *Charak Sanhita,* Part I, 2nd ed., Chaukhambha Sanskrit Sanathan, Varanasi, India, 1983, p. 281.
19. Shastri, S. (translator), *Madhav Nidanam Madhukosh Vyakhya,* Part I, Chaukhambha Sansrit Sansthan, Varanasi, India, 1985, p. 28.
20. Foster, W.R. and Burton, B.T., Health implications of obesity, *Ann. Intern. Med.,* 103, 1024, 1985.
21. Petrelli, J.M., Calle, E.E., Rodrigues, C., et al., Body mass index, height and post menopausal breast cancer mortality in a prospective cohort of US women, *Cancer Causes Control,* 13, 325, 2002.
22. Munshi, V.D., *Ashtang Hriday:* Sastum Sahityavardhak Mudranalaya, Ahmedabad, India, 1952, p. 132.
23. Mishra, B.S., *Bhavprakash of Shree Bhavmishra,* Part II, Chaukhambha Sanskrit Sansthan, Varanasi, India, 1988, p. 406.
24. Parekh, R., *Sharangadhar Sanhita,* Sastum Sahityavardhak Mudranalaya, Ahmedabad, India, 1955, p. 126.
25. Grunstein, R.R. and Widcox, I., Sleep-disordered breathing and obesity, *Clin. Endocrinol. Metab. Baillier's,* 8, 601, 1994.

26. Gislason, T. et al., Prevalence of sleep apnoea syndrome, *J. Clin. Epidemiol.*, 41, 571, 1988.
27. Daugero, K.D., A new perspective on glucocorticoid feedback: relation to stress, carbohydrate feeding and feeding behaviour, *J. Neuroendocrinol.*, 13, 1088, 2001.
28. Acharya, J.T., *Sushrut Sanhita of Sushrut*, Nirnay Sagar Press, Bombay, 1915, p. 98.
29. Shastri, P.K. (translator), *Charak Sanhita*, Part I, 2nd ed., Chaukhambha Sanskrit Sanathan, Varansi, India, 1983, p. 430.
30. Shastri, S., *Madhav Nidan-Madhukosh Vyukhya*, Part I, 15th ed., Chaukhambha Sanskrit Sansthan, Varanasi, India, 1985, p. 63.
31. Larsson, B. et al., Abdominal adipose distribution, obesity and risk of cardiovascular disease and death: 13 year follow up of participants in the study of men born in 1913, *Br. Med. J.*, 288, 1401, 1984.
32. Shringi, M.S., Vaidya, R.A., Vaidya, A.B., et al., Unpublished data, 2002.
33. Bray, G.A., Coherent, preventive and management strategies for obesity, in *The Origins and Consequences of Obesity*, Chadwick, D.J. and Cardea, G., Eds., John Wiley & Sons, London, 1996, p. 228.
34. Swoboda, R.E. (translator), *Prakriti: Your Ayurvedic Constitution*, 1st ed., Motilal Banarasidas, New Delhi, 1994, p. 132.
35. Shastri, P.K. (translator), *Charak Sanhita,* Part II, 2nd ed., Chaukhabha Sanskrit Sansthan, Varanasi, India, 1983, p. 189.
36. Ranade, S. and Paranjape, G.R. (translator), *Ashtang Sangraha-Sutrasthan*, 2nd ed., Anmol Prakashan, Pune, India, 1982, p. 307.
37. Kasture, H.S. (translator), *Ayurvediya Panchakarma Vidnyan*, 3rd ed., Shri Baidyanath Ayurved Bhavan Pvt. Ltd., Kolkata, India, 1985, p. 247.
38. Swoboda, R.E. (translator), *Prakriti: Your Ayurvedic Constitution*, 1st ed., Motilal Banarasidas, New Delhi, 1994, p. 108.
39. Parikh, R.J. (translator), *Sharangadhara Sanhita*, 1st ed., Sastum Sahityavardhak, Mudranalaya, Ahmedabad, India, 1955, p. 232.
40. Ranade, S. and Paranjape, G.R., *Ashtang Sangraha-Sutrasthan*, 2nd ed., Anmol Prakashan, Pune, India, 1982, p. 317.
41. Nityanand, S. and Kapoor, N.K., Hypocholesterolemic effect commiphora mukul resin (guggul), *Ind. J. Exp. Biol.*, 9, 376, 1971.
42. Paranjpe, P., Patki, P., and Patwardhan, P., Ayurvedic treatment of obesity: a randomised double blind, placebo-controlled clinical trial, *J. Ethnopharmacol.*, 29, 1–11, 1990.
43. Ranade, S. and Paranjape, G.R., *Asthangsangraha Sutrasthan*, 2nd ed., Anmol Prakashan Pune, India, 1979, chap. 3.
44. Shastri, G.M. (translator), *Charak Sanhita,* Part I, 1st ed., Sastum Sahitya Vardhak, Karyalaya, Ahmadabad, India, 1959, p. 543.
45. Dwivedi, V., Saidhantic vivaran, in *Aushadhi Vidnyan Shastra,* 1st ed., Baidyanath Ayurved Bhavan Pvt. Ltd., Kolkata, India, 1970, p. 161.
46. Shastri, G.M., Medoroga nidan, in *Yogratnakar*, Sastum Sahitya Vardhak, Karyalaya, Ahmadabad, India, 1971, p. 758.
47. Satyavati, G.V. et al., Experimental studies on the hypocholesterolemic effect of *Commiphora mukul* (guggul), *Ind. J. Med. Res.*, 57, 1950, 1969.
48. Sairam, T.B., *Home Remedies*, Vol. 2, Penguin Books, New Delhi, 1999, p. 132.
49. Munshi, V.D., *Ashtangahridaya*, 1st ed., Sanstum Satityavardhak, Mudranalaya, Ahmedabad, India, 1952, p. 134.
50. Bhavan's Swami Prakashananda Ayurveda Research Centre (SPARC), *Selected Medicinal Plants of India*, CHEMEXCIL, 1992, chap. 98.
51. Sairam, T.B., *Home Remedies*, Vol. 2, Penguin Books, New Delhi, 1999.
52. Shastri, P.K., *Charak Sanhita*, 2nd ed., Chaukhambha Sanskrit Santhan, Varanasi, India, 1983, p. 11.
53. Vaidya, A.B. et al., A double-blind clinical trial of Arogyawardhini — an Ayurvedic drug — in acute viral hepatitis, *Ind. J. Med. Res.*, 72, 588, 1980.
54. Godkar, P.B., Narayanan, P., and Bhide, S.V., Hypocholesterolemic effect of turmeric extract on swiss mice, *Ind. J. Pharmacol.*, 28, 177, 1996.

55. Bhavan's Swami Prakashananda Ayurveda Research Centre (SPARC), *Selected Medicinal Plants of India*, CHEMEXIL, 1992, p. 249.
56. Ranade, S. and Pranajpe, G., *Ashtangasangraha: Sutrastana*, 2nd ed., 1979, p. 280.
57. Svoboda, R.E., *Routine in Prakruti your Ayurvedic constitution*, 1st ed., 1994, pp. 18, 108.
58. Ranade, S., *Natural healing through Ayurveda*, Motilal Banarasidas, 1st ed., 1994, 66.
59. Kasture, H.S., *Ayurvediya Panchakarma: Vidnyana*, 3rd ed., Vaidyanath Ayurved Bhavan, Nagpur, India, 1985, p. 245.
60. Ranade, S. and Pranajpe, G., *Ashtangasangraha: Sutrastana*, 2nd ed., 1979, p. 283.
61. Bhavan's Swami Prakashananda Ayurveda Research Centre (SPARC), *Selected Medicinal Plants*, CHEMEXCIL, 1992, p. 103.
62. Satyavati, G.V., Guggulipid: a promising hypolipidaemic agent from gum guggul (*Commiphora wightii*). Economic and medicinal plant research, *Plants Traditional Med.*, 5, 47, 1991.

10

Rheumatoid Arthritis, Osteoarthritis, and Gout

Lakshmi Chandra Mishra

CONTENTS

0-8493-1366-X/04/$0.00+$1.50

10.1 Introduction

There are three basic types of musculoskeletal joint diseases described in Ayurveda, namely, *amavata, sandhivata,* and *vatarakta,* that are characterized by pain and swelling of the joints. In modern medicine, the diseases closely resembling *amavata, sandhigat vata,* and *vata rakta* are rheumatoid arthritis (RA), osteoarthritis (OA), and gouty arthritis, respectively. RA is described first followed by brief descriptions of OA, gout, and other *vataja* musculoskeletal diseases.

10.2 Rheumatoid Arthritis

Amavata (RA) is described in Ayurveda as a constitutional disorder with clinical manifestations of joint swelling, pain, and stiffness in the ankle, knee, hip joints, wrist, elbow, and shoulder. The incidence of RA ranges from 0.3 to 1.5% in most populations of the world and the rate is two to three times higher in females than in males. The peak incidence of onset of RA is in persons 30 to 60 years old, but no age is immune. The severity of RA may range from mild oligoarticular illness of a brief duration and very little or no joint damage to polyarthritis with marked functional impairment.

RA is commonly treated with nonsteroidal anti-inflammatory drugs (NSAIDs). These drugs do not modify disease progression.[1] They have a tendency to cause adverse gastrointestinal effects that may range from mild dyspepsia and heartburn to ulceration of the stomach and duodenum, and many produce fatal consequences.[2,3] Despite the popularity of NSAIDs, their use to treat OA has been controversial.[4] In one survey, 27% of the patients suffering from arthritis in the U.S. had used complementary alternative medicine therapies (CAM).[5] In a recent survey in India, 43% had used CAM therapies.[6] Disease-modifying therapies, such as methotrexate, leflunomide, sulfasalazine, gold salts, penicillamine, azathropine, cyclophosphamide, and chlorambucil, are used to modify the course of the disease but have serious toxic effects. These toxic effects include aplastic anemia (potentially life threatening), liver toxicity, gastrointestinal toxicity, leukopenia, and skin rashes.

The mechanism of action of NSAIDs is believed to be via inhibition of cyclooxygenase (COX) enzyme that is now known to exist in two separate isoforms. The COX-1 isoform is responsible for maintaining prostaglandin synthesis in the gastric mucosa, platelets, and kidney and its inhibition results in toxic effects in the organs. The COX-2 isoform is responsible for prostaglandin production in inflamed tissues, including RA synovium, and its inhibition results in beneficial effect in the effected tissues. Recently developed NSAIDs seem to offer some selective inhibition of COX-2 isoform resulting in less toxicity.[7] Corticosteroids are given to patients who are not responsive to NSAIDs, but corticosteroids may produce serious side effects, particularly after prolonged use. Dozens of therapies for RA have been used in Ayurvedic medicine for thousands of years. No serious side effect has been reported even after prolonged use of these therapies. For these reasons, interest in Ayurvedic management of RA is steadily growing around the world.

10.2.1 Pathogensis and Etiology (*Samprapti* and *Vyadhi Haitu*)

Pathogenesis of RA in Ayurveda is considered to be due to the formation of *ama* (metabolic toxic waste materials) in the intestine caused by poor digestive power. *Ama* physically resembles *kapha,* thus it tends to deposit in *kapha* locations, primarily the joints. When *ama* is vitiated (function impaired) by *vata, amavata* disease is produced.

The etiological factors in the pathogenesis of *amavata* are incompatible diet, poor digestion, and sedentary habits.[8] Poor digestion due to weak digestive power leads to the formation of *ama* in the intestine and is absorbed and distributed to all parts of the body. When *ama* is vitiated by the other three *dosas,* all types of diseases develop in the body.

An attempt has been made to determine if a relationship exists between the incidence of RA and other factors such as body constitution, lifestyle, and dietary habits of arthritis patients.[8] Patients positive for RA factor were of *vata-pittaja* body constitution. They had poor digestive power, a tendency to eat an incompatible diet, a high level of erythrocyte sedimentation rate (ESR), and low hemoglobin levels. This group has more patients with sedentary habits than the patients with negative RA factor. Patients with a negative RA factor were found to be of *vata-kaphaja* constitution. They had better digestive power, eating habits, a more active lifestyle, lower levels of ESR, and higher levels of hemoglobin than did the RA factor positive patients. The authors suggested that Ayurvedic pathology of RA based on body constitution seems to be of two types: *vata-pittaja* (RA positive) and *vata-kaphaja* (RA negative). They also concluded that RA-negative patients may have a better prognosis than do RA-positive patients. This is because immunity may be better developed by *rasayanas* in the RA-negative patients.

It is currently believed in conventional medicine that genetic susceptibility, primary exogenous arthritogen, autoimmune reactions in joint components, and mediators of the joint damage are the factors involved in pathogenesis of RA.[9] RA is believed to be an autoimmune disease. It is likely that *ama* contains some arthritogenic autoantigens that trigger the autoimmune reaction in a susceptible host, causing the development of RA. Although rheumatoid factors are found in 80% of the RA patients, these factors are not known to cause the disease.[1] Rheumatoid factors are also found to occur in other diseases that are characterized by chronic antigenic stimulation. These include bacterial endocarditis, tuberculosis, syphilis, *kala-azar,* viral infections, intravenous drug abuse, and liver cirrhosis.

10.2.2 Clinical Description (*Rog Vivaran)*

In Ayurvedic texts, the description of signs and symptoms of RA (*amavata*) includes pain (scorpionlike bite) and inflammation of one or more joints, particularly the hand, foot, thigh, sacrum, knees, and metatarsophalangeal (MTP). Joints develop swelling, tenderness, and reddish or bluish discoloration.

The characteristic feature of RA in conventional medicine is the persistent inflammation in the synovial membranes, usually of peripheral joints. Patients show loss of appetite, indigestion, constipation, occasionally low fever, malaise, fatigue, pain in different parts of the body, feeling of heaviness in the body, sleeplessness, and stiffness in the chest area. The seven criteria formulated by American Rheumatology Association[10] and the American College of Rheumatology[1] to classify RA are summarized as follows:

1. Morning stiffness in and around the joints for an hour or more, continuous for 4 weeks or more; swelling of soft tissue of three or more joints, continuous for 4 weeks or more
2. Swelling of soft tissue of three or more joints
3. Swelling of soft tissue of hand joints (proximal interphalangeal [PIP], metacarpophalangeal or [MCP], or wrist)
4. Symmetrical swelling of soft tissue
5. Subcutaneous nodules
6. Serum rheumatoid factor
7. Erosions or periarticular osteopenia in hand or wrist joints seen on radiograph

Criteria 1 to 4 must continue for 4 weeks or more, and criteria 2 to 5 must be observed by a physician.

The prominent clinical features of RA include swelling of the PIP; MCP in the hands; loss of motion in the wrists; pain in the thumb; synovial proliferation and effusion in the knees; painful deformities of the toes in the feet; and ankle or tarsal collapse, resulting in painful valgus deformities.

10.2.3 Clinical Examination and Diagnosis (*Nidan*)

The standard eight-point diagnosis of Ayurveda is used to diagnose RA and determine which *dosas* are vitiated as discussed in Chapter 2. Additionally, patients are examined for the classical signs of arthritis as discussed above. There is no specific laboratory diagnostic test for RA. Although only 80% of the patients are found to be positive for RA factor, the standard eight-point diagnosis is still one of the tests often used by physicians for diagnosis.

10.2.4 Clinical Course and Prognosis (*Sadhyata*)

RA is often considered a benign disease, but it may cause considerable disability, crippling, and death. Patients sometimes recover spontaneously and achieve complete remission. In most cases, the disease becomes chronic, resulting in functional deterioration of the joints and disability.

10.2.5 Strategy for Prevention

As previously mentioned, the major causative factors in the pathogenesis of RA are weak digestive power, leading to accumulation of *ama*, and a sedentary lifestyle. The strategy to prevent RA needs to include herbal formulas that improve digestion and clean the intestine from *ama* and a healthy active lifestyle as discussed in Ayurveda under daily

TABLE 10.1

Common Anti-Inflammatory Herbs Used in Ayurvedic Formulas

Sanskrit and Botanical Names
Ashwagandha (*Withania sosmnifera*)
Bhallataka (*Semecarpus anacardium*)
Bhutala (*Circuligo orchioides*)
Chitraka (*Plumbago zeylanica*)
Eranda (*Ricinus communis*)
Goraksa (*Vitex negundo*)
Guggulu (*Commiphora mukul*)
Haritika (*Terminalia chebula*)
Harsinger (*Nyctanthes arbor tristis*)
Karanja (*Pongamia glabra*)
Kirayat (*Andrographis paniculata*)
Kupilu (*Strychnos nux-vomica*)
Madhuka (*Basia latifolia*)
Madhuyasti (*Glycyrrhiza glabra*)
Punarnava (*Boerrhavia diffusa*)
Rasna (*Inula racemosa*)
Rasona (*Allium sativum*)
Sunthi (*Zinziber officinalis*)
Vatsanabha (*Aconimtum chasmenthum*)
Vidanga (*Embelia ribes*)
Yavasaka (*Alhagi pseudalhagi*)

routine. One must eat easily digestible food according to the body constitution and make sure that bowel movement is regular. Regular exercise is very important to prevent RA and arthritis.

10.2.6 Therapy (*Chikitsa*)

The basic strategy of treating RA is to reduce the accumulated *ama* in the body and balance *vata*, encourage proper exercise, maintain a normal healthy lifestyle, and provide adequate rest. First, the food intake is reduced to a bare minimum, giving only boiled rice and well cooked *mung dal* (lentil) soup for 1 to 2 months to help clean the body of *ama*. This diet is believed to increase metabolism and elimination of disease-producing *ama*. Herbs or herbal formulas (e.g., *Panchkola*, 2 g/day; equal parts of *Piper longum* root and fruits, *Piper chava*, *Plumbago zeylanica*, and *Zinziber officinale* powders) are given during this period to clean the body, improve the digestion, and reduce the inflammation (*Commiphora mukul*-containing formulas) and pain.[11]

Suitable herbal formulas are determined based on body constitution, disturbed *dosa*, and other disease conditions. For example, *Gokksharadi guggul* is recommended for patients who also suffer from kidney disorders, *Pushkarmoola guggul* is suggested for patients with heart problems, and *Kanchnar guggul* is recommended for patients with lymphadenopathy.[11] Some of the commercially available commonly used herbs and formulas are presented in Table 10.1 through Table 10.3. The patient is slowly brought back to a normal diet consisting of easily digestible light food, is given ghee (dehydrated butter), and may be asked to use a medicated sesame-oil enema to remove fat soluble toxic materials from the gastrointestinal tract. The patient is asked to do easy exercises and yoga. Body massage with oil, and hot fomentation may also be added to the treatment. Classic Panchakarma

TABLE 10.2

Formulas from Ayurvedic Formulary (AF) of India for Arthritis Treatment (1978)

Name	Dose	AF Section	Name	Dose	AF Section
Kanchnar guggul	3 g	5:1	*Rasa parpati*	250 mg	16:3
Goksharidi guggul	3 g	5:3	*Anand Bhaijarava rasa*	250 mg	20:3
Trayodashang guggul	3 g	5:4	*Mahalakshmi vilas rasa*	250 mg	20:27
Yograj guggul	3 g	5:7	*Sarvanabhupati rasa*	250 mg	20:51
Vyousadi guggul	3 g	5:9	*Rasnadi kvath curpa*	48 g	4:27
Vatari guggul	3 g	5:10	*Rasnadi kvath curpa maha*	48 g	4:28
Simhanad guggul	3 g	5:12	*Das-mula-haritiki*	12 g	3:14
Ajamodadi curpa	6 g	7:1	*Amrta ghrit*	12 g	6:1
Nimbadi curpa	3 g	7:20	*Brhat saindhavadya taila*	massage	8:40
Pancasma curpa	3 g	7:22	*Kotamuckkadi taila*	massage	8:10
Vaisvanara curpa	3 g	7:30	*Jiraka-modka*	3 g	3:12

TABLE 10.3

Miscellaneous Ayurvedic Formulas for the Treatment of RA

Name	Reference	Name	Reference
Brhat vata cintamani	BR[a]	*Maha rasnadi kvath*	SS[f]
Chandrprabha vati	SYS[b]	*Sunthi guduci kvath*	13[d]
Copper bhasma	RS[c]	*Puskarmoola guggul*	Shukla 1996
Gudici kvatha	20[d]	*Suvarna samirapannag rasa*	BR[a]
Gold bhasma	SYS[b]	*Rasnadi guggul*	YR[g]
Mrtyunjaya rasa	BR[a]	*Trailokya cintamani*	BR[a]
Maha Narayan taila	CD[e]	*Vatari guggul*	BR[a]
		Vatgajankush rasa	BR[a]

[a]BR = *Bhesajya Ratnavali.*
[b]SYS = *Sidha Yog Sangraha.*
[c]RS = *Rasayan Sar.*
[d]See References at end of chapter.
[e]CD = *Chakardatta.*
[f]SS = *Sarangdhar Samhita.*
[g]YR = *Yog Ratnakar.*

therapy described in Chapter 5 was evaluated in RA patients and was found to give encouraging results.[12]

Clinical trials based on the above basic strategy of treatment using a variety of Ayurvedic herbal formulas are summarized below.

10.2.6.1 *Zingiber officinale–Tinospora cordifolia* Decoction, *Vatagajanankusa Rasa*, and *Maharasnadi Kwath*

Z. officinalis–T. cordifolia decoction was given (50 ml three times/day) to 40 RA patients (group B) and *Yograj guggul* (1 g/day), *Vatagajanankusa rasa* (250 mg three times/day), and *Maharasnadi kwath* (50 ml three times/day) were administered to 37 arthritis patients (group A) for 6 to 8 weeks. There were a total of 48 males and 29 females. The diagnosis was confirmed based on 1959 American Rheumatism Association (ARA) criteria. All patients received a limited vegetarian diet without fish or chicken. Both treatments were effective in reducing pain and swelling, and the decoction treatment was found to be relatively more effective than the *Yograj guggul* combination.[13]

10.2.6.2 Dasmularista, Pippalyasava, and Vettumaran Gutika

Dasmularista, Pippalyasava, and *Vettumaran Gutika* were examined in 83 arthritis patients (1959 ARA criteria). Forty-three percent of the patients were unable to walk, and remaining cases showed varying degree of functional impairment of the joints. Measurements of swollen elbow, wrist, ankle, and knee joints were taken before and after treatment. An average of 90 days of treatment was found to be the minimum to obtain satisfactory improvements. Time taken for disappearance of RA ranged from 20 to 30 days. The results suggested that the combination of the above three formulas was effective in the acute stage of RA.[14]

10.2.6.3 Rasonadi Kvatha[15]

Rasonadi Kvatha was evaluated in 50 RA patients. The diagnosis was confirmed based on ARA 1959 criteria.[16] *Kvatha* is a decoction of equal parts of *Z. officinalis, Allium sativum,* and *Vitex negundo.* A dose of 25 ml of the decoction representing 25 g of each ingredient was given three times/day for 6 weeks. During the acute inflammatory stage of the disease, patients were treated with external application of poultice and *Baluka* hot sand fomentation. The participants' diet consisted of rice, bread, lentil soup, cream of wheat, and milk during the 6-week trial period. *Pippalyadi churna* or *Visatundika vati* was also administered during the acute phase to relieve pain. The results were assessed based on the degree of pain, swelling, tenderness, and restriction of affected joints. The change in functional capacity was measured by functional tests. Authors observed significant improvement in all the parameters. Most of the patients showed complete relief from pain.[16]

10.2.6.4 Withania somnifera, Boswellia serrata, Curcuma longa, and a Zinc Complex (Articulin-F)

A herbomineral formulation containing roots of *W. somnifera*, the stem of *B. serrata*, rhizomes of *C. longa*, and a zinc complex (Articulin-F) was evaluated in a randomized, double-blind, placebo-controlled, crossover study in 42 patients with OA. Clinical efficacy was evaluated every fortnight on the basis of severity of pain, morning stiffness, Ritchie, articular index, joint score, disability score, and grip strength. Other parameters like erythrocyte sedimentation rate and radiological examination were carried out on a monthly basis. Treatment with the herbomineral formulation produced a significant drop in the severity of pain ($p < 0.001$) and disability score ($p < 0.05$). Radiological assessment did not show any significant changes and no serious adverse effect was observed.[17]

10.2.6.5 Ginger (Zingiber officinale)

Ginger has been reported to be beneficial in seven arthritic patients.[18] In one study, ginger was given to 56 patients (28 with RA, 18 with OA, and 10 with muscular discomfort). More than 75% of the patients experienced varying degrees of relief from pain and swelling. All the patients with muscular discomfort experienced relief from pain. None of the patients reported adverse effects during the treatment period from 3 months to 2.5 years. The authors suggested that at least one of the mechanisms by which ginger shows its ameliorative effects could be related to inhibition of prostaglandin and leukotriene biosynthesis (dual inhibitor of eicosanoid biosynthesis).[19]

10.2.6.6 *Tinospora cordifolia, Balsamodendrom mukul, and Alpinia officinarum*

Tinospora cordifolia, Balsamodendrom mukul, and *Alpinia officinarum* were evaluated in 40 RA patients selected based on 1959 ARA criteria.[20] Forty patients (ages 10 to 65) were selected for the study on the basis of pain, swelling of multiple joints, and elevation of erythroicyte sedimentation rate. All patients were treated for the first 10 days as follows:

Day 1 — Fasting
Days 2–6 — *Panchkola* (2 g/day) to improve digestion and clean *ama* for days 2 to 6
Day 7 —*Ricinus communis* oil (30 ml) at 6 A.M. with hot water
Days 8–10 — *Panchkola* powder (2 g/day) with hot water

On day 11, the patients were separated randomly into 2 groups of 20 each. The first group was given 60 ml of *T. cordifolia* decoction, 1 ml of oil extract (*sneha*) of *T. cordifolia,* and 2 g of *B. mukul* three times/day. The second group received the same regimen except *B. mukul* was replaced by 2 g of *A. officinarum.*

The decoction consisted of one part of leaves and stem of the herb, boiled in four parts of water until one part of the water was left. The oil extract fortified three times consisted of 1 part herbal paste, 4 parts of sesame seed oil, and 16 parts of the decoction, boiled 6 to 8 h/day for 3 days to reduce the volume to one fourth of the total amount. It was filtered and the procedure was repeated three times.

A light diet was given in the first stage of 10 days and a normal hospital diet was given for rest of the treatment period. Criteria for assessment and classification of results followed were those adopted by American Medical Association (AMA). The authors stated that the improvement in signs and symptoms were highly encouraging and statistically significant at 0.1% level.

10.2.6.7 *Fasting*

Because *ama* is considered a major causal factor for RA, elimination of *ama* by fasting was studied in RA patients (1959 ARA criteria). The patients were subjected to total fasting for 2 days and partial fasting for the next 43 days. Notable clinical remission of signs and symptoms were observed, including a decrease in rheumatoid factor (RF) titer and chemically reactive proteins (CRP), which may be attributed to a decrease in *ama.*[21]

10.2.6.8 *Elimination of Ama by a Purgative (Gandharva hasta kashaya)*

The effect of eliminating *ama* by purgatives was evaluated in 60 arthritic patients. *Gandharva hastadi kvath* (50 ml), a purgative, was given three to four times/day for 21 days. The ingredients of the decoction were equal parts of *Gandharva hasta* (*Ricinus communis*), *Karavya* (*Pongamia glabra*), *Chitraka* (*Plumbago zeylanica*), *Shunti* (*Zinziber officinalis*), *Haritaka* (*Terminalia chebula*), *Punarnava* (*Boerrhavia diffusa*), *Yavasaka* (*Alhagi pseudalhagi*), and *Bhutala* (*Circuligo orchioides*). Of 60 patients, 46 were cured (complete disappearance of disease symptoms) and 14 showed significant relief in symptoms. Three patients had a relapse over a period of 1 year after observation. The study further confirms the hypothesis that the origin of arthritis is the formation of *ama* in the intestine.[22]

10.2.6.9 *Vatari Guggul (Bhasajya Ratnavali) and Maharasnadi Kvatha*

A dose of 1 g of *Vatari guggul* was given three times/day and *Maharasnadi kvatha* (*Sarangdhar samhita*) was given 20 ml three times/day in 24 RA patients. *Vatari guggul* consisted of castor oil, sulfur, *guggul* (*Commiphora mukul*), *haritiki* (*Terminalia chebula*), *amalki* (*Phyllanthus emblica*), and *vibhitiki* (*Terminalia belerica*). The major ingredient of *Maharasnadi kvath* was *rasna* (*Inula recemosa*). The results indicate a significant improvement in pain ($p < 0.001$) and a decrease in ESR levels ($p < 0.001$) in subjective and objective parameters ($p < 0.001$).[23]

10.2.6.10 Ashwagandha (Withania somnifera)

Ashwagandha (*Withania somnifera*) has been shown to have antiarthritic activity in animal models of RA.[24–28] In a recent clinical trial, 3 g of the drug was given three times/day with milk to 77 RA patients. The improvement in signs and symptoms of RA was good in 22.7%, moderate in 53.4%, and poor in 22.07%; there was no response in 2.59% of the patients.[29]

10.2.6.11 Purified Guggul and Guduchyadi Kvath

Purified *guggul* and *Guduchyadi kvath* were given to 34 RA patients for 6 weeks. Authors observed marked improvement in signs and symptoms in 27 patients, moderate improvement in 4 patients, and no improvement in 3 patients.

10.2.7 Scientific Basis for the Use of Ayurvedic Herbs in Arthritis

Ayurvedic herbs have been investigated in animal models of arthritis for anti-inflammatory effect in the same way as synthetic drugs have been for the past 30 years. The three most common animal models currently used to investigate anti-inflammatory effect of drugs are (1) adjuvant-induced, (2) streptococcal cell-wall induced, and (3) collagen-induced models.[30] Agents currently in clinical use or trials that are active in these models include corticosteroids, methotrexate, nonsteroidal anti-inflammatory drugs, cyclosporin A, leflunomide, interleukin-1 receptor antagonist, and soluble tumor necrosis factor receptors. Animal models of OA include mouse and guinea pig spontaneous OA, meniscotomy and ligament transection in guinea pigs, meniscotomy in rabbits, and meniscotomy and cruciate transection in dogs. None of these models have a proven track record of predictability in human disease presentation because none of the agents have been proven to provide anything other than symptomatic relief.[31]

The studies to assess anti-inflammatory activity and analgesic activity are evaluated, and the results supporting the use of Ayurvedic therapies in arthritis are summarized below.

10.2.7.1 Anti-Inflammatory Activity

10.2.7.1.1 *Vanda roxburghii*

Vanda roxburghii has been shown to have anti-inflammatory activity in albino rats.[32]

10.2.7.1.2 *Gum-Guggul from Commiphora mukul*

Anti-inflammatory activity of *guggul* has been reported by several investigators.[33–35] In another study, phenylbutazone, ibuprofen, and fraction "A" of gum-*guggul* from *Commiphora mukkul* were administered orally at a daily dose of 100, 100, and 500 mg/kg, respectively, for a period of 5 months. All three drugs decreased the thickness of joint swelling during the course of the drug treatment.[36]

The anti-inflammatory effect of extracts of *guggul* resins of four species of the Burseraceae plant family, *Boswellia dalzielli, Boswellia carteri* (gum olibanum), *Commiphora mukul,* and *Commiphora incisa,* were screened in arthritis models in rat. The aqueous extracts of the resins of *B. dalzielli, C. incisa,* and *C. mukul* significantly inhibited both the maximal edema response and the total edema response during 6 h of carrageenan-induced rat paw edema. The octanordammarane triterpenes, mansumbinone and mansumbinoic acid, were isolated from the resin of *C. incisa.* Prophylactical administration of mansumbinone proved to be more than 20 times less potent than indomethacin and prednisolone in inhibiting carrageenan-induced rat paw edema. The acid was able to reverse an established carrageenan-induced inflammatory response when administered 2 h after induction. Daily administration of mansumbinoic acid at 1.5×10^{-4} mol kg^{-1} dose level significantly reduced joint swelling in adjuvant-induced arthritic rats.[37]

New triterpenes, Myrrhanol A and Myrrhanone A, isolated from *guggul*-gum resins (*C. mukul*), were found to have a potent anti-inflammatory effect on adjuvant-induced air-pouch granuloma of mice. The study indicated that the anti-inflammatory effect of Myrrhanol A was greater than that produced by hydrocortisone and the 50% extract of the crude resin. Authors suggested that Myrrhanol A may be a potent anti-inflammatory agent.[38]

10.2.7.1.3 Harsinger (Nyctanthes arbor tristis)

The water-soluble portion of the alcoholic extract of the leaves of *Nyctanthes arbor tristis* (NAT) was screened for the presence of anti-inflammatory activity. NAT inhibited acute inflammatory edema produced by different phlogistic agents, such as carrageenin, formalin, histamine, 5-hydroxytryptamine, turpentine oil, and hyaluronidase, in the hindpaw of rats. It also inhibited the inflammation in adjuvant-induced arthritic models. In subacute models, NAT was found to check granulation tissue formation significantly in the granuloma pouch and cotton-pellet test. Acute and chronic phases of formaldehyde-induced arthritis were significantly inhibited. Anti-inflammatory activity in leaves of NAT supports its use in various inflammatory conditions by the followers of the Ayurvedic system of medicine.[39]

10.2.7.1.4 Semecarpus anacardium nut

A chloroform extract of *Semecarpus anacardium* nut was found to significantly reduce acute inflammation and was also active against the secondary lesions of adjuvant-induced arthritis in rats.[40]

A milk extract of *S. anacardium* nut was found to have anti-inflammatory effect in adjuvant-induced arthritis in rats at the dose level of 150 mg/kg.[41] The mechanistic studies indicated that the diseased state of adjuvant arthritis may be associated with augmented lipid peroxidation; the studies also concluded that the administration of the drug may exert its antiarthritic effect by retarding lipid peroxidation and causing a modulation in a cellular antioxidant (AO) defense system.[42]

10.2.7.1.5 Crataeva nurvala

The effect of triterpenes from stem bark was studied for its effect on lipid peroxidation in adjuvant induced arthritis in rats. Lupeol, a pentacyclic triterpene of *C. nurvala* stem bark, and its ester, lupeol linoleate, were synthesized and tested for anti-inflammatory activity in complete Freund's adjuvant-induced arthritic rats. The arthritic rats showed a significant increase in lipid peroxide level in plasma; a decrease of lipid peroxide in the liver; an increase in the AO enzymes, SOD, GPX, and catalase in both the liver and hemolysate; and a decrease in blood glutathione. Lupeol and lupeol linoleate at 50 mg kg^{-1} body weight daily for 8 days, from 11 to 18 days after the adjuvant injection brought back the alterations to normal levels. The effect of lupeol linoleate was found to be better in this respect when compared with lupeol.[43]

10.2.7.1.6 Hemidesmus indicus (HI)

The anti-inflammatory activity of the pure compound (2-hydroxy-4-methoxy benzoic acid) isolated and purified from anantamul root extract was investigated. 2-OH-4-MeO benzoic acid effectively neutralized inflammation induced by *Vipera russelli* venom in male albino mice and reduced cotton-pellet–induced granuloma in rats. The compound produced a significant fall in body temperature in yeast-induced pyrexia in rats but did not change the normothermic body temperature. The compound effectively neutralized viper-venom–induced changes in serum phosphatase and transaminase activity in male albino rats. It also neutralized free radical formation as estimated by thiobaraturic acid reactive substances (TBARS) and SOD activities.[44]

10.2.7.1.7 Andrographis paniculata

Andrographolide, a diterpenoid lactone isolated from *Andrographis paniculata* (anti-inflammatory herb), was investigated for the ability to prevent phorbol-12-myristate-13-acetate (PMA)–induced reactive oxygen species (ROS) production, as well as *N*-formyl-methionyl-leucyl-phenylalanine (fMLP)–induced adhesion by rat neutrophils. The study showed that PMA (100 ng/ml) induced rapid accumulation of H_2O_2 and O_2 in neutrophils within 30 min. Andrographolide (0.1 to 10 μM) pretreatment (10 min, 37°C) significantly reduced the accumulation of these two oxygen-radical metabolites. Administration of andrographolide also significantly prevented fMLP-induced neutrophils adhesion. These data suggest that the mechanism of anti-inflammatory action of andrographolide may be via preventing ROS production and neutrophils adhesion.[45]

10.2.7.1.8 Aglaia roxburghiana (AG)

Alcoholic extracts of aerial portions and fruits of AR and the triterpines, roxburghiadiol A and B, were studied in carrageenin-induced rat-paw edema, cotton-pellet granuloma, and mast-cell degranulation induced by compound 48/48. The extract and the triterpines were found to be effective anti-inflammatory agents in this study.[46]

10.2.7.2 Analgesic Activity

There are few data available on the analgesic activity of antiarthritic herbs. A p-quinone, embeline, derived from *Embelia ribes* was investigated for analgesic activity. The potassium salt of embeline was found to be effective by oral, i.m., and i.c. routes of administration and the results compared well with morphine. Although potassium embelate acts centrally to produce analgesia, its effect is not antagonized by naloxone indicating a different central site of action. It has no abstinence syndrome as observed with morphine and no demonstrable anti-inflammatory action. The anlagesic effect of the alkaloid provides a scientific basis for its use in arthritis. In addition, lack of any adverse effects, high therapeutic index, and absence of abstinence syndrome provide basis for long-term safety of embelate as an analgesic.[47]

10.2.7.3 Mechanism of Action

One of the mechanisms of anti-inflammatory activity of Ayurvedic herbs may the AO property. Andrographolide isolated from leaves of *Andrographis paniculata* has been shown to inhibit nitric oxide generation in endotoxin-stimulated macrophages.[48]

The AO activity of two polyherbal formulations, *Maharasnadhi quatha* (MRQ) and *Weldehi choornaya* (WC), used by Ayurvedic medical practitioners in Srilanka for the treatment of RA patients, was assessed on SOD, GPX and catalase, lipid peroxidation (as estimated by TBARS generation), concentrations of serum iron, hemoglobin (Hb), and the total iron-binding capacity (TIBC). The overall results of the study demonstrated that MRQ has greater AO potential than WC.[49]

In another study,[50] the mechanism of suppression of inducible nitric oxide synthase (iNOS) and (COX-2) by ergolide, a sesquiterpene lactone from *Inula Britannica,* was investigated. Ergolide markedly attenuated the iNOS activity in a cell-free extract of LPS/IFN-gamma-stimulated RAW 264.7 macrophages and markedly decreased the production of prostaglandin E(2) (PGE(2)) in cell-free extract of the macrophages in a concentration-dependent manner, without alteration of the catalytic activity of COX-2. Ergolide decreased the level of iNOS and COX-2 protein, and iNOS RNA caused by stimulation of LPS/IFN-gamma in a concentration-dependent manner and inhibited nuclear factor-kappaB (NF-kappaB) activation, a transcription factor necessary for iNOS and COX-2 expression in response to LPS/IFN-gamma. This effect was accompanied by the parallel reduction of nuclear translocation of the subunit p65 of NF-kappaB as well as IkappaB-alpha degradation. These effects were completely blocked by treatment with cysteine. This finding suggests that the inhibitory effect of ergolide may be mediated by alkylation of NF-kappaB or an upstream molecule of NF-kappaB. Ergolide also directly inhibited the DNA-binding activity of active NF-kappaB in LPS/IFN-gamma-pretreated RAW 264.7 macrophages. The authors suggested that the overall effect of ergolide is the suppression of the expression of iNOS and COX-2, which play important roles in the inflammatory-signaling pathway.

10.3 Osteoarthritis (*Sandhigat Vata*)

10.3.1 Introduction

Sandhigat Vata (*Krostuka-sirsa*) is primarily a disease of vitiated *vata* settling into bone and bone marrow without any involvement of *ama*. The disease is characterized by acute pain, stiffness of the joints, impairment of the function of the joints, loss of muscle strength, and sleeplessness. This disorder resembles OA, which is also characterized by acute pain, involvement of diarthroidial joints, and functional limitations. Sedentary lifestyle as a causative factor of amavata is scientifically valid.[51] Current experiments in rabbits have shown that short repetitive immobilization induces OA. Even a 4-day immobilization period had a cumulative effect in producing OA.[52]

10.3.2 Clinical Description

OA starts out with pain in one joint but subsequently spreads to other joints. The joints commonly involved are the big toe, fingers, hip, knees, and both lumbar and cervical spine. Ankles are generally spared except in the secondary form of OA. These joints in the advanced stage of the disease exhibit deformity. Patients do not show the presence of the RA factor.

10.3.3 Treatment

Because *ama* is not involved, the treatment of OA is simpler than RA. On the basis of the constitution and involvement of other *dosas*, herbs and herbal preparations that alleviate vitiated *vata* are selected to treat OA. Because muscle atrophy commonly accompanies OA, the treatment also involves an adequate exercise program. Both muscle strength and range of motion can be improved with appropriate physical exercise. Regular bench-press and leg-press exercises with a certain amount of weight may slow down or even stop the progress of OA in early stages and may even help in later stages in some patients. Adequate amount of rest is also an important adjunct and should be included in the daily routine of OA patients.

Basically, the drug treatments for OA and RA are very similar because both have a common cause, vitiated *vata*. Single herbs and formulas listed in Table 10.1 to Table 10.3 that are commonly used to treat RA are also applicable to treat OA. In addition, *Kishore guggul* from the Ayurvedic Formulary of India is also used for OA. Singh[53] reported a case study showing usefulness of *guggul* (*C. mukul*) in treating OA of the knee. In a larger study in 30 OA patients, *guggul* extract (500 mg, three times/day for 2 months) provided significant relief in signs and symptoms of OA.[54,11]

In conventional medicine, the treatment of OA includes a proper exercise program, rest, NSAIDs, and newer NSAIDs (COX-2 inhibitors). Intra-articular injections of steroids and hyaluronan and joint replacement surgery are also used to treat OA. It is interesting to note that the NSAIDs and newer NSAIDs are the drugs also used to relieve pain and inflammation in RA.

10.4 Gout (*Rakta Vata*)

10.4.1 General Description

In Ayurveda, the origin of gout is believed to be in blood. When functionally impaired (vitiated) *vata* invades the blood and bone joints, it produces gout. It is characterized by acute excruciating pain (worse at night) and inflammation of the joints, which generally begins from a toe or finger and then gradually spreads to the other joints of the body. The affected joints are warmer than the body, swollen, extremely tender with a burning sensation, and have shiny overlying skin and dilated veins. The other symptoms are excessive sweating, rigidity, numbness, and discoloration of the skin on the affected joints. The joints return to normal after a few days with desquamation of the overlying skin. An acute attack may cause fever, anorexia, and general malaise.

In conventional medicine, gout is known as an inflammatory arthritis induced by the pathogenic deposition of aggregated monosodium urate monohydrate crystals (*tophi*), which deposit in various tissues and joints. Urate crystals can also deposit in kidneys. Chronic high levels of uric acid in the blood are necessary for the development of gout, although some other factors may be involved. This etiology points in the direction of the Ayurvedic etiology that indicates that blood is involved in this disease. If untreated, it can cause painful, destructive arthropathy and urolithiasis resulting in renal failure.

10.4.2 Treatment

Ayurvedic treatments include the following:

1. *Guduchi* (*T. cordifolia*) decoction of 14 to 28 ml made from 6 to 8 g of powder of leaves and stem to be ingested with purified *guggul* (2 to 4 g, three times/day)
2. Decoction of equal parts of *vasa* (*Adhatoda vasica*) leaves, stem of *guduchi*, and fruit pulp of *Aaragvadha* (*Cassia*) of 14 to 18 ml taken with castor oil (7 to 14 ml two times/day)
3. *Kishora guggul* and *Punarnavadi guggul* (3 g/day)
4. Additional single herbs and formulas used for RA (see Table 10.1 to Table 10.3)

To apply the treatment on the affected joints, a poultice of black sesame seeds is prepared in milk.

Guda (*Jaggary*), rice, wheat, gram, pigeon peas, spinach, black coffee, ripe fruit of white gourd, *Guduchi*, *Deodar* (*Cidrus deodar)* are useful articles of diet. The food articles to avoid are seeds of *Masa* (black phaseolus bean), *Kulattha* (dolichos beans), pea, legumes, radish, sugarcane products, wine, and yogurt. Because uric acid is the end product of protein metabolism, it is important to avoid high-protein diet. Sleeping during the day, exposure to heat, and excessive exercising should be avoided.

10.5 Spasmodic Torticollis, Lockjaw (*Hanu-Stambha*), Lumbago (*Kati Shula*), and Fibromyalgia

10.5.1 General Description

Vitiated *vata* is the cause for torticollis (*Manya-stambha*), lockjaw (*Hanu-stambha*), and lumbago (*kati shula*). When the vitiated *vata* invades the neck muscles it causes muscle rigidity and immobility of the neck and pain in the neck muscles. Similarly, when it invades jaw muscles and joints, it causes lockjaw. When it invades the lower part of the back it causes lumbago, and when it invades all body muscles it causes fibromyalgia (*Sarvang shula*). Pain and stiffness of the muscles are the main features of these diseases.

Specific etiology of these diseases is not known at this time. Ayurvedic etiology of these diseases refers to food and lifestyle habits that can aggravate *vata*.

10.5.2 Treatment

Because the causative *dosa* is vitiated *vata*, single herbs and formulas for the treatment of RA listed in Table 10.1 to Table 10.3 for RA are applicable. Additional formulas not in these tables but also used for these diseases are *Kishora guggul* and *Triphala guggul* from the Ayurvedic Formulary of India. Both formulas are given at a dose of 3 g/day. It is interesting that there are so many choices of treatments in Ayurveda. A physician needs to assess the body constitution, diagnose accompanying diseases, and determine the predominance of other *dosas* in order to select suitable herbal formulas and other components of the management regimen.

10.6 Future Research on Ayurvedic Herbal Fomulas for Musculoskeletal Disorders

Because the efficacy of many Ayurvedic herbs has been shown in animal models, the next step is to investigate the mechanism of action so that effective combination of herbs can be formulated. It is likely that these herbs may have selective inhibitory activity on COX-2 because they have not been known to cause any toxicity in the stomach or intestine. Ergolide, a sequiterpine lactone from *Inula britanica,* has been shown to inhibit the COX-2 activity.[49] *Semicarpous anacardium* has been shown to bring back the levels of altered AO defense system in adjuvant-induced arthritic rats.[41]

These and other biochemical mechanisms of action of these herbs should be further investigated.

References

1. Arnett, F.C., Rheumatoid arthritis, in *Cecil Text Book of Medicine,* Goldman, L. and Bennett, J.C., Eds., W.B. Saunders, Philadelphia, 2000, chap. 21.
2. Insel, P.A., Analgesic-antipyretic and anti-inflammatory ageeents and drugs employed in the treatment of gout, in *Goodman & Gillman's The Pharacological Basis of Therapeutics,* Hardman, J.G., Limbird, L.E., Molinoff, P.B., Ruddon, R.W., and Gillman, A., Eds., McGraw-Hill, New York, 1996, chap. 27.
3. Hawkey, C.J., The gastroenterologist's case load: contribution of the rheumatologist, *Semin. Arthritis Rheum.,* 26, 11, 1997.
4. Brandt, K.D., Should nonsteroidal anti-inflammatory drugs be used to treat osteoarthritis, *Controversies Clin. Rheum.,* 19, 24, 1993.
5. Eisenberg, D.M., Davis, R.B., Ettner, S.L., Apple, S., Wilkey, S., Von Rompay, M., and Kessler, R.C., Trends in alternative medicine use in the United States, 1990–1997, *J.A.M.A.,* 280, 1569, 1998.
6. Chandrashekara, S., Anilkumar, T., and Jamuna, S., Complementary and alternative drug therapy in arthritis, *J. Assoc. Physicians India,* 50, 223, 2002.
7. Spangler, R.S., Cyclooxygenase 1 and 2 in rheumatic disease: implications for nonsteroidal anti-inflammatory drug therapy, *Semin. Arthritis Rheum.,* 26, 435, 1996.
8. Kumar, N. and Kumar, A., An applied aspect of rheumatoid arthritis: an ayurvedic approach, *J. Res. Ayurveda Siddha,* 16, 134, 1995.
9. Rosenberg, A., Bones, joints and soft tissue tumors, in *Robbins Pathologic Basis of Disease,* Cotran, R.S., Kumar, V. N., and Collins, T., Eds., W.B. Saunders, Philadelphia, 1999, chap. 28.
10. Harris, E.D., Clinical features in rheumatoid arthritis, in *Text Book of Rheumatology,* Kelley, W.N., Rudy, S., Harris, E.D., and Sledge, C.B., Eds., W.B. Saunders, Philadelphia, 1997, chap. 55.
11. Mishra, L.C., Singh, B.B., and Dagenais, S., Ayurvedic therapies for arthritis, *Top. Clin. Chiropractic.,* 7, 13–16, 2000.
12. Sudarsanan, P.K. and Sankarankutty, P., Evaluation of the efficacy of classical Sodhana therapy (Pancakarma) in the management of rheumatoid arthritis, *J. Res. Ayurveda Siddha,* 14, 115, 1993.
13. Prem Kishore, Pandey, P.N., and Ruhil, S.D., Role of sunthi-guduci in the treatement of amavata-rheumatoid arthritis, *J. Res. Ayurveda Siddha,* 1, 417, 1980.
14. Namboodiri, M.N.S., Sethu, K.S., Madhavikutty, P., Vijayan, N.P., and Namboodiri, P.K.N., Clinical study on the treatment of amavata with compound ayurvedic preparation, *J. Res. Ayurveda Siddha,* 5, 1, 1984.
15. Reddy, K.R.C. (Translator), *Aausadha Kalpana,* in *Bhasajya Ratnavali,* Chaukhambha Sanskrit Bhawan Charu Printers, Ghoghar, Varanasi-1, 1988.

16. Prem Kishore and Banerjee, S.N., Clinical evaluation of rasonadi kvatha in the treatment of amavata-rheumatoid arthritis, *J. Res. Ayurveda Siddha*, 9, 29, 1988.
17. Kulkarni, R.R., Patki, P.S., Jog, V.P., Gandage, S.G., Patwardhan, B., and Jeejeebhoy, B., Treatment of osteoarthritis with a herbomineral formulation: a double-blind, placebo-controlled, cross-over study, *J. Ethnopharmacol.*, 33, 91, 1991.
18. Srivastava, K.C. and Mustafa, T., Ginger (zingiber officinale) and rheumatic disorders, *Med. Hypotheses*, 29, 25, 1989.
19. Srivastava, K.C. and Mustafa, T., Ginger (zingiber officinale) in rheumatism and musculoskeletal disorders, *Med. Hypotheses*, 39, 342, 1992.
20. Bhattathiri, P.P.N., Sasidharan, S., Vijayan, M.P., and Nair, P.R.C., Management of Amavata with certain Ayurvedic preparations, *J. Res. Ayurveda Siddha*, 15, 115, 1994.
21. Reddy, K.P. and Singh, R.H., Clinical and immunological assessment of a relative langhana schedule in cases of amavata, *J. Res. Ayurveda Siddha*, 16, 15, 1995.
22. Srinivasulu, M., Role of virechana karma in amavata by Gandhara Hastadi Kwatha, *J. Res. Ayurveda Siddha*, 19, 132, 1998.
23. Swamy, G.K. and Bhattathiri, P.P.N., Vatari guggulu and Maharasnadi Kwatha in the management of Amavata: a clinical study, *J. Res. Ayurveda Siddha*, 19, 41, 1998.
24. Anbalagan, K. and Siddique, J., Influence of an Indian medicine (ashwagandha) on acute phase reactants in inflammation, *Indian J. Exp. Biol.*, 19, 245, 1981.
25. Anbalagan, K. and Siddique, J., Role of prostagandins in acute phase proteins in inflammation, *Biochem. Med.*, 31, 236, 1984.
26. Begum, V.H. and Sadique, J., Effect of withania somnifera on glycosaminoglycan synthesis in carragenin-induced air pouch granuloma, *Biochem. Med. Metab. Biol.*, 38, 272, 1987.
27. Begum, V.H. and Sadique, J., Long term effect of herbal drug withania somnifera on adjuvant induced arthritis in rats, *Indian J. Exp. Biol.*, 26, 877, 1988.
28. al Hindawi, M.K., Khafaji, S.H., and Abdul-Nabi, M.H., Anti-granuloma activity of Iraqi withania somnifera, *J. Ethnopharmacol.*, 37, 113, 1992.
29. Bikshapathi, T. and Kumari, K., Clinical evaluation of ashwagandha in the management of ama-vata, *J. Res. Ayurveda Siddha*, 20, 46, 1999.
30. Oliver, S.J. and Brahn, E., Combination therapy in rheumatoid arthritis: the animal model perspective, *J. Rheumatol.*, 23, 56, 1996.
31. Bendele, A., McComb, J., Gould, T., McAbee, T., Sennello, G., Chlipala, E., and Boulder, G.M., Animal models of arthritis: relevance to human disease, *Toxicol. Pathol.*, 27, 134, 1999.
32. Prasad, D.N. and Achari, G., A study of anti-arthritic action of vanda roxburghii in albino rats, *J. Indian Med. Assoc.*, 46, 234, 1966.
33. Gujaral, M.L., Sareen, K., Tangri, K.K., Amma, M.K.P., and Roy, A.K., Anti-arthritic and anti-inflammatory activity of gum (balsamodendron mukul hook), *Indian J. Physiol. Pharmacol.*, 4, 267, 1960.
34. Gujaral, M.L., Sareen, K., Reddy, G.S., Amma, M.K.P., and Kumari, G., Endocrinological studies on the loeoresin of gum guggul, *Indian J. Med. Sci.*, 16, 847, 1962.
35. Arora, R.B., Kapoor, S., Gupta, S.K., and Sharma, R.C., Isolation of a crystalline steroidal compound from Commiphora mukul and its anti-inflammatory activity, *Indian J. Exp. Biol.*, 9, 403, 1971.
36. Sharma, J.N. and Sharma, J.N., Comparison of the anti-inflammatory activity of commiphora mukul (an indigenous drug) with those of phenylbutazone and ibuprofen in experimental arthritis induced by mycobacterial adjuvant, *Arzneimittelforschung*, 27, 1455, 1977.
37. Duwiejua, M., Zeitlin, I.J., Waterman, P.G., Chapman, J., Mhango, G.J., and Provan, G.J., Anti-inflammatory activity of resins from some species of the plant family burseraceae, *Planta Med.*, 59, 12, 1993.
38. Kimura, I., Yoshikawa, M., Kobayashi, S., Sugihara, Y., Suzuki, M., Oominami, H., Murakami, T., Matsuda, H., and Doiphode, V.V., New triterpenes, myrrhanol A and myrrhanone A, from guggul-gum resins, and their potent anti-inflammatory effect on adjuvant-induced air-pouch granuloma of mice, *Bioorg. Med. Chem. Lett.*, 23, 985, 2001.

39. Saxena, R.S., Gupta, B., Saxena, K.K., Singh, R.C., and Prasad, D.N., Study of anti-inflammatory activity in the leaves of *nyctanthes arbor tristis linn:* an Indian medicinal plant, *J. Ethnopharmacol.*, 11, 319, 1984.
40. Saraf, M.N., Ghooi, R.B., and Patwardhan, B.K., Studies on the mechanism of action of semecarpus anacardium in rheumatoid arthritis, *J. Ethnopharmacol.*, 25, 159, 1989.
41. Vijayalakshmi, T., Muthulakshmi, V., and Sachdanandam, P., Effect of the milk extract of semecarpus anacardium nut on adjuvant arthritis: a dose-dependent study in Wistar albino rats, *Gen. Pharmacol.*, 27, 1223, 1996.
42. Vijayalakshmi, T., Muthulakshmi, V., and Sachdanandam, P., Salubrious effect of semecarpus anacardium against lipid peroxidative changes in adjuvant arthritis studied in rats, *Mol. Cell Biochem.*, 175, 65, 1997.
43. Geetha, T., Varalakshmi, P., and Latha, R.M., Effects of triterpines from crataeva nurvala stem bark on lipid peroxidation in adjuvant induced arthritis in rats, *Pharmacol. Res.*, 37, 191, 1998.
44. Alam, M.I. and Gomes, A., Viper venom-induced inflammation and inhibition of free radical formation by pure compound (2-hydroxy-4-methoxy benzoic acid) isolated and purified from anantamul (*Hemidesmus indicus* R. BR) root extract A, *Toxicon*, 36, 207, 1998.
45. Shen, Y.C., Chen, C.F., and Chiou, W.F., Suppression of rat neutrophil reactive oxygen species production and adhesion by the diterpenoid lactone andrographolide, *Planta Med.*, 66, 314, 2000.
46. Janaki, S., Vijaysekaran, V., Viswanathan, S., and Balkrishna, K., Anti-inflammatory activity of Aglaia roxburghiana var. beddomei extract and triterpines roxburghiadiol A and B, *J. Ethnopharmacol.*, 67, 45, 1999.
47. Atal, C.K., Siddiqui, M.A., Zutshi, U., Amla, V., Johri, R.K., Rao, P.G., and Kour, S., 1. J Non-narcotic orally effective, centrally acting analgesic from an Ayurvedic drug, *J. Ethnopharmacol.*, 11, 309, 1984.
48. Chiou, W.F., Chen, C.F., and Lin, J.J., Mechanisms of suppression of inducible nitric oxide synthase (iNOS) expression in RAW 264.7 cells by andrographolide, *Br. J. Pharmacol.*, 129, 1553, 2000.
49. Ira Thabrew, M., Senaratna, L., Samarawickrema, N., and Munasinghe, C., Antioxidant potential of two polyherbal preparations used in ayurveda for the treatment of rheumatoid arthritis, *J. Ethnopharmacol.*, 76, 285, 2001.
50. Whan Han, J., Gon Lee, B., Kee Kim, Y., Woo Yoon, J., Kyoung Jin, H., Hong, S., Young Lee, H., Ro Lee, K., and Woo Lee, H., Ergolide, sesquiterpene lactone from Inula britannica, inhibits inducible nitric oxide synthase and cyclo-oxygenase-2 expression in RAW 264.7 macrophages through the inactivation of NF-kappaB, *Br. J. Pharmacol.*, 133, 503, 2001.
51. Haapala, J., Arokoski, J.P., Ronkko, S., Agren, U., Kosma, V.M., Lohmander, L.S., Tammi, M., Helminen, H.J., and Kiviranta, I., Decline after immobilisation and recovery after remobilisation of synovial fluid, *Ann. Rheum. Dis.*, 60, 55, 2001.
52. Videman, T., Experimental osteoarthritis in the rabbit, *Acta. Orthop. Scand.*, 53, 339, 1982.
53. Singh, B.B., Mishra, L.C., Aquilina, N., and Kohlbeck, F., Usefulness of guggul (commiphora mukul) for osteoarthritis of the knee: an experimental case study, *Alternative Ther. Health Med.*, 7, 120, 2001.
54. Singh, B.B., Mishra, L.C., Vinjamury, S.P., Aquilina, N., Singh, V.J., and Shepard, N., The effectiveness of commiphora mukul for osteoarthritis of the knee: an outcomes study, *Alt. Ther. Health Med.*, 9, 74, 2003.

11

Ayurvedic Therapies of Sciatica (Gridhrasi)

Subhash Singh

CONTENTS

0-8493-1366-X/04/$0.00+$1.50

11.1 Introduction

Neuropathic pain due to injury or dysfunction of the nervous system is a difficult therapeutic challenge in the treatment of chronic pain. The pain of sciatica is typically a radiating pain that usually is related to a specific nerve root. Nerve dysfunction may be present in both motor and sensory modalities. The response of neuropathic pain to conventional analgesics has been in many cases disappointing. Several studies have suggested that spinal clonidine may be effective in treating some forms of neuropathic pain; some of the authors do not advocate such procedures because of its major complications. Thousands of years ago, Charaka, a great physician and Susruta (800 B.C.), the father of the surgery, identified the disease and named it *gridhrasi*. This recent research was aimed to establish the ancient ayurvedic therapeutic values among the people of modern era, evaluating fundamental principles by scientific parameters. In this chapter, the current knowledge about pathophysiologic mechanism, diagnosis, and management of sciatica is reviewed and discussed in relation to its prognosis.

11.2 Epidemiology

Lower back pain (LBP) is the most common presentation of lumbar spine disorders. Reports from various research institutes (Central Council for Research in Ayurveda and Siddha [CCRAS]), different modern class-three level hospitals, and referral centers show that 3 to 5% of the patients visiting annually in India present with LBP. Of them, 1.5% have features of sciatica, in which 62 to 69% are males and 31 to 38% are females. Sciatica affects mostly adult males, particularly those 41 to 60 years old. The ratio of incidence is similar in the people of low income as well as in higher income groups. It is more prevalent in the month from May to July (rainy season) in which *vata dosa* naturally gets vitiated and people become sick. People of *vataj prakriti* are more prone to the disease. Annual incidence of LBP in the U.S. is 2 to 5%, and annual cost of direct medical care for LBP has been estimated at $13 to $16 billion. Total annual societal costs are estimated at $20 to $50 billion.[1] Incidents are the same among heavy, light, and sedentary workers, although a higher proportion of heavy workers are incapacitated with LBP. Sciatic pain is common in people who either sit or stand for prolonged periods of time.

11.3 Definition

When tendons of the toes and heel become paralyzed due to vitiated *vata* and confine the extension of the leg, the disease is known as sciatica.[2,3] The pain arises in the gluteal region, gradually spreads and radiates down the back of the thigh and knee, and travels up to the leg and foot. Perception of numbness, excruciating pain, needling sensation, restrained movement, and muscle spasm repeatedly in the limb are the main characteristics of the disease. Patients sometime feel lassitude, heaviness in the body, and may also have lack of appetite.[4]

11.4 Clinical Description

Sciatica is a disease of the nerves. The sciatic nerve is the largest nerve in the body and has a long course. It is derived from fourth and fifth lumbar (L_4 and L_5) and first and second sacral (S_1 and S_2) roots. It provides motor innervation of the hamstring muscles and to all muscles below the knee. It carries sensory impulses from the posterior aspect of the thigh and the posterior and lateral aspect of the leg and entire sole. Any pathological process that impinges upon at this level may cause pain associated with sciatica. The mechanism involved in the disease process is distortion; stretching; and irritation or compression of the spinal root (most often central to the intervertebral foramen), which causes tingling, paresthesias and numbness or sensory impairment of the skin, soreness of the skin, and tenderness along the nerve. It usually accompanies radicular pain, loss of reflexes, weakness, atrophy, fascicular twitching, and occasionally stasis edema if motor fibers of the anterior root are involved.

Ayurveda divides this disease into two categories: *vataj* and *vat-kaphaj*. *Vataj* disease is caused by the vitiation of *vata dosa* alone and contains a needling sensation. The body becomes crooked and the joints of the thigh, knee, and hip are rendered stiff.[5] *Vata-kaphaj* disease is caused mainly by *vata* in company with *kapha dosa*. Numbness, excruciating pain, paresthesias, restrained movement, and repeated muscle spasms are distinguishing features of *vataj* sciatica. It is characterized by lassitude, heaviness in the body, and anorexia, along with associated symptoms of *vataj* sciatica. Patients suffer from dyspepsia and experience lassitude, anorexia, and excessive salivation.

11.5 Etiology (*Vyadhi Haitu*)

The potential causes of sciatica are myriad, but these account for only 15% of the total cases. The mechanisms of underlying neuropathic pain in 85% of the cases are still not clear. Sciatica is one of the many *vataj* diseases *(nanatmaj vyadhis)*. *Vata dosa* is the main culprit in the disease. The nucleus pulposus of intervertebral disc is probably not pain sensitive under normal circumstances but may induce some changes in the nerve root.[6]

The causes of sciatica may be classified in to two main categories: pathology based and injury based. Both categories are discussed below.

11.5.1 Pathology Based

The common causes of sciatica are *vata*-aggravating factors, such as grief, sorrowful thought and sickness, sitting or sleeping on uncomfortable beds, anger, day sleeping and night awakening, apprehension, suppression of natural urges, indigestion, injury, starvation, and systemic disorders (e.g., osteomalacia, hyperparathyroidism, hyperthyroidism, multiple myeloma, and glucocorticoid use). Osteoporosis may be associated with the causes of disk fracture. These degenerative changes may be considered under the cause described in Ayurveda in terms of *dhatu sanchhayat,* meaning the degeneration of essential constituents. Other causes of sciatica are spondylolisthesis (a degenerative spine disease), spinal stenosis resulting from bony encroachment by osteoarthritis, lumbar adhesive arachnoiditis (the result of a fibrotic process following an inflammatory response to local tissue injury within a subarachnoid space), systemic cancer with epidural metastases of tumor, diabetes mellitus (DM), and polyarteritis nodosa.

True sciatica or radicular pain related to nerve root compression occurs in a small percentage of patients with LBP, roughly 1%. Herniation of nucleus pulposus occurs in 95 to 98% of cases at the disc between the L_4 and L_5 vertebrae or between the L_5 and S_1; it sometimes plays an important role in developing sciatica. One third of the patients with undiagnosed LBP and known systemic cancer have epidural metastasis of tumor and one third have pain associated with vertebral metastasis alone.[7] Increased levels of circulating antibodies against one or more glycosphingo lipids were detected in 72% of patients with acute sciatica in 61% of sciatica patients at a 4-year follow-up visit (eight antigens analyzed) and in 54% in patients undergoing discectomy.[8] Nerve ischemia may constitute an important factor in the pathology of human peripheral nerve injury and neuropathy.[9,10] Studies on rats indicated that the circulating monocyte and macrophages are well involved in the development of hyperalgesia and wallerian degeneration after nerve injury.[11] The idiopathic mononeuropathy in young adults seems to occur in 6 to 10% of cases of microneuropathies of sciatic nerve.[12]

11.5.2 Injury Based

Common injury-related causes of sciatica are the unusual and excessive activities of the lower body and legs, such as jumping, climbing, stretching and other movements, and spinal fracture or dislocation resulting from compression (in 80%). The other causes are flexion injuries presenting the features of sciatica, neurologic impairment associated with the injuries caused by falling from height or sudden deceleration in an automobile accident, disk herniation, or spondylolysis as a bony defect of the pars interarticularis of the lower lumbar vertebrae (probably caused by stress fracture in the congenitally abnormal segment). The causes of arachnoiditis are myelography, multiple lumbar operations, chronic spinal infections, spinal cord injury, intrathecal hemorrhage, intrathecal injection of steroids, and anesthetics, and sometimes play an important role in producing sciatica. Overweight individuals, especially females who weigh >85 kg, occasionally present the features of sciatica recurrently due to abdominal muscle pressure on lumbosacral spine.

11.6 Pathogenesis

According to the *Ayurvedic* concept, vitiated *vata dosa,* by its own aggravating factors, strongly fills up the hollowed streams that produce many kinds of diseases pertaining to either all or one part of the body.[4,5,13] In this pathogenesis *vata dosa*, blood, muscle, bone, ligaments, and tendons are involved.

In conventional medicine, the lumbosacral nerve roots have been known for more than 6 decades to be intimately involved in sciatica. However, the basic pathophysiologic mechanisms are still not well understood. Intervertebral disk is a fibrocartilagenous structure that lies between two vertebral bodies. It consists of soft inner nucleus pulposus surrounded by thicker fibrous tissue wall, the annulus fibrosus. The nucleus pulposus is a gelatinous structure and acts as a shock absorber between adjacent vertebral bodies. As age advances, the entire disc structure becomes more susceptible to trauma and compression. Tears develop in the annulus fibrosus as a result of repeated minor trauma; eventually, if the tears become large enough, a portion of the soft nucleus pulposus herniates through the annulus. Asymptomatic herniation may occur into the center of the vertebral bodies bordering the disc. When disc material herniates into the vertebral canal, it can compress nerve endings and nerve roots, causing pain and other symptoms. Generally, the disc herniates lateral to the posterior longitudinal ligaments, compressing spinal roots as they enter the intervertebral foramen. Occasionally, the disc herniates more centrally, compressing either the spinal cord or the cauda equina.

An experimental study examined compression-induced impairment of vasculature. It was observed that sensory fibers are slightly more susceptible to compression than are the motor fibers and that nerve roots are more susceptible to compression injury than are the nerve fibers.[14] The study further suggests that nucleus pulposus has the potential to injure the nerve root. Proteoglycans and tumor necrosis factors present in disc cells may also be involved in early pathogenic process of the nerve root.[6]

11.7 Clinical Course and Prognosis

The clinical course of sciatic pain associated with systemic illness is that of the underlying disease. Excluding patients with local infections, congenital anomalies, metastatic neoplastic tumors, and cauda equina syndrome, whose prognosis depends on the specific cause and available treatment, the disease is left with the score of the typical patient with sciatica. From an Ayurvedic perspective, the prognosis is good in patients with *vataj* sciatica; 70% of patients are relieved of pain, enabling them to return to full activity within a 3- to 4-week period, and complete remission is observed in more than 90% of cases within a 6- to 8-week period. Among the patients who have the symptoms of *vat-kaphaj gridhrasi*, recurrence has been noted in 8% of cases 6 months to 5 years, after the treatment. Recurrence is also observed in those suffering from DM and herniated disc.

11.8 Clinical Examination and Diagnosis

11.8.1 History

History may provide a definite clue to set up the diagnosis of the patient. A patient presenting history of low back trauma with inability to move the legs strongly suggests either acute lumbar disc herniation or fracture. In more severe trauma, the patient may sustain a fracture, dislocation, or a burst fracture that involves not only the vertebral body but the posterior elements as well. Trauma caused by falling from a height may be associated with the fracture of pars interarticularis of L_5 vertebra. Pain after a pure flexion injury indicates a pathologic condition of the disc end plates, whereas pain after torsional is more often associated with disruption of posterior structures (i.e., facet joint and ligament injury). The duration, quality, severity and location of pain all are important in a detailed history.

An acute sciatic pain can last up to 6 weeks in 90% of patients; if it persists beyond 2 months, specific diagnosis in most cases is needed. Patients presenting a history of bowel and bladder dysfunction (incontinence or retention), perianal paresthesia, or pain are usually associated with cauda equina syndrome. Patients suffering from sciatica symptoms should be examined for the following conditions: spondylosis, osteomyelitis, osteoporosis, diskitis, spinal epidural abscess, herniated lumbar disk, DM, metastatic tumors, hyperparathyroidism, and neurological diseases. Occupational, social, and psychological factors also must be taken into account in history taking. For example, job dissatisfaction can sometimes adversely affect the prognosis. All factors should be considered in a proper manner.

11.8.2 Physical Examination

11.8.2.1 Spine Examination

A normal spine shows a thoracic kyphosis, lumbar lordosis, and cervical lordosis in sagital plain; exaggeration of these alignments may result in hyperkyphosis (*lameback*) of the thoracic spine or hyperlordsis (*swayback*) of the lumbar spine. A spasm of lumbar paravertebral muscles results in the flattening of the usual lumbar lordosis; examination may reveal lateral curvature of the spine (scoliosis) or an asymmetry in the appearance of paraspinal muscles, suggesting muscle spasm. Taut para spinal muscles limit the motion of the lumbar spine. Back pain of bony spine origin is often reproduced by palpation or percussion over the spinous process of the affected vertebrae. Nerve root compression is indicated by radicular pain, sensory disturbances, coarse twitching, fasciculation, muscle spasm, and the impairment of tendon reflexes. Motor abnormality may also occur but is usually less prominent than the pain and sensory disturbances.

Because the herniation of intervertebral lumbar disc most often occurs between L_4–L_5 and L_5–S_1 with irritation and compression of L_5 and S_1 root, respectively, it is important to recognize the clinical characteristics of lesions of these two roots. If a patient complains of pain in the hip region, groin, posterolateral thigh, lateral calf radiating to the external malleolus, or dorsal surface of the foot, the first or second and third toes indicate L_5 nerve root compression. Paresthesia may be in the entire territory or only in the lateral calf, foot, and toes. Tenderness is felt in lateral gluteal region and near the head of fibula. If there is muscle weakness, difficult dorsiflexion of the great toe and, less often, of the foot is shown. Moderately depressed ankle jerk may be observed in some patients. Generally, knee and ankle reflexes are not impaired but may be observed in rare cases.

Walking on the heel may be more difficult for a patient because of weakness of dorsiflexion of the foot. In S_1 root compression, the patient feels pain in the mid-gluteal region, posterior part of the thigh, posterior of calf to the heel, and the plantar surface of the foot and fourth and fifth toes. Tenderness is most pronounced over the mid-gluteal region (sacroiliac joint), posterior thigh area, and calf. It may sometimes extend to the rectum, testicles, or labia. The patient's complaint of paresthesia and loss of sensation is more likely in the lower leg and outer toes. If nerve weakness is present, there is difficulty in plantar flexion of the foot and toes. In this nerve involvement majority of cases show diminished or absent ankle reflex (Archilles tendon reflex); walking on the toes is more difficult because of the weakness of plantar flexors.

Disc may herniate into the adjacent vertebral body during the process of degeneration and may give rise to a Schmort's node. Such cases often show no signs of nerve root involvement, though the symptoms are same as in sciatica. The lumbar disc syndrome is usually unilateral. But sometimes massive derangements of disc or the extrusion of the large free fragment into the canal presents lateral symptoms and signs of sciatica that may be associated with the paralysis of the sphincters. The infrequent occurrence of L_3 and L_4 disk herniation with L_4 root compression is manifested as a diminished knee jerk (patellar tendon reflex), quadriceps weakness, and hypersthesia over the lateral aspect of the thigh.

11.8.2.2 Postural Examination

The fully developed syndrome of ruptured lumbar disc consists of backache, abnormal posture, and limitation of motion. Lateral bending to the side opposite the involved spinal element may stretch the affected tissue, worsen pain, and limit motion. Reduction of the lateral flexion is more suggestive of spondyloarthropathy. Hyperextension of the spine (with patient prone or standing) is limited in nerve root compression, ligamentous or facet joint injury, and bony spine disease. Increased discomfort with spinal extension indicates spinal stenosis. Forward bending in the standing posture with legs straight stretches the sciatic nerve and its root presenting pain. Flexion of the hip is normal in patients with lumbar spine diseases, but flexion of the lumbar spine is limited and sometimes painful. The manual internal and external rotation at the hip with the knee and hip in flexion (Patrick sign) may produce pain.

The most useful, simple maneuver in assessing nerve root impingement is the straight leg raising (SLR) test. In supine position, a passive straight leg raising (possible up to 80 to 90° in a normal individual without pain) or passive dorsiflexion of foot during the maneuver adds to the stretch of L_5 and S_1 nerve root and sciatic nerve, resulting in pain that is readily identified by the patient. If this is the case, the test is positive. To exclude false positive results, the physician should attempt repeated trials. The angle associated with pain should be reproducible when the physician passively flexes the patient's hip with the knee in flexion, then slowly extends the foreleg. An important supplement to the direct SLR is the *crossed SLR*. The crossed SLR is positive when performance of the maneuver on one leg reproduces pain in the opposite leg or buttock. The nerve root lesion is always on the side of the pain. The reverse SLR is a similar but less quantified provocative test that is performed to detect L_2 and L_4 nerve root lesion. This sign is elicited by making the patient stand next to the examination table and passively extending each leg while the patient continues to stand. This maneuver stretches the L_2 and L_4 nerve roots and the femoral nerve because the nerve passes anterior to the hip.

11.9 Diagnosis

After taking a detailed history and performing the complete physical examination of the patient, diagnosis is made on the basis of findings, subjective, and objective parameters preceding laboratory studies for mere confirmation. Examples of subjective parameters include radiating pain starting from the gluteal region toward the leg and foot, tenderness along the course of nerve, severe pain when squatting, sensory and motor changes, sphincteric tone, and positive SLR signs. Examples of objective parameters include pricking and pulling pain, stiffness, ankle and knee jerk, plantar and dorsal reflexes, pressing power, muscle wasting, walking speed, posture, and sensory impairment.

11.9.1 Laboratory Investigations

Investigations required for the patients are always guided by the history taken, examination performed, progress observed, and risk factors to the underlying disease. A physician has to decide what type of critical investigation is required for his or her patient. Exhaustive, hazardous, more expensive, and complication-creating tests should always be avoided. A patient having duration of illness less than 2 weeks and presenting history of no trauma or any serious disease without risk factors for underlying disease needs no investigation. Only conservative treatments are required. If the patient does not respond by the end of the second week, routine laboratory studies such as routine and microscopic urine examination; complete blood count; percentage of hemoglobin; erythrocyte sedimentation rate (ESR); chemistry panel; human leukocyte antigen (HLA) B-27; rheumatologic tests; immunoglobulin; calcium phosphate; alkaline phosphatase; and a plain x-ray of the lumbosacral part of the spine in anteroposterior, lateral, and oblique planes are required. Physician should keep in mind that the lumbosacral spine radiographs are abnormal in most persons over 50 years old and are rarely helpful.

If the pain still persists for more than 4 weeks and the causative factor is not elicited, the next option of choice is magnetic resonance imaging (MRI) and computed tomography (CT) scan-myelography. MRI is an excellent noninvasive imaging method for the lumbar spine. MRI elicites well the soft tissue such as disc, nerve roots, thecal sac, and paraspinous soft tissue. CT-myelography provides the greatest information about osseous lesions in the region of the lateral recess and intervertebral foramen. CT-myelography is particularly helpful in evaluating spondylolysis, infection, or tumor associated with bony destruction. Electromyography (EMG) is also useful to assess the functional integrity of the peripheral nervous system. In sciatica, sensory nerve conduction studies are normal. Sometimes a radionuclide bone scan is used to elucidate sinester cause for sciatica, including occult spondylolysis, primary and metastatic tumors, diskitis and vertebral osteomyelitis, but the technique is inferior to MRI and CT-myelography.

11.10 Therapy (*Chikitsa*)

A comprehensive treatment plan should be made keeping in view the duration, onset, risk factors of the disease, and a goal of early return of the patient to maximum routine functions. The treatment of sciatica in Ayurveda is based on a set of principles involving palliative purification as well as enema therapy (see Chapters 3 and 5). Preparations of

Commiphora mukul (guggul), Strychnos nuxvomica (vistinduk), Ricinus communis (erand), Allium sativum (garlic), and *Vitex negundo* Linn. *(nirgundi)* are extensively recommended for the treatment of *vat vyadhis* in general and sciatica in particular.

11.10.1 Shaman *Shodhan* Therapy

Palliative treatment (Shaman therapy) includes *guggul* and *vistinduk* preparations orally (Table 11.1) along with local massage and fomention. Complete bed rest for 4 to 5 days provides additional benefit to the patient. More than 65% of patients have been benefited within 2 to 3 weeks from this combination therapy. The response of steam fomention with *rasnasaptak* decoction has been proven better than poultice or fomentation with hot sand in bags. If the patient's bowels are constipated, he or she may be administered castor oil. Garlic, castor, and vitex act against the factors responsible for this disease. *Trayodashang* and *yogaraj* are better formulations in *guggul* preparations. *Punarnavadi guggul* is commonly prescribed in the patients with stasis edema. Common formulations used in the treatment of sciatica are listed in Table 11.1.

Most of the Ayurvedic classics recommend enema therapy in the management of sciatica. The enema is an important part of purification therapy that eliminates the waste materials from channels. Palliative treatment given after purification is believed to act more effectively and disease is not relapsed once cured. If the patient does not respond within 2 weeks of palliative treatment alone, purification therapy should then be included in the treatment. Purification procedures, in which oleation, fomentation, purgation, and enemas are used in the treatment of sciatica, have been found most effective (see Chapter 4 on *panchakarma* therapy).

When severe pain and neuromotor deficit from sciatica persist despite 4 to 8 weeks of appropriate conservative therapy, bloodletting therapy is advised. Bloodletting provides quick relief in pain and other inflammatory conditions. Details of the procedure are discussed in Chapter 4.

11.10.2 Cautery Therapy

If the pain and neurologic findings do not disappear on these prolonged conservative managements, or if the patient suffers frequently recurring acute episodes, cautery may be indicated. Cauterization stimulates the nerve briskly like transcutaneous electrical nerve stimulation (TENS) or percutaneous electrical nerve stimulation percutaneous electrical nerve stimulation (PENS). It is performed either between the tendo calcaneous and malleolus (in L_5 impingement) or at the plantar surface of the little toe (in S_1 impingement) in a peculiar marklike dot by a copper wire of 4 mm diameter. The burnt place is smeared with micro fine powders of *Pterocarpus santalinus* Linn. *(rakt chandan)* and *Glycyrrhiza glabra* Linn. *(yashtimadhu)*. Cauterization provides short-term relief to the patients. Occasionally, some patients may receive a permanent cure. In few studies, two to three burns on the limb along the course of nerve were found to be optimum. Cautery should be avoided in children, the elderly, apprehensive patients, patients with *pittaj prakriti*, pregnant women, hemoptytic or hematemetic, diarrheic, weakened, and leprotic patients.

A minor surgery for sciatica has been suggested by Datta (11th century A.D.),[16] but the details are not clear. Patients impaired by chronic sciatica pain also pose a special challenge. Alcoholism, depression, headaches, disruptions in family dynamics, unnecessary regular medications and job dissatisfaction, psychosocial issues, and narcotic addiction may cause chronic pain condition in sciatica. Attention must be focused on these factors. Lifestyle changes, reassurance, and education are important. If there is a

TABLE 11.1

Formulations Used in Therapy of Sciatica, Monoplegia, and Paraplegia

No.	Name (Manufacturer*)	Doses, Vehicle, and Duration	Ref.
1	*Dwatrinshak guggul*	3 g in the morning with cow's *ghrit* or honey (12 g)	13
2	*Punarnavadya guggul* (a, b, c)	3 g/day with lukewarm water	31
3	*Pathyadi guggul*	3 g/day with lukewarm water	32
4	*Rasnadya guggul* (a)	1 g three times/day with lukewarm water or milk	13
5	*Singhnad guggul* (a, b, c)	3 g/day with lukewarm water	16
6	*Trayodashang guggul* (a, b, c, d, e)	1 g three times/day with milk or lukewarm water	17
7	*Yograj guggul* (a, b, c, d, e)	1 g three times/day with lukewarm water	18
8	*Vatari guggul*	3 g/day with lukewarm water	34
9	*Gorochanadi gutika* (d)	250 mg three times/day for 60 days with *Ashwagandha* decoction (60 ml)	21
10	*Vistinduk vati* (b, e)	250 mg three times/day with water	17
11	*Ajamodadi churna* (b)	3 g three times/day with lukewarm water	35
12	*Krishna churna* (b)	500 mg/day in addition to cow's urine (50 ml) and castor oil (15 ml)	32, 33
13	*Dashmool, khireti, rasna* leaves, *guduchi*, and *shunthi* (powdered and mixed in equal proportion)	3 g twice/day with castor oil (15 ml/day)	16
14	*Mahanimb* stem bark kalk	3 g three times/day with water	13, 32
15	Purified *kupilu* seed powder	100 mg twice/day with water for 15 days	18
16	*Arusha, danti*, and *chirayata* (equal parts) decoction	25 ml twice/day with castor oil (15 ml)	32
17	*Erand mool twak, bilwagiri, brihati*, and *chhoti kateri kwatha* (equal parts)	25 ml twice/day with black salt (*kala namak* as per requirement)	32, 33
18	*Gridhrasi* decoction	20 ml twice/day with *pushkar moola* powder (3 g) and pure *hingu* powder (500 mg)	35
19	*Maharasnadi kwatha* (a, b, c, d, e)	50 ml twice/day with 1.5 g purified *guggul* or adding *shunthi/pippali* powder (500 mg), or with *ajamodadi* powder (3 g), or castor oil (15 ml)	35
20	*Nirgundi* leaves decoction	20 ml twice/day with *dashmoola* powder (3 g) and pure *hingu* powder (500 mg)	16
21	*Panchmooli* decoction	50 ml/day with castor oil (15 ml) or *nishoth mool* (bark) powder (3 g)	13
22	*Rasnasaptak kwatha*	20 ml twice/day with *shunthi* powder (1 g)	32
23	*Shefalika* leaves decoction	50 ml/day in two divided doses with castor oil (12 ml)	33
24	*Lahshun kalk*	12 g with erand *mool twak kwatha* (25 ml/day) for 1 month	13, 16
25	*Bala ashwagandha lakshadi taila* (b, d)	Apply to the affected parts of the leg	21
26	*Hingu triguna taila* (d)	5 ml two to three times/day orally with water for 3 to 4 weeks	36
27	*Mahavishagarbh taila* (a, c, e)	Apply to the affected parts of the leg	13

TABLE 11.1 (continued)

Formulations Used in Therapy of Sciatica, Monoplegia, and Paraplegia

No.	Name (Manufacturer*)	Doses, Vehicle, and Duration	Ref.
28	*Mahamash taila* (a, b, c, d, e, f)	Apply to the affected parts of the leg	16
29	*Narayan taila* (c, d, e, f)	Apply to the affected parts of the leg	35
30	*Prasarini taila* (a, f)	Apply to the affected parts of the leg	34
31	*Prabhanjan vimardanam taila* (d)	Apply to the affected parts of the leg	20
32	*Saindhavadya taila* (a, b)	Apply to the affected parts of the leg	13
33	*Erand phal payas*	Oral, once/day (12 g/day) for 1 month (*Note*: *Payas* made of 30 to 50 uncoated cooked castor seeds in 350 ml cow's milk)	13, 33
34	*Vrihachhagaladya ghrit* (d)	Oral (12 g/day)	31
35	*Gunja phal/gunja pistadi lepa*	Apply once/day	13, 35
36	*Ekang vir ras* (a, c, e, f)	125 mg three times/day for 60 days with milk	37
37	*Khanjanikari ras* (a)	250 mg three times/day for 90 days	33
38	*Lashun ksheer pak* made of *Rason kalk* (15 g) in cow's milk (200 ml)	200 ml/day	4

* (a) Baidyanath Pharmaceuticals;
(b) Indian Medicines Pharmaceutical Corporation Ltd. (IMPCL);
(c) Unjha Pharmaceuticals;
(d) Indian Medical Practitioners Co-operative Pharmacy & Stores (IMPCOPS);
(e) Zandu Pharmaceuticals;
(f) Dabur Pharmaceuticals.

progressive neurologic deficit with increasing weakness after 12 weeks of conservative management with or without clinical evidences of epidural abscesses, malignancy, hematoma, nerve root compression with persistent pain, spondylolysthesis or spinal stenosis, surgery may be considered. Surgery should be considered only in patients who have clearly defined anatomic structural abnormality and have failed from other therapeutic treatments.

11.11 Strategy for Prevention of Sciatica

Changed dietary habits, rapid industrialization, stress, pollution, and altered lifestyle have made people prone to many serious diseases. Sciatica may be one of them. Preventive measures include avoiding fast food (little food), starvation, regular and unnecessary medication, frequent use of cold materials, sleeping during the day and staying awake at night, and strenuous stretching exercises. The recurrences of pain can be reduced and chronic disability can be prevented in patients with mechanical sciatica due to lumbosacral strain or sprain by using a properly supervised exercise program, avoiding prolonged sitting, prolonged standing, and improper lifting.

11.12 Scientific Basis for the Use of Ayurvedic Drugs in Sciatica

11.12.1 Clinical Studies

1. In one study, 52 sciatica patients were given *Trayodashang guggul* (2 g) and *vistinduk vati* one tab three times/day for 3 weeks. The patients were also treated with *Nirgundi taila* massage and poultice for 3 weeks.[17] In another study, 60 sciatica patients were given *Yograj guggul* (1 g) three times/day plus purified *Nuxvomica* seed powder (100 mg) in one capsule twice/day for 15 days. The patients were also treated with *Mahavisgarbha taila* massage and steam fomentation of *Rasnasaptak* decoction.[18] The criteria for assessment of the results were based on pricking and pulling pain, stiffness, tenderness over sciatic nerve, SLR, knee and ankle jerks, plantar reflexes, muscle wasting, pressing power, walking speed, sensory impairment, and posture, as per global score method. In both studies, results were significant ($p < 0.05$) in more than 70% of the patients in terms of relief from the symptoms.
2. *Nirgundi* oil and dehydrated butter prepared as per the *Ayurvedic Formulary of India* were administered classically under purification therapy on 66 sciatica patients along with purified *guggul* (1 g) and *Vitex negundo* decoction (60 ml) three times/day for 45 days. The results showed complete cure in 76% of sciatica patients.[19]
3. Sixty-eight sciatica patients were distributed equally in four groups at random: (1) palliation, (2) placebo, (3) purification, and (4) purification with palliation. They were given *Prabhanjan vimardanam taila* as per classical schedule. Although the results of treatment were highly encouraging in both purification and purification cum palliation groups, the results were better in the purification cum palliation than the purification group.[20]
4. In a clinical trial conducted on 80 patients with paraplegia, a group of 40 patients received *panchakarma* therapy with *Moorchhit Sesamum indicum* (til) oil as per classical schedule, and the other group was treated with one tablet of *Gorochanadi gutika* (250 mg) after *Ashwagandha* decoction (60 ml) three times/day. Both groups were given massage with 50 ml of *bala ashwagandha lakshadi taila* for 60 days. Results of both the groups were quite significant ($p < 0.001$). The group with *panchakarma* therapy showed better results than did the *ashwagandha* group, even after a 6-month follow-up. The progress in relief was judged on the basis of pain, bladder control, rectum control, sensory changes, muscle powers, fasciculations, deep tendon reflexes, plantar reflexes, wasting, and walking speed, as per global score method.[21]

11.12.2 Animal Studies for Anti-Inflammatory Activity

11.12.2.1 Yograj Guggul and Rasnasaptak Decoction

The aqueous extract of *yograj guggul* and *rasnasaptak* decoction were administered intraperitoneally (i.p.) in albino rats 30 min prior to carrageenin challenge, in combination and alone at the doses of 1 g/kg. Test drugs produced significant inhibition of paw edema. Phenylbutazone was taken for standard comparison in the study.[22]

11.12.2.2 Commiphora mukul (Hook. ex stocks) (Burseraceae)

Phenylbutazone (100 mg/kg), hydrocortisone acetate (20 mg/kg i.p.), ibuprofen (50 mg/kg orally), acetylsalicylic acid (300 mg/kg orally), or steroidal compound from C. *mukul* (100 mg/kg i.p.) were given 1 h before the carrageenin challenge to groups of 6 rats. No treatment was given to a control group of six rats. The steroid isolated from C. *mukul* showed a pronounced anti-inflammatory ($p < 0.001$) in paw edema as compared to phenylbutazone ($p < 0.001$), hydrocortisone acetate ($p < 0.005$), ibuprofen ($p < 0.01$), and acetylsalicylic acid ($p < 0.001$).[23]

11.12.2.3 Vitex negundo Linn. (Verbenaceae) and Withania somnifera Linn. (Solanaceae)

The aqueous extract of *Vitex negundo* Linn. at the dose of 1 g/kg i.p. produced anti-inflammatory activity by 45, 60, and 44% at 2, 3, and 4 h of treatment in the carrageenin-induced rat's paw edema model. *W. somnifera* also exhibited anti-inflammatory activity in carrageenin induced rat's paw edema. The inflammation was recorded as 61, 56, and 27% at the first, second, and third hour of treatment, respectively. The study further revealed that *W. somnifera* acts by blocking histamine h_1 and h_2 receptors in early phase followed by inhibition of prostaglandin in delayed phase of acute inflammatory reaction. However, anti-inflammatory activity of *V. negundo* is mediated through histamine and 5-HT, which is further maintained during delayed phase.[24]

11.12.2.4 Ricinus communis Linn. (Euphorbiaceae)

Petroleum ether extract of *R. communis* exhibited significant anti-inflammatory activity against formaldehyde and adjuvant-induced rat's paw arthritis.[25]

11.12.2.5 Pluchea lanceolata (DC) Clarke (Compositae) and Allium sativum Linn. (Liliaceae)

The water-soluble portion of the 90% alcoholic extract of *P. lanceolata* administered orally in the dose of 2000 mg/kg/day produced significant anti-inflammatory activity in formalin induced albino rat's hind paw arthritis and granuloma pouch in comparison with betamethasone. The pharmaceutical preparation allisatin, a concentrated formulation of fresh *Allium sativum,* was suspended in water and administered in the dose of 2000 mg/kg/day. The results showed slight anti-inflammatory activity against formalin-induced arthritis but not against granuloma pouch.[26]

11.12.2.6 Sida cordifolia Linn. (Malvaceae)

An aqueous extract of *S. cordifolia* was administered orally at a dose of 400 mg/kg body weight. The results showed a significant inhibition of carrageenin induced rat's paw edema but did not block the edema induced by arachiodonic acid.[27]

11.12.2.7 Tinospora cordifolia (willd.) Miers. (Ex Hook. f.) and Thoms. (Menispermaceae)

Water extract of stem of *T. cordifolia* (neem giloe) at the dose of 500 mg/kg given orally and i.p. inhibited acute inflammatory response evoked by carrageenin, significantly ($p < 0.05$). Analgesic and antipyretic actions have also been observed in the study.[28]

11.13 Discussion

Although sciatica is not a terminal disease, lack of proper treatment may lead to difficulty in walking and other movements. The most often prescribed drugs in the treatment of sciatica are nonsteroidal anti-inflammatory drugs (NSAIDs), acetaminophen, muscle relaxants, and opioids. Several randomized double-blind studies demonstrate that NSAIDs are superior to placebo, but they provide short-term relief to patients.[1] Allergic reactions have also been reported by the use of drugs. The use of opioids, benzdiazepines, and tricyclics may be helpful, but in many cases drug dependence, tolerance, and drowsiness have been observed. Muscle relaxants provide short-term relief, but drowsiness often limits their day-time use.[7] Using chymopapain to dissolve herniated disc material proved most effective in relieving sciatica, but severe neurologic complications restrict its use. Traction, acupuncture, and exercise programs have failed to show benefits of these therapies in sciatica.

In spite of the fact that the spinal diseases are difficult to cure, the Ayurvedic concept of treatment for sciatica is more effective and suitable as compared with the modern mode of treatment. The therapies can be used for prolonged periods of time without any toxic side effects. Oleation is considered the most effective remedy in the treatment of *vata* diseases. Medicated oils either given orally or applied externally, or both, help in the restoration of muscle strength. Massage increases circulation, prevents nerve degeneration, and promotes tissue building. It renders the body soft and helps in the elimination of accumulated waste materials that obstruct the channels causing vitiation of *vata*. Oleation followed by fomentation liquefies *dosas* adhered in the channels and brings them to the gastrointestinal tract *(kostha)* where they are expelled by the downflow action of purgation. Hemoglobin levels increased in one study in both albino rats and humans after oleation.[29] Heat applied by steam, poultice, hot sandbags, or other means reduces the stiffness and muscle spasms by decreasing efferent activity, improving tissue flexibility, and hastening tissue healing by increasing the blood flow and nutrients to the injured area. Heat application has a vasodilatory effect that can lead to edema; therefore, it should be used cautiously.[30] The role of bloodletting in the management of sciatica has also proved to be significant.

11.14 Monoplegia and Paraplegia

11.14.1 Definition

When vitiated *vata* situated in the low back region hurts the tendons of single lower limb *(sakthi)*, the person is considered affected by monoplegia. When both the limbs are paralyzed, the disease is called paraplegia.

11.14.2 Etiology

Monoplegia and paraplegia both are *vata*-predominant diseases. Degeneration of essential constituents, trauma (especially on the oscoccygis bone [*kukunder marma*]), and obstructions caused in normal passage are the basic factors causing vitiating *vata.* According to conventional medicine, monoplegia is usually caused by lower motor neuron diseases. A small thoracic cord lesion, tumor, or demyelinative plaque may result in upper motor neuron diseases. Paraplegia results from injuries at T_1 vertebra and below. Compression in the low thoracic and lumbar region causes a conus medularis or cauda equina syndrome. Upper motor neuron and occasionally lower motor neuron diseases, epidural metastases, and spinal cord ischemia may be associated with monoplegia. Acute onset of paraplegia results from diseases of cerebral hemisphere (i.e., anterior cerebral artery ischemia, superior sagital sinus thrombosis, and cortical venous thrombosis). Gradual onset over weeks or months is almost always due to multiple sclerosis, intraparenchymal tumor, and chronic spinal cord compression from degenerative diseases of the spine.

11.14.3 Clinical Course and Prognosis (*Sadhyasadhyata*)

The overall prognosis of monoplegia and paraplegia can be improved by the use of *panchakarma* therapy. In acute onset these therapeutic modalities produced a remission in the number of patients. Prognosis is poorer in epidural metastases, intraparenchymal tumor, lumbar intraspinal metastases, and in patients ages 60 and over with acute onset. Over time, the disease fails to respond to Ayurvedic therapy. Disease usually requires prolonged course of treatment if the condition is more chronic and the prognosis is not good.

11.14.4 Diagnosis

Monoplegia with acute onset presenting sensory loss or pain is usually caused by lower motor neuron diseases. A localized lower motor neuron disease presents progressive weakness with atrophy in one limb that develops over weeks or months. Distribution of weakness is commonly localized to a single nerve root or peripheral nerve within one limb. EMG and nerve conduction studies confirm the diagnosis in such cases. Monoparesis of distal and nonantigravity muscle without sensory loss or pain indicate an upper motor neuron lesion. Weakness of one limb with numbness is generally due to an involved peripheral nerve, spinal nerve root, or lumbosacral plexus. If numbness is absent, segmental anterior horn cell disease is likely. Paraplegia with numbness, frequent micturition, and fecal incontinence results from acute spinal cord disease. Drowsiness, confusion, and seizures present the disease with cerebral origin. Gradual onset over weeks or months indicates spinal cord compression due to degenerative diseases of the spine, intraparenchymal tumor, or multiple sclerosis. MRI of the spinal cord or brain may be helpful in diagnosis.

11.14.5 Therapy *(Chikitsa)*

Treatment plan advised in Ayurveda for the management of monoplegia and paraplegia involves oleation, fomentation, purgation, and enema along with *guggul* orally. *Khanjanikari ras, Ekangvir ras,* and *Gorochanadi gutika* are the some Ayurvdic formulas that have shown better results in studies.[21] These formulas are listed in Table 11.1. Recent controlled trials have documented the efficacy of *Sirovasti* and *nasya (*refer *panchakarma)* in monoplegia and paraplegia with cerebral or motor neuron disease origin.

References

1. Haffernan, J.J., *Textbook Of Primary Care Medicine,* 3rd ed., Noble, J. et al., Eds., C.V. Mosby, St. Louis, 2001, chap. 127.
2. Susruta, *Susruta Samhita,* Part 1, 8th ed., commentary by Shastri, K., Ambikadatta, Chowkhamba Sanskrit Sansthan, Chowkhamba, Varanasi, India, Samavat 2038, 1981, nidan sthanam 234, 1993, chap. 1.
3. Vagbhatta, *Ashtang Hridayam,* 4th ed., commentary by Gupta, K., Atrideva, Chowkhamba Sanskrit Series Office, Varanasi, India nidan sthanam 279, 1970, chap. 15.
4. Charaka, *Charak Samhita,* Part 2, 3rd ed., commentary by Shastri, K. and Chaturvedi, G.N., Chowkhamba Vidya Bhavan, Varanasi, India, chikitsa sthanam 787, 1970, chap. 28.
5. Madhavkar, *Madhav Nidanam,* Purvardham, 4th ed., madhukosh commentary by Shastri, S.S., Chowkhamba Sanskrit Series Office,Varanasi, India, 1970, 437, chap. 22.
6. Olmarkar, K., Radicular pain: recent pathophysiologic concepts and therapeutic implications, *Schmerz,* Dec. 15(6), 425–429, 2001.
7. Engstrom, J.W., *Harrison's Principles of Internal Medicine,* 15th ed.,Vol. 1, Braunwald, E. et al., Eds., McGraw-Hill, Medical Publishing Division, New Delhi, 1999, chap. 16.
8. Brisby, H. et al., Glyco sphingolipid antibodies in serum in patients with sciatica, *Spine,* 27, 380, 2002.
9. Hao, J.X. et al., Development of a mouse model of neuropathic pain following photochemically induced ischemia in the sciatic nerve, *Exp. Neurol.,* 163, 231, 2000.
10. Hao, J.X., Xu, X.J., and Wiesenfeld-Hallin, Z., Effects of intrathecal morphine, clonidine and baclofen on allodynia after partial sciatic nerve injury in the rat, *Acta Anaesthesiol. Scand.,* 43, 1027, 1999.
11. Tao, L. et al., Depletion of macrophages, reduces axonal degeneration and hyperalgesia following nerve injury, *Pain,* 86, 25, 2000.
12. Sawaya, R.A., Idiopathic sciatic mononeuropathy, *Clin. Neurol. Neurosurg.,* 101, 256, 1999.
13. Yogratnakar, *Yogratnakarah purvardham,* 3rd ed., commentary by Shastri, V.L., Chowkhamba Sanskrit Sansthan, Varanasi, India, 1983, pp. 502 and 515.
14. Olmarkar, K. and Rydevik, B.J., Pathophysiology of spinal nerve roots as related to sciatica and disc herniated, *The Spine,* 4th ed., Vol. 1, Herkowitz, H.N. et al., Eds., W.B. Saunders, Philadelphia, 1999, p. 159.
15. Susruta, *Susrut Samhita,* Part I, 8th ed., sira vyadh vidhi shariram, commentary by Shastri, K. Ambikadatta, Chowkhamba Sanskrit Sansthan Varanasi, samvat 2038, 1981, Sharir sthanam, 65, 1993, chap. 8.
16. Datta, C., *Chakradatta,* 3rd ed., commentary by Tripathi, S.J.P., Chowkhamba Sanskrit Series Office, Varanasi, India, Vata vyadhi chikitsa, 1961.
17. Nanda, G.C. et al., Effect of trayodashang guggul and vistinduk vati along with abhyanga and svedan in the management of gridhrasi, *J. Res. Ayurveda Siddha,* 19, 116, 1998.
18. Singh, S. et al., Effect of siravedha in gridhrasi, *J. Res. Ayurveda Siddha,* 22, 173, 1999.
19. Nair, P.R. et al., The effect of nirgundi panchang and guggul in shodhan cum shaman treatment, *JRIMYH,* 13, 14, 1978.
20. Nair, P.R. et al., Clinical evaluation of prabhanjan vimardanam taila and shodhan therapy in the treatment of gridhrasi, *J. Res. Ayurveda Siddha,* 12, 41, 1991.
21. Madhavi, K.P. et al., Shaman therapy versus panchkarma therapy in the management of pangu, *J. Res. Ayurveda Siddha,* 19, 112, 2000.
22. Maurya, Singh, D.P. and Acharya, M.V., Anti inflammatory activity of yograj guggul and rasna saptak decoction in albino rat's hind paw induced arthritis, under publication.
23. Arora, R.B. et al., Isolation of a crystalline steroidal compound from *Commiphora mukul* and its anti inflammatory activity, *Ind. J. Exp. Biol.,* 9, 403, 1971.

24. Srivastava, D.N., Sahni, Y.P., and Gaidhani, S.N., Anti inflammatory activity of some indigenous medicinal plants in albino rats, *J. Med. Aromatic Plant Sci.*, 22–23, 73, 2000–2001.
25. Banarjee, S. et al., Further studies on the anti inflammatory activities of *Ricinus communis* in albino rats, *Indian J. Pharmacol.*, 23, 149, 1991.
26. Prasad, D.N., Bhattacharya, S.K., and Das, P.K., A study of anti inflammatory activity of some indigenous drugs in albino rats, *Indian J. Med. Res.*, 54, 582, 1966.
27. Franzotti, E.M. et al. Anti inflammatory, analgesic activity and acute toxicity of *Sida cordifolia* L.(Malva-branca), *J. Ethnopharmacol.*, 72, 273, 2000.
28. Pendse, V.K. et al., Anti inflammatory, immuno suppressive and some related pharmacological actions of the water extract of neem giloe (tinospora cordifolia), a preliminary study, *Indian J. Pharmacol.*, 9, 221, 1977.
29. Nair, P.R. et al., Effect of snehapan on haemoglobin: a serendipitous find, *J. Res. Ayurveda Siddha*, 10, 125, 1989.
30. Ekbot, S.V. and Kher, S.S., *Recent Advances in Orthopedics*, Kulkarni, G.S., Ed., Jaypee Brothers, Medical Publishers (O.) Ltd., Daryaganj, New Delhi, 1997, chap. 19.
31. Anon., *Ayurvedic Formulary of India*, Part II, (1st English ed.), Ministry of Health and Family Welfare, Government of India, 5(2), 94; 6(3), 102; 8(3), 138, 2000.
32. Mishra, Bhava, *Bhav Prakash Uttarardham*, commentary by Pt., Shri Brahmashankar Mishra, Chowkhamba Sanskrit Sansthan, Varanasi, India, 1980, chap. 24.
33. Das, S.G., *Bhaisajya Ratnavali*, 3rd ed., commentary by Shastri, Ambikadatta, Chowkhamba Sanskrit Series Office Varanasi, India, 1969, chap. 26.
34. Anon., *Ayurvedic Formulary of India*, Part 1, 1st ed., Ministry of Health and Family Planning, Deptartment of Health, Government of India, 5(2), 60; 5(10), 59; 8(32), 111, 1976.
35. Sharngdharacharya, *Sharngdhar Samhita*, commentary by Sharma, Shri Prayagdatta, Chowkhamba Amar Bharati Prakashan, Varanasi, India, 1981, pp. 152, 188, 235, 239, 430.
36. Prem Kishore and Padhi, M.M., The role of hingu triguna taila in the treatment of gridhrasi, *J. Res. Ayurveda Siddha*, 6, 36, 1985.
37. Nair, P.R. et al., A comparative study on ekang vir rasa and mahamash taila with shodhan therapy in khanj and pangu, *J. Res. Ayurveda Siddha*, 15, 98, 1994.

12

Allergic Reaction

Lakshmi Chandra Mishra

CONTENTS

12.1 Introduction

Allergic reaction illnesses (ARIs), drug allergies, or hypersensitivities are considered *kapha*-dominated diseases in Ayurveda. Examples are asthma and eczema. In Allopathic medicine, the treatment of these diseases clusters around the use of steroids, antihistamines, and bronchodilators (beta-adrenergic blockers). Ayurveda has approaches worth investigating for the management of ARI. These approaches and available studies on herbs are discussed.

12.2 Definition and Clinical Description

There is no specific definition of ARI given in Ayurveda, but these disorders fall under the broad category of *kaphaja* diseases. In the conventional system of medicine, ARIs are characterized as disorders of the immune system. Clinical signs and symptoms of ARI differ according to organs involved. For example, an allergic reaction occurring in the upper respiratory tract would show an inflammation of the tract and congestion (allergic rhinitis). An allergic reaction occurring in the lungs would show the symptoms of an asthma attack. If it occurs in the skin, it may show the signs and symptoms of urticaria, eczema, psoriasis, or contact dermatitis. One common ARI is allergic rhinitis, which

0-8493-1366-X/04/$0.00+$1.50

accounts for at least 2.5% of all physician's office visits and costs about $2.4 billion on prescriptions and on counter medication and $1.1 billion physician billings per year in the U.S.[1] Other common ARI are allergic asthma and skin reactions.

12.3 Etiology

No specific etiology of ARI is available in ancient Ayurvedic texts. ARI in Ayurveda is described as intolerance developed in the body due to a variety of unwanted toxic materials generated inside the body; this intolerance is either caused by poor digestion of food materials, inadequate metabolism of nutrients (*ama-visa*), or exposure to environmental pollutants (*dushi-visa*).

Ayurvedic etiology of ARI is related to a decrease in immunity or *vyadhiksamatva* (resistance to diseases) that protects a person from diseases. Immunity is recognized as natural as well as acquired. This resistance is associated with or due to a biological material present in humans called *ojas*. Ayurveda has a number of herbs and herbal formulas called *rasayanas* or dietary supplements that are used to strengthen immunity and improve resistance to diseases.

ARIs are currently known in conventional medicine to be mediated by the immune system. Allergic reactions are described as adverse reactions caused by a second exposure of a subject to the same chemical or a structurally similar chemical or an organic material after the subject has been sensitized earlier with the chemical or the organic material. The reactions are invoked not only by exposure to exogenous antigens but also by endogenous (intrinsic to the body) antigens. This etiology of ARI is similar to that stated in classic Ayurvedic texts. Intrinsic antigens are known to be responsible for many of the important immune diseases, such as autoimmune diseases (immune reaction against the individual's own tissue, e.g., rheumatoid arthritis, systemic lupus erythematosus), immunologic deficiency syndrome, and amyloidosis.

12.4 Pathogenesis

Ayurveda includes all body tissues as possible targets of ARI. The pathogenesis of ARI involves invasion of various organs by vitiated *kapha*. The pathology in general consists of inflammation and excessive secretion of fluid.

In conventional medicine, the pathology of allergic reactions in general is also similar to that described in Ayurveda with respect to inflammation of the tissue and excessive secretion of fluid. On the basis of the immunologic mechanisms mediating the disease, ARI has been categorized in four types.[2] Type I reactions, also called anaphylactic shock, are mediated by immunoglubulin E (IgE) antibodies. The examples are food allergies, skin allergies (urticaria and atopic dermatitis), allergic rhinitis, asthma, and anaphylactic shock. Type II or cytolytic reactions are mediated by immunoglobulins G and M (IgG and IgM), and the common examples of this reaction are penicillin-induced hemolytic anemia, quinidine-induced thrombocytopenic purpura, sulfonamide-induced granulocytopenia, and procainamide-induced systemic lupus erythematosus. Type III reactions, or serum sickness, are primarily mediated by IgG. It involves antigen-antibody complex formation that deposits in the vascular epithelium, causing inflammation of the tissue, urticarial skin eruptions, arthritis, lymphadenopathy and fever. Type IV reactions (delayed sensitivity) are mediated by previously sensitized T-lymphocytes and macrophages. An example of this type of reaction is contact dermatitis caused by poison ivy.

12.5 Diagnosis and Prognosis

Diagnosis is made based on the history of occurrence of the reaction and possible association with certain chemicals or organic materials. Skin tests are used to determine specific allergens. An ARI may be discomforting and may take weeks to subside. The acute phase involving lungs may be fatal, although rare, if not treated appropriately.

12.6 Therapy

The treatment of allergic reactions in Ayurveda essentially consists of identifying the allergens, avoiding the exposure to them, using drugs to relieve acute symptoms, improving digestion, and cleaning the intestine of toxic materials in the gut (*ama*). Emesis is recommended to treat allergy and asthma because ARI are considered *kaphaja* disease. Dietary recommendations include diet that suppresses *kapha* as discussed in Chapter 3. *Sitopaldi churn* is useful in upper respiratory tract ARI. The following single herbs are commonly used in ARI and scientific studies in support of the use are listed below:

1. *Clerodendrum seratum*[3]
2. *Benincasa hispida*[4]
4. *Aquilaria agallocha*[5]
4. *Albezia lebbeck*[6]
5. *Curcuma longa*[7]
6. *Inula racemosa*
7. *Galphimia glauca*
8. *Picrorhiza kurora*
9. *Adhatoda vasica*

Treatment specific to skin diseases and asthma are discussed in Chapters 17 and 18.

12.7 Scientific Basis

The herbs listed in the previous section have been investigated primarily in type I hypersensitivity models. The studies summarized here appear to support the use of these herbs in Ayurvedic therapies of ARI.

Prolonged administration of a saponin from the *Clerodendron serratum* plant has been reported to exhibit antihistaminic and antiallergic activity.[3] Alcoholic extract of the root of *Inula racemosa*, prepared by continuous heat extraction, was studied for its antiallergic effect in experimental models of type I hypersensitivity (egg-albumin–induced passive cutaneous anaphylaxis [PCA] and mast cell degranulation) in albino rats.[8] LD_{50} of this extract was found to be 2100 ± 60 mg/kg intraperitoneally (i.p.). The extract was given orally for 7 days or once only. As a positive control for mast cell degranulation, compound 48/80 was given with the same dosage schedule. Remarkable protection against egg-albumin–induced PCA was observed on the extract treated group after a single dose. The extract also protected against compound 48/80-induced mast cell degranulation, and the protection was similar to that of an antiallergic drug disodium cromoglycate. The 7-day drug treatment schedule showed greater protection than did disodium cromoglycate intraperitoneally. The results suggest that *I. racemosa* possesses potent antiallergic properties in rats.

The methanol extract of wax gourd, the fruits of *Benincasa hispida* (*Kooshamanda*),[4] was found to show inhibitory activity on the histamine release from rat exudate cells induced by an antigen-antibody reaction. Four known triterpenes and two known sterols were isolated as active components based on the bioassay. The other constituents isolated were flavonoid C-glycoside, an acylated glucose, and a benzyl glycoside. Two triterpenes, alnusenol and multiflorenol, were found to be potent inhibitors of histamine release.

An aqueous extract of stems of *Aquilaria agallocha* (*agaru*) has been investigated on the immediate hypersensitivity reactions.[5] The aqueous extract of stems showed inhibitory effects on passive cutaneous anaphylaxis, anaphylaxis induced by compound 48/80, and histamine release from rat peritoneal mast cells (RPMC). The extract also prevented the degranulation of RPMC in rats. The authors concluded that the aqueous extract inhibits the immediate hypersensitivity reaction by the inhibition of histamine release from mast cells.

Decoction of *Albizzia lebbeck* bark has been investigated to determine its possible antiallergic activity.[6] The effect of the decoction on the degranulation rate of sensitized peritoneal mast cells of albino rats challenged with antigen (horse serum) was studied. Triple vaccine was used as an adjuvant and disodium cromoglycate (DCG) and prednisolone were used for comparison. Drugs were given during the first or second week of sensitization and the mast cells were studied at the end of the second or third week. Serum from these rats was used to passively sensitize recipient rats whose peritoneal mast cells were then studied. The effects of *A. lebbeck* and DCG on the degranulation rate of the sensitized mast cells were also studied *in vitro*. The results show that *A. lebbeck* had a significant cromoglycate-like action on the mast cells. In addition, it appears that it inhibited the early processes of sensitization, and synthesis of reaginic-type antibodies. If the decoction were given during the first week of sensitization, it markedly inhibited the early sensitizing processes; if given during the second week, it suppressed antibody production during the period of drug administration. The active ingredients of the bark appear to be heat stable and water soluble.

Several plants used in traditional medicine for the treatment of bronchial asthma have been investigated.[9] Thiosulfinates and cepaenes have been identified as active antiallergic compounds in onion extracts. They exert a wide spectrum of pharmacologic activities, both *in vitro* and *in vivo*. Tetragalloyl quinic acid from *Galphimia glauca*, suppressed allergen- and platelet-activating factor (PAF)-induced bronchial obstruction, PAF-induced bronchial hyperreactivity (5 mg/kg orally) *in vivo*, and thromboxane biosynthesis *in vitro*. *Adhatoda vasica* alkaloids (not identified) showed pronounced protection against allergen-induced bronchial obstruction in guinea pigs (10 mg/ml aerosol). Androsin from *Picrorhiza kurroa* prevented allergen- and PAF-induced bronchial obstruction (10 mg/kg orally; 0.5 mg inhalative). Histamine release *in vitro* was inhibited by other unidentified chemical constituents of the plant extract.

Compound 73/602 (AA) is a structural analogue of vasicinone, an alkaloid, present in the leaves and roots of *Adhatoda vasica* (acanthaceae); this compound was found to possess potent anti-allergic activity in mice, rats, and guinea pigs.[10] The immunologic effect of curcumin, a natural product of plants obtained from *Curcuma longa* (turmeric), has been reported in animal models.[7,11]

12.8 Summary

Ayurvedic management of ARI is basically similar to conventional medicine — identify the allergen and avoid the exposure to it. In addition, the Ayurvedic approach includes dietary *kapha*-suppressing foods, herbs, and herbal formulas for treatment.

References

1. deShazo, R.D., Allergic rhinitis, in *Cecil Text Book of Medicine,* Goldman, L. and Bennett, J.C., Eds., W.B. Saunders, Philadelphia, 2000, chap. 274.
2. Coombs, R.R.A. and Gell, P.G.H., Classification of allergic reactions responsible for clinical hypersensitivity and disease, in *Clinical Aspects of Immunology,* Gell, P.G.H., Coombs, R.R.A., and Lachman, P.J., Eds., Blackwell Scientific, Oxford, 1975, p. 761.
3. Gupta, S.S., Development of antihistamine and anti-allergic activity after prolonged administration of a plant saponin from Clerodendron serratum, *J. Pharm. Pharmacol.,* 10, 801, 1968.
4. Yoshizumi, S., Murakami, T., Kadoya, M., Matsuda, H., Yamahara, J., and Yoshikawa, M., Medicinal foodstuff. XI. Histamine release inhibitors from wax gourd, the fruit of Benincas hispida, *Yakugaku Zasshi,* 118, 188, 1998.
5. Kim, Y.C., Lee, E.H., Lee, Y.M., Kim, H.K., Song, B.K., Lee, E.J., and Kim, H.M., Effect of the aqueous extract of Aquilaria agallocha stems on the immediate hypersensitivity reactions, *J. Ethnopharmacol.,* 58, 31, 1997.
6. Tripathi, R.M., Sen, P.C., and Das, P.K., Studies on the mechanism of action of Albizzia lebbeck, an Indian indigenous drug used in the treatment of atopic allergy, *J. Ethnopharmacol.,* 1, 385, 1979
7. Madan, B., Gade, W.N., and Ghosh, B., Curcuma longa activates NF-kappaB and promotes adhesion of neutrophils to human umbilical vein endothelial cells, *J. Ethnopharmacol.,* 75, 25, 2001.
8. Srivastava, S., Gupta, P.P., Prasad, R., Dixit, K.S., Palit, G., Ali, B., Misra, G., and Saxena, R.C., Evaluation of antiallergic activity (type I hypersensitivity) in rats, *Indian J. Physiol. Pharmacol.,* 43, 235, 1999.
9. Dorsch, W. and Wagner, H., New antiasthmatic drugs from traditional medicine?, *Int. Arch. Allergy Appl. Immunol.,* 94, 262, 1991.
10. Paliwa, J.K., Dwivedi, A.K., Singh, S., and Gutpa, R.C., Pharmacokinetics and in-situ absorption studies of a new anti-allergic compound 73/602 in rats, *Int. J. Pharm.,* 197, 213, 2000.
11. Kang, B.Y., Song, Y.J., Kim, K.M., Choe, Y.K., Hwang, S.Y., and Kim, T.S., Curcumin inhibits Th1 cytokine profile in CD4+ T cells by suppressing interleukin-12 production in macrophages, *Br. J. Pharmacol.,* 128, 380, 1999.

13

Bronchial Asthma

Rakesh Lodha and Sushil K. Kabra

CONTENTS

0-8493-1366-X/04/$0.00+$1.50

13.1 Introduction

Bronchial asthma is a common global health problem. Individuals of all ages are affected by this chronic airway disorder that can be severe and occasionally fatal. The prevalence of asthma is increasing worldwide, especially in children.[1]

Over the past few decades, there have been significant scientific advances leading to improved understanding of the disease and better management. However, the current modes of therapy in conventional medicine do not cure the disorder but control the symptomatology. There is a need to explore safe alternative therapies, such as Ayurvedic medicine, so that they can be successfully integrated with conventional therapy to provide maximal benefits to patients.

13.2 Definition

Ayurveda: *Svasa* (increased or difficult breathing, dyspnea) refers to the disorders of the respiratory system. There are five kinds: *ksudraka, tamaka, chchinna, mahan,* and *urdhava*. Of these, *tamaka svasa* refers to asthma.[2–5]

Modern medicine: Asthma is a chronic inflammatory disorder of the airway in which many types of cells and cellular elements play a role. The chronic inflammation causes an associated increase in airway hyperresponsiveness that leads to recurrent episodes of wheezing, breathlessness, chest tightness, and coughing, especially at night or in the early morning. These episodes are usually associated with widespread but variable airflow obstruction that is often reversible either spontaneously or with treatment.

13.3 Epidemiology

Asthma is currently a worldwide problem, and there is evidence that the prevalence has been increasing in many countries.[1] There are no clear-cut data from the Ayurvedic texts about the extent of the problem in ancient times. It is likely that the prevalence of the disorder was much less in ancient India because of factors discussed later in the chapter.

13.3.1 Children

The prevalence of asthma symptoms in children may be as high as 30%. The differences among various populations may be consequences of responses to environment, industrialization, or different allergen loads.[1] Asthma may develop less frequently in children who are exposed to infections and parasitic infestations early in life.[6,7]

13.3.2 Adults

The prevalence of asthma symptoms in adults varies from 1 to 25%.[8–11] Similar symptoms from cardiac failure and chronic obstructive pulmonary disease make accurate estimates of asthma in older individuals difficult.[8–11]

Mortality data from developed countries show that the rates vary from 0.1 to 0.8 per 100,000 persons aged 5 to 34.[12–14]

13.4 Etiology

According to Ayurveda, the general etiology of *svasa roga* is that all things, materials, and conditions that could help increase *vata dosa* and *kapha dosa* are causally responsible for *tamaka svasa*. This develops from an increase in cough (*kasa*), undigested materials (*ama*), diarrhea, vomiting (*vamathu*), poison (*visa*), anemia (*pandu*), and fever (*jvara*); coming into contact with air containing dust, irritant gases, pollens, or smoke; injuring vital spots; using very cold water; and residing in cold and damp places.[2–5] Excessive use of dry food and astringent food and irregular dietary habits may also trigger an attack. In addition, constipation, excessive fasting, excessive use of cold water, excessive sexual indulgence in adults, exposure to extremes of temperature, anxieties, grief, disturbance of peace of mind, and debility may all precipitate an attack. Cough and coryza have also been implicated as etiologic agents. The habitual use of lablab-bean, black gram, *til* preparations, irritant spicy food, and *kapha*-producing diet may also be involved in development of the disease.[2–5]

In modern medicine the risk factors for asthma are classified under two categories: host factors and environmental factors.

The host factors include genetic predisposition, atopy, airway hyperresponsiveness, gender, and ethnicity. Asthma can be considered to be a heritable disorder.[15,16] More boys than girls develop asthma during childhood; this difference disappears by age 10.[17,18] Subsequently, females are at greater risk for developing asthma. Environmental factors influence the susceptibility to developing asthma in predisposed individuals, precipitate asthma exacerbations, and cause persistence of asthma. The important allergens that play a role in asthma are domestic mites, cockroach allergens, animal allergens, various fungi, and pollen.[19–22] Exposure to tobacco smoke and various pollutants may play a role in enhancing symptoms in susceptible individuals.[23] Infections do cause exacerbations in asthmatic individuals.[24,25] Severe viral respiratory infections in early childhood have been shown to be associated with the development of asthma.[26,27]

According to the hygiene hypothesis, improvement in hygiene and reduced incidence of common infections is associated with increased prevalence of asthma and atopy in developed countries.[28] This may explain the apparent low prevalence of the disorder in the ancient era.

Risk factors for acute exacerbations trigger inflammation or cause bronchoconstriction or both. There is a wide interindividual variation in triggers. The triggers include exposure to various allergens and irritant gases, exercise, cold air, various drugs, and emotional changes. Various indoor and outdoor allergens and air pollutants are implicated in precipitating acute exacerbations. There is strong evidence linking acute viral respiratory infections to acute exacerbations of asthma; the most common are rhinovirus and respiratory synticial virus infections. They are particularly important in children. Emotional stress can trigger an asthma exacerbation. These possibly act via hyperventilation, which can cause airway narrowing.[29] Other conditions, like sinusitis, can be associated with exacerbations. In children, gastroesophageal reflux may lead to the exacerbation of asthma.

From the above it is clear that even in the ancient era there was an excellent understanding of the etiologic factors of bronchial asthma.

13.5 Pathology and Pathogenesis

The pathogenesis of asthma, according to Ayurvedic texts, appears to arise from an abnormal interaction between *vata* and *kapha*. The initial step is the increase in *vata*. Because of the obstruction to normal movements of *vata* by *kapha*, *vata* begins to move in all directions. This disturbs the channels of respiration (*prana*), food (*anna*), and water (*udaka*) located in the chest, and produces dyspnea (*svasa*) originating from the stomach (*amasaya*). This suggests that the root cause of asthma is related to the digestive tract.[2–4]

Modern medicine recognizes the inflammatory processes in the airway as the key pathogenetic mechanism for asthma. Current evidence shows that the T-lymphocytes have an important role in regulating the inflammatory response through the release of various cytokines. Eosinophils and mast cells are the key effector cells; these cells secrete a wide range of chemicals that act on airways both directly and indirectly through neural mechanisms.[30,31] There is a continuum of disease: acute inflammation, persistent disease, and remodeling.[32]

Asthma is frequently found in association with atopy (the production of abnormally high amounts of immunoglobin E [IgE] directed against common environmental allergens such as animal proteins, dust mites, pollen and fungi).[33] Because of this, mast cells are sensitized and upon activation lead to inflammation. Atopy is one of the strongest risk factors for asthma. The process of sensitization may begin *in utero*. The potential for allergic sensitization and risk for wheezing appears to be influenced by many factors in early life, including viral respiratory infections, exposure to endotoxin, exposure to tobacco smoke, use of antibiotics, house dust-mite sensitization, and diet.[34]

Airway hyperresponsiveness and acute airflow limitation are the two major manifestations of abnormalities of lung function in asthma. Hyperresponsiveness is the presence of an exaggerated bronchoconstrictor response to a wide variety of endogenous and exogenous stimuli. Airway inflammation is the key factor for hyperresponsiveness.

Airflow limitation is produced by acute bronchoconstriction, swelling of the airway wall, chronic mucus plug formation, and airway remodeling. Allergen-induced bronchoconstriction results from the IgE-dependent release of histamine, prostaglandins, and leukotrienes by the mast cells.[35]

The lungs of individuals who died of asthma were hyperinflated; the small and large airways were filled with plugs formed by mucus, serum proteins, inflammatory cells, and debris. The microscopy (both autopsy material and now on endobronchial biopsies) reveals extensive infiltration by eosinophils and lymphocytes in the airway wall and lumen.[36,37] In addition, there are features of microvascular leakage, epithelial disruption, and airway remodeling.

13.6 Clinical Features

The prodromal symptoms described in the Ayurvedic texts include pain in the region of the chest and flanks, movement of *prana* (*vata*) in an upward direction, distension of abdomen, and cutting pain in temples. Other premonitory symptoms are pain in the temporal region, restlessness, anorexia, abnormality in taste, flatulence, and pain.

There are several symptoms of *tamaka svasa*. *Vata*, undergoing an increase, travels in an upward direction in the passages, causes increase of *kapha*, and seizes the head and neck.

There is pain in the chest and flanks, a noisy cough (from the throat and the chest), an increase in breathing effort, and wheezing (*ghur ghur* sounds). An acute attack may lead to delusions, loss of appetite, nasal discharge, and thirst. With increasing intensity of bouts, the patient may become unconscious. The patient finds relief for a few moments after expectoration of sputum, breathes with great difficulty while lying down, and finds comfort while sitting. The patient's eyes are wide open, and he or she perspires from the forehead, suffers dryness of mouth, gets bouts of dyspnea (often with shivering), and desires additional warmth. The disease greatly increases on cloudy days and in rain, cold, or direct breeze and other factors that may cause an increase of *kapha*. In addition there is throat irritation, vomiting, and anorexia. This description is quite similar to what we understand today.

Tamaka svasa has been classified into two varieties: *Tamaka svasa vatapradhan* (*vata dosa* is predominant) and *Tamaka svasa shlesma pradhan* (*kapha dosa* is predominant). The indicators of the former are highly painful breathing with high frequency of noisy sounds, little expectoration, difficulty in expectoration, and insomnia. The latter is characterized by high vibrating noise in throat while breathing, coryza, easy and copious expectoration, and painful fast breathing.

The clinical manifestations of asthma as we see it today include episodes of shortness of breath, cough, wheezing, and chest tightness. Patients with more severe cases are likely to have persistent symptoms, worsening at night and early mornings. Often the chest congestion takes more than 10 days to clear up. The symptoms may be precipitated by exposure to the various stimuli discussed above. Very often, exacerbations occur in the absence of any well-defined exposure, particularly in patients with persistent disease. These symptoms usually respond to bronchodilators; this response supports the diagnosis of asthma.

The practitioners of Ayurveda confirm the diagnosis by a detailed case history of the patient and objective examination to determine the imbalances between various constituents. An evaluation is made about the patient's body constitution, state of digestion, and level of activity through interrogation. Interrogation also includes questions on precipitating and pacifying factors and lifestyle. A detailed physical examination of all systems, including checking the pulse and tongue, is done to identify the specific type of *dosa* involved in the pathology. Diagnosis is finally made based on the symptoms, which are dependent on the location of morbid *dosa* and nature of pathology.

Currently, many practitioners use the modern techniques such as auscultation of the chest with a stethoscope for confirming the diagnosis. As there is progress toward holistic medicine, the Ayurvedic practitioners will benefit from the advances made in the diagnosis of asthma.

In modern medicine, the diagnosis can often be made convincingly on the basis of clinical history and physical examination. However, the examination of respiratory system may be normal as the symptoms are variable. A physical examination is more likely to be fruitful if the individual is examined in the symptomatic period.

Measurement of pulmonary function has an important place in diagnosis especially if history and physical examination are inconclusive. In addition, there can be inaccuracies in assessment of severity of symptoms by both patient and physician.

Measurement of airflow limitation (such as peak expiratory flow rate [PEFR] and forced expiratory volume [FEV_1]) and its reversibility are important in establishing a clear diagnosis of asthma. Newer guidelines recommend serial measurements for monitoring the course of asthma. The tests can be performed with ease in individuals older than 5 years.

On the basis of the symptomatology and the result of spirometry, asthma can be classified into intermittent, mild persistent, moderate persistent, and severe persistent types (Table 13.1).

TABLE 13.1

Classification of Asthma According to Severity

Severity	Symptoms	Nighttime Symptoms	PEFR
Severe persistent	Continuous, limited physical activity	Frequent	≤60% predicted; variability >30%
Moderate persistent	Daily use of beta-2 agonist, daily attack affects activity	>One time/week	>60–80% predicted; variability >30%
Mild persistent	>One time/week but < one time/day	>Two times/month	≥80% predicted; variability 20–30%
Intermittent	<One time/week, asymptomatic and normal PEFR between attack	≤Two times/month	≥80% predicted; variability <20%

13.7 Clinical Course and Prognosis

According to Ayurveda, of all the significant *svasa* disorders, *tamaka svasa* (asthma) is *yapya* (i.e., controllable).[1] It is not curable and symptoms are likely to persist. The only exceptions to this may be disease of short duration in strong, healthy, young individuals and if the disease severity is mild.

In the past few decades, a lot of research has been conducted to determine the natural history of asthma. Asthma symptoms may disappear in one third to one half of children at puberty.[38,39] Even though symptoms may be absent, abnormalities in lung function can be demonstrated. However, symptoms may appear later in adulthood. Nearly two thirds of children continue suffering from the disorder through adolescence and adulthood.

Asthma may have onset in adult life.[40] The exact proportion of such patients is not known. It is likely that exposure to allergens and development of atopy later in life are responsible for late onset of asthma. The role of viral infections in causation in adults is not clear; they may be a trigger for acute exacerbation.

The overall description of the prognosis of asthma in Ayurveda and the current practice appear to be similar.

13.8 Management

13.8.1 Ayurvedic Approach

Management of asthma in Ayurveda judiciously encompasses herbal and herbomineral drugs in addition to advising a healthy lifestyle and diet that are contrary to the cause of disease and the disease itself. As the pathogenesis of this disorder involves an imbalance between the *vata* and *kapha*, the therapy is directed at correcting this imbalance. In addition, there are a few therapies for controlling the acute symptoms.

The texts recommend that the patients should be given sudation and steaming therapy (*svedana*) after anointing their bodies with oils processed with salt.[2–5] With this method, the solidified phlegm (*kapha*) adhering inside the channels gets liquefied and comes into the alimentary tract. The channels become soft and *vata* attains its normal downward movement. After sweating, the patient is advised to eat food rich in fats and food that improves the secretion of mucus. In order to eliminate the pathological *kapha*, a therapeutic emesis is induced with herbs such as *Piper longum* (*pippali*). With this, channels are cleared and *vata* moves without any hindrances. Purgation therapy (*virechana*) may also help in a few patients. Because of the nature of these therapies, they should be avoided in young children and pregnant women.

The purification (*shodhan*) can also be achieved by a more elaborate process: *panchakarma*. *Panchakarma* involves therapeutic vomiting and emesis (*vamana*), purgation (*virechan*), enema (*basti*), elimination of toxins through the nose (*nasya*), and purification of the blood (*rakta mokshana*). *Rakta mokshana* may be useful in patients with allergies. This purification therapy should not be performed in debilitated individuals, the elderly, young children, pregnant women, and frail women.

Various medications are described in Ayurveda.[2–5] These include single drugs and compound formulations (see Tables 13.2 and 13.3).[5,41] Some of them are listed below the table.

1. *Krsnadi churna* — Powder of *Piper longum* (*pippali*), *Emblica officinalis* (*amlaka*), and *Zingiber officinalis* (*sunthi*) with honey and sugar added
2. *Bharangyadi churna — nagaradi churna* — Powder of *bharangi* (*Clerodendrum serratum*) and *sunthi* (*Zingiber officinalis*) with hot water or powder of *sunthi*, sugar, and *sauvarcala*
3. *Srangydi churna — Pistacia chinensis* (*karkatasrngi*), *trikatu* (combination of ginger root, pippali berry, black pepper), *triphala* (combination of *Emblica officinalis, Terminalia chebula,* and *Terminalia bellirica*), *Solanum xanthocarpum* (*kantakari*), *Clerodendrum serratum* (*bharangi*), *Inula racemosa* (*puskarmula*), and five salts
4. *Parnasapancaka* — Decoction of *Tinospora cordifolia* (*guduci*), *Zingiber officinalis* (*sunthi*), *Rivea hypocrateriformis* (*phanji*), *Solanum xanthocarpum* (*kantakari*), and *Ocimum sanctum* (*parnasa, tulsi*) mixed with *Piper longum* (*pippali*) powder
5. Decoction of *dasamula* (a combination of ten roots: *shonyaka, patala, kasmari, agnimantha, brhati, mahabalam, guduci, kakoli, ananta*) added with *Inula racemosa* (*puskaramula*)
6. Decoction of *Dolichos biflorus* (*kulattha*), *Zingiber officinalis* (*sunthi*), *Solanum xanthocarpum* (*kantakari*), and *Adhatoda vasica* (*vasa*) added with *Inula racemosa* (*puskuramala*)
7. Use of jaggery with equal mustard oil
8. Powder of *Pistacia chinensis* (*karkatasrngi*), *Zingiber officinalis* (*sunthi*), *Piper longum* (*pippali*), *Cyperus rotundus* (*musta*), *Inula racemosa* (*puskarmula*), *Hedychium spicatum* (*sati*), *Piper nigrum* (*marica*), and sugar taken with a decoction of *Tinospora cordifolia* (*guduci*), *Adhatoda vasica* (*vasa*), and *pancamulla*
9. Linctus made from *Curcuma longa* (*haridra*), *Piper nigrum* (*marica*), *Vitis vinifera* (*draksa*), jaggery, *Pluchea lanceolata* (*rasna*), *Piper longum* (*pippali*), and *Hedychium spicatum* (*sati*)
10. The powder of *Terminalia bellirica* (*bibhitaka*) fruit mixed with honey
11. Preparation made from ghee, milk, and the paste of *Capparis sepiaria* (*himsra*); *Embelia ribes* (*vidanga*), *Mentha spicata* (*putika*); *trikatu*; *triphala*; and *Plumbago zeylanica* (*citraka*)
12. Preparation made from ghee and paste of *tegovati*, *Terminalia chebula* (*haritaki*), *Piper longum* (*pippali*), *Strychnos potatorum* (*katuka*), *bhutika*, *Inula racemosa* (*puskara-*

TABLE 13.2

Single Drugs Used in Ayurvedic Anti-Asthmatic Preparations

Adhatoda vasica
Aegle marmelos
Alangium salviifolium
Aquilaria agallocha
Arsenic rubrum
Benincasa hispida
Bhasma of horn of stag
Boerhavia diffusa
Calotropis procera
Cedrus deodara
Garcinia pedunculata
Clerodendrum serratum
Curcuma longa
Curcuma zedoria
Datura stramonium
Dolichos biflorus
Elettaria cardamomum
Fagonia cretica
Ferula narthex
Glycyrrhiza glabra
Gypsum
Honey
Inula racemosa
Jaggery
Leptadenia reticulata
Mica
Mucuna pruriens
Ocimum sanctum
Phyllanthus embica
Phyllanthus urinaria
Piper longum
Piper nigrum
Rhus succedanea
Solanum xanthocarpum
Terminalia bellirica
Vitis vinifera
White arsenic

Source: Modified from Goyal, H.R., *Tamaka Shwasa (Bronchial Asthma): A Clinical Study*, Central Council for Research in Ayurveda and Siddha, New Delhi, 1997.

mula), *Butea monosperma* (*palasa*), *Plumbago zeylanica* (*citraka*), *Hedychium spicatum* (*sati*), *sauvarcala*, *Cinnamomum tamala* (*tamalaki*), rock salt, *Aegle marmelos* (*bilva*), *Abies webbiana* (*talisapatra*), *Leptadenia reticulata* (*jivanti*), *Acorus calamus* (*vaca*), and *Ferula foetida* (*hinga*)

13. Preparation made from *Clerodendrum serratum* (*bharangi*) and *dasamula*, *Terminalia chebula* (*haritaki*), jaggery, honey, *trikatu*, and *trijata* (powdered) and *yavakasra*
14. Preparation made from *Dolichos biflorus* (*kulatha*), *dasamula*, *Clerodendrum serratum* (*bharangi*), jaggery, honey, *Bambusa arundinacea* (*vamsalocana*), *Piper longum* (*pippali*), and *trijata*

The above medications are likely to have both therapeutic and preventive effects. It is advised to continue any of these for a prolonged duration.

TABLE 13.3

Compound Preparations for the Management of Asthma

Name	Instructions
Eladi churn	1–3 with 4–6 g of honey twice/day
Sitopalidi churn	1–3 with 4–6 g of honey twice/day
Srangydi churn	1–3 with 4–6 g of honey twice/day
Talisadi churn	1–3 with 4–6 g of honey twice/day
Dashmula kvath	14–28 ml twice/day
Kantaryadi kvath	14–28 ml twice/day
Srmgyadi kvath	14–28 ml twice/day
Vasadi kvath	14–28 ml twice/day
Agastya haritiki avaleha	12–24 g twice/day
Chavanprash avaleha	12–24 g twice/day
Chitraka haritiki avaleha	12–24 g twice/day
Vasa avaleha	12–24 g twice/day
Vyaghriharitiki avaleha	12–24 g twice/day
Draksharishta	14–28 ml with equal quantity of water twice/day after meals
Vasarishta	14–28 ml with equal quantity of water twice/day after meals
Kanakasva	5–10 ml with equal quantity of water twice/day after meals (due to its potency, caution is advised)
Abhraka bhasma (plain)	120–150 mg with honey twice/day
Maygrapuccha bhasma	1–2 g with honey twice/day
Apamarga ksara	1 g with warm water twice/day
Arka lavana	1 g with warm water twice/day
Khadiradi vati	2–4 vati three times/day
Lavangadi vati	1 vati six times/day

Source: Modified from *Swas roga,* in *Handbook of Domestic Medicine and Common Ayurvedic Remedies,* Central Council for Research in Ayurveda and Siddha, 1999. These preparations may be obtained from major Ayurvedic pharmaceutical companies in India.

For controlling acute symptomatology, inhalation of medicated smoke from the following preparations have been described in Ayurveda[2–4]:

1. Inhalation of the smoke of the fruit, the stem, and leaves of *Dhatura fastuosa* from a *hooka*. A paper dipped in water in which saltpetre has been dissolved is dried in the sun and rolled up in the form of a cigar.
2. Paste of *Cedrus deodara, Sida cordifolia,* and *Nardostachys jatamansi* is dried in sun, laced in ghee. Patient inhales the smoke from a hollow stick made out of this.
3. Leaves of *haridra*, root of *Ricinus communis* (*eranda*), *Cocculus lack* (*laksa*), *Psidium guajava* (*manassial*), *Cedrus deodara* (*devadaru*), *Elettaria cardamomum* (*ela*), and *mamsi* are all macerated and made into cigarette, which is smeared with ghee and smoked.

After alleviating the intensity of asthmatic breathing, the following syrups may be used:

1. Peacock feathers are reduced to ashes in a slow fire. They are mixed with a quantity of fruit of *Piper longum* reduced to powder. A syrup is then made with the aid of honey. If licked occasionally, it alleviates the intensity of asthmatic breathing.
2. Turmeric (*Curcuma longa*), black pepper (*Piper nigrum*), *Uvoe passae*, old molasses, *Vanda roxburghii*, *Piper longum*, and *Circuina zerumbet* are reduced to a powder and mixed with mustard oil.
3. A decoction of *Tinospora cordifolia*, dry ginger, *Siphonanthus indica*, *Solanum xanthocarpum*, and *Ocimum sanctum* mixed with powdered *Piper longum* is made.

4. *Parnasapancaka* — A decoction of *guduci, sunthi, phanji, kantakari,* and *parnasa (tulsi)* mixed with *pippali* powder is made.
5. A syrup made out of *Curcuma zedoria (kachur), Inula racemosa (pushkarmool), Citrus decumona (amla vetas), Elettaria cardamomum (choti Elaichi), Ferula narthex (hingu), Ocimum sanctum (tulsi), Aquilaria agallocha (agar), Phyllanthus urinaria (bhumyamalki), Leptadenia* reticulata *(jeewanti),* and *Santalum album (chanda)* is recommended as a bronchial antispamodic.

Although inhaling the smoke of various herbs may cause relief through the bronchodilatory effect of the constituents such as *dhatura,* this practice has not been evaluated scientifically to recommend its routine usage. In addition, the smoke may actually worsen the bronchospasm. This form of therapy is neither feasible in children nor advisable.

13.8.1.1 Precautions

The drugs, diet, and practices that aggravate the disease should be avoided. These include dust, smoke, residing in cold places, excessive use of cold water, seasonal changes, excessive walking, excessive use of dry foods, astringent food, irregular dietary habits, indigestion, trauma to vital organs, and habitual use of *lablab*-bean, black gram, til paste, and other *kapha*-producing articles.

13.8.1.2 Diet

Foods and drinks that restore the normal course of *vata* are useful in treating asthma. If the *vata* is greatly excited, syrup made up from old tamarind pulp is helpful. Sugar candy with lemon (*Citrus medica*) juice is beneficial. Light foods should be eaten at night. Heavy and rich foods, which are difficult to digest, foods that are dry, curds, fish, and chillies should all be avoided.

13.8.1.3 Lifestyle

Staying awake at night, exercising, labor, exposing oneself to the heat of the sun or fire, and anxieties, grief, wrath, and everything that disturbs peace of mind should be avoided. A healthy lifestyle would have a preventive role.

13.8.1.4 Breathing Exercises

Breathing exercises, particularly *pranayam,* reduce the frequency and severity of symptoms,[42–44] improve exercise tolerance, and enhance lung function. Two systematic reviews have highlighted the need for studying the beneficial aspects of various breathing exercises.[45,46]

13.8.1.5 Meditation

Meditation helps in reducing the stress and may check recurrence. *Sahaja* yoga is an Indian system of meditation based on traditional yogic principles, which may be used for therapeutic purposes. Clinical trials of this therapy in patients with asthma have found evidence of improvement in lung function and reduced frequency of exacerbations.[47]

Some commercial Ayurvedic formulas are also available that may be useful in asthma. Examples include Asmon (Herbochem Remedies, Kolkata) and Asmakure (Herbicure Pvt. Ltd., Bishanpur, West Bengal).

TABLE 13.4

Stepwise Treatment of Asthma

Steps	Long-Term Prevention
Step 4: Severe persistent	Inhaled short-acting beta-agonist as required; inhaled corticosteroids: Budesonide and Beclomethasone (400 μg twice/day) increase up to 2000 μg/day in selected cases; long-acting bronchodilator: long-acting inhaled β_2-agonist or sustained release theophylline; corticosteroids tablets: low dose on alternate days (if no relief with above treatment)
Step 3: Moderate persistent	Inhaled short-acting beta-agonist as required; inhaled corticosteroids: Budesonide and Beclomethasone (400–800 μg divided twice/day); long-acting bronchodilator (if needed): long-acting inhaled β_2-agonist salmeterol (50 μg once or twice/day or sustained release theophylline)
Step 2: Mild persistent	Inhaled short-acting β-agonist as required; inhaled corticosteroids: Budesonide and Beclomethasone (200–400 μg) or cromolyn or sustained release theophylline or leukotriene modifiers
Step 1: Intermittent	Inhaled short-acting β-agonist as required for symptoms relief; if they are needed more than three times/week, move to step 2

Note: If Fluticasone is used, the dose is half that of Budesonide/Beclomethasome.

13.8.2 Conventional Medicine Approach

There is no cure available for asthma in Western medicine. However, appropriate management leads to control of the disorder. The goals of management are to:

1. Control the symptoms.
2. Prevent acute exacerbations.
3. Maintain normal or near normal pulmonary functions.
4. Maintain normal levels of activity.
5. Avoid adverse effects from medications.
6. Prevent mortality due to asthma.

Currently, therapy of asthma is guided by the fact that it is a chronic inflammatory airway disorder; the control of airway inflammation is the key to effective control. Except for mild intermittent asthma, the therapy includes regular use of anti-inflammatory medication and bronchodilators (as required). In addition, environmental control to avoid exposure to certain risk factors should improve the control of symptoms.

The first step in management after the diagnosis is made is the correct assessment of severity of asthma (Table 13.1).

The pharmacological therapy of bronchial asthma involves the use of drugs that relax smooth muscle and dilate the airways and drugs that decrease inflammation and prevent exacerbations. The medications used for long-term treatment of asthma include bronchodilators, steroids, mast-cell stabilizers, leukotriene modifiers, and theophylline.[48–75] Table 13.4 shows the treatment plan according to disease severity. The use of bronchodilators alone in persistent asthma is not recommended, as this does not control the airway inflammation and there is a false sense of security.

13.8.2.1 Immunotherapy

This therapeutic mode consists of gradually giving increasing quantities of an allergen extract to a clinically sensitive subject to ameliorate the symptoms associated with subsequent exposure to a causative allergen. This is considered only occasionally in highly selected children who are sensitive to a specific allergen such as grass pollen, mites, etc. It is done only under specialist supervision and must usually be given for 3 years.[76] Some studies suggest that specific immunotherapy may induce a diminution of nonspecific bronchial hyperresponsiveness and enable reduction of symptomatic treatment.[77,78]

13.8.2.2 Management of Acute Exacerbation

Severe exacerbations of asthma are life-threatening medical emergencies requiring hospital-based care. The aims of treatment are to reverse airflow obstruction and hypoxemia as rapidly as possible. The severity of an acute exacerbation can be judged by clinical symptoms and signs, lung function tests, and arterial blood gas analysis. Rapid-acting inhaled bronchodilators, early introduction of systemic glucocorticoids, and supplemental oxygen are the mainstay of treatment of acute exacerbations. Close monitoring of the patient's condition and response to therapy are mandatory. In addition, a plan should be formulated to prevent future relapses.

13.8.2.3 Complications of Therapy

Use of systemic (oral, parenteral) steroids over a prolonged period is associated with significant side effects. However, the current day management relies more on inhalation drugs. The main concern with the use of inhalation steroids is the effect on growth. An approximate 20% reduction in the growth velocity during the first year of treatment with inhaled steroids is reported. Subsequently, the growth velocity recovers and children ultimately attain predicted adult height.[56,57] Studies have also reported that children treated with inhaled steroids were more likely to reach predicted adult height than children whose asthma was not treated with preventive medication.[57,58] These findings show that the concern about adverse effect of inhaled steroids on growth is inappropriate.

The complications associated with beta-2 agonists are cardiovascular stimulation, skeletal muscle tremor, hypokalemia, and irritability. These adverse effects are more commonly seen with oral drugs than with inhaled medications.

If asthma severity is assessed properly and inhaled medications are used judiciously, the benefits far outweigh the risks.

13.9 Scientific Basis

A large number of single drugs have been described for use in asthma (Table 13.2).[4] In addition there are quite a few compound preparations available (Table 13.3).[41] There is a great deal of scientific literature available that supports the use of Ayurvedic preparations in the management of asthma. Most of the data are experimental. These studies highlight the anti-inflammatory and bronchodilatory activity in various medications. The following list shows the evidence available for various herbs:

1. *Picrorrhiza kurroa* — *P. kurroa* is a widely used herb in the Ayurvedic system. It belongs to the Scrophulariaceae family, and the active constituents are obtained from the root and rhizomes.[79] It is traditionally used in treatment of respiratory conditions such as asthma and bronchitis. Studies on an alcoholic extract have shown antioxidant and anti-inflammatory effects.[80] In animal studies, antiallergic,

antianaphylactic, anti-inflammatory, and immunomodulatory activities have been demonstrated. The active ingredients include pikuroside II, picroliv (containing iridoid glycoside fraction), and androsin.[81–86]

2. *Adhatoda vasica* — This is widely used in treatment of respiratory tract ailments. Alkaloids from this herb have been shown to possess anti-inflammatory and antiallergic properties.[85,87,88] In addition, its extract has an antitussive effect.[89]
3. *Albizzia lebbek* — The decoction of the bark of *A. lebbek* is used in treatment of asthma and eczema. Studies on animals show that *A. lebbek* has a significant cromoglycate-like action on the mast cells. It also appears to inhibit the early processes of sensitization and synthesis of reaginic-type antibodies.[90,91]
4. *Solanum* species — Powder of or a decoction made from the whole dry plant of *Solanum xanthocarpum* or *Solanum trilobatum* is used in the treatment of asthma and other respiratory disorders. The mechanism of action in asthma may involve bronchodilation, reduction of bronchial mucosal edema, and reduction of airway secretions.[92–94]
5. *Tylophora indica* — *T. indica* is widely used in Ayurvedic medications to provide relief to patients with bronchial asthma. Studies have shown that alkaloids of *Tylophora indica* suppress cellular immune response.[95]
6. *Cedrus deodara* — The wood oil of *C. deodara* has been shown to have anti-inflammatory activity. This can be attributed to its mast-cell stabilizing activity and the inhibition of leukotriene synthesis.[96]
7. *Boswellia serrata* — The gum resin of *B. serrata* contains boswellic acids which have been shown to inhibit biosynthesis of leukotrienes.[97]
8. *Phyllanthus urinaria* — The extracts of the stems, leaves, and roots have been shown to have a relaxant effect on the respiratory tract smooth muscle; involvement of adenosine tri-phosphate- (ATP) sensitive potassium channels is postulated.[98]
9. *Aquilaria agallocha* — Aqueous extracts of stems of *A. agallocha* have been shown to inhibit immediate hypersensitivity reaction by inhibition of histamine release from mast cells.[99]
10. *Calotropis procera* — The latex of *Calotropis procera* has anti-inflammatory property demonstrated in a rat paw edema model.[100]
11. *Elettaria cardamomum* oil — Anti-inflammatory and antispasmodic properties have been demonstrated in a study on rats.[101]
12. *Ocimum sanctum* — Extracts of this widely used plant have been shown to possess immunomodulatory potential and antioxidant and cyclooxygenase inhibitory properties.[102,103] Its fixed oils can inhibit enhancement of the vascular and capillary permeability and leukocyte migration after inflammatory stimulus.[104]
13. *Piper longum* — Piperine, isolated from this plant, has anti-inflammatory potential.[105]

13.9.1 Review of Clinical Trials

13.9.1.1 Picrorrhiza kurroa

Doshi et al.[106] studied the efficacy of *P. kurroa* in a randomized, crossover, double-blind trial. They enrolled 72 patients (ages 14 to 60) for a 14-week study. The patients were given either *P. kurroa* root powder (300 mg three times/day) or an identical placebo. The study had three arms: (1) group A had a long duration of 12 weeks and an active drug was given from week 3 to week 14, (2) group B had a short duration of 3 weeks and an active drug was given from week 3 to week 6 with placebo during the rest of the period, and (3) group C had an intermediate duration of 6 weeks and an active drug was given from week 3–6 and 9–12 with a placebo during intervening periods. The patients were asked to maintain a symptom diary. Weekly pulmonary function tests were performed. The authors did not observe any significant reduction in clinical exacerbation, need for bronchodilators, or improvement in pulmonary function. Fifty patients dropped out of study at different points during the trial. Significant side effects were seen in ten patients — four experienced vomiting, three had anorexia, two had diarrhea, two experienced itching, one had a skin rash, and one experienced giddiness. As this preparation is used frequently, there is need for further studies.

13.9.1.2 Solanum spp.

Govindan et al.[107] studied the efficacy of this herb in bronchial asthma. They enrolled 60 adults with bronchial asthma. Twenty patients each received 300 mg of dry powder of *S. xanthocarpum* or *S. trilobatum,* whereas 10 patients each received salbutamol 4 mg or deriphylline 200 mg. Pulmonary function tests were performed before and 2 h after drug administration. *S. xanthocarpum* and *S. trilobatum* increased FEV_1 by 65 and 67%, respectively, at 2 h. This effect was less than that with salbutamol or deriphylline. Subjective relief lasted 6 to 8 h.

Similar results have been reported in other studies as well; the response rates were poor.[108,109] In these studies the duration for which the drug was given was small; these results may lead to an underestimation of the effects because most Ayurvedic herbal preparations have their best action after about 2 weeks.

13.9.1.3 Tylophora indica

Shivpuri et al.[110] conducted a double-blind, crossover study in 110 patients over 10 years old. Fifty-three patients in the control group ate one spinach leaf daily. At the end of week 1, 62% in the *T. indica* group had moderate to complete relief of symptoms compared with 28% in the control group. At the end of the 12-week study period, improvements in the two groups were 16 and 0%, respectively.

In another double-blind, crossover study,[111] 195 asthmatic patients received either alcoholic tincture of *T. indica* or a placebo for 12 weeks. A daily dairy of symptoms scores was maintained. After a week, 56% of the patients in *T. indica* group had moderate to complete improvement in symptoms compared with 31.6% in the placebo group. After the crossover, 34.2% had improved with *T. indica* and 13.5% with placebo. At the end of study period, 14.8% in the *T. indica* group and 7.2% in the placebo group improved.

The efficacy of alkaloids extracted from *T. indica* was studied in a double-blind trial of 123 patients.[112] The study group received alkaloid extract from *T. indica* in glucose, whereas the control group received glucose colored with spinach. Lung-function tests were evaluated along with symptom scores. The percentage of patients in whom FEV_1 improved by more than 15% was significantly greater in the study group than the control at 1, 2, 4, 8, and 12 weeks, peaking at 4 weeks. The symptom scores were significantly better in the study group, with the peak at 1 week.

Thiruvengadam et al.[113] studied the efficacy of dried *T. indica* in 30 asthmatic patients. The patients were enrolled into a four-arm, double-blind randomized clinical trial for 16 days. Dried *T. indica* powder was compared with standard drugs and a placebo. Pulmonary function tests and symptom scores were evaluated. Among all the parameters, nocturnal dyspnea was the only one that showed significant improvement with *T. indica*.

A placebo-controlled double-blind study[114] on 135 asthmatic patients was conducted to evaluate the efficacy of powdered *T. indica*. The drug or placebo was given for 1 week with another 2 weeks of follow-up. Pulmonary function tests and symptoms scores were evaluated. There were no differences between the two groups.

13.9.1.4 Boswellia serrata

The gum resins of *B. serrata* (*salai guggul*) have been used in asthma. Gupta et al.[115] compared the effect of gum resins of *B. serrata* with placebo in a double-blind, randomized trial on 80 adult asthmatic patients. Pulmonary function tests were evaluated serially. A significant increase in FEV_1 was reported in the test group compared with the placebo group.

13.9.1.5 Miscellaneous Herbs

Iyenger et al.[116] studied the effect of a combination of five plants — *Adhatoda vasica, Solanum xanthocarpum, Albizzia lebbek, Glycyrrhiza glabra,* and *Picrorrhiza kurroa* — in 14 adult patients with asthma. All the patients showed clinical improvement with prevention of recurrence and reduction in severity of symptoms. However, the medication was not effective during acute exacerbation.

Shanker et al.[117] conducted a clinical trial on 15 patients with bronchial asthma using *Gardenia turgida* and *Gardenia latifola*. The results were unimpressive.

Sharma et al.[118] reported significant improvement in one third of the 15 patients they treated with *Euphorbia prostrata* for a period of 2 weeks.

Swamy et al.[119] evaluated the efficacy of *sirisa twak kvatha (Albizzia lebbek)* in 19 patients with asthma. They reported significant improvement in symptoms in most patients.

Trivedi et al.[120] reported bronchodilatory, antispasmodic, and antiasthmatic effects of *vibhitakphal churna* (*Terminalia bellirica*) in a trial on 93 patients.

In another trial,[5] 240 cases of bronchial asthma were administered *naradeeya lakshmi vilas rasa* and *godanti bhasma* in a dose of 0.5 and 1.0 g, respectively, three times/day with honey for a varying period of 4 to 12 weeks. Ninety-six patients received 100% relief, 27 patients received 75% relief, 50 patients received 50% relief, 18 cases received 25% relief, and 28 remained unchanged; 21 cases left against medical advice. In the second group of this study, 210 cases received *shvasa kesari* tablets (500 mg) made from *Solanum xanthocarpum* and *Godanti bhasma* three times/day for 2 to 12 weeks. Seventy-five cases showed complete relief, 49 cases showed 75% relief, 26 cases showed 50% relief, 25 cases showed 25% relief, and 24 did not respond to therapy; 10 cases left against medical advice.

As can be judged from these studies, most trials have demonstrated some benefit. When analyzing the available literature and Ayurvedic texts, we conclude that more clinical research is still required before these therapies can be routinely used. Although there are good experimental data to justify use of Ayurvedic preparations in asthma, issues about doses, combinations, and duration of therapy are still to be resolved. In addition, these preparations do not seem to offer effective medications for acute exacerbations of asthma, which can be life threatening. There are plenty of Ayurvedic preparations with anti-inflammatory and immunomodulatory effects (vide supra). Further research is required to determine the optimal combinations that will help in reducing the airway inflammation and therefore lead to better control of symptoms. It appears that a judicious mix of Ayurvedic medications and modern medicine may be able to improve the control of this common respiratory disorder.

13.10 Areas of Research

Further research is needed to:

1. Establish efficacy of various Ayurvedic preparations used in asthma by good quality randomized controlled trials.
2. Determine the active principles in various Ayurvedic medications.
3. Evaluate the impact of Ayurvedic medications on the natural history.
4. Evaluate the role of immunomodulator medications available in Ayurveda.

13.11 Conclusions

The review of literature highlights need for more research in utility of Ayurvedic preparations in bronchial asthma. At present, the medications and the management are not well standardized. As a large number of experimental studies have documented the presence of anti-inflammatory properties in various Ayurvedic preparations, there is potential for discovering new compounds useful in the management of asthma.

References

1. International Study of Asthma and Allergies in Childhood (ISAAC) Steering Committee, Worldwide variation in prevalence of symptoms of asthma, allergic rhinoconjunctivitis, and atopic eczema: ISAAC, *Lancet*, 351, 1225, 1998.
2. Murthy, K.R.S., *Astanga Samgraha of Vagbhata*, Vol. 2, Chaukhmba Orientalia, Varanasi, 1986, p. 326.
3. Sharma, P.V., *Cakradatta: A Treatise on Principles and Practices of Ayurvedic Medicine*, Chaukhambha Orientalia, Varanasi, 1994, p. 145.
4. Sengupta, N.N., *The Ayurvedic System of Medicine*, Vol. 1, Neeraj Publishing, New Delhi, 1984, p. 198.
5. Goyal, H.R., *Tamaka Shwasa (Bronchial Asthma): A Clinical Study*, Central Council for Research in Ayurveda and Siddha, New Delhi, 1997.
6. Weiss, S.T., Parasites and asthma/allergy: what is the relationship?, *J. Allergy Clin. Immunol.*, 105, 205, 2000.
7. Masters, S. and Barrett-Connor, E., Parasites and asthma-predictive or protective?, *Epidemiol. Rev.*, 7, 49, 1985.
8. Haahtela, T., Lindholm, H., Bjorksten, F., et al., Prevalence of asthma in Finnish young men, *Br. Med. J.*, 301, 266, 1990.
9. Veale, A.J., Peat, J.K., Tovey, E.R., et al., Asthma and atopy in four rural Australian aboriginal communities, *Med. J. Aust.*, 165, 192, 1996.

10. European Community Respiratory Health Survey (ECRHS), Variations in the prevalence of respiratory symptoms, self-reported asthma attacks, and use of asthma medication in the European Community Respiratory Health Survey (ECRHS), *Eur. Respir. J.*, 9, 687, 1996.
11. Devereux, G., Ayatollahi, T., Ward, R., et al., Asthma, airways responsiveness and air pollution in two contrasting districts of northern England, *Thorax*, 51, 169, 1996.
12. Burney, P.G., Luczynska, C., Chinn, S., et al., The European Community Respiratory Health Survey, *Eur. Respir. J.*, 7, 954, 1994.
13. Asher, M.I., Keil, U., Anderson, H.R., et al., International Study of Asthma and Allergies in Childhood (ISAAC): rationale and methods, *Eur. Respir. J.*, 8, 483, 1995.
14. Beasley, C.R.W., Pearce, N.E., and Crane, J., Worldwide trends in asthma mortality during the twentieth century, in *Fatal Asthma*, Sheffer, A.L., Ed., Marcel Dekker, New York, 1998, p. 13.
15. Holgate, S.T., Genetic and environmental interaction in allergy and asthma, *J. Allergy Clin. Immunol.*, 104, 1139, 1999.
16. Wiesch, D.G., Meyers, D.A., and Bleecker, E.R., Genetics of asthma, *J. Allergy Clin. Immunol.*, 104, 895, 1999.
17. Gissler, M., Jarvelin, M.R., Louhiala, P., et al., Boys have more health problems in childhood than girls: follow-up of the 1987 Finnish birth cohort, *Acta Paediatr.*, 88, 310, 1999.
18. Sears, M.R., Burrows, B., Flannery, E.M., et al., Atopy in childhood. I. Gender and allergen related risks for development of hay fever and asthma, *Clin. Exp. Allergy*, 23, 941, 1993.
19. Platts-Mills, T.A., Role of allergens in asthma and airway hyperresponsiveness: relevance to immunotherapy and allergen avoidance, in *Asthma: Its Pathology and Treatment*, Kaliner, M.A. and Persson, C.G., Eds., Marcel Dekker, New York, 1991.
20. Sporik, R., Holgate, S.T., Platts-Mills, T.A., et al., Exposure to house-dust mite allergen (Der p I) and the development of asthma in childhood: a prospective study, *N. Engl. J. Med.*, 323, 502, 1990.
21. Pearce, N., Douwes, J., and Beasley, R., Is allergen exposure the major primary cause of asthma?, *Thorax*, 55, 424, 2000.
22. Lau, S., Illi, S., Sommerfeld, C., et al., Early exposure to house-dust mite and cat allergens and development of childhood asthma: a cohort study, Multicentre Allergy Study Group, *Lancet*, 356, 1392, 2000.
23. Gold, D.R., Environmental tobacco smoke, indoor allergens, and childhood asthma, *Environ. Health Perspect.*, 108(Suppl. 4), 643, 2000.
24. Jones, A.P., Asthma and the home environment, *J. Asthma*, 37, 103, 2000.
25. Johnston, S.L., Viruses and asthma, *Allergy*, 53, 922, 1998.
26. Gern, J.E., Viral and bacterial infections in the development and progression of asthma, *J. Allergy. Clin. Immunol.*, 105, S497, 2000.
27. Sigurs, N., Bjarnason, R., Sigurbergsson, F., et al., Respiratory syncytial virus bronchiolitis in infancy is an important risk factor for asthma and allergy at age 7, *Am. J. Respir. Crit. Care Med.*, 161, 1501, 2000.
28. Keeley, D.J., Neill, P., and Gallivan, S., Comparison of the prevalence of reversible airways obstruction in rural and urban Zimbabwean children, *Thorax*, 46, 549, 1991.
29. Sandberg, S., Paton, J.Y., Ahola, S., et al., The role of acute and chronic stress in asthma attacks in children, *Lancet*, 356, 982, 2000.
30. Vignola, A.M., Chanez, P., Campbell, A.M., et al., Airway inflammation in mild intermittent and in persistent asthma, *Am. J. Respir. Crit. Care Med.*, 157, 403, 1998.
31. Bousquet, J., Chanez, P., Lacoste, J.Y., et al., Eosinophilic inflammation in asthma, *N. Engl. J. Med.*, 323, 1033, 1990.
32. Bousquet, J., Jeffery, P.K., Busse, W.W., et al., Asthma: from bronchoconstriction to airways inflammation and remodeling, *Am. J. Respir. Crit. Care Med.*, 161, 1720, 2000.
33. Lampinen, M., Rak, S., and Venge, P., The role of interleukin-5, interleukin-8 and RANTES in the chemotactic attraction of eosinophils to the allergic lung, *Clin. Exp. Allergy*, 29, 314, 1999.
34. Humbert, M., Menz, G., Ying, S., et al., The immunopathology of extrinsic (atopic) and intrinsic (non-atopic) asthma: more similarities than differences, *Immunol. Today*, 20, 528, 1999.
35. Chung, K.F. and Barnes, P.J., Cytokines in asthma, *Thorax*, 54, 825, 1999.

36. Dunnill, M.S., The pathology of asthma with special reference to changes in the bronchial mucosa, *J. Clin. Pathol.*, 13, 27, 1960.
37. Wenzel, S.E., Szefler, S.J., Leung, D.Y., et al., Bronchoscopic evaluation of severe asthma: persistent inflammation associated with high dose glucocorticoids, *Am. J. Respir. Crit. Care Med.*, 156, 737, 1997.
38. Kelly, W.J., Hudson, I., Raven, J., et al., Childhood asthma and adult lung function, *Am. Rev. Respir. Dis.*, 138, 26, 1988.
39. Martin, A.J., Landau, L.I., and Phelan, P.D., Asthma from childhood at age 21: the patient and his disease, *Br. Med. J.* (Clin. Res Ed.), 284, 380, 1982.
40. Lange, P., Prognosis of adult asthma, *Monaldi. Arch. Chest. Dis.*, 54, 350, 1999.
41. Central Council for Research in Ayurveda and Siddha (CCRAS), *Handbook of Domestic Medicine and Common Ayurvedic Remidies*, Ministry of Health and Family Welfare, Government of India, New Delhi, Documentation and Publication Division, CCRAS, 61-65 Institutional Area, Janakpuri, New Delhi, 1999, chap. Swasa roga.
42. Vedanthan, P.K., Kesavalu, L.N., Murthy, K.C., et al., Clinical study of yoga techniques in university students with asthma: a controlled study, *Allergy Asthma Proc.*, 19, 3, 1998.
43. Jain, S.C. and Talukdar, B., Evaluation of yoga therapy programme for patients of bronchial asthma, *Singapore Med. J.*, 34, 306, 1993.
44. Singh, V., Wisniewski, A., Britton, J., et al., Effect of yoga breathing exercises (pranayama) on airway reactivity in subjects with asthma, *Lancet*, 335, 1381, 1990.
45. Ernst, E., Breathing techniques: adjunctive treatment modalities for asthma? A systematic review, *Eur. Respir. J.*, 15, 969, 2000.
46. Holloway, E. and Ram, F.S., Breathing exercises for asthma, *Cochrane Database Syst. Rev.*, 3, CD001277, 2000.
47. Manocha, R., Marks, G.B., Kenchington, P., et al., Sahaja yoga in the management of moderate to severe asthma: a randomised controlled trial, *Thorax*, 57, 110, 2002.
48. Lenney, W., Boner, A.L., Ebbutt, A., et al., Efficacy and safety of salmeterol in childhood asthma, *Eur. J. Pediatr.*, 154, 983, 1995.
49. Blake, K., Pearlman, D.S., Scott, C., et al., Prevention of exercise induced bronchospasm in pediatric asthma patients. Comparision of Salmeterol powder with salbutamol, *Ann. Allergy Asthma Immunol.*, 82, 205, 1999.
50. Greening, A.P., Ind, P.W., Northfield, M., et al., Added salmeterol versus higher dose corticosteroids in asthma patients with symptoms on existing inhaled corticosteroids, *Lancet*, 344, 219, 1994.
51. Bartow, R.A. and Brogdem, R.N., Formeterol: an update of its pharmacologic properties and therapeutic efficacy in the management of asthma, *Drugs*, 55, 303, 1998.
52. Mitchell, J.A., Belvisi, M.G., Mon, R.A., et al., Induction of cyclooxygenase 2 by cytokines in human pulmonary epithelial cells regulation by dexamethasone, *Br. J. Pharmacol.*, 113, 1008, 1994.
53. Scarfone, R.J., Fuchs, S.M., Nager, A.L., et al., Controlled trial of oral prednisone in the emergency department treatment of children with acute asthma, *Pediatrics*, 92, 513, 1993.
54. Dahl, R. and Johansson, S.A., Importance of duration of treatment with inhaled budesonide on the immediate and late bronchial reaction, *Eur. Respir. J.*, 63(Suppl. 122), 167, 1998.
55. Ferguson, A.C., Spier, S., Manjra, A., et al., Efficacy and safety of high-dose inhaled steroids in children with asthma: a comparison of fluticasone propionate with budesonide, *J. Pediatr.*, 134, 422, 1999.
56. Agertoft, L. and Pedersen, S., Effect of long-term treatment with inhaled corticosteroids on growth and pulmonary function in asthmatic children, *Respir. Med.*, 88, 373, 1994.
57. Agertoft, L. and Pedersen, S., Effect of long-term treatment with inhaled budesonide on adult height in children with asthma, *N. Engl. J. Med.*, 343, 1064, 2000.
58. The Childhood Asthma Management Program Research Group, Long-term effect of budesonide or nedocromil in children with asthma, *N. Engl. J. Med.*, 343, 1054, 2000.
59. Allen, D.B., Mullen, M.C., and Mullen, B., A meta analysis of the effect of oral and inhaled corticosteroid on growth, *J. Allergy Clin. Immunol.*, 93, 967, 1994.

60. Szefler, S.J., A review of Budesonide inhalation suspension in the treatment of pediatric asthma, *Pharmacotherapy,* 21, 195, 2001.
61. Furukawa, C.T., Shapiro, G.G., Bierman, C.W., et al., A double blind study comprising the effectiveness of cromolyn and sustained release theophylline in childhood asthma, *Pediatrics,* 74, 453, 1984.
62. Croce, J., Negreiros, E.B., Mazzei, J.A., et al., A double blind, placebo-controlled comparison of sodium cromoglycate and ketotifen in the treatment of childhood asthma, *Allergy,* 50, 524, 1995.
63. Yasuhiro, K., Kae, M., Michiko, F., et al., Disodium cromoglycate use in children and adolescents with asthma: correlation between plasma concentrations and protective effects for various inhalation methods, *Ann. Allergy Asthma Immunol.,* 83, 553, 1999.
64. de Benedictis, F.M., Tuteri, G., Bertotto, A., et al., Comparison of the protective effects of cromolyn sodium and nedocromil sodium in the treatment of exercise induced asthma in children, *J. Allergy Clin. Immunol.,* 94, 684, 1994.
65. Cherniack, R.M., Wasserman, S.I., Ramsdell, J.W., et al. A double blind multicentre group comparative study of the efficacy of nedocromil sodium in management of asthma, *Chest,* 101, 1292, 1990.
66. Childhood Asthma Management Program Research Group, Long-term effects of budesonide or Nedocromil in children with asthma, *N. Engl. J. Med.,* 343, 1054, 2000.
67. Kabra, S. K., Pandey, R.M., Singh, R., et al., Ketotifen for asthma in children aged 5 to 15 years: a randomized placebo-controlled trial, *Ann. Allergy Asthma Immunol.,* 85, 46, 2000.
68. Legg, J. and Warner, J., Asthma: the changing face of drug therapy, *Indian J. Pediatr.,* 67, 147, 2000.
69. Romanet, S., Stremler-Lebel, N., Magnan, A., et al., Role of leukotriene inhibitors in the treatment of childhood asthma, *Arch. Pediatr.,* 7,969, 2000.
70. Weisberg, S.C., Pharmacotherapy of asthma in children, with special reference to leukotriene receptor antagonists, *Pediatr. Pulmonol.,* 29, 46, 2000.
71. Knorr, B., Holland, S., Rogers, J.D., et al., Montelukast adult (10-mg film-coated tablet) and pediatric (5-mg chewable tablet) dose selections, *J. Allergy Clin. Immunol.,* 106 (Suppl. 3), S171, 2000.
72. Kemp, J.P., Dockhorn, R.J., Shapiro, G.G., et al., Montelukast once daily inhibits exercise-induced bronchoconstriction in 6 to 14-year old children with asthma, *J. Pediatr.,* 133, 424, 1998.
73. Berkowitz, R., Schwartz, E., Bukstein, M.D., et al., Albuterol protects against exercise-induced asthma longer than metaproterenol sulfate, *Pediatrics,* 77, 173, 1986.
74. Green, C.P. and Price, J.F., Prevention of exercise-induced asthma by inhaled salmeterol xinafoate, *Arch. Dis. Child.,* 67, 1014, 1992.
75. Knorr, B., Matz, J., Bernstein, J., et al., Montelukast for chronic asthma in 6-to 14-year-old children. *J.A.M.A.,* 279, 1181, 1998.
76. Bousquet, J., Hejjaove, A., and Michel, F.B., Specific immunotherapy in asthma, *J. Allergy Clin. Immunol.,* 86, 292, 1990.
77. Pichler, C.E., Helbling, A., and Pichler, W.J., Three years of specific immunotherapy with house-dust-mite extracts in patients with rhinitis and asthma: significant improvement of allergen-specific parameters and of nonspecific bronchial hyperreactivity, *Allergy,* 56, 301, 2001.
78. Pajno, G.B., Morabito, L., Barberio, G., et al., Clinical and immunological effect of long term sublingual immunotherapy in asthmatic children sensitized to mites: a double blind, placebo-controlled study, *Allergy,* 55, 842, 2000.
79. Anon., Picrorrhiza kurroa, monograph, *Altern. Med. Rev.,* 6, 319, 2001.
80. Russo, A., Izzo, A.A., Cardile, V., et al., Indian medicinal plants as antiradical and DNA cleavage protectors, *Phytomedicine,* 8, 125, 2001.
81. Jia, Q., Hong, M.F., and Minter, D., Pikuroside: a novel iridoid from Picrorrhiza kurroa, *J. Nat. Prod.,* 62, 901, 1999.
82. Baruah, C.C., Gupta, P.P., Nath, A., et al., Anti-allergic and anti-anaphylactic actively of picroliv-a standardized iridoid glycoside fraction of Picrorrhiza kurroa, *Pharmacol. Res.,* 38, 487, 1998.

83. Simons, J.M., Haart, L.A., Van Dijk, H., et al., Immunomodulatory compounds from Picrorrhiza kurroa: isolation and characterization of two anti complementary polymeric fractions from an aqueous root extract. *J. Ethnopharmacol.*, 26, 169, 1989.
84. Dorsch, W., Stuppner, H., Wagner, H., et al., Anti asthmatic effects of Picrorrhiza kurroa: androsin prevents allergen and PAF induced bronchial obstruction in guinea pigs, *Int. Arch. Allergy Appl. Immunol.*, 95, 128, 1991.
85. Dorsch, W. and Wagner, H., New antiasthmatic drugs from traditional medicine?, *Int. Arch. Allergy Appl. Immunol.*, 94, 262, 1991.
86. Mahajani, S.S. and Kulkarni, R.D., Effect of disodium cromoglycate and Picrorrhiza kurroa root powder on sensitivity of guinea pigs to histamine and sympathomimetic amines, *Int. Arch. Allergy Appl. Immunol.*, 53, 137, 1977.
87. Claesan, U.P., Malmfors, T., Wikman, G., et al., Adhatoda vasica: a critical review of ethnopharmacological and toxicological data, *J. Ethnopharmacol.*, 72, 1, 2000.
88. Gupta, O.P., Sharma, M.L., Ghatak, B.J., et al., Pharmacological investigations of vasicine and vasicinone – the alkaloids of Adhatoda vasica, *Indian J. Med. Res.*, 66, 680, 1977.
89. Dhuley, J.N., Antitussive effect of Adhatoda vasica extract on mechanical or chemical stimulation-induced coughing in animals, *J. Ethnopharmacol.*, 67, 361, 1999.
90. Tripathi, R.M., Sen, P.C., and Das, P.K., Studies on the mechanism of action of Albizzia lebbek, an Indian indigenous drug used in the treatment of atopic allergy, *J. Ethnopharmacol.*, 1, 385, 1979.
91. Tripathi, R.M. and Das, P.K., Studies on antiasthmatic and anti-anaphylactic activities of Albizzia lebbek, *Indian J. Pharmacol.*, 9, 189, 1977.
92. Gupta, S.S. and Gupta, N.K., Effect of Solanum xanthocarpum and Clerodendron serratum on histamine release from tissues, *Indian J. Med. Sci.*, 21, 795, 1967.
93. Gupta, S.S., Verma, S.C., Singh, C., et al., Chemical and pharmacological studies on Solanum xanthocarpum (Kantakari) in chronic bronchitis, bronchial asthma and non-specific unproductive cough, *Indian J. Med. Res.*, 55, 723, 1967.
94. Bector, N.P. and Puri, A.S., Solanum xanthocarpum (Kantakari) in chronic bronchitis, bronchial asthma and non specific unproductive cough, *J. Assoc. Phy. India*, 19, 741, 1971.
95. Ganguly, T. and Sainis, K.B., Inhibition of cellular immune responses by Tylophora indica in experimental models, *Phytomedicine*, 8, 348, 2001.
96. Shinde, U.A., Kulkarni, K.R., Phadke, A.S., et al., Mast cell stabilizing and lipooxygenase activity of Cedrus deodara Loud. wood oil, *Indian J. Exp. Biol.*, 37, 258, 1999.
97. Ammon, H.P.T., Mack, T., Singh, G.B., et al., Inhibition of LT B4-formation in rat peritoneal neutrophils by an ethanolic extract of the gun resin extract of Boswellia serrata, *Planta Med.*, 57, 203, 1999.
98. Paulino, N., Cechinel-Filho, V., Yunes, R.A., et al., The relaxant effect of extract of Phyllanthus urinaria in the guinea pig isolated trachea: evidence for involvement of ATP-sensitive potassium channels, *J. Pharm. Pharmacol.*, 48, 1158, 1996.
99. Kim, Y.C., Lee, E.H., Lee, Y.M., et al., Effect of the aqueous extract of Aquilaria agallocha stems on the immediate hypersensitivity reactions, *J. Ethnopharmacol.*, 58, 31, 1997.
100. Kumar, V.L., Basu, N., Anti-inflammatory activity of the latex of Calotropis procera, *J. Ethnopharmacol.*, 44, 123, 1994.
101. al-Zuhair, H., el-Sayeh, B., Ameen, H.A., et al., Pharmacological studies of cardamom oil in animals. *Pharmacol. Res.*, 34, 79, 1996.
102. Mediratta, P.K., Sharma, K.K., and Singh, S., Evaluation of immunomodulatory potential of Ocimum sanctum seed oil and its possible mechanism of action, *J. Ethnopharmacol.*, 80, 15, 2002.
103. Kelm, M.A., Nair, M.G., Strasburg, G.M., et al., Antioxidant and cyclooxygenase inhibitory phenolic compounds from Ocimum sanctum Linn., *Phytomedicine*, 7, 7, 2000.
104. Singh, S. and Majumdar, D.K., Effect of Ocimum sanctum fixed oil on vascular permeability and leucocytes migration, *Indian J. Exp. Biol.*, 37, 1136, 1999.
105. Mujumdar, A.M., Dhuley, J.N., Deshmukh, V.K., et al., Anti-inflammatory activity of piperine, *Jpn. J. Med. Sci. Biol.*, 43, 95, 1990.
106. Doshi, V.B., Shetye, M., Mahashur, A.A., et al., Picrorrhiza kurroa in bronchial asthma, *J. Postgrad. Med.*, 29, 89, 1983.

107. Govindan, S., Vishwanathan, S., Vijayashekaran, et al., A pilot study on the efficacy of Solanum xanthocarpum and Solanum trilobatum in bronchial asthma, *J. Ethnopharmacol.*, 66, 205, 1999.
108. Jain, J.P., A clinical trial of Kantakari (Solanum xanthocarpum) in cases of Tamak Swasa (some respiratory diseases), *J. Res. Ayurveda Siddha*, 1, 447, 1980.
109. Gupta, P.P., Dubey, S.D., Mishra, J.K., et al., A comparative study on brihati and kantakari in *svasa* and *kasa*, *J. Res. Ayurveda Siddha*, 20, 191, 1999.
110. Shivpuri, D.N., Menon, M.P.S., and Prakash, D., Preliminary studies an Tylophora indica in the treatment of asthma and allergic rhinitis, *J. Assoc. Physicians India*, 16, 9, 1968.
111. Shivpuri, D.N., Singal, S.C., and Parkash, D., Treatment of asthma with an alcoholic extract of Tylophora indica: a cross over, double blind study, *Ann. Allergy*, 30, 407, 1972.
112. Mathew, K.K. and Shivpuri, D.N., Treatment of asthma with alkaloids of Tylophora indica: a double blind study, *Aspects Allergy Appl. Immunol.*, 7, 166, 1974.
113. Thiruvengadam, K.V., Harnath, K., Sudarsan, S., et al., Tylophora indica in bronchial asthma, *J. Indian Med. Assoc.*, 71, 172, 1978.
114. Gupta, S., George, P., Gupta, V., et al., Tylophora indica in bronchial asthma: a double blind study, *Indian J. Med. Res.*, 69, 981, 1979.
115. Gupta, I., Gupta, V., Parihar, A., et al., Effects of Boswellia serrata gum resin in patients with bronchial asthma: results of a double blind, placebo-controlled, 6 week clinical study, *Eur. J. Med. Res.*, 3, 511, 1998.
116. Iyenger, M.A., Jambaiah, K.M., Kamath, M.S., et al., Studies on an anti-asthmatic kada — a proprietary herbal combination. I. Clinical study, *Indian Drugs*, 31, 183, 1994.
117. Shankar, A., Parsai, M.R., Naqvi, S.M.A., et al., A clinical trial of Bharangi in cases of Tamaka Swasa (bronchial asthma), *J. Res. Ayurveda Siddha*, 1, 470, 1980.
118. Sharma, G.D., Upadhyay, B.N., and Tripathi, S.N., A clinical trial of Euphorbia prostrata and Euphorbia thymifolia in the treatment of bronchial asthma, *J. Res. Ayurveda Siddha*, 3, 109, 1982.
119. Swamy, G.K., Bhattathiri, P.P.N., Rao, P.V., et al., Clinical evaluation of Sirisa Twak Kvatha in the management of Tamaka Shwasa (bronchial asthma), *J. Res. Ayurveda Siddha*, 18, 21, 1997.
120. Trivedi, V.P., Nesamany, S., and Sharma, V.K., A clinical study of the anti-tussive and anti-asthmatic effects of Vibhitakphal churna (Terminalia belerica) in the cases of Kasa-swasa, *J. Res. Ayurveda Siddha*, 3, 1, 1982.

14

Hepatic Disorders

Premalatha Balachandran and Rajgopal Govindarajan

CONTENTS

0-8493-1366-X/04/$0.00+$1.50

14.1 Introduction

In Ayurvedic texts (or Ayurveda), the liver is called *yakrut* or *yakruta* or *yakrit*. The word *yakrut* has two verbs, "ya" and "krut." *Ya* denotes activity and *krut* denotes several meanings such as "to breakdown" or "to be instrumental" in performing any activity. The liver is an organ that is continuously engaged in the activity of breaking down various stimuli (e.g., food, water, air, or other sensory stimuli) and is instrumental in sustaining the process of life. In some instances, the word *yakrut* is also used as a synonym to the word "restoration" because it helps bring back damaged body tissues to a normal physiological state.[1] Ayurveda describes the liver as a center of origin (*mula sthana*) of the circulatory system (*raktavaha srotas*).

In Ayurveda, the role of liver is explained in relation to pathogens (*dosa*), tissues (*dhatu*) and its development, muscle (*mamsa*), heart (*hridroga*), blood (*rakta*), respiration (*pranavaha srotas*), and excretion (*mala*). The liver may be affected in the diseases involving these systems.

In conventional medicine, the liver is known to play a central role in the maintenance of metabolic homeostasis by its involvement in carbohydrate, lipid, and protein metabolism. It converts sugar into glycogen, carbohydrates and proteins into fats, toxic ammonia into nontoxic urea, etc. It produces bile, blood coagulating and anti-coagulating factors, proteins, and enzymes. It stores critical trace elements and vitamins and is responsible for detoxification and elimination of various toxins, carcinogens, nitrogen-containing waste products, and alcohol.

The maintenance of a healthy liver is vital to overall health and well-being. Unfortunately, environmental toxins, poor eating habits, alcohol consumption, and therapeutic drug use often abuse this vital organ, and as a consequence there is an overall decline in metabolic functions of the liver. This hepatotoxicity eventually leads to serious diseases like hepatitis, cirrhosis, alcoholic liver disease, and ultimately results in hepatic cancers (liver tumors).

Hepatic diseases like acute or chronic hepatitis and cirrhosis are some of the major causes of significant human mortality, which may result from a wide variety of viral infections and a range of toxins including alcohol. Although the etiology and pathology of hepatic disorders are not clearly defined in detail in Ayurvedic texts, symptoms of hepatic diseases are well described. The symptoms include increased serum bilirubin (*pittavriddhi*), decreased hepatic uptake (*yakruta dhatwagni manya*), decreased hepatic conjugation (*saman vikruti*), hepatocellular damage (*yakruta shotha*), biliary stasis (*sang*), steostasis (*medomay, yakrut medoj siragranthi*), and cirrhosis (*yakrutshosh*).[2] Modern diagnostic tools presented in Table 14.1 are widely used by Ayurvedic practitioners currently for accurate and speedy diagnosis of hepatobiliary disorders and to understand the underlying mechanisms of the diseases.

The aim of this chapter is to provide information on the Ayurvedic treatment of hepatitis, hepatic coma, ascities, cirrhosis, and liver cancer. Scientific information available on Ayurvedic treatments is summarized.

14.2 Hepatitis (*Kamala*)

According to Ayurveda, hepatitis is a disease of the circulatory system and is categorized under biliary (*pitta*) diseases; *ranjaka pitta* is the type of biliary fluid involved in this

TABLE 14.1

Tests for Hepatobiliary Disorders

Test (Reference Range)	Diagnosis
Biochemical Analysis	
Alanine aminotransferase (up to 35 IU/l)	Elevation indicates degree of inflammation and possible causes for the disease
Aspartate aminotransferase (6–38 IU/l)	
Alkaline phosphatase (53–128 IU/l)	Elevation suggestive of obstructive liver diseases and liver cancer
Gamma glutamyl transpeptidase (<50 IU/l)	γ-GT is an indicator of alcohol usage
Total bilirubin (0.2–1.0 mg/dl)	Elevation indicates diseases of the liver and bile ducts
Direct bilirubin (0–0.2 mg/dl)	
Albumin (3.5–5.0 g/dl)	Decreased level suggests chronic liver disease and liver cancer, particularly worse cases, though a decrease is also noticed in generalized protein deficiency conditions (e.g., kwashiokar and marasmus)
Alphafetoprotein (up to 10 ng/ml)	Specifically rises to 500 ng/ml during hepatocarcinoma
Abnormal clotting studies	Suggestive of worsening chronic liver disease
Antibody test (blood sample)	Indicates hepatitis A, B, or C
Hepatitis B DNA (blood sample)	Indicates hepatitis B
Hepatitis C RNA (blood sample)	Indicates hepatitis C
Bile duct imaging	Indicates primary biliary cirrhosis
HFE gene analysis for C282Y mutation	Indicates hemochromatosis
Liver biopsy	Indicates nonalcoholic steatohepatitis, chronic hepatitis B or C, primary biliary cirrhosis, autoimmune hepatitis, alcoholic liver disease
Imaging Modalities[a]	
Plain abdomen x-ray	Detects gallstones, calcification
Oral cholecystography	Gives size, shape, position, and function of gall bladder
IV cholangiography	Visualizes bile duct
Percutaneous transhepatic cholangiography	Detects obstructive jaundice
Endoscopic retrograd cholangiography	Confirms obstructive jaundice
Ultrasound scanning	Diagnoses cysts, abscesses, neoplasm, degenerative changes, and metastatic deposits
CT scanning	Diagnoses malignant tumors, focal nodular hyperplasia, hemangioma, cysts, and abscesses
Radionucleotide or isotope scanning	Detects and estimates metastatic lesions
MRI scanning	Produces images of gall bladder and biliary duct

[a]Dole, V.A., *Ayurved and Hepatic Disorders*, Sri Satguru Publications, Delhi, 2001, 71.

pathogenesis.[3] The liver secretes *Pachaka pitta* (more than 500 cc in a day) and is stored in the gall bladder (*pittashaya*). The stored bile gets reabsorbed and leaves a fraction of original bile (*tyakta drava pitta*). The concentration of original bile in the circulation is critical and any derangement leads to diseases arising out of weak digestive and metabolic activity (*agni vaishamya*). The more dilution of bile in the gall bladder results predominantly in symptoms like nausea, vomiting, and fever. When the concentration is too high, it leads to symptoms like burning sensations, thirst, profused sweating, giddiness, and hemorrhagic conditions (Figure 14.1).[1]

Ayurveda classifies two basic types of hepatitis: hemolytic jaundice *(kostashakhasrita kamala, paratantra kamala,* or *bahupittaja kamala*) and obstructive jaundice (*shakhasrita kamala).* Hepatitis could also be intrahepatic (*swatantra*) or extrahepatic jaundice (*paratantra*). The other minor types of hepatitis are chronic hepatic failure (*kumba kamala*), fulminant hepatic failure (*halimaka*), and hepatorenal syndrome (*panaki*).[3] Hemolytic hepatitis is associated with moderate to severe anemia. Accelerated destruction of red blood cells and hemoglobin (increased *malaroopa ranjaka pitta*), due to the diet and lifestyle that increase *pitta* (*pittavardhaka ahara* and *vihara*), leads to enhanced bilirubin formation. The obstructive hepatitis is due to the obstruction in the biliary flow. Water (*kapha*) or fluid accumulation obstructing the passage channels of biliary system results in this manifestation. The stools will be clay colored (*tilapista nibha*) until bile comes to the intestine (*kosta*).[3]

Conventional medicine considers hepatitis as one of the most common liver diseases. Hepatitis is caused by agents like viruses (hepatitis A, B [HBV], C [HCV], D, E, G, cytomegalovirus [CM virus], Epstein-Barr virus [EB virus], yellow fever), parasites (*E. histolytica*), bacteria (leptospirosis, cholangitis, septicemia), drugs, and toxins. Although these agents can be distinguished by their antigenic properties, clinically they all are generally manifested as jaundice along with some associated constitutional symptoms. Hepatitis may be contacted through the intake of viral contaminated food stuff, virus-infected blood, serum, saliva, sexual contact, urine or feces, blood transfusion, or fecal-contaminated food stuff.

Viral infection in liver causes destruction of parenchymal cells at the deoxyribonucleic acid (DNA) level, which leads to hepatocellular failure, disturbances in nitrogen metabolism, inflammation, necrosis, and cirrhosis resulting in the obstruction of bile-canaliculi. This obstruction leads to resorbtion of bile into the peripheral bloodstream through the hepatic vein and lymphatics.The process then causes the serum bilirubin level to rise above 2 mg% and is sufficient to be termed clinically as jaundice.[4]

14.2.1 Treatment

Removing biliary tract blockade during hepatitis by purgatives forms the basis for its treatment. The elimination of vitiated pathogens (*shodana* approach of *panchakarma*), preceded by curative along with liver regenerative therapy (*snehana*), forms the primary treatment protocols. Supplementary treatment includes the administration of a daily dose of purgatives, chologogue drugs like *katuki*, and medicated ghees. *Samprapti vighatana* treatment strikes at the root of the disease process by destroying and neutralizing the inflammation, removing the obstruction, and bringing the pathogens to the intestine. Viral hepatitis patients were treated with *pancha gavyam ghritam* (5 g B.D.) and *Katuka rohini* (1 g) daily in the morning with milk and *bhumi amla swarasa* (50 ml/day). For nasal infiltration (*nasya karma*), *katu tumbi jal* was used. *Netranjan* has been used as *jyotishmati swarasa.* After 4 to 6 weeks of treatment, encouraging results were obtained and clinical symptoms of jaundice completely disappeared.[4]

This *panchakarma* treatment is more appropriate for hemolytic jaundice than hepatocellular jaundice. This is because a patient with a poor appetite and general disability would not be able to tolerate the above-mentioned exhaustive procedures.[3] In such cases, hepatoprotective drugs would be beneficial.

14.2.2 Herbal Treatment of Hepatitis

Two reviews have been published so far on hepatoprotective Ayurvedic drugs. The first one gives extensive review of the experimental and clinical research on the

TABLE 14.2

Hepatoprotective Ayurvedic Herbal Therapies

Botanical Name	Liver Disorders	Type of Study	Ref.
Acacia catechu	Viral hepatitis	Clinical	47
Adhatoda vasica	Liver diseases	Clinical	47
Aegle marmelos	Hepatitis B	Clinical	7
Aloe vera	Hepatoma	Yoshida AH-130 ascite hepatoma cell line	48
Anacardium occidentale	Hepatoma	Hepatoma 129 cell line	49
Azadirachta indica	Hepatitis B	Clinical	47
Bacopa monnieir	Viral hepatitis	Clinical	7
Chichorium intybus	Chronic hepatitis	Clinical	50
Citrullus lanthus	Viral hepatitis	Clinical	7
Emblica officinalis	Hepatomegaly hepatitis C	Clinical	51
Fummaria parviflora	Hepatitis C	Clinical	52
Glycyrrhiza glabra	Hepatoma	*In vitro*	53
Gynandropis pentaphylla	Hepatoma	Hepatoma 129 cell line	49
Phyllanthus niruri	Hepatitis B	*In vitro*	54
Plumbago zeylanica	Hepatoma	Animal studies	55
Saussurea lappa	Hepatoma	HepG2 cell line (human hepatoma cell line)	56
Solanum nigrum	Viral hepatitis	Clinical	47
Sphaeramthus indicus	Viral hepatitis	Clinical	7
Tephrosia purpurea	Viral hepatitis	Clinical	7
Vitex nigundo	Hepatitis B	Clinical	50
Withania somnifera	Hepatoma	*In vitro*	49

hepatoprotective effects of medicinal plants and their preparations.[5] The second review gives a compilation of the information on various studies on these plant medicines.[6] The herbs with their scientifically proven hepatoprotective property are discussed in the end of the chapter and also listed in Tables 14.2 and 14.3. These herbs also possess one or more properties, including antiviral, cholerectic, regeneration of hepatocytes, antifibrotic, etc.[7] Individual treatment profiles for various types of hepatitis presented in Table 14.4 will help practitioners choose a better drug for these dreadful diseases. Classical Ayurvedic formulations for diseases related to circulatory system, liver ailments, and jaundice are listed in Table 14.5. The Ayurvedic formulas commercially available for the treatment of hepatic disorders are presented in Table 14.6.

14.3 Ascites (*Udaram, Jalodhar, Asadhya*)

According to Ayurveda, the accumulation of abnormal toxic fluids around the liver creates blockage (*srotorodh*) that inhibits the secretion of bile resulting in liver enlargement. Impaired digestive power (*agni*) has been considered the basic etiological factor for this disease and clinical features include abdominal distension, weakness, sluggish passage of feces, and flatus. The successful treatment depends on the treatment of underlying causes. *Phalatrikadi kasaya* formula has the potential to remove a toxic blockage of the liver. The herbs *triphala, katuki,* and *chira* have the properties to clear off the abnormal pathogens. Constipation associated with ascites may be relieved by *Katuki.* Necessary detoxification

TABLE 14.3

Ayurvedic Herbs Shown to Have Antitumor Activity

Research Protocol	Therapeutic Hepatoprotective Properties	Ref.
Andrographis paniculata (Kalmegh) *Active constituent: Andrographolide*		
Paracetamol-induced toxicity on isolated rat hepatocytes	Increases the viability percentage of the hepatocytes; antagonizes the toxic effects of paracetamol on liver function enzymes	57
Carbon tetrachloride (CCl_4) and galactosamine toxicity in rats	Stimulates hepatic regeneration and increases resistance to damage by toxins; activates reticuloendothelial system	58
Animal tumors	Antihepatocarcinogenic and enhances carcinogen detoxification by the regulation of antioxidant defense system and microsomal drug metabolism	59
Annona atemoya/muricata (Sitaphala) *Active constituent: Bullatacin*		
In vitro studies in 2.2.15 cells, human hepatocarcinoma cell line	Induces cell death due to apoptosis, preceded by cell blebbing, chromatin margination, and condensation	60
Animal studies	Inhibits mitochondrial electron transport and NADH oxidase activity; arrests abnormal cell growth by inhibiting oxidative phosphorylation and lowering ATP levels	61
Boerhavia diffusa (Punarnava) *Active constituent: Punarnavine alkaloid*		
CCl_4 -induced toxicity in rats	Shows strong choleretic activity and increases normal bile flow	62
Animal studies	Pharmacological potency depends on the morphological features and time of collection of herb; plant roots of 1–3 cm diameter, collected in the summer, exhibited very high hepatoprotective effect	63
Eclipta alba (Bhringaraj) *Active components: Wedelolactone and demethyl-wedelolactone*		
In vitro studies in rat hepatocytes	Anti hepatotoxic and stimulates liver cell regeneration	64
CCl_4-induced hepatotoxicity in rats	Regulates GSH levels, hepatic drug metabolism, and activities of lysosomal enzymes	54
Clinical trials — hepatitis patients	Used as a cholagogue and as deobstruent; down regulates HBAg	
Piper longum (Pippali) *Active constituent: Piperine*		
CCl_4-induced toxicity in animals and culture	Reduces lipid peroxidation by increasing glutathione levels	59
Terminalia chebula (Haritaki) *Active constituent: Tannins*		
Cholesterol-induced hypercholesterolemia in rabbits	Hypocholesterolemic effect	65
Clinical trials	Used in many anticancer formulations for the treatment of liver enlargement	

TABLE 14.3 (continued)

Ayurvedic Herbs Shown to Have Antitumor Activity

Research Protocol	Therapeutic Hepatoprotective Properties	Ref.
Semecarpus anacardium Linn. (Bhallataka)		
Animal studies — Aflatoxin-induced hepatocellular carcinoma in rats	Gradual increase in body weight; decreases bilirubin and abnormal nucleic acid content; normalizes cancer marker activities, lysozomal enzymes, glycoprotein content, immunosuppression, and hyperlipidemia; reduces alpha-fetoprotein to normal range and regulates abnormal mineral metabolism; cures hypoglycemia by activating gluconeogenic enzymes, thereby increasing the synthesis of glucose; controls abnormal lipid peroxidation and maintains antioxidant defense status of the host; as a bifunctional inducer induces both phase I and phase II biotransformation enzymes and causes carcinogen detoxification; prevents tumor initiation by the metabolic activation of carcinogens; replaces necrotic tissues by newly regenerated hepatocytes	66–73
Clinical trial — *Anacartin forte* an Ayurvedic preparation containing *Semecarpus anacardium* nuts and seeds in the proportion of 1:200 (90 g/day of divided doses for 3 months)	Gives subjective and objective improvement, alleviates troublesome symptoms, increases survival time and causes complete regression of hepatocarcinoma; patient recovers by gaining weight and appetite; normalizes liver abnormalities like tenderness and enlargement; blood count and liver function tests become normal	74
		75
Ayurvedic formulation containing *Semecarpus anacardium* nuts, *Amura rohitaka, Glycyrrhiza glabra* Linn., and *Tamra bhasma*		
Animal studies — C_3H jax strain breast tumor-bearing mice	Inhibits tumor development and increases survival period; tumor specific γ-amino butyric acid level decreases to normal	
Clinical studies — cancer patients (1.5 g of divided doses)	Response to this formulation was higher than conventional chemotherapy and combined chemo- and radiotherapy; reduces the toxic effects of other chemotherapeutic agents, prolongs the drug efficiency, and increases the body's resistance to cancer; normalizes γ-aminobutyric acid levels and glutamic acid decarboxylase activities	

and blood purification are carried out by *nimba* and *vasa* because they have the detoxification properties and often are used as blood purifiers. *Guduchi* and *triphala* are used to restore health.[8]

14.4 Hepatic Coma

Ayurveda does not have a clear description and diagnosis of hepatic coma except that it resembles an advanced stage of *kumbha kamala.* Viral-, toxic-, or drug-induced hepatocel-

TABLE 14.4

Therapeutic Modalities for Hepatitis

Disease	Comment and Treatment	Ref.
Hemolytic jaundice	Bilirubin seldom exceeds 6 mg% and more than 80% is indirect bilirubin Treatment modalities include antibiliary measures, internal oleation, *virechana*, hepatoprotective drugs, *ghritha*, and *rasayana* drugs (e.g., *Brahmarasayana, Indukantha ghritha, Panchathiktha ghritha, Rohitakarista,* and *Suvarnamalini vasantha*)	3, 50
Hepatitis B	Annual incidence in U.S.: 140,000–320,000 Mild cases: *Virechaka* like *Phalatrikadi kashaya* and viricidal agent, *Phyllanthus niruri* Moderate: *Arogyavardhini* with viricidal and *virechaka* drugs Severe cases (serum bilirubin exceeds 20 mg%): *Kamalihara rasa* (0.3 g), *Tapyadi lauha* (0.25 g), *Arogyavardhini* (0.5 g), *Nirgundi sallaki* (3 g), and *Guduchi* (3 g) are used in three divided doses/day for 3 to 4 weeks; minerals like *tapyadi lauha* and *srothoshodhaka* drugs like *shilajithu, nirgundi,* and *Semecarpus anacardium* are additionally used	10, 50
Acute viral hepatitis (HBAg negative)	*Arogyavardini* (500 mg), hepax (500 mg), *valiliv* (250 mg), *kamalahar forte* (250 mg) and Liv.52 (275 mg); *Arogyavardini* and hepax are more beneficial Decrease in total serum bilirubin was evident from the 4th day of treatment; stimulates either hepatic or extra hepatic clearance of bilirubin; normalizes HDL cholesterol and other lipid levels	76
Acute viral hepatitis (HBAg positive)	*Swarasa* composed of *P. kurroa, Azadirachta indica, Amrita, Eclipta alba,* and *P. niruri* is beneficial in 17/20 patients in 30 days *Suvarnamalini vasantha, P. niruri,* and *R. emodi* (100 mg 2 times/day for 3 to 6 months)	50, 77
Hepatitis C	Complicates into hepatic cirrhosis followed by liver failure *N. stellata* seeds (250 mg), *abhrak bhasma* (250 mg), *P. longum* (100 mg), *Fummaria parviflora* (100 mg), *Tinospora cordifolia* (100 mg), *Boerhavia diffusa* (100 mg), *Emblica officinalis* (100 mg) (total 1 g three times/day dose)	52
Amebic hepatitis	Combination of *Shankhabhasma vati, Laghusutshekhar vati, Indrayav vati* (250 mg 3 times/day for 15 days) *Shankhabhasma vati* has the property of *ushna, laghu, ruksha,* and *teekshna* and described as *Grahanirognashan* *Indrayav vati* is a combination of *tridoshaghna, sangrahi,* and *katu*; it acts as *deepan, shoolnashak, jwarnashak, atisarnashak,* and *krumighna*	78
Drug- or alcohol-induced hepatitis	*Eclipta alba, Andrographis paniculata, P. kurroa, Tephrosia purpurea,* and *trikatu* in combinations or Liv.52 (275 mg twice daily)	
Chronic hepatitis	Hepatoprotective drugs (*Arogyavardini, E. alba, Solanum nigrum, Chichorium intybus, P. kurroa*), anti-inflammatory drugs (*Vitex nigundo, P. longum,* sallaki, *Tephrosia purpurea*), *rasayani* drugs (*Vardhamana, P. longum, rasayana*), and immunomodulators (*Amritha, Semecarpus anacardium, Punarnava mandoora*) are used in combinations	50

lular necrosis results in a hepatic coma — a clinical syndrome due to neuropsychiatric complications. This kind of hepatocellular failure and portal systemic shunts contributes to the genesis of hepatic encephalopathy. This process occurs by allowing nitrogenous products of bacterial fermentation in the colon (e.g., ammonia) to reach the brain, which is sensitive to their toxic actions. The aromatic amino acids formed from the conversion of branched chain amino acids act as weak neurotransmitters and may displace normal neurotransmitters (adrenaline and dopamine) in the brain, producing hepatic coma. It is accompanied by jaundice, gynecomastia, hepatomegaly, splenomegaly, and ascites. Because hepatic coma is not a single disease but a complication resulting from various

TABLE 14.5

Classic Ayurvedic Formulations for Diseases Related to *Raktavaha srotas* (e.g., Liver Ailments, Jaundice [Kamala])

Formulation, Manufacturer, and Ingredients	Indications and Dose	Ref.
Abhrak bhasma (UNJHA, UAP Pharma Pvt. Ltd.) *Abhra, Ravi ksira, Vata ksira, Snuhi ksira, Kakamaci, Goksura, Kharamanjari, Vata praroha, Gomutra, Tulasi, Kadali sipha*	Viral hepatitis (250 mg)	52
Bhallataka vati (Imis Pharmaceuticals Pvt. Ltd.) *Bhallataka, tila bija, Haritaki, Guda*	Cancer (1–3 pills after food)	
Brahmarasayana (Nagarjuna Herbal Concentrates Ltd.) *Pathya, Dhatri, Bilva, Ganikarika, Salaparni, Prasniparni, Brhati, Kantakari, Goksura, Bala, Punarnava, Eranda, Masaparni, Mudgaparni, Satavari, Meda, Jivati, Jivaka, Rsabhaka, Sali, Kasa, Sara, Darbha, Iksu, Tvak, Ela, Musta, Rajani, Pippali, Agaru, Candana, Mandukaparni, Kanaka, Sankhapuspi, Vaca, Plava, Yastyahvaya, Vidanga, Sitopala, Sarpi, Taila, Ksaudra*	Hemolytic jaundice (12 g)	50
Candanabalalaksadi taila (Dabur Ayurvedic Specialties Ltd.) *Candana, Bala mula, Laksa, Lamajjaka, Taila, Usira, Nisa Madhuka, Satahva, Aguru, Katurohini, Devadaru, Bala, Kustha, Manjistha, Balaka, Asvagantha, Darvi, Murva, Musta, Mulaka, Ela, Tvak, Naga kusuma, Rasna, Laksa, Sugundhika, Campaka, Pitasara, Sariva, Sauvarcala, Saindhava, Ksira*	Hepatitis (6 g)	
Draksadi arkom (Nagarjuna Herbal Concentrates Ltd.) *Vitis vinifera, Madhuca latifolia, Glycyrrhiza glabra, Symplocos racemosa, Cyperus Rotundus*	Liver diseases (15–30 ml)	79
Gudapippali (SRI Dhanwantari Matam Ayurvedics Pvt. Ltd.) *Embelia ribes, Piper longum, Zingiber officinale, Piper nigrum, Plumbago rosea, Nigella sativa*, salt, and mineral additives	Liver diseases	79
Indukantha ghritha (Nagarjuna Herbal Concentrates Ltd.) *Ptia, daru, Bilva, Agniatha, Syonaka, Gambhari, Patala, Salaparni, Prsniparni, Brhati, Kantakari Goksura, Ksira, Ghrta, Pippali, Pippalimula, Cavya, Citraka, Sunthi, Saindhava*	Hemolytic jaundice (12 g)	50
Kutajavaleha (Zandu Pharmaceutical Works Ltd.) *Kutaja tvak, Guda, Rasanjana, Mocarasa, Sunthi, Marica, Pippali, Haritaki, Bibhitaka, Amalaki, Lajjalu, Citraka, Patha, Bilva, Indrayava, Vaca, Bhallataka, Prativisa, vidanga, Balaka Ghrta, Madhu*	Hepatic diseases (6–12 g)	
Laghusutshekhar vati (Gary and Son, U.S.A.) *Svarna gairika, Sunthi, Nagavalli svaras*	Amebic hepatitis (1 to 2 tablets)	78
Pancha Gavyam Ghritam (Imis Pharmaceuticals Pvt. Ltd.) *Gomaya svarasa, Dadhi, Gomtra, Goghta*	Hepatitis (12 g)	4
Panchathiktha ghritha (Vyas Pharmaceuticals) *Nimba, Patola, Vyaghri, Guduci, Vasaka, Haritaki, Bibhitaka, Amalaki, Ghrta*	Hemolytic jaundice (6 g)	50
Patolakaturohinyadi arkom (Nagarjuna Herbal Concentrates Ltd.) *Trichosanthus cucumarina, Picrorrhiza kurroa, Santalum album, T. cordifolia, Chonemopha fragrans*	Liver diseases (15–30 ml)	79
Phalatrikadi kasaya (Rajashree Ayurvedic Pharmacy) *Haritaki Bibhitak, Amalaki, Amruta, Vasa, Katuki, Nimb, Kirattikta*	Cirrhosis, ascites (20 ml)	80
Punarnavasava (Nagarjuna Herbal Concentrates Ltd.) *Sunthi, Marica, Pippali, Haritaki, Bibhitaka, Amalaki, Darvi, Svadamstra, Brhati, Kantakari, Vasa, Eranda mula, Katuki, Gajapippali, Sothaghni, Picumarda, Guduci, Suska mulaka, Duralabha, Patola, Dhataki, Draksa, Sita, Maksika*	Hepatic diseases (12–24 ml)	
Rohitakarista (UNJHA, UAP Pharma Pvt. Ltd.) *Rohitaka, Guda, Dhataki, Pippali mula, Cavya, Citraka, Sunthi, Tvak, Ela, Patra, Haritaki, Bibhitaka, Amalaki*	Hemolytic jaundice (12–24 ml)	50

TABLE 14.5 (continued)

Classic Ayurvedic Formulations for Diseases Related to *Raktavaha srotas* (e.g., Liver Ailments, Jaundice [Kamala])

Formulation, Manufacturer, and Ingredients	Indications and Dose	Ref.
Shankhabhasma vati (UNJHA, UAP Pharma Pvt. Ltd.) *Sanka, Kanjika*	Amebic hepatitis (250 mg)	78
Suvarnamalini vasantha (UNJHA, UAP Pharma Pvt. Ltd.) *Mauktika bhasma, Hingula, Marica, Kaphari, Svarna bhasma*	Hemolytic jaundice (10 g)	50
Tapyadi lauha (*Vyas Pharmaceuticals*) *Haritaki, Amalaki, Vibhitakaki, Sunthi, Marica, Pippali, Vidanga, Citraka mula, Musta, Pippalimula, Devadaru, Daruharidra, Dalcini, Cavya, Silajitu, Svarnamaksika bhasma,Raupya bhasma, Lauha bhasma, Mandura bhasma*	Viral hepatitis (250–500 mg)	50
Vasagulu chyadi kvatha (Vaidyaratnam Oushadhasala) Adhatoda vasica, T. cordifolia, Glycyrrhiza glabra, Strychnos potatorum, Melia azadirachta	Liver diseases (15–30 ml)	79

disorders, the choice of treatment depends on symptoms of individual patients. Treatment profile includes the combination of the following drugs and a vegetarian diet:

1. *Nasya of haridra* and *daru haridra quath* reduce ammonia saturation in encephalopathy.
2. *Basti* (a type of enema) with *dashmool quath* and *saindhava* can reduce toxicity in guts.
3. Sugarcane juice maintains electrolyte balance.
4. *Vasa* prevents gastrointestinal bleeding.
5. *Guduchi* is an antibiotic.
6. *Triphala* and *katuki* manage constipation.
7. *Bhunimb* and nimb help in regeneration of liver cells.[9]

14.5 Cirrhosis

Ayurveda does not have a clear description and diagnosis of cirrhosis. According to conventional medicine, the etiology of the liver cirrhosis is due to the diffuse degeneration and infiltration of parenchyma that results in the structural alteration of fat lobules, dense perilobular connective tissue formation, and development of regeneration areas. Cirrhosis is the seventh leading cause of death in the U.S., with 4000 annual deaths.[10] Advanced cirrhosis leads to ammonia toxicity, hepatic coma, gastrointestinal hemorrhage, and kidney failure. It is not a primary disease but the end result of a diffuse liver injury secondary to poor nutrition, anorexia and action of toxins, alcoholism, hepatitis C, or biliary obstruction. As liver cells are destroyed, they are systematically replaced by scar tissue. Hepatic cirrhosis occurs following one or more clinical manifestations such as the loss of appetite, hepatomegaly, splenomegaly, ascites, edema of the legs, fever, diarrhea, hematemesis, jaundice, portal hypertension, and anemia.

TABLE 14.6

Patent Ayurvedic Formulas for Hepatobiliary Disorders

Formulation, Manufacturer, and Ingredients	Indications and Dose	Ref.
ARKA LIV Tablet (Ayurvedeeya Arkashala Ltd.) *Guduchi, Rohitaka, Daruharidra, Amalaki, Katuki, Shankha, Karpardika, Dagadiber bhasma*	Hepatitis, jaundice, hepatoprotective (2–3 tablets two times/day with honey)	
Arogyavardhini (Zandu Pharmaceutical Works Ltd.) *Mercury, Sulfur, Lohabhasma, Tamrabhasma, Abhrakbhasma, Triphala churna, Shilajit-, Guggul, Chitrakamal Churna, Kutaki churna,* decoction of *A. indica*	Hepatitis (500 mg/day)	80
Ayu Liv Tablet (AYUDRUGS) *Kalamegha, Sharpunkha, Chitraka, Punarnava, Triphala, Kakmachi, Senai* leaves, *Arjuna, Rohitakarishta, Kutaja tvak, Mandoora bhasma, Ajamoda, Khus-Khus,* bile salt	Liver diseases, sluggish liver, jaundice (1–2 tablets/day)	
Hepabex (Swastik Formulations Pvt. Ltd.) *Solanum nigrum, Tephrosia pupurea, Picrorrhiza kurroa, Ipmoea tupethum, Eclipta alba, Phyllanthus niruri, Tecomella undulata, Boerhaavia diffusa, Tinospora cordifolia, Glycyrrhiza glabra*	Hepatoprotective, hepatitis B, and jaundice (2 tsp two times/day)	
Hepa Cap (Capro Labs Exports India Ltd.) *Zizyphus jujuba, Terminalia chebula, Aegle marmelos, Calcium oximum, Berberis aristata, Vitis vinifera, Ipomoea digitata, Emblica officinalis*	Jaundice, cirrhosis, infective hepatitis (2 capsules two to three times/day)	81
Hepajun (Phyto Pharma Pvt. Ltd.) *Bhringaraja, Madayantika, Daruharidra, Kalamegha, Punarnava, Nimba, Chitraka, Mandura bhasma, Shankha bhasma, Kasamarda, Pathari, Nishothara, Katuki, Kharavath, Kapardika*	Impaired liver function, hepatitis, hepatobiliary disorders (2 capsules/day)	
Hepatovit (Millenium Herbal Care Ltd.) *Phyllanthus niruri, Terminalia chebula, Terminalia belerica, Embilica officinalis, Eclipta alba, Berberis aristata, Fumaria parviflora, Boerhaavia diffusa, Zingiber officinale, Plumbago zeylanica, Tinospora cordifolia, Andrographis paniculata, Picrorrhiza kurroa, Piper longum*	Hepatitis, hepatobiliary dysfunction, enlarged liver, cirrhosis (1–2 capsules/day)	
Hepax (Anglo-French Drugs and Industries Ltd.) *Chitraka, Katuki, Maricha, Ardraka, Sarjikakshara, Amalaki, Yavakshara, Chuna, Haritaki*	Chronic hepatitis, cirrhosis, infective hepatitis (2 tablets three times/day)	76
Hepin (Nupal Remedies Pvt. Ltd.) *Yashthimadhu, Daruharidra, Pippali, Bhumyamalaki, kakamachi, Gudardrakam, Musali, Ela, Tripadi, Kandasari*	Hepatitis A and B, non-A and non-B hepatitis (2 tablets three times/day)	82
Herboliv (Vyas Pharmaceuticals) *Arogyavardhini vati, Punarnava mandura,Bhumyamalaki, Bhringaraja, Punarnava,Vidanga, Haridra, Haritaki, Guduchi, Rohitaka, Nishothara, Mehandi, Varuna, Arjuna, Parpata Sugar*	Anemia, hepatitis, hepatomegaly, anorexia (1–2 tablets/day)	
Liv.52 (The Himalaya Drug Company) *Himsra, Kasani, Mandur bhasma, Kakamachi, Arjuna, kasamarda, Biranjasipha, Jhavuka; processed in Bhringaraja, Bhumyamalaki, Punarnava, Guduchi, Daruharidra, Mulaka, Amalaki, Chitraka, Vidanga, Haritaki, parpata*	Viral hepatitis, cirrhosis, hepatotoxicity (2–3 tablets/day)	76
Livotrit (Zandu Pharmaceutical Works Ltd.) *Arogyavardhini rasa, Eclipta alba, Mandura bhasma, Boerhaavia diffusa, Andrographis paniculata*	Infectious hepatitis, liver dysfunctions (2 tablets two times/day)	
Livshield syrup (Bajaj Consumer Care Ltd.) *Bhumyamalaki, Bhringaraja, Guduchi, Gokshura, Kasamarda, Chitraka, Kantakari, Krishna tulasi, Palasha pushpa, Punarva, Arjuna twak, Triphala, Karanaja, Maricha, Methika beeja, Nagavalli, Trivrut, Pippali, Ativisha, Ajamoda satva*	Liver dysfunction, jaundice (2 tsp three times/day)	

TABLE 14.6 (continued)

Patent Ayurvedic Formulas for Hepatobiliary Disorders

Formulation, Manufacturer, and Ingredients	Indications and Dose	Ref.
Stimuliv (Fraco-Indian Pharmaceuticals Ltd.) *Kalamegha, Bhringaraja, Parpata, Bhumyamalaki*	Viral hepatitis, hepatomegaly, loss of appetite, constipation (2 tablets/tsp two times/day)	83
Vasuliv (Vasu Pharmaceuticals Ltd.) *Bringaraj, Punarnava, Sharapunkha, Kasni, Bjumyamlaki, Kalamegh, Katuki*	Liver dysfunction, hepatomegaly, jaundice, viral hepatitis, alcoholic liver diseases (2 tablets three times/day)	84

In a case report of early hepatic cirrhosis due to biliary obstruction, patients with moderate jaundice and anorexia with a tender, enlarged liver were treated with *arogyavardhini* and *phalatrikadi kasaya* with milk on empty stomachs for 3 months. No other food was allowed. The main symptoms and signs were relieved completely in 3 months, and the patients' appetites increased. The liver regained normal morphology, jaundice disappeared, blood pressure became normal, and ascites were not detected. Hepatomegaly and splenomegaly were reduced. Although the cirrhotic changes in the liver are irreversible, the hepatic functions can be maintained with the rest of the healthy tissues by this treatment.[11]

14.6 Liver Cancer

In Ayurveda, tumors are discussed under the names *granthi* and *arbuda* to designate basic common neoplasms, which can appear in any tissue or organ of the body. *Granthi*, or minor neoplasm, is a localized small swelling within the subcutaneous fat tissue, muscle, or blood veins; it is round, erect, and knotted. *Arbuda*, or major neoplasm, is a spherical, stable, massive, painless swelling occurring at one site; it expands slowly with deeper roots. Immobile recurrence of *arbuda* at the site of previous swelling is called *ashyarbuda*. When two *arbudas* appear simultaneously the condition is known as *dvirarbuda*, which indicates their malignant nature.[12, 13]

The different abnormal growths of pre- and postcancerous states and malignant and nonmalignant stages arising from various organs are grouped and known as cystic growths (*gulma*), benign growths (*apaci*), lymphatic growths (*gandamala*), bone tumor (*asthila*), cystic tumors (*mutragranthi*), vaginal tumors (*yonikarnini*), and systemic tumors (*granthivisarpa* and *balmika*). These growths represent morbid anatomy as neoplasm.[13] Both allopathic and Ayurvedic systems generally refer to neoplasms as the uncoordinated abnormal cell growth found within particular organs or body tissues.

The words *vataja, pittaja,* or *kaphaja* tumors (adenoma) or *medhaja* (lipoma) or a combination of any two of them is used to signify a benign neoplasm where one or two of the three major bodily systems (*tridosas*) are out of control. Benign tumors are not very harmful because there is still coordination among the systems, which to some extent controls the damage. Malignant abnormal growth has been indicated as *tridosaja* neoplasm (metastatic tumors), because the three major bodily systems have lost mutual coordination and cannot prevent damage to tissues, resulting in a deadly morbid condition.[13]

According to conventional medical pathology, primary malignant hepatic tumors may arise from any constituent cells of the liver. Cancer arising from two types of cells are very common: liver cell cancer (hepatocellular carcinoma) and carcinoma of the biliary epithelium (cholangiocarcinoma). Other rare tumors that arise from the liver tissue include fibrolamellar carcinoma, squamous cell carcinoma, epithelial hemangioendothelioma, angiosarcoma, Kaposi's sarcoma, hepatoblastoma, and hepatocellular adenoma. In addition to these malignant primary liver cancers, metastatic involvement of the liver is also very common because of the extreme chance of spreading cancer from several parts of the body to the liver.

14.6.1 Hepatocellular Carcinoma

Hepatocellular carcinoma (HCC), also referred to as a fatal malignancy, is regarded as one of the most aggressive tumors with poor prognosis. It has a worldwide incidence of 250,000 to 1,000,000 patients annually.[14] HCC is prevalent in Asia and Africa where annual incidence of 500 cases occurs per 100,000 population.[15] In China, HCC was the third cancer killer, and annual deaths from HCC have exceeded 110,000, accounting for approximately 45% of the total HCC deaths in the world.[16] According to 1996 annual statistics, in the U.S. there have been more than an estimated 19,500 new cases of HCC and 15,200 deaths due to this cancer. This estimate is based on incidence rates of the Service, Epidemiology, and End Results (SEER) program from 1979 to 1992.[17]

14.6.1.1 Etiology of Liver Cancer

According to Ayurvedic texts, cancer is a disease resulting from the derangement of bodily systems due to dietary constituents (chemical carcinogenesis). It differs according to each person's pathogens (exogenous) and constitutions (genetic, *bijadosa*).[13] Sushruta called the sixth layer of the skin *Rohini* (the skin layer with the nature of growth), which represents the Western medical word *epithelium*, the layer of cells forming the epidermis of the skin and the surface layer of the mucous membranes where most cancers originate. Pathogenic injuries to the inner layer of the dermis can be caused by the imbalances of three bodily systems or lifestyle errors, such as unhealthy foods, poor hygiene, or behavioral habits and physical trauma resulting in ulcerous conditions. Because of the fast-growing nature of these tissues, the process of healing often leaves tiny scars. These slow-healing ulcers may develop into early neoplasms, which are complicated and difficult to cure.[13]

HCC is a multifactorial and multistage process whose precise etiology is not known. Both chronic hepatitis and cirrhosis are considered major precipitating factors. HBV or HCV infection results in tumor initiation.[14] Other factors include the ingestion of high amounts of aflatoxins, occupational exposure to vinyl chloride or similar toxic chemicals, and alcoholism. Long-term use of oral contraceptives and angiogenic therapy have also been found to cause liver cancer development in fewer cases.

14.6.1.2 Pathogenesis of Liver Cancer

In Ayurveda, *Sushruta* has proposed six stages of pathogenesis, which apply more to the neoplasms (especially liver tumors) because of their metastatic nature:

1. Localization of growth (*sanchaya*)
2. Transformation of growth into metastatic tumors (*prakopa*)

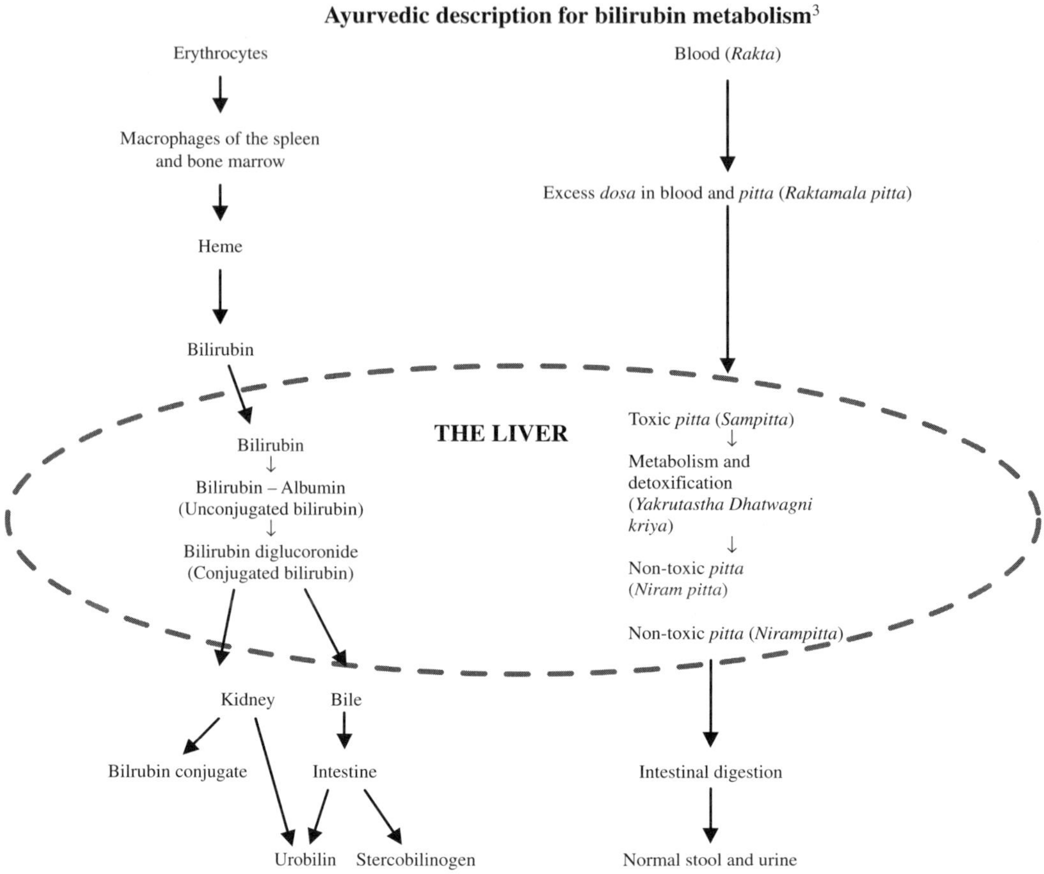

FIGURE 14.1
Ayurvedic description for bilirubin metabolism. (From Mali, M.D. and Kulkarni, P.H., *Ayurved and Hepatic Disorders*, Sri Satguru Publications, Delhi, 2001.)

3. Metastasis (*prasara*)
4. Secondary growth (*sthana samsraya*)
5. Expression of symptoms (*vyakti*)
6. Histopathological differentiation (*bheda*)

On the basis of *tridosas* concept, *pitta* present in each and every cell is responsible for digestion and metabolic function. In liver cancer, the decreased state of deranged metabolism (*dhatwagni* imbalance) results in the excessive growth of the liver tissue and creates metabolic crisis where anabolic phase exceeds the catabolic phase (aggravation of *vatha* forces and suppression of *kapha* forces) resulting in proliferation. It is clearly stated that liver enlargement (*ekadesavriddhi*) is accompanied by weight loss (*anyasthaniyakshaya*) in liver cancer.[18]

14.6.1.3 Diagnosis of Liver Cancer

In early stages, liver cancer usually has no noticeable symptoms. Hepatomegaly (*yakrutodara)*, with moderate pain (*ruk*) or tenderness (*sparsahsnutwam*) that is localized to the upper abdomen or the right upper quadrant, is often the major complaint from the HCC patients.[19] Macroscopically, the tumor may be a solitary mass with multiple necrotic (*kotham*) nodules or may present diffusely, which infiltrates the liver and usually is cirrhotic. On microscopical examination, several abnormal architectural patterns of malignancy (e.g., trabecular, pseudoglandular, solid, etc.) exist, and these tumors are mitotically active. In certain cases, abdominal swelling (*sopham*) due to liver enlargement with or without ascites also occurs. Pyrexia, pain, or fractures due to bone metastasis are some of the rare presentations of preneoplastic syndromes. Anorexia (*aruchi*), weight loss, hypercalcemia, hypoglycemia, hyperlipidemia, hemotologic, and neurologic syndromes are also clinical manifestations that occur during HCC (see Figure 14.1).

Although serum alpha-fetoprotein (AFP) is a highly specific marker in HCC cases, ultrasonographic screening is also recommended because AFP levels are not always elevated in the early stages of HCC (in 30% of cases). Presence of alkaline phosphatase isoenzymes, carcinoembryonic antigen, and human chorionic gonadotropin are other associated complications in HCC patients. Bleeding of esophageal varices may present as a terminal sequele.

14.6.1.4 Treatment

HCC is an important cause of morbidity and mortality worldwide. The course of clinically apparent disease is rapid, and if untreated, most patients die within 3 to 6 months of diagnosis. Individual prognostic factors such as the extent of the disease, the site of metastasis, histological condition of the tumor, and the biochemical abnormalities have to be considered in selection of a therapy.

14.6.1.4.1 *Ayurvedic Treatment Modalities*

In Ayurvedic classical texts, specific treatment protocols for liver cancer were not mentioned. Ayurvedic practitioners are taking the advantage of available knowledge of treatment on cancer from the old classical texts and are applying those methods in liver cancer management. Empowerment, participation in the healing process, relief of cancer symptoms, time and personal attention, and reduced cost of care are essential elements in the Ayurvedic management of liver cancer.

The fundamental principles of Ayurveda are finding the cause of an illness and restoring the balance between the three major bodily systems by supplying deficient substances and by reducing the excessive ones (*tridosa siddhanta*). Anticancer therapeutic approach can be divided into four categories:

1. Restoration of balance (*prakritisthapani chikitsa*)
2. Curative therapy (*roganashani chikitsa*)
3. Restoration of normal function (*rasayana chikitsa*) and spiritual therapy (*naishthiki chikitsa*)
4. Surgery (considered only as a last resort)

Unlike Western medicine, which mostly epitomizes the one symptom–one disease–one drug paradigm, Ayurvedic medicines are holistic and go a long way to substantiate the defects and deficiencies of medical practices.

14.6.1.4.2 *General Line of Treatment*

1. Purification process (*sodhana chikitsa* including *panchakarma*) using internal and external medications which can eliminate pathogens (*dosas*)

2. Curative therapy (*samana chikitsa)* pacifies pathogens (*dosas*)
3. Correction of metabolic defects (*dhatwagni chikitsa*)
4. Immunotherapy (*rasayana prayoga*)
5. Anticancerous drugs (*vyadhipratyanika chikitsa*)
6. Symptomatic treatment (*lakshanika chikitsa*)
7. Surgical treatment with herbal and mineral medicines (*Sastra chikitsa*)[18]

The herbal treasure chest of ancient Ayurveda offers a host of new phytochemicals that can be used both preventively and clinically to manage a spectrum of liver-related imbalances, including hepatocarcinoma. Tables 14.2 and 14.3 describes not only efficient and effective therapies for liver diseases, but also their underlying scientific principles based on an extensive literature search of Ayurvedic texts and research reports on hepatoprotective herbs with anticancerous property. Ayurvedic practitioners are using Ayurvedic text preparations that utilize the recent research outcomes on anticancer herbs (Table 14.5). Many Ayurvedic drug manufacturers are designing their own appropriate drug formulations (Table 14.6). These herbal formulas contain multiple chemical agents as active ingredients; these agents may operate synergistically, producing tremendous therapeutic benefits, lowering risks on adverse effects, and avoiding unnecessary supplemental therapy. The benefit of an herbal formula is that it can nourish the body as a whole by supporting various organ systems, yet its main focus will be on nourishing the liver and its functions. These formulations are reported to work on multiple biochemical pathways and are capable of influencing several organ systems simultaneously. This kind of orientation makes the Ayurvedic approach to liver cancer especially attractive.

14.6.1.4.3 Allopathic Treatment

Among allopathic treatment modalities, surgery is seldom of value for hepatic metastases nor is hormonal therapy. In radiotherapy using intraarterial ^{131}iodine-lipiodol[20] or ^{90}yttrium, microspheres,[21] the clinical benefits are of modest value because of side effects like fibrosis, pneumonitis, neurological abnormalities, colitis, enteritis, malabsorption, and sterility. Although chemotherapy is an essential component of an effective multidisciplinary cancer treatment program, current systematic therapies with 5-fluorouracil, floxuridine, doxorubicin, mitomycin-C, and cisplatin are less effective and responses are partial (5 to 25% range) and short lived.[22]

Radiotherapy and chemotherapy also damage adjacent healthy cells and increase the possibility of developing a secondary cancer; many times, the mortality increases by the toxicity of the drug or radiation rather than the disease. Other approaches, namely, hepatic artery embolization with chemotherapy, alcohol ablation, ultrasound guided cryoablation, immunotherapy with monoclonal antibodies, and gene therapy with retroviral vectors, are also of only minimal benefit. Liver transplantation may be considered as another therapeutic option, but again the recurrence of tumor or metastases after transplantation has limited its usefulness. The major drawback with the treatment of HCC is that it has a significant propensity to develop metastases with major sites spreading to other parts of the liver, lymph nodes, lungs, bones, adrenal glands, and the peritoneal cavity.[23] Multifocal HCC is a very difficult neoplasm to treat due to the lack of efficacy of chemotherapeutic regimes and the inaccessibility of this tumor to surgical procedures. The World Health Organization (WHO) also categorized hepatic cancers under group 3 tumor, for which there are no effective drugs.[24]

Given the lack of useful therapies for this disease, there is a great need to discover drugs that are selectively cytotoxic only to hepatic cancer cells without damaging the body's other normal cells. Because Ayurvedic herbal therapies have the potential to inhibit cancer cells without damaging normal cells, liver cancer patients who already are crippled with the disease and burdened by chemotherapy-induced toxic side effects are often turning to seek help from Ayurvedic physicians. Patients hope for a better cure without adverse side reactions from Ayurvedic therapies. The high cost of conventional medicine is also driving the search for alternatives in other medical systems such as Ayurveda.

14.7 Prevention of Hepatic Diseases

Prevention is a preferred strategy than cure, especially for chronic hepatic diseases such as liver cancer. Regular intake of hepatoprotective herbal tonics would be beneficial in this strategy. It may also be argued reasonably that prevention of viral infection by HBV vaccine may help prevent HCC. The antifibrotic agents prolyl 4-hydroxylase inhibitor (HOE 077), sho-saiko-to (TJ-9), and interferon can also reduce the risk of development of HCC.[25]

14.8 Scientific Basis

14.8.1 *Phyllanthus niruri/amarus* (*Bhumyamalaki*)

14.8.1.1 Clinical Trials

In a clinical study[26] conducted on 55 patients with chronic viral hepatitis, all the 30 patients under *P. amarus* treatment were cured within 3 months with remarkable recovery of liver functions and inhibition of HBV replication. Another study[27] indicated that 59% of the *P. amarus*-treated patients became HBAg negative.

14.8.1.2 In Vivo and In Vitro Studies

The aqueous extract of *P. amarus* not only increased the life span of the *N*-nitrosodiethylamine-induced HCC-bearing rats from 33 to 52 weeks, but also normalized gamma glutamyl transpeptidase and serum HCC marker activity.[28] The ethanolic extract exhibited a hepatoprotective effect on alcohol toxicity in rats and in carbon tetrachloride and galactosamine-induced cytotoxicity in primary cultured rat hepatocytes.[29] *P. amarus* extract inhibited HBAg secretion in Alexander, a human hepatocellular carcinoma cell line, because of its ability to down-regulate HBV messenger ribonucleic acid (mRNA) transcription and up-regulate HBV enhancer I activity.[30] It also inhibited HBV polymerase activity and decreased episomal HBV DNA content.[31]

14.8.2 *Picrorrhiza kurroa* (*Katuki*)

14.8.2.1 Clinical Trials

The active principle of *katuki* is *kutkin*. The standardized preparation used in studies is Picroliv. In a placebo-controlled trial[32] with acute viral hepatitis patients, *P. kurroa* (375 mg three times/day for 14 days) normalized liver function test (LFT) parameters with quicker clinical recovery and 100% clinical and biochemical clearance.

14.8.2.2 In Vivo and In Vitro Studies

P. kurroa acts as a direct viricidal agent and alters biotransformation of the toxins. In several studies[33,34] it inhibited the uncoupling between respiration and oxidative phosphorylation and aflatoxin-induced lipid peroxidation in rats. In addition, it caused the reversal of low-density lipoprotein binding to paracetamol and lowered bilirubin level by biliary flow stimulation. It also showed a protective role against ethanol and carbon tetrachloride-induced toxicity in rat hepatocytes.[35] During *Plasmodium berghei* infection in *Mastomys caucha*, it showed hypolipidemic property by regulating lipolytic enzymes.[36] As an effective inhibitor of hepatocarcinogenesis, it normalized liver function enzymes and reduced liver enlargement and hepatic nodular formation in N-nitrosodiethylamine-induced hepatocarcinoma conditions.[37]

14.8.3 *Podophyllum hexandrum* Linn. (*Giriparpata, Vanatrapusi*)

14.8.3.1 Clinical Studies

P. hexandrum (active constituent: Podophyllotoxin) is a hepatic stimulant, blood purifier, and *raktaarbudanasna* (anticancer drug). Etoposide (VP-16), a semisynthetic derivative of podophyllotoxin, has been used against HCC for several years. P-glycoprotein, an energy-dependent drug efflux pump that reduces intracellular concentration of drugs in tumor cells, seems to be less effective in reducing VP-16 concentration in hepatoma cell lines; this drug is found to be more efficient in hepatocarcinoma.[38] In a phase II study on anticancer effectiveness of VP-16 in combination with epirubicin, 3% of 36 HCC patients achieved complete response, 36% had partial response, and 31% exhibited stable disease; the disease progressed in another 31% of patients.[39]

14.8.3.2 In Vivo and In Vitro Studies

P. hexandrum has the property of karyoplastic and causes mitotic arrest, nuclear fragmentation, and impaired spindle formation dispersing the chromosomes. Necrosis and rapid reduction of the cytochrome oxidase are suggested mechanisms for its antitumor property.[40]

14.8.4 *Tinospora cordifolia* (*Guduchi*)

14.8.4.1 Clinical Trials

In a study[41] with malignant obstructive jaundice patients, *T. cordifolia* decreased morbidity and mortality due to liver cell failure. In addition, a 92.4% survival rate after treatment without blood poisoning was noticed when compared with only a 40% survival rate on conventional treatment. As an immunomodulator, it strengthened host defense and normalized phagocytic and killing capacities of neutrophils. In another study[42] with hepatitis patients, the treatment showed symptomatic relief with improvement in yellow discoloration of urine and body and reduction of LFT parameters. Of a total of 20 cases, 75% were cured and 25% improved from their illness.

14.8.4.2 In Vivo and In Vitro Studies

T. cordifolia prevented fibrosis by hepatic tissue regeneration, membrane stabilization, and activation of kupffer cells in carbon tetrachloride-induced liver damage in rats.[43] In experimental animal tumors, it increased IgG antibodies and enhanced humoral- and cell-mediated immunity.[44] It not only stimulated the proliferation of stem cells and increased white blood and bone marrow cells, but also reduced tumor volume by 58.8%, which was comparable with cyclophosphamide.[45]

Scientific basis for other hepatoprotective Ayurvedic herbs are continued in Table 14.3.

14.9 Summary and Conclusion

The complete cure of liver diseases such as HCC is one of the biggest challenges in the medical world. Scientific researchers in medical sciences are conducting multidirectional research on various aspects of hepatic disorders in order to determine useful remedies for these dreadful diseases. New findings discussed are a result of the development of Ayurvedic science through the ages and their accomplishments in modern cancer therapeutics. The details of experimental and clinical studies conducted on single and compound Ayurvedic preparations for their efficacy against liver cancer and other hepatic ailments are also important; they strongly emphasize Ayurvedic therapy as a scientifically feasible medical practice and an unconventional entity. Research in this field should be sustained and strengthened in order to better understand its scientific merit and determine its utility for a heterogenous population. Hepatic diseases are no longer inevitable and can be prevented and effectively treated. Ayurvedic medicine now has an opportunity to contribute to the end of liver cancer's long scourge of mankind.

Acknowledgments

The authors are highly thankful to the authorities and staff of the literary research and documentation department, Central Research Institute (Siddha), Chennai, India for permitting the use of their library facilities.

References

1. Nanal, V., Liver disorders and their Ayurvedic management, in *Ayurved and Hepatic Disorders,* Kulkarni, P.H., Ed., Sri Satguru Publications, Delhi, 2001, p. 142.
2. Mali, M.D. and Kulkarni, P.H., Clinical interpretation of LFT with ayurvedic point of view, in *Ayurved and Hepatic Disorders,* Kulkarni, P. H., Ed., Sri Satguru Publications, Delhi, 2001, p. 59.
3. Madikonda, P.K. and Singh, R.H., The concept of kamala, *Ayurmedline-Hepatitis,* 17, 2002.
4. Srinivasarao, T., Panchakarma approach to physiological problems of hepatitis (yakritdalyodar), in *Ayurved and Hepatic Disorders,* Kulkarni, P.H., Ed., Sri Satguru Publications, Delhi, 2001, p. 101.
5. Vaidya, A.B. et al., Selected medicinal plants and formulations as hepatobiliary drugs: an overview, *Indian J. Clin. Pharmacol. Ther.,* 12, 7, 1996.
6. Bhatt, A.D. and Bhatt, N.S., Indigenous drugs and liver disease, *Indian J. Gastroenterol.,* 15, 63, 1996.
7. Acharya, M.V. and Bansal, P., A proposed hepato-immunomodulating drug regimen for hepatitis, in *Ayurved and Hepatic Disorders,* Kulkarni, P.H., Ed., Sri Satguru Publications, Delhi, 2001, p. 176.
8. Wali, A.G. and Mulye, M., Hepatitis induced ascites: a clinical study, in *Ayurved and Hepatic Disorders,* Kulkarni, P. H., Ed., Sri Satguru Publications, Delhi, 2001, p. 125.
9. Sane, M.D., Hepatic coma: Ayurvediya management, in *Ayurved and Hepatic Disorders,* Kulkarni, P.H., Ed., Sri Satguru Publications, Delhi, 2001, p. 196.
10. Sastry, J.L.N., Augustine, J., and Eeswarymma, L., Management of chronic hepatitis B carriers, *Ayurmedline-Hepatitis,* 160, 2002.
11. Nachiket, W. and Neha, W., Clinical evaluation of phalatrikadi kwath and arogyavardhini in early hepatic cirrhosis: a case report, in *Ayurved and Hepatic Disorders,* Kulkarni, P.H., Ed., Sri Satguru Publications, Delhi, 2001, p. 79.
12. Charak Samhita (700 B.C.), translated by Sharma, P.V., Choukhamba Orientalia, Varanasi, India, 1981.
13. Sushruta samhita (early 1000 B.C.), translated by Bhishagratna, K.L., Choukhamba Orientalia, Varanasi, India, 1991.
14. Haydon, G.H. and Hayes, P.C., Hepatocellular carcinoma, *J. Appl. Medicine,* 21, 425, 1995.
15. Isselbacher, K.J. and Dienstay, J.L., Tumors of the liver and biliary tract, in *Harrisons Principles of Internal Medicine,* Fauci, J.B., Braunwald, E., and Isselbacher, K.J., Eds., Mc-Graw-Hill, New York, 1998, p. 579.
16. Zhaoyou, T., Small hepatocellular carcinoma: past, present and future, *Chin. Med. J.,* 109, 21, 1996.
17. Parker, S.L. et al., Cancer statistics, *CA Cancer J. Clin.,* 46, 5, 1996.
18. Sastry, J.L.N., *Introduction to Oncology, Cancer in Ayurveda,* Chaukhambha Orientalia, Varanasi, India, 2001.
19. Isselbacher, K.J. and Dienstay, J.L., Tumors of the liver and biliary tract, in *Harrisons Principles of Internal Medicine,* Fauci, J.B., Braunwald, E., and Isselbacher, K.J., Eds., Mc-Graw-Hill, New York, 1998, p. 579.
20. Lau, W.Y. et al., Adjuvant intra-arterial lipiodol iodine-131 for respectable hepatocellular carcinoma: a prospective randomized trial, *Lancet,* 353, 797, 1999.
21. Ho, S. et al., Combating hepatocellular carcinoma with an integrated approach, *Chin. Med. J. (English),* 112, 80, 1999.
22. O'Reilly, E.M. et al., A phase II study of Irinotecan in patients with advanced hepatocellular carcinoma, *Cancer,* 91, 101, 2001.
23. Lee, Y.T. and Gheere, D.A., Primary liver cancer: pattern of metastasis, *J. Surg. Oncol.,* 36, 26, 1987.
24. World Health Organization Consultation, Essential drugs for cancer chemotherapy, *Bull. WHO,* 72, 693, 1994.

25. Okita, K., Sakaida, I., and Hino, K., Current strategies for chemoprevention of hepatocellular carcinoma, *Oncology*, 62, 24, 2002.
26. Xin-Hua, W. et al., A comparative study of *Phyllanthus amarus* compound and interferon in the treatment of chronic viral hepatitis B, *J. Trop. Med. Public Health*, 31, 140, 2001.
27. Mehrotra, R. et al., In vitro effect of *Phyllanthus amarus* on hepatitis B virus, *Indian J. Med. Res.*, 93, 71, 1991.
28. Rajeshkumar, N.V. and Kuttan, R., *Phyllanthus amarus* extract administration increases the life span of rats with hepatocellular carcinoma, *J. Ethnopharmacol.*, 73, 215, 2000.
29. Prabhakar, S., Hepatoprotective activity, *Ayurmedline-Hepatitis*, 29, 2002.
30. Jayaram, S. and Thyagarajan, S.P., Inhibition of HBsAg secretion from Alexander cell line by *Phyllanthus amarus*, *Indian J. Pathol. Microbiol.*, 39, 211, 1996.
31. Lee, C.D. et al., *Phyllanthus amarus* down-regulates hepatitis B virus mRNA transcription and replication, *Eur. J. Clin. Invest.*, 26, 1069, 1996.
32. Vaidya, A.B. et al., *Picrorrhiza kurroa* Royle ex Benth as a hepatoprotective agent experimental and clinical studies, *J. Postgrad. Med.*, 42, 105, 1996.
33. Anandan, R., Prabhakaran, M., and Devaki, T., Biochemical studies on the hepatoprotective effect of *Picrorrhiza kurroa* on changes in liver mitochondrial respiration and oxidative phosphorylation in D-galactosamine induced hepatitis in rats, *Fitoterapia*, 70, 548, 1999.
34. Rastogi, R., Srivastava, A.K., and Rastogi, A.K., Long term effect of aflatoxin B_1 on lipid peroxidation in rat liver and kidney: effect of picroliv and silymarin, *Phytother. Res.*, 15, 307, 2001.
35. Santra, A. et al., Prevention of carbon tetrachloride induced hepatic injury in mice by *Picrorrhiza kurroa*, *Indian J. Gastroenterol.*, 17, 6, 1998.
36. Ramesh, C., Khanna, A.K., and Dhawan, B.N., Picroliv regulates lipid metabolism in Plasmodium berghei induced liver damage in Mastomys caucha, *Indian J. Pharmacol.*, 29, 39, 1997.
37. Rajeshkumaran, N.V. and Kuttan, R., Inhibition of N-nitrosodiethylamine induced hepatocarcinogenesis by Picroliv, *J. Exp. Clin. Cancer Res.*, 19, 459, 2000.
38. Park, J.G. et al., MDR1 gene expression its effect on drug resistance to doxorubicin in human hepatocellular carcinoma cell lines, *J. Natl. Cancer Inst.*, 86, 700, 1994.
39. Pallavacini, E.B. et al., Epirubicin and etoposide combination chemotherapy to treat hepatocellular carcinoma patients: a phase II study, *Eur. J. Cancer*, 33, 1784, 1997.
40. Pandey, G., *Anticancer Herbal Drugs of India with Special Reference to Ayurveda*, Sri Satguru Publications, Delhi, 2002.
41. Rege, N. et al., Immunotherapy with *Tinospora cordifolia*: a new lead in the management of obstructive jaundice, *Indian J. Gastroenterol.*, 12, 5, 1993.
42. Prakash, S. and Rai, N.P., Role of *T. cordifolia* (WILLD.) MIERS. (Guduchi) in the treatment of infective hepatitis, *J. Res. Ayurveda Siddha*, 17, 58, 1996.
43. Nagarkatti, D.S. et al., Modulation of kupffer cell activity by *Tinospora cordifolia* in liver damage, *J. Postgrad. Med.*, 40, 65, 1994.
44. Kapil, A. and Sharma, S., Immunopotentiating compounds from *Tinospora cordifolia*, *J. Ethnopharmacol.*, 58, 89, 1997.
45. Matthew, S. and Kuttan, G., Immunomodulatory and antitumor activities of *Tinospora cordifolia*, *Fitoterapia*, 70, 35, 1999.
46. Dole, V.A., Hepatic disorders and imaging, *Ayurved and Hepatic Disorders*, Kulkarni, P.H., Ed., Sri Satguru Publications, Delhi, 2001, p. 71.
47. Lalitha, B.R., Awareness of hepatotoxicity and protectivity, in *Ayurved and Hepatic Disorders*, Kulkarni, P.H., Ed., Sri Satguru Publications, Delhi, 2001, p. 97.
48. Corsi, M.M. et al., The therapeutic potential of Aloe vera in tumor-bearing rats, *Int. J.Tissue React.*, 20, 115, 1998.
49. Dhar, M.L. et al., Screening of Indian plants for biological activity. I, *Indian J. Exp. Biol.*, 9, 91, 1968.
50. Shripathi, R., Management of medical jaundice, *Ayurmedline-Hepatitis*, 21, 2002.
51. Kapoor, L.D., *CRC Handbook of Ayurvedic Medicinal Plants*, CRC Press, Boca Raton, FL, 1990.
52. Khajgiwale, D.J., Introduction to hepatitis C and its ayurvedic management, in *Ayurved and Hepatic Disorders*, Kulkarni, P.H., Ed., Sri Satguru Publications, Delhi, 2001, p. 67.

53. Arase, Y. et al., The long-term efficacy of glycyrrhizin in chronic hepatitis C patients, *Cancer*, 79, 1494, 1997.
54. Thygarajan, S.P. et al., In vitro inactivation of HBsAg by Eclipta alba Hassk and *Phyllanthus niruri* Linn., *Indian J. Med. Res.*, 76, 124, 1982.
55. Parimala, R. and Sachdanandam, P., Effect of Plumbagin on some glucose metabolizing enzymes studied in rats in experimental hepatoma, *Mol. Cell. Biochem.*, 125, 59, 1993.
56. Chen, H.C. et al., Active compounds from Saussurea lappa Clarke that suppress hepatitis B virus surface antigen gene expression in human hepatoma cells, *Antiviral Res.*, 27, 99, 1995.
57. Visen, P.K. et al., Andrographolide protects rat hepatocytes against paracetamol-induced damage, *J. Ethnopharmacol.*, 40, 131, 1993.
58. Handa, S.S. and Sharma, A., Hepatoprotective activity of andrographolide against galactosamine and paracetamol intoxication in rats, *Indian J. Med. Res.*, 92, 284, 1990.
59. Trivedi, N. and Rawal, U.M., Effect of aqueous extract of *Andrographis paniculata* on liver tumor, *Indian J. Pharmacol.*, 30, 318, 1998.
60. Chih, H. et al., Bullatacin, a potent antitumor annonaceous acetogenin, inhibits proliferation of human hepatocarcinoma cell line 2.2.15 by apoptosis induction, *Life Sci.*, 69, 1321, 2001.
61. Morre, J.D. et al., Mode of action of bullatacin, A potent antitumor acetogenin: inhibition of NADH oxidase activity of HeLa and HL-60, but not liver, plasma membranes, *Life Sci.*, 56, 343, 1995.
62. Chandan, B.K., Sharma, A.K., and Anand, K.K., *Boerhavia diffusa*: a study of its hepatoprotective activity, *J. Ethnopharmacol.*, 3, 299, 1991.
63. Rawat, A.K. et al., Hepatoprotective activity of *Boerrhavia diffusa* roots: a popular Indian ethnomedicine, *J. Ethnopharmacol.*, 56, 61, 1997.
64. Saxena, A.K., Singh, B., and Anand, K.K., Hepatoprotective effects of *Eclipta alba* on subcellular levels in rats, *J. Ethnopharmacol.*, 40, 155, 1993.
65. Thakur, C.P. et al., The Ayurvedic medicines Haritaki, Amla and Bahira reduce cholesterol-induced atherosclerosis in rabbits, *Int. J Cardiol.*, 21, 167, 1988.
66. Premalatha, B. and Sachdanandam, P., Effect of *Semecarpus anacardium* nut extract against aflatoxin B_1 induced hepatocellular carcinoma, *Fitoterapia*, 70, 484, 1999.
67. Premalatha, B., Muthulakshmi, V., and Sachdanandam, P., Anticancer potency of the milk extract of *Semecarpus anacardium* Linn. nuts against aflatoxin B_1 mediated hepatocellular carcinoma bearing Wistar rats with reference to tumor marker enzymes, *Phytother. Res.*, 13, 183, 1999.
68. Premalatha, B. and Sachdanandam, P., Immunomodulatory activity of *Semecarpus anacardium* Linn. Nut milk extract in Aflatoxin B_1 induced hepatocellular carcinoma in rats, *Pharm. Pharmacol. Commun.*, 4, 507, 1998.
69. Premalatha, B. and Sachdanandam, P., Effect of *Semecarpus anacardium* nut milk extract on rat serum alpha-fetoprotein level in aflatoxin B_1 mediated hepatocellular carcinoma, *Fitoterapia*, 70, 279, 1999.
70. Premalatha, B. and Sachdanandam, P., Regulation of mineral status by *Semecarpus anacardium* Linn. nut milk extract in aflatoxin B_1 induced hepatocellular carcinoma, *J. Clin. Biochem. Nutr.*, 25, 63, 1998.
71. Premalatha, B., Sujatha, V., and Sachdanandam, P., Modulating effect of *Semecarpus anacardium* Linn. nut extract on glucose metabolizing enzymes in aflatoxin B_1 induced experimental hepatocellular carcinoma, *Pharmacol. Res.*, 36, 187, 1997.
72. Premalatha, B. and Sachdanandam, P., *Semecarpus anacardium* L. nut extract administration induces the in vivo antioxidant defense system in aflatoxin B_1 mediated hepatocellular carcinoma, *J. Ethnopharmacol.*, 66, 131, 1999.
73. Premalatha, B. and Sachdanandam, P., Potency of *Semecarpus anacardium* Linn. nut milk extract against aflatoxin B_1 induced hepatocarcinogenesis: reflection on microsomal biotransformation enzymes, *Pharmacol. Res.*, 42, 161, 2000b.
74. Vad, B.G., Study of complete regression in four cases of cancer, *Indian Pract.*, 26, 253, 1973.
75. Prasad, G.C., Studies on cancer in Ayurveda and its management, *J. Res. Ayurveda Siddha*, 3, 147, 1987.

76. Dange, S.V. et al., Comparative efficacy of five indigenous compound formulations in patients of acute viral hepatitis, in *Ayurved and Hepatic Disorders,* Kulkarni, P.H., Ed., Sri Satguru Publications, Delhi, 2001, p. 155.
77. Nayak, S., Management of Shakhashrita kamala vis-a-vis hepatitis B, *Ayurmedline-Hepatitis,* 194, 2002.
78. Yawatkar, P.C., Clinical Assessment of Shankhabhasma vati (Rasashala) + Laghusutshekhar vati and Indrayav vati in amoebic hepatitis, in *Ayurved and Hepatic Disorders,* Kulkarni, P.H., Ed., Sri Satguru Publications, Delhi, 2001, p. 105.
79. Nair, R.B. et al., Hepatoprotective effect of Gudapippali, Vasagulu chyadi arkom, Patolakaturohinyadi arkom, Draksnadi arkom and Madantha decoction on rats: a comparative study, *J. Res. Ayurveda Siddha,* 19, 49, 1998.
80. Nachiket, W. and Neha, W., Clinical evaluation of Phalatrikadi kwath and arogyavardhini in early hepatic cirrhosis: a case report, in *Ayurved and Hepatic Disorders,* Kulkarni, P.H., Ed., Sri Satguru Publications, Delhi, 2001, p. 79.
81. Ashalatha, A., clinical study on Hepacap, *Ayurmedline-Hepatitis,* 438, 2002.
82. Nayak, B., Efficacy of Hepin in HBsAg positive patients — a clinical study, *Ayurmedline-Hepatitis,* 444, 2002.
83. Kagali, M., Effect of 'Stimuliv' in Viral hepatitis, in *Ayurved and Hepatic Disorders,* Kulkarni, P.H., Ed., Sri Satguru Publications, Delhi, 2001, p. 114.
84. Shah, D.S. and Shah, B.K., Acute toxicity studies of 'Vasuliv tablets': a herbal preparation for liver disorders, *Ayurmedline-Hepatitis,* 440, 2002.

15

Antimutagenic Effect of Ayurvedic Therapies

Satwinderjeet Kaur

CONTENTS

0-8493-1366-X/04/$0.00+$1.50

15.1 Introduction

The purpose of this article is to explore the antimutagenic effect of Ayurvedic therapies, as this effect may be an underlying mechanism of their therapeutic uses. Also, these products may act to supplement antimutagens in our diets which have now become essential in order to combat the unavoidable environmental mutagens to which we are constantly exposed.

15.2 Background

A technologically advanced society creates an environment that warrants exposure to different types of genotoxic substances. The deoxyribonucleic acid (DNA) from living organisms is continuously exposed to exogenous or endogenous damaging agents as a result of which there is a substantial level of DNA damage. It has been hypothesized that DNA damage contributes to organismal senescence and the increased risk for specific age-related diseases.[1–4] DNA lesions can interfere with most DNA metabolisms, including replication, transcription, and recombination as well as other important cell functions (e.g., cell-cycle regulation or cell division). Cancer initiation is classically associated with the induction of mutations on specific oncogenes or tumor suppressor genes due to the presence of unrepaired DNA lesions produced by endogenous or exogenous genotoxic agents. The somatic mutation theory proposes that changes in DNA are responsible for changes that bring about senescence and death.

Exposure to mutagens and carcinogens either endogenously or exogenously is unavoidable. Cigarette smoking, diet, infection, and chronic inflammation account for a large proportion of cancers. Epidemiological studies have indicated that cigarette smoking significantly elevates the risk of tumor development in the upper-aerodigestive tract and in other organs.[5,6] Polycyclic aromatic hydrocarbons, N-nitrosamines, and many mutagens and carcinogens and their precursors have been detected from cigarette smoke condensate.[5,6] The total calorie intake and fat intake appear strongly associated with enhancement of human cancer development.[7–10] Lipid peroxidation yields exocyclic propano-, etheno-, and malondialdehyde adducts in DNA to induce mutation.[11,12] The mutagens and carcinogens may be present as microcomponents in various foodstuffs.[13,14] The compounds include naturally occurring pyrrolizidine alkaloids, ptaquiloside, and cyasin. Mycotoxins like aflatoxin B_1, sterigmatocystin, and fumonisin exist as contaminants in food. Hepatocarcinomas developed in people who are living in areas where alfatoxin B_1 is highly contaminated in diet show a characteristic mutation in the p53 gene, namely, change of G to T at the third position of codon 249.[15,16]

It is practically difficult to completely eliminate mycotoxin contamination of food materials. Heterocyclic amines (HCAs) are produced under normal cooking conditions, especially in the overcooked fish and meat. HCAs are metabolized by the cytochrome P450 family, especially by CYP1A2 to *N*-hydroxyamino derivatives, and are then esterified to the ultimate forms that produce DNA base adducts.[17,18] Infection and chronic inflammation may produce oxidative agents in addition to cytokines and chemokines that enhance cell proliferation, increasing the chance of replication error and genetic change.

15.3 Mechanism of Mutagenic Activity

The generation of reactive oxygen species (ROS) in biological systems, either by normal metabolic pathways or as a consequence of exposure to chemical carcinogens, has been extensively studied.[19] Free radicals generate oxidative damage to main cellular components such as DNA, lipids, carbohydrates, and proteins; they have been implicated in the aging phenomena, ischemia,[20] cancer,[21] autoimmune diseases,[22] and neural cell death.[23] It is now universally agreed that the ROS generation contributes to the multistage process of carcinogenesis.[19,24] Evidence has accumulated that lack of protection against free-radicals and lack of repair of oxidative damage in biological macromolecules have a significant role in mutagenesis and carcinogenesis. Kawanishi and co-workers[25] reported that sequence-specific oxidative damage to DNA may play an important role not only in carcinogenesis but also in aging.

15.4 Prevention

There are two complementary strategies for preventing chronic degenerative diseases. The first one is avoidance of exposure to recognized risk factors which evolves through risk assessment and risk management. The risk management is based either on risk communication and health education for controlling lifestyle risk factors or on suitable regulations for controlling environmental risk factors. The other strategy is to favor the intake of protective factors and to modulate the host defense mechanisms. This approach is more practical and is referred to as chemoprevention. It is based on dietary and pharmacological interventions, has already found extensive application in the field of cardiovascular disease, and is encountering a growing interest in cancer prevention.

Food is a complex mixture that may contain mutagenic or carcinogenic compounds such as polycyclic aromatic hydrocarbons and heterocyclic amines present in meat.[26,27] On the other hand, food may contain protective antimutagenic or anticarcinogenic substances that are mostly present in plants. It is important to maintain a varied nutritionally balanced diet in which food antimutagens outweigh the mutagens. Inhibition of mutagenesis or carcinogenesis is generally not based on one mechanism. Protection against cancer can occur at different stages of the complicated processes of carcinogenesis. Compounds and complex mixtures with antimutagenic activity have different modes of action and act in parallel at different levels. As inhibitors, they may prevent the formation of mutagens, such as the endogenous formation of nitrosamines. As blocking agents, they can prevent the biotransformation of promutagens into reactive metabolites by inhibiting metabolic activation, stimulating detoxification enzymes, or scavenging reactive molecules. As suppressing agents, they may modulate intracellular processes, which are involved in DNA repair mechanisms, tumor promotion, and tumor progression.[28] Discovery and exploration of compounds possessing antimutagenic and anticarcinogenic properties are of great importance.

15.5 Ayurvedic Herbs as Antimutagens

Phytochemicals are secondary metabolic products produced by plants in response to environmental stresses. Thousands of these phytochemicals have been identified and, when consumed in human diet, may affect chronic disease risk.[29] Of well over 2000 preparations known to the modern practitioner of Ayurveda, nearly 1500 are of plant origin. *Susruta Samhita* refers to 700 drugs including a small number which were not available in the country in that time. The list has grown substantially since then. Ancient Indian medical literature has references not only to plants that cure difficult and incurable diseases, but also to some endowed with many magical properties. Times have changed and people are looking at logical causes and effects. India has been exposed for well over a century to the application of allopathic medicines with their definite merits as well as failings.

There is a return to some kind of natural healing and to Ayurveda and Siddha medicines. The blind superstitious belief of the past has prompted extensive testing of several ancient medicines. Out of the known 1500, well over 100 medicines have qualified for entry in the Indian and British pharmaceutical Codex and the U.S. dispensatory. The investigations have involved clinical and pharmacological testing of principal components, such as phenolics and alkaloids, extracted from the herbs. Studies carried out on antimutagenic effects of the Ayurvedic therapies were critically reviewed, their protocol studied, and the significant results have been pointed out, as this effect may account for their therapeutic effect to great extent. The Ayurvedic herbs discussed here with respect to their antimutagenic and antiviral activity occupy an important place in the Ayurvedic system of medicine and are used in the treatment of various ailments either alone or from a part of various formulations.

15.6 Scientific Basis of Antimutagenic and Antiviral Activity of Ayurvedic Therapies

Antimutagenic and antiviral activities of the herbs used in Ayurveda are presented. The review indicates that the use of these herbs may be protective from exposure to environmental mutagens.

15.6.1 *Terminalia arjuna*

With a view to explore Ayurvedic plants for chemopreventive activities, *T. arjuna* was selected for testing of antimutagenic activity in our laboratory. *T. arjuna* is an important cardiotonic plant described in Ayurveda and is widely used in the preparation of important Ayurvedic formulations like *Arjunaristam, Cintamanirasam, Laksagulgulu,* Liv.52, etc.

15.6.1.1 Antimutagenic and Antitumor Activity

Ellagic acid was isolated from *T. arjuna* and its antimutagenic potential was evaluated in TA98 and TA100 strains of *Salmonella typhimurium* against direct- and indirect-acting mutagens. It was found to be quite effective against promutagen 2-aminofluorene.[30] Various other fractions were also isolated and were tested in Ames assay, comet, and micronucleus (MN) tests, which indicate that the bark harbors constituents with promising antimutagenic and anticarcinogenic potential.[31–33] Gallic acid, ethyl gallate, and luteolin were reported to be active cancer-cell growth inhibitory constituents from *T. arjuna* by Pettit and co-workers[34] using bioassay-guided separation methods. Kandil and Nassar[35] have reported an ellagitannin from the leaves of *T. arjuna* to be an anticancer promoter. The effects of acetone and methanol extracts of *T. arjuna* were investigated on the growth of human normal fibroblasts (WI-38), osteosarcoma (U2OS), and glioblastoma (U251) cells *in vitro*.[36] It was found that both extracts inhibited the growth of human U251 and U2OS at 30 to 60 μg/ml. It was also discovered that the extracts contained components that can induce growth arrest of transformed cells by p53-dependent and independent pathways.

15.6.1.2 Antiviral Activity

Casuarinin, a hydrolysable tannin isolated from the bark, has been shown to possess antiherpes virus activity.[37]

15.6.2 *Ocimum sanctum*

Different parts of *O. sanctum* are traditionally used in Ayurveda and Siddha systems for treating diverse ailments. Examples include infections, skin diseases, hepatic disorders, common cold and cough, and malarial fever. *O. sanctum* is also used as an antidote for snake bite and scorpion sting.[38]

15.6.2.1 Antimutagenic and Antitumor Activity

O. sanctum was one of the nine plant products that significantly decreased the incidence of both benzo[a]pyrene (B[a]P)-induced neoplasia in the stomachs of Swiss mice and 3'-methyl-4-dimethylaminoazobenzene (3'MeDAB)-induced hepatomas in Wistar rats.[39] The topical treatment of the ethanolic leaf extract of *O. sanctum* significantly reduced the values of tumor incidence, the average number of tumors per tumor bearing mice, and the cumulative number of papillomas in 7,12-dimethylbenz[a]anthracene (DMBA)-induced skin papillomagenesis in male Swiss albino mice at the periinitiational, postinitiational, or continuously at both the peri- and postinitiational stages of papillomagenesis as compared with the corresponding control group.[40] There was also significant twofold elevation of reduced glutathione content in the skin of mice ($p < 0.05$) and an elevation of glutathione S-transferase activity by 25% compared with the control group ($p < 0.05$) after 15 days of the treatment.

In a study carried out by Banerjee et al.,[41] oral treatment with the alcoholic leaf extract at 400 and 800 mg/kg body weight given to mice for 15 days significantly elevated the activities of cytochrome P450 ($p < 0.05$), cytochrome b5 ($p < 0.01$, $p < 0.001$), aryl hydrocarbon hydroxylase ($p < 0.05$), and glutathione S-transferase ($p < 0.05$, $p < 0.01$), all of which are important in the detoxification of carcinogens as well as mutagens. The reduced glutathione level in liver, lung, and stomach tissues was also elevated ($p < 0.01$, $p < 0.001$) by treatment with the leaf extract.

O. sanctum leaf extract was also reported by Prashar and coworkers[42] to block or suppress the events associated with chemical carcinogenesis by inhibiting metabolic activation of the carcinogen. They treated the primary cultures of rat hepatocytes with up to 500 μg of *O. sanctum* extract for 24 h and then with DMBA (10 or 50 μg) for 18 h. A significant reduction in the levels of DMBA-DNA adducts was observed in all cultures pretreated with *O. sanctum* extract. *O. sanctum* also showed chemopreventive activity against DMBA-induced hamster buccal pouch carcinogenesis.[43] *O. sanctum* in the form of fresh leaf paste, aqueous extract, and ethanolic extract were topically applied and the extracts were orally administered to buccal pouch mucosa of animals exposed to 0.5% of DMBA. There was significant reduction in the incidence of papillomas and squamous cell carcinomas. In addition, there was an increase in the survival rate in the topically applied leaf paste and orally administered extracts to animals. From the observations, it was suggested that the orally administered extract of *O. sanctum* may have the ability to prevent the early events of carcinogenesis.

Antiproliferative activity of seed oil of *O. sanctum* against HeLa cells in culture has also been reported.[44] Prakash and Gupta[45] tested the chemopreventive activity of the seed oil of *O. sanctum* against subcutaneously injected 20-methylcholanthrene-induced fibrosarcoma tumors in the thigh region of Swiss albino mice. Supplementation of maximal tolerated dose of 100 μl/kg body weight of the oil significantly reduced the 20-methylcholanthrene-induced tumor incidence and tumor volume. In liver enzymatic and nonenzymatic antioxidants and lipid peroxidation end product, malondialdehyde levels were significantly modulated with oil treatment as compared with untreated 20-methylcholanthrene-injected mice. The potential chemopreventive activity of the oil was partly attributed to its antioxidant properties.

15.6.2.2 Antiviral Activity

O. sanctum is an ingredient of *tefroli*, which is used in condition of viral hepatitis. Rajalakshmi and co-workers[46] have reported *O. sanctum* to show highly significant clinical and biochemical clearance of viral hepatitis (*manjal kamalai*) when used as a single drug within 2 weeks of treatment. Patients for the above study were screened and selected from the outpatient department of the Central Research Institute (Siddha) [C.R.I], Chennai, India, based on the symptoms such as fever, dull ache in the right costal margin, yellow tint of the sclera, anorexia, nausea and vomiting, dark-colored urine, clay-colored stools, and enlarged and tender liver. Clinical diagnosis was confirmed by laboratory parameters such as bile salts, bile pigment level in urine, and liver function test along with additional laboratory parameters. Serum alkaline phosphatase, serum amylase, choleocystogram, and stool tests were done to rule out the cases of surgical jaundice, neoplasm in the abdominal cavity, obstruction in the biliary tract due to stone, and infestation with worms, respectively. Twenty cases were screened and admitted in the inpatient department of CRI for trial.

All the cases were assessed once a week with both clinical and biochemical parameters. The leaves of *O. sanctum* were ground into paste and given in the dose of 10 g/day in two divided doses. A diet of fat, tamarind, and spices with plenty of glucose was given throughout the period of treatment. Within a week, anorexia, nausea, and vomiting disappeared and stool regained its normal color. After 2 weeks of treatment, 50% of the cases showed clearance of conjunctiva and dark-colored urine was seen only in 15% cases. The reduction in the icteric index level was observed to be slow when compared with reduction in serum bilirubin level. After 3 weeks of treatment, all the symptoms had cleared except liver enlargement, which was persistent in 10% of the cases.

15.6.3 *Glycyrrhiza glabra*

The root of *G. glabra* is extensively used in traditional medicine and in food products as a sweetening and flavoring agent.

15.6.3.1 Antimutagenic and Antitumor Activity

Zani et al.[47] investigated the effects of *G. glabra* extract, glycyrrhizinic acid, and 18α- and 18β-glycyrrhetinic acids on the mutagenicity of ethylmethanesulfonate (3 μl/plate), *N*-methyl-*N*'-nitro-*N*-nitrosoguanidine (1 μl/plate), and ribose-lysine (25 μl/plate) Maillard model systems in TA100 tester strain of *S. typhimurium* with the *S. typhimurium* and microsome reversion assay. The compounds tested were also found to exhibit des-mutagenic activity, where the compound exerted its effect by direct interaction with the mutagen, and antimutagenic activity, where the compound acted at the cellular level suppressing the process of mutagenesis. All the compounds showed des-mutagenic activity only against ribose-lysine mutagenic browning mixture. *G. glabra* extract showed antimutagenic activity against ethylmethanesulfonate and ribose-lysine.

Glycyrrhizin, the main water-soluble constituent of licorice, was shown to possess considerable antitumorigenic activity in Sencar mice. In this study, Agarwal et al.[48] showed that oral feeding of glycyrrhizin to Sencar mice resulted in substantial protection against skin tumorigenesis caused by DMBA initiation and 12-*O*-tetradecanoylphorbol-13-acetate (TPA) promotion. The latent period prior to the onset of tumor development was considerably prolonged in glycyrrhizin-fed animals compared with animals not fed by glycyrrhizin. Results showed a significant decrease in the number of tumors per mouse both during and at the termination of the experiment. Oral feeding of glycyrrhizin in drinking water also resulted in inhibition in the binding of topically applied [^{3}H]B[*a*]P and [^{3}H]DMBA to epidermal DNA. The possible mechanism(s) of the antitumor-initiating activity was attributed to the possible involvement of glycyrrhizin as an inhibitor of the carcinogen metabolism followed by DNA adduct formation.

15.6.3.2 Antiviral Activity

Pompei et al.[49] studied the effect of glycyrrhizic acid on the growth of vaccinia, herpes simplex type 1 (HSV-1), Newcastle disease, vesicular stomatitis, and polio type 1 viruses in cultures of human aneuploid HEp2 cells. Twenty-four-hour-old cell monolayers (10^7 cells per sample) were infected with five infectious units per cell of each virus at 20°C for 1 h, washed three times in Hank's balanced saline solution (BSS), and incubated at 37°C for 18 h in Eagle's essential medium supplemented with 2% calf serum (pH 7.4). Infectious virus yield was determined by the Dulbecco and Vogt technique and slightly modified for vaccinia and HSV-1 viruses. Cytopathic effects were evidenced by observing Giemsa-stained cells with a light microscope and by measuring spectrophotometrically at 530 nm the amount of neutral red incorporated by cell cultures (100 μg/ml, 1-h pulses in drug-free medium) after solubilization in 1% sodium deoxycholate in BSS. It was reported that addition of 8mM glycyrrhizic acid after incubation completely inhibited both growth and cytopathic effects of viruses except poliovirus type 1. It produced irreversible inactivation of HSV-1 virus as the suspensions of this virus suffered a loss of infectivity of 10^5 when incubated at 37°C with 8 m*M* glycyrrhizic acid for only 15 min. It was hypothesized that glycyrrhizic acid interacted with sensitive virus proteins both at virionic stage and later, when these are synthesized in host cells.

Glycyrrhizin was reported to inhibit varicella-zoster virus (VZV) in human embryonic fibroblast (HEF) cells *in vitro*.[50] On treatment of HEF with glycyrrhizin after inoculation of virus (posttreatment), the average 50% inhibitory dose (ID_{50}) for five VZV strains was 0.71 m*M*, and the selectivity index (ratio of ID_{50} for host-cell DNA synthesis to ID_{50} for VZV replication) was 30. Glycyrrhizin was also effective against VZV replication when HEF cells were treated 24 h before the inoculation (pretreatment). Furthermore, at a concentration of 2.4 m*M* glycyrrhizin inactivated more than 99% of virus particles within 30 min at 37°C. Glycyrrhizin was reported to show a dose-dependent inhibition of the replication of human immunodeficiency virus type 1 in MOLT-4 (clone No. 8) cells within the concentration range of 0.075 to 0.6 m*M*.[51] Within this concentration range, glycyrrhizin also effected a dose-dependent reduction in the protein kinase C (PKC) activity of MOLT-4 cells. PKC inhibition was considered as one of the mechanisms by which glycyrrhizin inhibited human immunodeficiency virus type-1 (HIV-1) replication as a PKC inhibitor, 1-(5-isoquinolinesulfonyl)-2-methylpiperazine dihydrochloride, also proved inhibitory to HIV-1 replication in MOLT-4 cells.

Badam[52] reported that indigenously purified glycyrrhizin was a more potent antiviral agent than licorice from *G. glabra* and ammonium salt of glycyrrhizic acid (Sigma) in inhibiting Japanese encephalitis virus (JEV) *in vitro*. Glycyrrhizin was found to inhibit plaque formation in all the three strains of JEV — Nakayama, P-20778, and 821564 XY48 — at a concentration of 500 µg/ml at 96 h, whereas licorice and ammonium salt of glycyrrhizic acid inhibited at 1000 µg/ml concentration. A daily injection of glycyrrhizin (stronger neo-minophagen C [SNMC] containing 40 mg glycyrrhizin in a 20-ml ampoule) was reported to lower alanine aminotransferase (ALT) levels in patients with chronic viral hepatitis.[53] The therapeutic effects of intermittent administration of SNMC three times/week for 12 weeks were evaluated and compared between two doses (40 and 100 ml) in a randomized clinical trial. The therapeutic response was better in the 53 patients allocated 100 ml than in the 59 who were allocated to have 40 ml of SNMC. At the completion of SNMC treatment, ALT levels decreased more extensively in the patients on 100 ml than in those on 40 ml of SNMC. Minor side effects occurred in both the patients on 100 ml of (20%) and in those on 40 ml (12%) but did not require any therapies. It was suggested that intermittent SNMC would be efficient in suppressing ALT levels in patients with chronic viral hepatitis in a dose-dependent manner.

15.6.4 *Semecarpus anacardium*

S. anacardium Linn. of the family Anacardiaceae has many applications in the Ayurvedic and Siddha systems of medicine. It is popularly known as multipurpose medicine (*ardha vaidya*).

15.6.4.1 Antimutagenic and Antitumor Activity

Water, alcohol, and oil extracts of *S. anacardium* were found to be antimutagenic against B[a]P-induced mutagenicity in TA98 and TA100 tester strains of *S. typhimurium*.[54] Methanol extract, resinous fraction, and *Bhilawanol* isolated from *S. anacardium* showed antitumour activity against P388 lymphocytic leukemia in BDF1 mice as judged by their median survival time.[55] Smit and co-workers[56] studied 14 specimens from the list of Ayurvedic herbal drugs and collected from various parts of India and Nepal for cytostatic activity.

The ethanolic (70% v/v) extracts were tested for cytotoxicity on COLO 320 tumor cells, using the microculture tetrazolium assay. The nuts of *S. anacardium* displayed a cytotoxic effect with a IC_{50}-value of 1.6 μg/ml.

Premalatha et al.[57] have reported the modulating effect of the extract of SA against aflatoxin B_1-induced experimental hepatocellular carcinoma. Anticancer property was attributed to its strong antioxidant capacity and its capability to induce *in vivo* antioxidant system.[58] In a study,[59] the beneficial effect of SA in the treatment of hepatocellular carcinoma was attributed to the stabilization of biomembranes by *S. anacardium* nut extract. *S. anacardium* nut milk extract was administered orally at a dose of 200 mg/kg/day for 14 days to normal rats as well to animals whose biomembranes were rendered fragile by the induction of hepatocellular carcinoma with aflatoxin B_1, where the discharge of lysosomal enzymes increased significantly with a subsequent increase in glycoprotein components. The nut extract administration reversed these adverse changes to near normal in treated animals. The administration of the same dose to male albino rats with aflatoxin B_1-induced hepatocellular carcinoma was found to be highly effective in inducing phase I and phase II biotransformation enzymes.[60]

The administration of *S. anacardium* nut extract has also been reported to cause a significant decrease in the activity of glycolytic enzymes and an increase in gluconeogenic enzymes activities to near normal values in drug-treated animals.[61] *Anacartin forte*, an Ayurvedic preparation, exhibited not only a broad spectrum of anticancer properties in clinical and animal studies, but also a wide margin of safety in therapeutic dosage even when used for long periods. It showed satisfactory results in cases of cancer of the esophagus, liver, urinary bladder, liver, and chronic leukemia by giving subjective and objective improvement, alleviation, or disappearance of troublesome symptoms and clinical benefit with extension of survival time. The preparation has selective action, attacking only the cancer cells without harming the normal cells.[62]

15.6.5 *Terminalia chebula*

T. chebula is a *rasayana* to *vata*, increasing awareness, and has a tonic effect on the central nervous system. It improves digestion, promotes the absorption of nutrients, and regulates colon function. *T. chebula* is most useful in prolapsed organs, improving the strength and tone of the supporting musculature.

15.6.5.1 Antimutagenic and Antitumor Activity

Water extract of *T. chebula* was shown to significantly reduce 4-nitro-*o*-phenylenediamine (NPD) as well as 2-AF induced his^+ revertants in Ames assay.[63] A tannin fraction (TC-E) obtained from the dried fruit pulp of *T. chebula* was subjected to column chromatography to yield four fractions — TC-EI, TC-EII, TC-EIII, and E-IV — which were evaluated for their antimutagenic potential. The fractions were quite effective in inhibiting the mutagenicity of 2-AF. The monomeric fraction (TC-EI) was the least effective in comparison with other oligomeric fractions.[64] A 70% methanol extract of *T. chebula* fruit was studied for its effects on growth in several malignant cell lines including a human (MCF-7) and mouse (S115) breast cancer cell line, a human osteosarcoma cell line (HOS-1), a human prostate cancer cell line (PC-3), and a nontumorigenic immortalized human prostate cell line (PNT1A) by using assays for proliferation, cell viability, and cell death. In all cell lines studied, the extract decreased cell viability, inhibited cell proliferation, and induced cell death in a dose-dependent manner.[65]

15.6.5.2 Antiviral Activity

Badmaev and Nowakowski[66] tested a multicomponent herbal formula, ledretan-96, consisting of 23 components on an epithelial tissue culture cell line (MDCK) for its protective activity against cytopathic effects caused by influenza A virus. The whole formula and each of its 23 individual components were tested in the same system. The results indicated that the formula, when prepared according to established procedure, in the form of decoction was active in protecting epithelial cells against damage caused by influenza A virus used at different dosages. Of the 23 components tested, only *T. chebula* showed a significant protective effect when applied to the epithelial cells individually. The bioassay-directed isolation of *T. chebula* fruits afforded four HIV-1 integrase inhibitors, gallic acid, and three galloyl glucoses.[67] The galloyl moiety played a major role for inhibition against the 3'-processing of HIV-1 integrase.

T. chebula has also been reported to show a significant inhibitory activity on human immunodeficiency virus reverse transcriptase.[68] Anti-HSV-1 activity of *T. chebula* has been reported by Kurokawa et al.[69] *T. chebula* reduced virus yield in the brain and skin more strongly than acyclovir alone and exhibited stronger anti-HSV-1 activity in the brain than in the skin, in contrast to acyclovir treatment by itself. A group[70] from Japan showed *T. chebula* to possess anticytomegalovirus (CMV) activity. Shiraki et al.[71] reported *T. chebula* as one of the medicinal plants to inhibit replication of human CMV and murine CMV *in vitro* and suggested it to be beneficial for the prophylaxis of CMV diseases in immunocompromized patients.

15.6.6 *Terminalia bellerica*

T. bellerica is also a strong rejuvenator of the body and is recommended as a daily supplement.

15.6.6.1 Antimutagenic Activity

Two polyphenolic fractions isolated from *T. bellerica* were significantly effective against mutagenic effects in *S. typhimurium.* Interaction of the polyphenols with S9 proteins may be the probable cause of the inhibitory effect.[72]

15.6.6.2 Antiviral Activity

Suthienkul et al.[73] reported the extract of *T. bellerica* to show retroviral reverse transcriptase inhibitory activity. Hot water and methanol extracts of 57 Thai herbs and spices were examined for their retroviral reverse transcriptase inhibitory activity with Moloney murine leukemia virus reverse transcriptase. Hot water extract of *T. bellerica* at a concentration of 125 μg/ml showed relative inhibitory ratio of 75%, whereas its methanol extract exhibited an inhibitory ratio (IR) value of 83%. An extract of *T. bellerica* showed significant inhibitory activity on HIV-1 reverse transcriptase, with $IC_{50} \leq 50$ μg/ml.[68] Four lignans isolated possessed demonstrable anti-HIV-1 activity *in vitro.*[74]

15.6.7 *Emblica officinalis*

E. officinalis is an important traditional medicine with broad prospects. The fruits of the plant have been used in Ayurveda as potent *rasayanas* and form the major constituent of *chyavanprash awaleha* and *triphala.*

15.6.7.1 Antimutagenic and Antitumor Activity

Water, acetone, and chloroform extracts of *E. officinalis* fruit were reported to significantly reduce the mutagenicity of sodium azide and NPD in TA100 and TA97a strains, respectively, of *S. typhimurium.*[75] *E. officinalis* extract was reported to show a pronounced protective effect in counteracting the genotoxicity induced by aluminium and lead.[76,77] Oral administration of *E. officinalis* extract for 7 consecutive days before the exposure of mice to the metals by intraperitoneal injections reduced the frequencies of sister chromatid exchanges and micronuclei-induced in bone marrow cells by both metals. Aqueous extract of *E. officinalis* was reported to be quite effective in inhibiting mutagenicity of S9-dependent mutagens, aflatoxin B_1 (0.5 μg/plate), and B[a]P (1 μg/plate) in TA98 and TA100 tester strains of *S. typhimurium* in Ames assay.[78]

Dietary supplementation with extract of fruit of *E. officinalis* to Swiss albino mice significantly reduced the cytotoxic effects of 3,4-B[*a*]P *in vivo.*[79] Age-matched Swiss albino mice were fed by gavaging the fruit extract daily for 28 days, and one dose of the carcinogen was given on alternate days up to a total of eight doses from day 9. On day 29, all mice were transferred to normal diet. Control sets received the extract alone, the carcinogen alone, and olive oil alone. All mice were sacrificed at 12 weeks and 14 weeks after the end of the experiment. Chromosome preparations were made from bone marrow after the usual colchicine-hypotonic-fixative-airdrying-Giemsa staining schedule. The end points screened were the frequencies of chromosomal aberrations and damaged cells that were induced, which clearly pointed toward the modulation of B[*a*]P-induced cytotoxic effects by the fruit extract.

Sharma and co-workers[80] studied the effect of *E. officinalis* extract administration on the *in vivo* genotoxicity of B[*a*]P and cyclophosphamide (CP) using bone marrow chromosomal aberration and micronucleus induction tests in mice. Three doses (50, 250, and 500 mg/kg body weight) of the plant extract were administered orally for 7 consecutive days prior to the administration of single dose of mutagens (B[*a*]P 125 mg/kg oral; CP 40 mg/kg intraperitoneal). It was found that administration of 250 and 500 mg/kg of *E. officinalis* extract significantly inhibited the genotoxicity of B[*a*]P as well as CP in both the assay systems. There was a significant induction in the levels of glutathione content (GSH) and of antioxidant and detoxification enzymes. Extract of *E. officinalis* significantly inhibited hepatocarcinogenesis induced by N-nitrosodiethylamine (NDEA) in a dose-dependent manner.[81] Its anticarcinogenic activity was evaluated by its effect on tumour incidence, levels of carcinogen metabolizing enzymes, levels of liver cancer markers, and liver injury markers, which clearly indicated its protection against chemical carcinogenesis.

In a study,[82] *in vitro* antiproliferative activity of extracts from medicinal plants were compared with human tumor cell lines, including human erythromyeloid K562, B-lymphoid Raji, T-lymphoid Jurkat, and erythroleukemic HeLa cell lines. Extracts from *E. officinalis* were the most active in inhibiting *in vitro* cell proliferation and contained pyrogallol as an active component. Aqueous extract of *E. officinalis* has also been reported by Jose et al.[83] to be cytotoxic to L929 cells in culture in a dose-dependent manner. The concentration needed for 50% inhibition was found to be 16.5 μg/ml. *E. officinalis* and chyavanaprash extracts were also found to reduce ascites and solid tumors in mice induced by Dalton's lymphoma ascites (DLA) cells. Animals treated with 1.25 g/kg body weight of *E. officinalis* extract increased the life span of tumor-bearing animals by 20%, whereas animals treated with 2.5 g/kg body weight of *chyavanaprash* produced a 60.9% increase in the life span. Antitumor activity of *E. officinalis* extract was attributed partially to its interaction with cell cycle regulation as was found to inhibit cell cycle-regulating enzymes.

15.6.7.2 Antiviral Activity

A bioassay-guided fractionation of a methanol extract of the fruit of *E. officinalis* yielded Putranjivain A (1) as a potent inhibitory substance on the effects of HIV-1 reverse transcriptase with $IC_{50} = 3.9$ μM, together with (2) 1,6-di-*O*-galloyl-β-D-glucose, (3) 1-*O*-galloyl-β-D-glucose, (4) kaempferol-3-*O*-β-D-glucoside, (5) quercetin-3-*O*-β-D-glucoside, and (6) digallic acid. The inhibitory mode of action by 1, 2, and 6 was noncompetitive with respect to the substrate but competitive with respect to a template-primer.[68]

15.6.8 *Cinnamomum cassia*

C. cassia is known as *dalchini* in the Indian subcontinent. The bark of *C. cassia* is frequently used in Ayurveda and Unani preparations.

15.6.8.1 Antimutagenic Activity

Sharma et al.[84] evaluated the antimutagenic effect of *C. cassia* against two mutagens, B[*a*]P and CP, by *in vivo* chromosomal aberration and micronuclei tests after pretreatment with the extract orally for 7 consecutive days and with Ames assay. *C. cassia* pretreatment decreased cytochrome P450 content but increased GSH content and the activity of glutathione-dependent antioxidant enzymes. These results indicate its modulatory effect on the xenobiotic bioactivation and detoxification processes. 2'-Hydroxycinnamaldehyde isolated from *C. cassia* was found to strongly inhibit *in vitro* growth of 29 kinds of human cancer cells and *in vivo* growth of SW-620 human tumor xenograft without the loss of body weight in nude mice.[85] It prevented adherence of SW-620 cells to the culture surface but did not inhibit oncogenic K-Ras processing, implying its antitumor mechanisms at the cellular level. Kwon et al.[86] found the key functional group of the cinnamaldehyde-related compounds in the antitumor activity to be in the propenal group.

15.6.8.2 Antiviral Activity

C. cassia was one of the many medicinal plants possessing potent anti-HIV activity. Premanathan et al.[87] studied the inhibitory effect of plant extracts on HIV replication in terms of the inhibition of virus-induced cytopathogenicity in MT-4 cells. The MT-4 cells were infected with HIV. The HIV-infected MT-4 cells were incubated at 37°C in a CO_2 incubator in the presence of the plant extracts. After 5 days, cell viability was measured by a tetrazolium-based colorimetric assay.

15.6.9 *Withania somnifera*

W. somnifera is one of the Indian medicinal plants having a remarkable reputation, as a factor of health care, among the indigenous medical practitioners. Several studies over the past few years have indicated that *W. somnifera* has anti-inflammatory, antitumor, antistress, antioxidant, mind-boosting, and rejuvenating properties.

15.6.9.1 Antitumor Activity

The alcoholic extract of the dried roots of the plant, as well as the active component withaferin A isolated from the extract, showed significant antitumor and radiosensitizing effects in experimental tumors *in vivo*, without any noticeable systemic toxicity.[88] Russo et al.[89]reported the effect of methanolic extract of *W. somnifera* in reducing the hydrogen peroxide-induced cytotoxicity and DNA damage in human nonimmortalized fibroblasts. The extract showed dose-dependent free radical scavenging capacity and a protective effect on DNA cleavage.

The chemopreventive activity of a hydroalcoholic extract of *W. somnifera* roots against 20-methylcholanthrene induced fibrosarcoma tumors in Swiss albino mice was reported by Prakash et al.[90] A single subcutaneous injection of 200 μg 20-methylcholanthrene in 0.1 ml of dimethyl-sulphoxide into the thigh region of mice produced a high incidence (96%) of tumors. Oral treatment of animals with 400 mg/kg body weight of extract (1 week before injecting 20-methylcholanthrene and continuing until 15 weeks thereafter) significantly reduced the tumor incidence and tumor volume and enhanced the survival of the mice, compared with 20-methylcholanthrene–injected mice. Liver biochemical parameters revealed a significant modulation of reduced glutathione, lipid peroxides, glutathione-S-transferase, catalase, and superoxide dismutase in extract-treated mice. The extract was also quite effective in preventing DMBA-induced squamous cell carcinoma of skin in Swiss albino mice.[91] The skin lesions were induced by the twice-weekly topical application of DMBA (100 nmol/100 μl acetone) for 8 weeks on the shaved backs of mice. The extract was administered at the maximal tolerated dose of 400 mg/kg body weight three times/ week on alternate days 1 week before DMBA and continued for 24 weeks thereafter. The chemopreventive activity was also linked to the antioxidant and free radical-scavenging constituents of the extract.

15.6.10 *Centella asiatica*

Centella asiatica (Umbelliferae) syn. *Hydrocotyl asiatica* has been used in various parts of India for different ailments. Examples include headaches, body aches, insanity, asthma, leprosy, ulcers, eczemas, and wound healing.

15.6.10.1 Antimutagenic and Antitumor Activity

The researchers at the Amala Cancer Research Centre in Kerala, India, tested both crude extract of *C. asiatica* and its partially purified fractions (AF) for their antitumor activity. AF inhibited the proliferation of the transformed cell lines significantly more than the crude extract and other solvent fractions in dose-dependent manner. Fifty percent effective doses of AF on its 3-h exposure for Ehrlich ascites tumor cells (EAC) and DLA were reported to be 17 and 22 μg/ml, respectively. AF also significiantly suppressed the multiplication of mouse lung fibroblast (L-929) cells at a concentration of 8 μg/ml in long-term culture. Oral administration of the extracts retarded the development of solid and ascites tumors and increased the life span of these tumor-bearing mice. Tritiated thymidine, uridine, and leucine incorporation assay suggested that the fraction acted directly on DNA synthesis.[92] Yen et al.[93] reported the inhibitory effect of *C. asiatica* against the mutagenicity of 2-amino-3-methyl-imidazole (4,5-f) quinoline.

15.6.10.2 Antiviral Activity

Aqueous extract of *C. asiatica* was one of the 500 herbs tested that showed significant anti-HSV-II action as determined by the virus inhibition logarithm.[94] Yoosook et al.[95] reported asiaticoside from *C. asiatica* to be an active constituent against antiherpes simplex virus. It showed both anti-HSV-1 and 2 activities in plaque inhibition assay.

15.7 Conclusion

A search of the literature on Ayurvedic herbs revealed ten herbs that have studies showing antimutagenic and antiviral activity: *T. arjuna, O. sanctum, G. glabra, S. anacardium, T. chebula, T. bellerica, E. officinalis, C. cassia, W. somnifera,* and *C. asiatica*. The data are indicative of their possible protective effect against the environmental mutagens. Future research is needed to further confirm their antimutagenic and antiviral effects in animals and humans.

References

1. Ames, B.N., Shigenaga, M.K., and Hagen, T.M., Oxidants, antioxidants and the degenerative diseases of aging, *Proc. Natl. Acad. Sci. U.S.A.*, 90, 7915, 1993.
2. Holmes, G.E., Bernstein, C., and Bernstein, H., Oxidative and other DNA damages as the basis of aging: a review, *Mutat. Res.*, 275, 305, 1992.
3. Lyras, L. et al., An assessment of oxidative damage to proteins, lipids and DNA in brain from patients with Alzheimer's disease, *J. Neurochem.*, 68, 2061, 1997.
4. Culter, R.G., Human longevity and aging: possible role of reactive oxygen species, *Ann. N.Y. Acad. Sci.*, 621, 1, 1991.
5. Schottenfeld, D. and Fraumani, J.F., Jr., *Cancer Epidemiology on Prevention*, Oxford University Press, New York, 1996.
6. Doll, R. and Peto, R., The causes of cancer: quantitative estimates of avoidable risks of cancer in the United States today, *J. Natl. Cancer Inst.*, 66, 1191, 1981.
7. Tannenbaum, A., The genesis and growth of tumors. III. Effect of high-fat diet, *Cancer Res.*, 2, 468, 1942.
8. Kritchevsky, D., Weber, M.M., and Klurfeld, D.M., Dietary fat versus caloric content in initiation and promotion of 7,12-dimethylbenz[a] anthracene-induced mammary tumorigenesis in rats, *Cancer Res.*, 44, 3174, 1984.
9. Willet, W.C. et al., Dietary fat and the risk of breast cancer, *N. Engl. J. Med.*, 316, 22, 1987.
10. Willet, W.C. et al., Relation of meat, fat and fibre intake to the risk of colon cancer in a prospective study among women, *N. Engl. J. Med.*, 323, 1664, 1990.
11. Nath, R.G. and Chung, F.L., Detection of exocyclic 1, N^2-propanodeoxyguanosine adducts as common DNA lesions in rodents and humans, *Proc. Natl. Acad. Sci. U.S.A.*, 91, 7491, 1994.
12. Chaudhary, A.K. et al., Detection of endogenous malondialdehyde-deoxyguanosine adducts in human liver, *Science*, 265, 1580, 1994.
13. Ames, B.N., Dietary carcinogens and anti-carcinogens, *Science*, 221, 1256, 1983.
14. Sugimura, T., Mutagens, carcinogens and tumor promoters in our daily food, *Cancer*, 49, 1970, 1982.
15. Hsu, I.C. et al., Mutational hotspot in the p53 gene in human hepatocellular carcinomas, *Nature*, 350, 427, 1991.
16. Bressac, B. et al., Selective G to T mutations of p53 gene in hepatocellular carcinoma from Southern Africa, *Nature*, 350, 429, 1991.
17. Kato, R. and Yamazoe, Y., Metabolic activation and covalent binding to nucleic acids of carcinogenic heterocyclic amines from cooked foods and amino acid pyrolysates, *Jpn. J. Cancer Res.*, 78, 297, 1987.
18. Aoyama, T., Gonzalez, F.J., and Gelboin, H.V., Mutagen activation by cDNA expressed P_1 450, P_3 450 and P $_4$50a, *Mol. Carcinog.*, 1, 253, 1989.
19. Wattenberg, L.W., Inhibition of carcinogenesis by naturally occurring and synthetic compounds, in *Antimutagenesis and Anticarcinogenesis Mechanisms II*, Kuroda, Y., Shankel, D.M., and Waters, M.D., Eds., Plenum Publishing, New York, 1990, p. 155.

20. McCord, J.M., Oxygen-derived radicals: a link between reperfusion injury and inflammation, *Fed. Proc.*, 46, 2402, 1987.
21. Trus, M.A. and Kensler, T.W., An over-review of the relationship between oxidative stress and chemical carcinogenesis, *Free Radic. Biol. Med.*, 10, 201, 1991.
22. Halliwell, B., Production of superoxide, hydrogen peroxide and hydroxyl radicals by phagocytic cells: a cause of chronic inflammatory disease, *Cell. Biol. Int. Rep.*, 6, 529, 1982.
23. Reiter, R.J., Oxidative processes and anti-oxidative defence mechanisms in the ageing brain, *FASEB J.*, 9, 526, 1995.
24. Agarwal, R. and Mukhtar, H., Oxidative stress in skin chemical carcinogenesis, in *Oxidative Stress in Dermatology*, Fuchs, J. and Packer, L., Eds., Marcel-Dekker, New York, 1993, p. 207.
25. Kawanishi, S., Hiraku, Y., and Oikawa, S., Mechanism of guanine-specific DNA damage by oxidative stress and its role in carcinogenesis and aging, *Mutat. Res.*, 488, 65, 2001.
26. Phillips, D.H., Polycyclic aromatic hydrocarbon in the diet, *Mutat. Res.*, 443, 139, 1999.
27. Sugimura, T., Overview of carcinogenic heterocyclic amines, *Mutat. Res.*, 376, 211, 1997.
28. Bailey, G. and Williams, D., Potential mechanisms for food-related carcinogens and anticarcinogens, *Food Technol.*, 47, 105, 1993.
29. Messina, M. and Messinia, V., Nutritional implication of dietary phytochemicals, in *America Institute for Cancer Research*, (Ed.), *Dietary Phytochemical in Cancer Prevention and Treatment*, Plenum Press, New York, 1996, p. 207.
30. Kaur, S.J., Grover, I.S., and Kumar, S., Antimutagenic potential of ellagic acid isolated from *Terminalia arjuna*, *Indian J. Exp. Biol.*, 35, 478, 1997.
31. Kaur, S.J., Grover, I.S., and Kumar, S., Modulatory effect of tannin fraction isolated from *Terminalia arjuna* on the genotoxicity of mutagens in *Salmonella typhimurium*, *Food Chem. Toxicol.*, 38, 1113, 2000.
32. Kaur, S.J., Grover, I.S., and Kumar, S., Antimutagenic potential of extracts isolated from *Terminalia arjuna*, *J. Environ. Path. Toxicol. Oncol.*, 20, 9, 2001.
33. Scassellati-Sforzolini, G. et al., Antigenotoxic properties of *Terminalia arjuna* bark extracts, *J. Environ. Path. Toxicol. Oncol.*, 18, 119, 1999.
34. Pettit, G.R. et al., Antineoplastic agents 338: the cancer cell growth inhibitory constituents of *Terminalia arjuna* (Combretaceae), *J. Ethnopharmacol.*, 53, 57, 1996.
35. Kandil, F.E. and Nassar, M.I., A tannin, anti-cancer promotor from *Terminalia arjuna*, *Phytochemistry*, 47, 1567, 1998.
36. Nagpal, A. et al., Growth suppression of human transformed cells by treatment with bark extracts from a medicinal plant, *Terminalia arjuna*, in vitro, *Cell. Dev. Biol. Anim.*, 36, 544, 2000.
37. Cheng, H.Y., Lin, C.C., and Lin, T.C., Antiherpes simplex virus type 2 activity of casuarinin from the bark of *Terminalia arjuna* Linn., *Antiviral Res.*, 55, 47, 2002.
38. Satyavati, G.V., Gupta, K.A., and Tandon, N., Eds., Ocimum Linn, in *Medicinal Plants of India*, Vol. II, Indian Council of Medical Research, New Delhi, 1987, p. 354.
39. Aruna, K. and Sivaramakrishnan, V.M., Anticarcinogenic effects of some Indian products, *Food Chem. Toxicol.*, 30, 953, 1992.
40. Prashar, R. et al., Chemopreventive action by an extract from *Ocimum sanctum* on mouse skin papillomagenesis and enhancement of skin glutathion-S-transferase activity and acid soluble sulfhydryl level, *Anticancer Drugs*, 5, 567, 1994.
41. Banerjee, S. et al., Modulatory influence of alcholic extract of Ocimum leaves on carcinogen-metabolising enzyme activities and reduced glutathione levels in mouse, *Nutr. Cancer*, 25, 205, 1996.
42. Prashar, R. et al., Inhibition by an extract of *Ocimum sanctum* of DNA-binding activity of 7, 12-dimethylbenz [a] anthracene in rat hepatocytes *in vitro*, *Cancer Lett.*, 128, 155, 1998.
43. Karthikeyan, K., Ravichandran, P., and Govindasamy, S., Chemopreventive effect of *Ocimum sanctum* on DMBA-induced hamster buccal pouch carcinogenesis, *Oral Oncol.*, 35, 112, 1999.
44. Prakash, J., Gupta, S.K., and Joshi, S., Antiproliferative studies on *Ocimum sanctum*, *Indian J. Pharmacol.*, 31, 79, 1999.
45. Prakash, J. and Gupta, S.K., Chemopreventive activity of *Ocimum sanctum* seed oil, *J. Ethnopharmacol.*, 72, 29, 2000.

46. Rajalakshmi, S.G., Sivanandam, G., and Veluchamy, G., Role of Tulsi (*Ocimum sanctum* Linn.) in the management of Manjal Kamalai (viral hepatitis), *J. Res. Ayurveda Siddah,* 9, 118, 1986.
47. Zani, F. et al., Inhibition of mutagenicity in *Salmonella typhimurium* by *Glycyrrhiza glabra* extract, glycyrrhizinic acid, 18α- and 18β-glycyrrhetinic acids, *Planta Medica,* 59, 502, 1993.
48. Agarwal, R., Wang, Z.Y., and Mukhtar, H., Inhibition of mouse skin tumor-initiating activity of DMBA by chronic oral feeding of glycyrrhizin in drinking water, *Nutr. Cancer.,* 15, 187, 1991.
49. Pompei, R. et al., Glycyrrhizic acid inhibits virus growth and inactivates virus particles, *Nature,* 281, 689, 1979.
50. Baba, M. and Shigeta, S., Antiviral activity of glycyrrihizin against varicella-zoster virus *in vitro, Antiviral Res.,* 7, 99, 1987.
51. Ito, M., Mechanism of inhibitory effect of glycyrrhizin on replication of human immunodeficiency virus (HIV), *Antiviral Res.,* 10, 289, 1988.
52. Badam, L., *In vitro* antiviral activity of indigenous glycyrrhizin, licorice and glycyrrhizic acid on Japanese encephalitis virus, *J. Commun. Dis.,* 29, 91, 1997.
53. Miyake, K. et al., Efficacy of Stronger Neo-Minophagen C compared between two doses administered three times a week on patients with chronic viral hepatitis, *J. Gastroenterol. Hepatol.,* 17, 1198, 2002.
54. Kothari, A.B. et al., *In vitro* studies on antimutagenicity of water, alcoholic and oil extracts of *Semecarpus anacardium, Indian J. Pharmacol.,* 29, 301, 1997.
55. Indap, M.A., Ambaye, R.Y., and Gokhale, S.V., Antitumor and pharmacological effects of the oil from *Semecarpus anacardium* Linn., *Indian J. Physiol. Pharmacol.,* 27, 83, 1983.
56. Smit, H.F. et al., Ayurvedic herbal drugs with possible cytostatic activity, *J. Ethnopharmacol.,* 47, 75, 1995.
57. Premalatha, B. et al., Protective role of *Serankottai nei,* a siddhi preparation on cell membranes in aflatoxins B_1 induced hepatocellular carcinoma bearing rats, *Indian Drug,* 34, 384, 1997.
58. Premalatha, B. and Sachdanandam, P., Pharmacological effects of *Semecarpus anacardium* Linn. nut extract against aflatoxin B1 induced hepatocellular carcinoma, *Fitotherapia,* 70, 484, 1999.
59. Premalatha, B. and Sachdanandam, P., Stabilization of lysosomal membrane and cell membrane glycoprotein profile by *Semecarpus anacardium* Linn. nut milk extract experimental hepatocellular carcinoma, *Phytother. Res.,* 14, 352, 2000.
60. Premalatha, B. and Sachdanandam, P., Potency of *Semecarpus anacardium* Linn. nut milk extract against aflatoxin B(1)-induced hepatocarcinogenesis: reflection on microsomal biotransformation enzymes, *Pharmacol. Res.,* 42, 161, 2000.
61. Premalatha, B., Sujatha, V., and Sachdanandam, P., Modulating effect of *Semecarpus anacardium* Linn. nut extract on glucose metabolizing enzyme in aflatoxin B_1 induced experimental hepatocellular carcinoma, *Pharmacol. Res.,* 36, 187, 1997.
62. Vad, B.G., Study of complete regression in four cases of cancer, *Indian Practit.,* 26, 253, 1973.
63. Grover, I.S. and Bala, S., Antimutagenic activity of *Terminalia chebula* (myroblan) in *Salmonella typhimurium, Indian J. Exp. Bio.,* 30, 339, 1992.
64. Kaur, S. et al., Antimutagenicity of hydrolysable tannins from *Terminalia chebula* in *Salmonella typhmurium, Mutat. Res.,* 419, 169, 1998.
65. Saleem, A. et al., Inhibition of cancer cell growth by crude extract and the phenolics of *Terminalia chebula* Retz. fruit, *J. Ethnopharmacol.,* 81, 327, 2002.
66. Badmaev, V. and Nowokewski, M., Protection of epithelial cells against influenza A virus by a plant derived biological response modifier Ladretan-96, *Phytother. Res.,* 14, 245, 2000.
67. Ahn, M.J. et al., Inhibition of HIV-1 integrase by galloyl glucose from *Terminalia chebula* and flavonol glycoside gallates from *Euphorbia pekinensis, Planta Medica,* 68, 457, 2002.
68. El-Mekkawey, S. et al., Inhibitory effects of Egyptian folk medicines on human immunodeficiency virus (HIV) reverse transcriptase, *Chem. Pharm. Bull.,* 43, 641, 1995.
69. Kurokawa, M. et al., Efficacy of traditional herbal medicines in combination with acyclovir against herpes simplex virus type1 infection *in vitro* and *in vivo, Antiviral Res.,* 27, 19, 1995.
70. Yukawa, T.A. et al., Prophylatic treatment of cytomegalovirus infections with traditional herbs, *Antiviral Res.,* 32, 63, 1996.
71. Shiraki, K. et al., Cytomaglovirus infection and its possible treatment with herbal medicines, *Nippon. Rinsho.,* 56, 156, 1998.

72. Padam, S.K., Grover, I.S., and Singh, M., Antimutagenic effects of polyphenols isolated from *Terminalia bellerica* myroblan in *Salmonella typhimurium*, *Indian J. Exp. Biol.*, 34, 98, 1996.
73. Suthienkul, O. et al., Retrovirus reverse transcriptase inhibitory activity in Thai herbs and spices: screening with Moloney murine leukemia viral enzyme, *South East Asia J. Trop. Med. Pub. Health*, 24, 751, 1993.
74. Valsaraj, R. et al., New anti-HIV-1, antimalarial, and antifungal compounds from *Terminalia bellerica*, *J. Natl. Prod.*, 60, 739, 1997.
75. Grover, I.S. and Kaur, S., Effect of *Emblica officinalis* Gaertn. (Indian goose berry) fruit extract on sodiumazide and 4-nitro-o-phenylenediamine induced mutagenesis in *Salmonella typhimurium*, *Indian J. Exp. Biol.*, 27, 207, 1989.
76. Dhir, H., Roy, A.K., and Sharma, A., Relative efficiency of *Phyllanthus emblica* fruit extract and ascorbic acid in modifying lead and aluminium-induced sister-chromatid exchanges in mouse bone marrow, *Environ. Mol. Mutagen.*, 21, 229, 1993.
77. Roy, A.K., Dhir, H., and Sharma, A., Modification of metal-induced micronuclei formation in mouse bone marrow erythrocytes by Phyllanthus fruit extract and ascorbic acid, *Toxicol. Lett.*, 62, 9, 1992.
78. Sharma, N. et al., *In vitro* inhibition of carcinogen-induced mutagenicity by *Cassia occidentalis* and *Emblica officinalis*, *Drug Chem. Toxicol.*, 23, 477, 2000.
79. Nandi, P., Talukder, G., and Sharma, A., Dietary chemoprevention of clastogenic effects of 3,4-benzo[a] pyrene by *Emblica officinalis* Gaertn. fruit extract, *Br. J. Cancer*, 76, 1279, 1997.
80. Sharma, N. et al., Inhibitory effect of *Emblica officinalis* on the *in vivo* clastogenicity of benzo[a]pyrene and cyclophosphamide in mice, *Hum. Exp. Toxicol.*, 19, 377, 2000.
81. Jeena, K.J., Joy, K.L., and Kuttan, R., Effect of *Emblica officinalis*, *Phyllanthus amarus* and *Picrorrhiza kurroa* on N-nitrosodiethylamine induced hepatocarcinogenesis, *Cancer Lett.*, 136, 11, 1999.
82. Khan, M.T. et al., Identification of pyrogallol as an antiproliferative compound present in extract from the medicinal plant *Emblica officinalis*: effect on *in vitro* cell growth of human tumor cell lines, *Int. J. Oncol.*, 21, 187, 2002.
83. Jose, J.K., Kuttan, G., and Kuttan, R., Antitumor activity of *Emblica officinalis*, *J. Ethnopharmacol.*, 75, 65, 2001.
84. Sharma, N. et al., Inhibition of benzo[a]pyrene- and cyclophosphamide-induced mutagenicity by *Cinnamomum cassia*, *Mutat. Res.*, 480, 179, 2001.
85. Lee, C.W. et al., Inhibition of human tumor growth by 2'-hydroxy-2'-benzoyloxycinnamaldehydes, *Planta Medica*, 65, 263, 1999.
86. Kwon, B.M. et al., Synthesis and *in vitro* cytotoxicity of cinnamaldehydes to human solid tumor cells, *Arch. Pharm. Res.*, 21, 147, 1998.
87. Premanathan, M. et al., A survey of some Indian Medicinal Plants for anti-human immunodeficiency virus (HIV) activity, *Indian J. Med. Res.*, 112, 73, 2000.
88. Devi, P.U., *Withania somnifera* (Ashwagandha) potential plant source of a promising drug for cancer chemotherapy and radio sensitization, *Indian J. Exp. Biol.*, 34, 927, 1996.
89. Russo, A. et al., Indian medicinal plants as antiradicals and DNA cleavage protectors, *Phytomedicine*, 8, 125, 2001.
90. Prakash, J. et al., Chemopreventive activity of *Withania somnifera* in experimentally induced fibrosarcoma tumors in Swiss albino mice, *Phytother. Res.*, 15, 240, 2001.
91. Prakash, J., Gupta, S.K., and Dinda, A.K., *Withania somnifera* root extract prevents DMBA-induced squamous cell carcinoma of skin in Swiss albino mice, *Nutr. Cancer*, 42, 91, 2002.
92. Babu, T.D., Kuttan, G., and Padikkala, J., Cytotoxic and anti-tumour properties of certain taxa of Umbelliferae with special reference to *Centella asiatica* (L.) urban, *J. Ethnopharmacol.*, 48, 53, 1995.
93. Yen, G.C., Chen, H.Y., and Peng, H.H., Evaluation of the cytotoxicity, mutagenicity and antimutagenicity of emerging edible plants, *Food Chem. Toxicol.*, 39, 1045, 2001.
94. Zheng, M.S., An experimental study of the anti-HSV-II action of 500 herbal drugs, *J. Trad. Chem. Med.*, 9, 113, 1989.
95. Yoosook, C. et al., Anti-herpes simplex virus activity of crude mater extract of Thai medicinal plants, *Phytomedicine*, 6, 411, 2000.

16

Benign Growths, Cysts, and Malignant Tumors

Manoranjan Sahu and Lakshmi Chandra Mishra

CONTENTS

0-8493-1366-X/04/$0.00+$1.50

16.1 Introduction

Approximately 1.2 million new cases of invasive cancer are confirmed each year in the U.S., and about 500,000 people die from the disease each year.[1] The second most deadly disease is cancer and is expected to be the first in the early 21st century. Over the past century there have been tremendous changes in the environment, both dietary and lifestyle, resulting in the increase of lung cancer in both men and women. Melanoma, non-Hodgkin's lymphoma, and brain tumors have also increased, particularly among the elderly. The overall mortality, esspecially with people under the age of 65, has declined mostly due to increasingly effective therapy for cancers of fetal and hematopoietic origin.[1]

In spite of progress in the science of medicine, the understanding of the cancerous condition is still not complete. Although the knowledge has expanded considerably about the etiology and treatments, the exact cause of the disease and an effective management of cancer in general is still an unresolved mystery to the scientists. Cancer has been recognized and characterized by the science of Ayurveda. The descriptions regarding this disease are available in a scattered form under the context of various diseases. Compilation of this information collectively, in a systemic manner, may help us in understanding the etiology and the pathology of the disease in a better way. Numerous drugs have been mentioned for the management of this condition; if evaluated methodically, they may generate some curative or supportive remedy for the sufferers of this disease. The present era of modern sciences has undergone many folds of technical advancement for the diagnosis and confirmation of cancer by histopathological studies under light and electron microscopes. Before this, doctors and researchers had to depend entirely on various clinical symptomatology with *dosa* theory.

The purpose of this chapter is to review and summarize the available information on Ayuravedic management of benign growths, cysts, and malignant tumors.

16.2 Historical Perspective

Cancer is derived from the Greek word meaning a crab, presumably because a cancer "adheres to any part that it seizes upon in an obstinate manner like the crab." The large veins surrounding a malignant growth, which to the ancients suggested the claws of a crab, medically inspired the use of this term.

The identification and description of malignant diseases are available in the literature of ancient India and Ayurveda. The earliest and foremost records are cited in *Atharva Veda* (2200 B.C.). During this period, the disease was probably described under the heading of *apachi* or *apachit*, which refers to the present knowledge of various types of lymph node swellings. In a later period, Sushruta (400 B.C.), in his classic *Sushruta Samhita*, described this apachi as multiple lymph node swellings that may arise at different places such as the neck, axilla, and groin.

The ancient Indian clinicians were aware of the malignant diseases and presented their views regarding neoplasia as follows:

1. As a swelling on the body surface or situated in deeper structure in relation to various systems and organs
2. As a chronic nonhealing ulcer

In classical texts of Ayurveda, the superficial swellings have been categorized under the heading of tumors (*arbuda*), whereas nonhealing ulcers listed as incurable ulcers (a*sadhya vrana*).

The word *arbuda* has been derived from the root "Arb" with suffix "Ena" along with augmentation of "Nd," which means "to destroy" (particularly *mamsa dhatu*). Grammatically, it denotes the fleshy outgrowths. *Arbuda* has various meanings such as swelling, number of 10 billions, a mountain, a fleshy mass, a serpent, clouds, or a demon (i.e., a serpent). During the *Vedic* period, *arbuda* was considered as a serpentlike demon that was conquered by "Lord Indra," whereas the literary meaning of *arbuda* is a lump or a mass or a polyp. According to Sushruta, *arbuda* are gradually increasing, big, globular, slightly painful, fixed, deep-seated, fleshy masses that usually do not suppurate. They can arise from any part of the body surface. They are caused by the derangement of *mamsa* and *rakta* vitiated by *tridosa.*

The malignant lesions of deeper structures have been described in various contexts, such as intra-abdominal lesions having been described in the name of *gulma*. *Gulma* literally means a shrub (i.e., it can be understood as a lump or a mass in the abdomen and many of these lumps have been described to be incurable). The description of neoplastic growths is also available under the heading of *granthi*. The characteristic features of *arbuda* and *granthi* are similar. *Granthi* literally means a knotty growth. The etiology and clinical features of both *granthi* and *arbuda* are similar, with a difference that on breaking open, the *granthi* gives various discharges based on the involvement of the *dosas*. Thus, it can be understood that *granthi* may actually represent cystic growths.

The phenomenon of the spread of tumors or metastasis (*dwirarbuda*) was well known to the ancient Hindu physicians and surgeons. Several references are available regarding the local and distal spread of the tumor as well as its recurrence. Sushruta has described metastasis (i.e., distal spread of tumor under the heading of *dwirarbuda*), and the recurrence of tumor has been mentioned as *adhyarbuda*. Metastasis of tumors was described as an occurrence of a couple of similar types of tumors simultaneously serially. When a tumor arises on a preexisting site or near a primary tumor, it is called *adhyarbuda*. There are several other descriptions available in Ayurveda regarding distal spread and recurrence of tumor. While describing the treatment of tumors, Sushruta mentioned that all efforts should be made for the complete removal of tumors, as incomplete removal causes recurrence and ultimately destroys the person. To explain the graveness of recurrence, he gave an example that a small remnant tumor can destroy the body just as a small spark of fire can destroy a house. Distal spread of a tumor has also been described in connection with malignant ulcer (*asadhya vrana*).

16.3 Etiology

Sushruta has considered trauma and irritation precipitating or activating the formation of tumors as one of the etiological factors of soft-tissue tumor (*mamsarbuda*) and diseases of external genitalia (*sukaroga*) due to the use of irritants. Overeating of meat may lead to vitiation of muscle tissue and soft tissue (*mamsa*), considered an important factor for development of *mamsarbuda*. For the enlargement of external genitalia, local application of certain irritable medicines has been advised. Although this condition is rare, improper uses of these drugs used for the enlargement of external genitalia of male (*lingavridhikara yoga*) may lead to development of soft-tissue tumors (*mamsarbuda*) in external genitalia. The external application of irritable medicines and certain other internal medications have both been advised for enlarging the external genitalia. These medications may shed some light on the etiology of neoplasia, particularly the role of hormones in the development of tumors.

Vagbhata, another famous exponent of Ayurveda, also emphasizes that factors responsible for excessive formation of muscle and soft tissue (*mamsa dhatu*) may lead to the development of tumors and other pathological conditions. Examples include thyroid swelling (*galaganda*), cervical lymphadenopathy (*gandamala*), cysts (*granthi*), and fleshy growths (*adhimamsa*).

The genetic cause for the manifestation of cancer is also well documented in Ayurveda. In the etiology of familial polyposis coli (*sahaja arsha*), *Sushruta* has described that defects in ovum (*sonita*) and sperm (*shukra*) are responsible for the development of this disease.

From the above description, the factors responsible for the development of tumors may be categorized under the following headings:

1. Unwholesome diet (*mithya ahara*)
2. Unwholesome regimen (*mithya vihara*)
3. Trauma (*abhigata*)
4. Irritation
5. Genetic (*anuvanshaja*)

It can be concluded that unwholesome diet and lifestyle (*mithya ahara* and *vihara*) cause local and systemic biochemical changes. At the same time, these factors may alter the hemodynamics at the site of origin of tumors.

In conventional medicine, the common pathway in the induction (initiation) of cancer is a cellular genetic mutation that converts normal cells to cancer cells. The genes controlling normal cellular processes become mutated by a variety of chemical interactions with the dexoribonucleic acid (DNA) initiation process. These initiated genes promote cancer and are called promoter genes (oncogenes). The other normal genes suppress cancer and are called suppressor genes. Oncogenes produce cancer by encoding proteins that are further activated to induce cancer. The tumor suppressor genes cause cancer when their normal tumor suppressor function is blocked. Chemical agents, physical agents, chronic irritation, biologic agents, and even dietary factors contribute to carcinogenesis. Regulatory agencies in the U.S. and other countries infect, monitor, and regulate environment and dietary sources of carcinogens.[2] The single most important agent known to contribute to increased incidence of cancer in the U.S. and Europe is tobacco, because it contributes to one third of all cancers, primarily cancers of the lung, esophageal, head, neck, and bladder.[1] Because genes define the cellular phenotype, this indicates that the mutational profile of a cancer cell may predict the clinical outcome, and this has become a reality.[1]

16.4 Pathogenesis

In contemporary medicine, cancer is considered essentially as a disturbance of normal cell growth. Tumors of any cell type may show a wide range of behavior in their rate of growth, power and mode of spread, and degree of toxic effects on the host. There are tumors that grow slowly, remain quite localized, and do not invade the neighboring structures. They usually cause no harm and are known as benign tumors or harmless tumors. The other groups of tumors grow rapidly, penetrate the surrounding tissues, and spread to distant areas. They are invariably fatal and are termed cancerous tumors or malignant tumors.

The pathogenesis of tumors has been described in Ayurveda based on the theory of three *dosa* (*tridosa*). The vitiated *dosa* affects the local tissues (*dhatu* or *dushya*). *Vata, pitta,* and *kapha* are considered as *dosas*; muscle and soft tissue (*mamsa*), adipose tissue (*meda*), and blood (*rakta*) are termed *dushyas* (that which can be vitiated). Due to excess of *kapha* and adipose tissue, tumors usually do not suppurate. It is justified to suggest that excess of *kapha* might be responsible for the development of tumors. Moreover, as a tumor is a disorder of growth and as *kapha* is an essential factor for growth, it can also be postulated that preponderance of vitiated *kapha* is an essential factor for the manifestation of tumors.

TABLE 16.1
Clinical Features of Various Tumors in Ayurveda

Symptom	*Vataja Arbuda*	*Pittaja Arbuda*	*Kaphaja Arbuda*	*Medaja Arbuda*	*Mamsaja Arbuda*	*Raktaja Arbuda*
Pain	Variable	Burning	Mild pain with itching	Mild pain with itching	Painless or mild pain	—
Consistency	Hard or soft (variable)	—	Stony or hard	Soft	Stony	—
Mobility	Mobile	—	—	Freely mobile	Fixed	—
Skin over the tumor	Black	Red, yellowish	No change in color	Glossy	Normal or covered by prominent veins	—
Surface	Nodular	Smooth	Smooth	Smooth	Smooth	Covered with fleshy projections
Discharge	Nil	Nil	Nil	Nil	Nil	Blood
Shape and size	Raised above the surface like bladder	—	Large globular	Large	Large	Elevated fleshy growth
Growth rate	—	—	Slow	—	Slow	Rapid
Prognosis	Curable	Curable	Curable	Curable	Incurable	Incurable

In the etiopathogenesis of *raktaja tumors,* vitiated *dosa* cause the derangement of blood, and as a consequence the vessels (*siras*) of the local site become constricted. This results in a rapidly growing fleshy growth known as *raktarbuda* (ulcerated malignant tumor).

16.5 Clinical Manifestations of Tumors

Ayurveda has six major clinical manifestations of tumors. See Table 16.1 for an overview:

16.5.1 Benign Neoplasia of Fibrous Tissue and Hematoma (*Vataja* Tumor)

Various types of pain, such as pricking, stretching, and cutting, characterize *vataja* tumor. The growth assumes a black color, appears rough, and is elevated like a bladder. These tumors are mobile, soft in consistency, and change in size without reason.

16.5.2 Inflammatory State of Benign Neoplasia (*Pittaja* Tumor)

Pittaja arbuda are red or yellow and characterized by severe burning, fuming, and sucking or throbbing pain. They undergo early suppuration.

Like neoplastic growth, tumors usually do not suppurate due to excess *kapha* and *meda*. However, due to secondary infections, inflammatory changes may occur and cause suppuration.

16.5.3 Benign Neoplasia of Osseous, Other Soft Tissues, and Adenomas (*Kaphaja* Tumor)

These swellings are cold to the touch, relatively painless, stony in consistency, and develop very slowly. The color of the tumor is similar to the color of the surrounding skin or is slightly glossy.

Based on the signs and symptoms, *vataja, pittaja,* and *kaphaja* tumors can be correlated to benign neoplastic conditions, irrespective of site. Examples include fibroma, hematoma, and neurofibroma (*vataja* tumors); inflammatory state of any benign neoplasia (*pittaja* tumor); and benign neoplasm of epithelial tissue, lymphoid tissue, and soft-tissue osteoma (*kaphaja* tumors).

16.5.4 Benign Conditions of Mesenchymal Tissues Like Lipoma (*Medaja* Tumor)

This tumor is slow growing, arises with slight pain, and is associated with itching. The tumor is freely mobile with a glossy appearance. The size varies according to the contents of adipose tissue (*medas*) in the body. If the content of adipose tissue in the body increases, the size of this tumor also increases and vice versa.

16.5.5 Ulcerated Malignant Lesions (*Raktaja* Tumor)

Raktaja tumors are very rapidly growing, slightly suppurated, exudating tumors covered with projectile small fleshy masses. The person affected by this tumor becomes pale due to continuous exudation of blood from this growth. This type of tumor is incurable.

16.5.6 Tumors of Muscle and Soft Tissues Like Breast Tissue (*Mamsaja* Tumor)

External trauma vitiates the soft tissues (*mamsa*) of any part of the body and gives rise to a smooth, large, painless, nonsuppurative, stony, skin-colored, fixed swelling called a *mams* tumor. Such swellings are usually covered with prominent veins. This is also an incurable tumor.

16.5.7 Tumors of Mixed Variety (*Tridoshaja* Tumor)

This type of tumor is incurable. It has mixed features of *vataja, pittaja,* and *kaphaja* tumor varieties.

16.6 Classification of Tumors

Based on the predominance of the vitiated *dosa* involved, tumors have been classified as *vataja arbuda, pittaja arbuda, kaphaja arbuda, tridoshaja arbuda, raktaja arbuda, mamsaja arbuda,* and *medaja* tumors. It is very difficult to give a specific modern nomenclature of each tumor mentioned in Ayurveda. In one study, 50 patients with various types of tumors and clinical features of different swellings mentioned in Ayurveda were compared with *vataja, pittaja,* and *kaphaja* benign neoplastic conditions irrespective of site. It was observed that

TABLE 16.2

Classification of Tumors According to Conventional Medicine

	Type of Tumor	
Tissue of Origin	**Benign**	**Malignant**
Tumors of Connective Tissue		
Fibrous tissue	Fibroma	Fibrosarcoma
Cartilage	Chondroma	Chondrosarcoma
Bone	Osteoma	Osteosarcoma
Adipose tissue	Lipoma	Liposarcoma
Blood vessels	Hemangioma	Hemangiosarcoma
Sinovial tissue	Sinovioma	Sinoviosarcoma
Smooth muscle	Leomyoma	Leomyosarcoma
Striated muscle	Rhabdomyoma	Rhabdomyosarcoma
Reticulo-Endothelial Tissue		
Lymphoid tissue		Hodgkin's lymphoma Non-Hodgkin's lymphoma
Granulocytes		Myeloid leukemia
Plasma cell		Myeloma
Tumor of Epithelial Tissue		
Sqamous	Papilloma	Sqamous cell carcinoma
Transitional	Papilloma	Transitional cell carcinoma
Glandular		
Papillary	Papilloma	Papillary carcinoma
Solid	Adenoma	Adenocarcinoma
Cystic	Cystadenoma	Cystadinocarcinoma
Mixed	Papillary cystadenoma	Papillary cystadinocarcinoma
Neural Tissue		
Glial tissue		Glioma
Nerve sheath	Neuroleimoma	Neurogenic sarcoma
Meningis	Meningioma	Meningeosarcoma
Other Tissues		
Placenta	Hydatidiform mole	Choriocarcinoma
Pigmented cells	Nevus	Malignant melanoma
Germ cell	Benign teratoma	Malignant teratoma

the *kaphaja* tumor is benign neoplasm of epithelial tissue, lymphoid tissue, and soft tissue; the *medaja* tumor is benign conditions of mesenchymal tissues like lipoma, fibrolipoma, and hemangioma. A *raktaja* tumor is an ulcerated malignant lesion and includes carcinoma of integument and other ulcerated malignant growth. The *mamsaja* tumor is a testicular tumor, ductal carcinoma of breast, lymphoid tumor, follicular carcinoma of thyroid, and soft-tissue sarcoma.[3] Tumors classified according to conventional medicine are listed in Table 16.2.

Tumors may arise from any part of the body; no site is exempt. Tumors of the eye, ear, nose, oral cavity, and external genitalia have been dealt with separately (Table 16.3).

TABLE 16.3

Tumors of the Head and Neck in Ayurveda

Name of the Tumor	Site	*Dosa*	Clinical Presentation	Prognosis
Tumors of the eyelid (*vartmarbuda*)	Inner side of the eyelid	*Pitta* and *rakta*	Irregular, knotty, reddish mass with mild pain	May be curable
Tumors of the ear (*karnarbuda*)	External ear	Involvement of any one of the three *dosas* or in combination	Features based on the involved *dosa*	May be curable
Tumors of the nose (*nasa arbuda*)	Nasal cavity	Involvement of any one of the three *dosas* or in combination	Features based on the involved *dosa*	May be curable
Tumors of Lips (oshtarbuda)				
Cystic growths of lips (*jalarbuda*)	Lips	*Vata* and *kapha*	The growth appears like a water bubble	Fatal
Ulcerated malignant growths of lips (*raktarbuda*)	Lips	*Rakta*	Lips become red and swollen and discharge blood	Fatal
Tumors of the palate (*talu arbuda*)	Palate	*Rakta*	Swelling resembling the shape of lotus	Fatal
Tumors of the oral cavity (*mukharbuda*)	Inner surface of the mouth	*Kapha*	Pale, blackish mass that persists even after various surgical treatments	Fatal
Tumors of the throat (*galarbuda*)	Root of the tongue or in the middle of the throat		Nonuppurating, painless, hard, fixed and reddish tumor	Incurable
Tumors of the head (*shiro arbuda*)	*Shiras*		General features of *arbuda*	May be curable

16.6.1 Tumor of the Lip (*Mamsaja Oshta Roga*)

The lip becomes a heavy and thick projection of fleshy mass, subsequently leading to the formation of an ulcer, which may be infested with maggots.

16.6.2 Tumor of the Floor of the Mouth (*Alas*)

This tumor is a deep-seated mass on the under surface of the tongue due to vitiation of blood (*rakta*) and *kapha*. It is considered an incurable tumor, which increases gradually in size, fixes the tongue, and may suppurate. The tumor ultimately destroys the surrounding structures and exudates discharge with fishy odor.

Carcinoma of the floor of the mouth may give rise a similar picture like that of *alas*. Adenocystic and mucoepidermoid tumors of the salivary gland present themselves as an ulcerated growth that gradually holds the tongue and leads to progressive difficulties in speech. These malignant lesions are usually complicated with secondary infection. Foul-smelling discharge and destruction of the surrounding tissue are very often found in these diseases.

16.6.3 Tumor of the Hard Palate (*Mamsa Kacchapa*)

The tumor develops on the palate because of vitiation of *kapha* and appears like a shell of a tortoise. It is a slow growing, painless, and considered an incurable tumor.

The tumors of the hard palate are characterized by slow growth and are usually not associated with pain. The tumors are smooth and hemispherical in shape, comparable with the convex shell of a tortoise. Similarly, carcinoma of the maxillary antrum may present as a convex mass in the hard palate.

16.6.4 Tumor of the Throat (*Galugha*)

This is considered an incurable tumor that is caused by vitiation of blood and *kapha*. The disease is characterized by a large swelling that develops on the inner and outer sides of the throat. It interferes with the functions of *udana vata*, resulting in the obstruction of food and air passages. The disease is also characterized by feeling of heaviness in the head, excessive salivation, and fever.

The oropharynx is the key structure for swallowing, breathing, and speaking. A malignant growth at the oropharynx may give rise to the obstructive features like that of throat tumor (*galugha*). Tumors at the oropharynx, palatine arch, and ulcerate become infected easily, causing pain in this nerve-rich area. Headache and otalgia are also common due to referred pain as the ninth cranial nerve supplies both the sites. Moreover, patients with carcinoma of the base of the tongue or primary malignant lesions of the oropharynx present with metastasis at the neck gland and may present only with neck gland swelling. The above features of oropharyngeal cancer can be corelated with the features of *galugha*.

16.6.5 Tumor of the Oropharynx (*Balaya*)

This is considered a malignant tumor of the throat that develops due to deranged *kapha*. The tumor is widespread and painless and ultimately obstructs the food passage.

These tumors could be malignant lesions of a deeper part of the oropharynx, which ulcerate later. Pain is less because of fewer nerve endings. The features of food-passage obstruction are found much earlier than the symptoms of airway obstruction due to their close vicinity to the esophagus.

16.6.6 Tumor of the Thyroid (*Asadhya Galaganda*)

Thyroid swellings (*galaganda*) of long duration (more than a year) lead to breathing difficulty, emaciation, anorexia, weakness, and hoarseness of the voice. This tumor is considered an incurable and may be due to malignant lesion of the gland.

The first symptom of thyroid carcinoma is the enlargement of the thyroid gland. It develops slowly, and choking attacks may occur due to pressure effect on the trachea. Hoarseness may be caused by the displacement of the larynx or involvement of the recurrent laryngeal nerve, which is found in a good proportion of cases. Weight loss and anorexia are seldom present.

16.6.7 Intra-Abdominal Malignant Tumors (*Tridoshaja* and *Asadhya Gulma*)

Intra-abdominal malignant tumors (*tridoshaja gulma*) are characterized by an intra-abdominal stony mass with severe burning pain. Such patients loose mental peace, strength, and appetite.

Intra-abdominal malignant tumors (*asadhya gulma*) are gradually increasing, widespread, and fixed. They have a tortoise shell-like mass associated with weakness, anorexia, cough, vomiting, fever, and thirst. Multiple prominent veins usually cover the skin over the mass. Both of the above varieties are considered incurable.

In contemporary medicine, these conditions can be correlated with intra-abdominal malignant tumors, especially with tumors of liver. In hepatoma the lump is usually solitary, big, fixed, and convex; it may be comparable with the convex shell of the tortoise. The patient's general condition, physical and mental strength, and appetite decrease. Prominent abdominal veins may be due to portal hypertension or obstruction of the inferior vena cava. Cough and painful respiration are common symptoms that may result from pulmonary metastasis. Except primary hepatic carcinoma, a number of other abdominal conditions, such as retroperitoneal malignancies, ovarian and uterine carcinomas, lymphoma, and carcinoma of the stomach and bowels, may give rise to similar features.

16.6.8 Malignant Ascites (*Asadhya Udara Roga*)

This is considered an incurable ascites associated with flank pain, marked anorexia, generalized edema, and diarrhea. The recurrence of ascites is very fast even after removal of ascitic fluid by paracentesis. This very early recurrence of ascitic fluid in *asadhya udara roga* suggests the possibility of malignancy.

16.6.9 Familial Adenomatous Polyposis Coli (*Sahaja Arsha*)

The disease originates from defects in the genetic material (i.e., sperm and ovum). Such fleshy masses (*arsha*) are hardly visible (high enough), rough, painful, yellowish in color and directed inward.

The patients are emaciated and irritable, have a feeble voice and poor digestion, and tend to develop diseases of head and neck. Cracking sounds and shiny skin are the other symptoms of familial adenomatous polyposis. It is also considered an incurable disease.

Considering the etiology and clinical features of *sahaja arsha*, the disease can be compared with familial adenomatous polyposis coli. It has been described in the texts of contemporary medicine as a hereditary disease that is characterized by a large number of adenomatous polyps in the colon and rectum; if left untreated, it will almost certainly change in to adenocarcinoma of the large bowel. Here again the disease originates from defects in the sperm and ovum. Bleeding, anemia, diarrhea, partial obstruction, pain in abdomen, and indigestion are the presenting symptoms. It is similar to the symptoms mentioned under *sahaja arsha*.

16.6.10 Tumor of the Lungs (*Kshayaja Kasa*)

This is considered an incurable tumor and may mimic other lung diseases (e.g., *kshayaja kasa*). It initially starts with a dry cough and becomes complicated with hemoptysis after a while. The patient feels a severe pricking pain in the chest and throat and suffers from malaise and fever. The patient also experiences difficulty breathing, choking, and wheezing during coughing. The disease is frequently associated with generalized body ache, fever, and a burning sensation. The patient gradually becomes emaciated and thin, devoid of fleshes and vitality. The person spits mucus, blood, and pus.

The symptomatology and the sequence of symptoms of *kshayaja kasa* is similar to the symptomatology of carcinoma of the lungs. It has been described in the texts of conventional medicine that the cough initially is nonproductive but subsequently becomes productive with increasing amounts of mucoid expectoration, sometimes tinged with blood and a possible development of hemoptysis. Chest pain is severe and pleuritic, characterized by pinching pain. Paroxysmal hyperpnea may develop due to the presence of mucus buildup in the secondary and tertiary bronchi. Pleural effusion and empyema may cause dyspnea. Wheezing occurs when mucus partially obstructs the bronchus. Attacks of fever are common because of repeated obstructive pneumonia. Weight loss is a rather constant symptom of anorexia and metastasis.

16.6.11 Tumor of the External Genitalia of the Male (*Lingarsha*)

These lesions are ordinarily nonmalignant and do not grow like malignant tumors. Vitiated *dosas* affect the local flesh and blood of external genitalia, causing an itching sensation and ulceration. Such an ulcer usually grows over the foreskin or glans of the penis and is covered with papillomatous growth. The ulcer discharges slimy blood, ultimately destroys the penis, and halts the reproductive activity of the patients.

Penile neoplasms are very limited in number. Only two conditions, papilloma and carcinoma, produce new growth. The description of *lingarsha* is very close to the clinical features of carcinoma of the penis mentioned in conventional medicine. The patients with penile carcinoma usually present with a papillomatous growth in the glans with delayed features such as pain, hemorrhage, and discharge. The lesion initially is papillary, but gradually ulcerates and subsequently the ulcerative process destroys the entire penis, leaving a hornlike structure (penile horn) behind. Based on clinical presentation, course, treatment, and prognosis, the diseases listed in Table 16.4 can be considered malignant.

16.7 Prognosis of Tumors and Ulcers

The prognosis of tumors has been explained based on the response to various treatment modalities. Depending upon the modality, the tumors that respond or are cured are considered *sadhya* or benign. Those that do not respond or are incurable are considered *asadhya* or malignant. *Vataja*, *pittaja*, and *kaphaja* tumors (benign neoplastic conditions) and benign conditions of mesenchymal tissue (*medaja* tumors) of any site are curable (*sadhya*). Tumors of muscle and soft tissue (*mamsarbuda*), ulcerated malignant growths (*raktaja* tumors), mixed type of tumors (*tridoshaja* tumors) of any site, cystic growths of lips, tumors of the palate and throat, and tumors of the oral cavity are considered incurable. Any tumor

TABLE 16.4

Neoplastic Diseases in Ayurveda

Arbuda (Neoplasia)	*Asadhya-Vrana* (Incurable Ulcers)	*Arbudavat Anya Vyadhi* (Diseases Comparable with Malignancy)
Tumors of muscle and soft tissue (*mamsarbuda*)		Head and neck
		Tumors of the lip (*mamsaja oshta roga*)
		Tumors of the floor of the mouth (*alas*)
Ulcerated malignant lesions (*raktarbuda*)		Tumors of the hard palate (*mamsakacchapa*)
		Tumors of the throat (*galugha*)
Mixed types of tumors (*tridosaja arbuda*)		Tumors of the oropharynx (*balaya*)
		Tumors of the thyroid (*asadhya galaganda*)
Tumors of the palate (*talu arbuda*)		
		Gastrointestinal tract
Tumors of the oral cavity (*mukharbuda*)		Intra-abdominal malignant tumors (*tridoshaja gulma, asadhya gulma*)
Tumors of the throat (*galarbuda*)		Malignant ascites (*asadhya udara roga*)
		Familial adenomatous polyposis coli (*sahaja arsha*)
		Respiratory system
		Tumors of the lungs (*kshayaja kasa*)
		External genitalia of male
		Tumors of the penis (*lingarsha*)

that reaches the stage of recurrence (*adhya* tumors) or metastasis (*dwiraar* tumor) is also considered incurable.

Almost all clinical presentations of incurable class of ulcers described by Sushruta can be included under malignant ulcers. Some of their specific features are:

1. Ulcers cropping up like a fleshy mass
2. Edges raised like those of external genitalia of a mare
3. Ulcers containing soft fleshy masses like the horn of a cow
4. Base of the ulcer being raised above the margins
5. Ulcers secreting various fluids, including vitiated blood and other substances similar to fatty (*vasa*) substance, adipose tissue (*meda*), bone marrow (*majja*), or brain matter
6. Ulcers manifested in an emaciated patient with discharge of blood and pus and the patient's condition being complicated by indigestion, cough, painful respiration, and anorexia
7. An ulcer that does not heal in spite of proper medication

In modern medicine, the description of malignant ulcers is similar. For example, the margins are raised above the base, rolled up, and hard in consistency; multiple fleshy masses develop (as seen in fungating basal cell carcinoma); and the base is raised above the margins many times. Cauliflowerlike ulcerative growths are an example of this type of malignant ulcer. Malignant ulcers bleed severely even with slight trauma. In addition, varieties of discharges are seen in malignant lesions. Painful respiration, cough, and

TABLE 16.5

Diagnosis

History/Interrogation	Signs and Symptoms[a]	Investigation
Family history	Change in wart or mole	Hemogram
Occupational history	Lump in the breast	TLC, DLC, Hb%, ESR, GBP, LFT, etc.
Dietary habits	Nonhealing sore	Radiogram
Geographical relation	Persistent cough	Plain x-ray
History of previous illness (may be predisposing factor etc.)	Unusual bleeding or discharge from any source	Barium contrast
		IVP, USG
	Indigestion or difficulty in swallowing	CT scanning
		MRI etc.
	Change in bowel and urinary habits	Histopathological and biochemical
		Aspiration
		Cytology
		Biopsy
		Enzyme
		Hormone
		Immunity factor
		Certain tumor markers
		Endoscopy
		Gastroscopy
		Colonoscopy
		Cystoscopy
		Bronchoscopy
		Laparoscopy
		Mediastinoscopy
		Histeroscopy

[a] Seven danger signals by the American Cancer Society.

anorexia are additional symptoms of malignant ulcers that suggest metastasis of the tumor in the lungs.

16.8 Principles of Diagnosis

Ayurvedic diagnosis of tumors is carried out based on clinical manifestations, physical examination, and systemic examination. Apart from these methods, various diagnostic methods used by physicians of contemporary medicine are also adopted for a correct diagnosis.

The general condition of the patient (*rogi*) is examined after the standard eight-point examination procedures (i.e., pulse, feces, urine, various auscultatory findings, palpation, skin, eyes, and body strength).

Additional examinations includes history, type of pain, specific signs and symptoms, size and shape of the tumor (*akriti of arbuda*), consistency, color, tissue involved, site, and stage of the tumor (Tables 16.1 and 16.5).

In conventional medicine, the first principle of diagnosis is that adequate tissue for a biopsy be obtained from the tumor to establish the specific diagnosis and type of cancer. The second diagnostic principle is to establish the extent of the disease through physical examination, laboratory tests, and diagnostic imaging. In solid tumors, surgery is required to determine the extent of the disease or the stage of the tumor.[1]

Early detection of cancer is very helpful in treating cancers. The following procedures and tumor markers have been proven useful as a secondary strategy in an attempt to reduce cancer mortality:[1]

Procedures	Tumor markers
Sigmoidoscopy	Colorectal — CEA
Fecal occult blood test	Ovary — Ca-125
Digital rectal exam	Testicle — hCG, AFP
Prostate exam	Prostate — PSA
Papanicolaou test	Breast — CA15-2, CEA
Pelvic exam	Non-Hodgkin's lymphoma — LDH
Breast self-exam	Myeloma — Beta$_2$-M
Mammography	Hepatoma — AFP

Ayurvedic physicians also use these detection procedures and tumor markers for diagnosing and assessing the effect of therapeutic agents.

16.9 Management

16.9.1 Principle of Cancer Therapy

In Ayurveda, detoxification (*shodhana* therapy) is a major part of the treatment not only for *arbuda*, but also for all other diseases. The main principle of this procedure is to eliminate vitiated *dosas* to maintain their equilibrium, preserving the immunity (*rogibala*) of the patients. Detoxification is the pretherapy in the actual line of management, but not all patients are fit to undergo these procedures. The procedures are contraindicated in emaciated and severely ill patients who cannot tolerate therapeutic emesis or purgation.

The role of detoxification therapies on cancer patients as pretherapy to conventional line of treatment has been studied.[3,4] The study showed that these procedures increased body weight, improved serum immunoglobulins, increased hemoglobin levels, and normalized liver functions. It was found helpful in minimizing the adverse effects of chemotherapeutic agents. The study concluded that the following procedures were helpful:

1. Oleation therapy (*snehana*) using medicated ghee prepared with *triphala* (*Terminalia chebula, Terminalia bellerica, Emblica officinalis*) in patients with breast cancer
2. Therapeutic purgation (*virechana*) in malignant conditions of hepatobiliary system
3. Medicated enema (*basti karma*) in malignancy of the genitor-urinary system

Sushruta has indicated that a patient's natural resistance or immunity to the disease (i.e., *rogibala*) is one the essential factors that should be preserved for the arrest of the progress of the disease. Fasting (*langhana*) is one of the principles of treatment for *kapha*-predominant diseases but has not been recommended because it may reduce the ability to defend

TABLE 16.6

Common Ayurvedic Formulations to Treat Tumors

Name of the Formulation	Main Constituents	Indication	Dose	Ref.
Rudra rasa (arbudahara rasa)	Mercury and sulphur ground with the decoctions of betel leaf, boerhavia, cow's urine, *Piper longum*, and amaranthus	Mentioned in all types of cancer	125–250 mg twice/day	58
Lokanatha rasa (brihat)	Mercury, sulphur, mica, aloe, iron oxide ground with *Solanum nigrum*	Mentioned in liver and spleen disorders	125–250mg twice/day	59
Tamra basma	Colloidal copper	Used in all types of intra-abdominal swellings (*gulma*)	15–125 mg[a]	60
Abhraka basma	Mica	Mentioned in all types of debilitating diseases	125–250 mg[a]	61
Suvarna basma	Gold dust	Used to improve immunity, strength, and body weight	2.5–6.0 mg[a]	62
Manashila	Arsenic disulphide	For external application on tumors	Quantity sufficient	63

[a] As directed by the physician.

against the disease process (*rogibala*). Various drugs and formulations have been mentioned in Ayurveda for the management of tumors, but they have not been proven to have a direct cytotoxic effect on humans (Table 16.6).

16.9.2 General Treatment

The following treatments are used according to the involvement of *dosa* and the type of the tissues:

1. Detoxification therapies (*samshodhana chikitsa*) are advocated for the management of tumors based on the involvement of *dosa*. Oleation (*snehana*) is advised for *vata dosa*, purgation (*virechana*) is advised for *pitta dosa*, and emesis (*vamana*) is advised for *kapha dosa*.
2. After detoxification, administration of *dosa* subsiding drugs (*samshamana oushadha*) is advised as per involvement of *dosa*.
3. Local treatments like medicated poultice (*upanaha*), sudation (*swedana*), and local application of various drugs (*lepana*) are also indicated.
4. Parasurgical measures such as bloodletting (*raktamokshana*), application of caustics (*kshara karma*), and cauterization (*agnikarma*) are also mentioned.
5. Surgical excision (*shastrakarma*) of the tumor is performed.
6. Postoperative wound management by various Ayurvedic drugs is conducted.
7. Parasurgical approaches include bloodletting (*raktamokshana*), therapeutic cautery (*agnikarma*), application of caustics (*ksharakarma*), and maggotification.

16.9.3 Specific Treatments

In vivo and *in vitro* studies have been carried out on different Ayurvedic drugs in various institutions all over the world. The purpose of these studies is to evaluate drugs' cytotoxic action, their role in improving the hemopiesis, and level of immunity. Studies have also been used to show how drugs reduce the toxic effects of conventional therapies and improve the well-being of the patient, as an adjuvant to chemotherapy and radiotherapy.

1. A compound Ayurvedic drug containing *bhallataka* (*Semicarpus anacardium*), *rohitaka* (*Amoora rohitaka*), and *yastimadhu* (*Glyceriza glabra*) along with other conventional treatment modalities plays an important role in immunological alteration in cancer. This compound helps in terms of increases in mean lymphocyte count, improvements in cell-mediated immunity, increases in T-cell count, decreases in positivity to C-reactive protein, and increases in the levels of serum immunoglobulins (Ig) such as IgA, IgG, and IgM.[5]
2. *Rohitaka* and *bhallataka* reduce the hepatotoxicity induced by chemotherapy in hepatobiliary, gastrointestinal malignancy,[6] and squamous cell carcinoma.[7] These drugs normalize the liver functions after chemotherapy.
3. Various other clinical and experimental investigations have been done to evaluate the role of various Ayurvedic drugs as an adjuvant therapy. They were found effective in reducing the chemotherapy- and radiotherapy-induced toxicities in various types of cancers.[8]
4. Studies indicate that *Withania somnifera* (*ashwagandha*) could reduce the cyclophosphamide induced toxicity and hence be useful in cancer therapy.[9] *W. somnifera* produces immunopotentiating and myeloprotective effects, as seen from the enhancement of cytokine production and stem-cell proliferation and its differentiation.[10]
5. The tablet Cystone, a polyherbal Ayurvedic preparation, protects against cisplatin-induced nephrotoxicity without interfering with its antitumor activity.[11]
6. Certain vegetable oils rich in linoleic acid (e.g., sesame oil) that are recommended for topical use by Ayurveda may contain selective antineoplastic properties; these properties are similar to those demonstrated for essential polyunsaturated fatty acids and their metabolites. This suggests that vegetable oils may have potential clinical usefulness.[12]

16.9.3.1 Treatment of Vataja Tumors

Vataja tumors are treated locally by medicated poultice (*upanaha*), fomentation with steam (*nadi sweda*), and bloodletting (*raktamokshana*). They are treated systemically by medicated dehydrated butter and herbal formulations.

16.9.3.2 Medicated Poultice

Various medicated poultices are mentioned for the management of *vataja* tumors. *Kushmanda* (*Benincasa cerifera*), *ervaruka* (*Cucumis utilissimus*), *narikela* (*Cocos nucifera*), *priyala* (*Buchanania lanzan spreng*), and *eranda* (*Ricinus communis*) seeds that are boiled with milk, water, and ghee and mixed with oil should be applied. Another medicated poultice made up of boiled meat has also described as effective.[13]

TABLE 16.7

Drugs Having a *Vata* Mitigating Effect (*Vatahara Dravya*)

Name of Plant	Botanical Name	Family Name	Parts Used
Devadaru	*Cedrus deodara* Roxb.	Pinaceae	Heart wood
Kusta	*Saussurea lappa* C.B Clarke.	Compositae	Root
Haridra	*Curcuma longa* Linn.	Zingiberaceae	Tuber
Varuna	*Crataeva nurvala* Buch-Ham.	Capparidaceae	Bark
Meshashrungi	*Gymnema sylvestre* R.Br.	Asclepiadaceae	Leaf, root
Bala	*Sida cordifolia* Linn.	Malvaceae	Root, seed
Atibala	*Abutilon indicum* Linn.	Malavaceae	Root, seed
Kacchura	*Curcuma zedoaria* Rose.	Zingiberaceae	Tuber
Sallaki	*Boswellia serrata* Roxb.	Burseraceae	Bark, latex
Kuberaksha	*Caesalpina crista* Linn.	Caesalpinioideae	Seed
Arjuna	*Termenalia arjuna* Roxb.	Combretaceae	Bark
Sahachara	*Barleria prionitis* Linn.	Acanthaceae	Whole plant
Kulattha	*Dolichos biflorus* Linn.	Papillionatae	Seeds
Kola	*Zizyphus jujuba* Lam.	Rhamnaceae	Leaf, fruit
Shatavari	*Asparagus racemosus* Wild.	Lilliaceae	Tuber
Punarnava	*Boerhavia diffusa* Linn	Nyctaginaceae	Root, seed, whole plant
Eranda	*Ricinus communis* Linn.	Euphorbiaceae	Root, leaf
Arka	*Calotropus procera* R.Br.	Asele piadaceae	Root bark, flower, leaf

Source: Ganekar, B.G. and Vaidya, L.C., *Samshodhana samshamaneeya Adhyaya in sutrasthana of Sushruta Samhita by Acharya Sushruta*, 5th ed., 1994, chap. 40, p. 142, verse 7. With permission.

16.9.3.3 Fomentation

Fomentation of local part in the form of *nadi sweda* is advised. Drugs such as moringa pterygosperma (*shigru*) and the juice of meat (*mamsa rasa*) are boiled and steam is to be passed through a tube over the site.[14]

16.9.3.4 Bloodletting (Raktamokshana)

Bloodletting with the help of horns (*shringa*) has been described to be effective in the treatment of *vataja* tumors.[14]

16.9.3.5 Systemic Treatment

Medicated ghee boiled with decoction of drugs that fix the aggravated *vata* (Table 16.7)[64] is given with milk or *kanji.*

16.9.3.6 Treatment of Pittaja Tumors

The local treatment of the tumor includes rubbing with the leaves of udumbara (*Ficus glomerata* Linn.) or other leaves having a rough surface. This is followed by sprinkling of fine dust of *sarjarasa* (*Viteria indica*), *priyangu* (*Callicarpa macrophylla*), *raktachandana* (*Pterocerpus santalinus*), *arjuna* (*Terminalia arjuna*), and *yastimadhu* (*Glycyrhiza glabra*) mixed with honey.

A plaster composed of *aragvadha* (*Cassia fistula*), *soma* (*Sarcostemma acidum*), and *shyama* (*Callicarpa macrophylla*) is also prescribed. The above local application of medicaments is usually advised after bloodletting (*raktamokshana*).

16.9.3.7 Systemic Treatment

Medicated ghee prepared with *madhuyasthi* (*Glycyrhiza glabra*), *draksha* (*Vitis venifera*), *shyama* (*Callicarpa macrophylla*), *girihwa* (*Clitoria ternatea*), *anjanaki* (*Strychnus colubrina*), and *yavatikta* (*Erythraea roxburgii*) is given internally.

16.9.3.8 Treatment of Kaphaja Tumors

Local application of various medicated pastes are used after detoxification (*samshodhana chikitsa*) especially after emesis (*vamana*). The paste of the drugs used for emesis (*vamana*) and purgation (*virechana*) may also be applied locally to arrest the disease.

Caustics (*kshara*) in a cow's urine are also prescribed as a local application for *kaphaja* tumors after the bloodletting procedure.

16.9.3.9 Treatment of Medaja Tumors

Surgical and parasurgical approaches for the management of *medaja* tumors are emphasized in Ayurveda. Nevertheless, medicated paste containing *haridra* (*Curcuma longa*), *lodhra* (*Symplocos recemosa*), *patanga* (*Caesalpinia sappan*), *manashila* (real gar), and *haritala* (opiment) mixed with honey is also used as a local application.

16.9.3.10 Bloodletting (Raktamokshana)

Bloodletting is indicated after detoxification in the management of *vataja, pittaja, kaphaja,* and *medaja* tumors. The use of cow's horn, nonpoisonous leeches, and gourd (*Lagenaria vulgaris*) for bloodletting has been advised in *vataja, pittaja,* and *kaphaja* tumors, respectively. In *medaja* tumors, bloodletting has been advised after making an incision over the tumor.

16.9.3.11 Use of Cautery and Application of Caustics (Agnikarma and Ksharakarma)

Thermal cauterization (*agnikarma*) and application of caustics (*ksharakarma*) is used alone or in combination with surgery for the management of *kaphaja* tumors, *medaja* tumors, and tumors that do not respond to medical treatment.

The recurrence of a tumor after surgical excision was recognized by Sushruta. His idea was that even the last particle of *dosa* of a tumor left over would lead to a fresh growth and bring death, just like the last spark of an unextinguished fire. A radical excision was advised to avoid recurrence. Because it may not be possible to remove an entire tumor mass by surgery, therapeutic cautery and the application of caustics (*ksharakarma*) have been advised especially after surgery.

16.9.3.12 Maggotification

Maggotification (currently not practiced) is another important parasurgical treatment of tumors that was practiced by early Ayurvedic practitioners. In this unique technique, the gradual destruction of a tumor mass was achieved by maggotification of tumor. To attract the flies, *kulattha* (*Dolichos biflorus*), oil cakes of sesamum, and powder of dry meat are mixed with curd. This solution should be applied over the *arbuda* so that worms and parasites either grow locally or are attracted toward the tumor. They feed upon the tumor, and when only a small part of the tumor remains, the worms and the paste should be washed off the area and the remnant mass should be treated with cautery.

Local treatments mentioned in Ayurveda, like medicated poultice (*upanaha*), sudation (*swedana*), application of medicated pastes (*lepana*), and bloodletting (*raktamokshana*), are being practiced by Ayurvedic physicians in cancer as well as various other disorders. However, there is a lack of *in vitro* or *in vivo* trials and scientific studies to support their role in different types of cancer.

16.9.4 Surgical Management

16.9.4.1 Indications

If a tumor (*arbuda*) does not resolve or respond to proper medical treatment, it should be treated surgically. The main surgical treatments of tumors are excision (*chhedana*) and excision with scrapping (*lekhana*).

Sushruta has described certain principles of the excision of tumors as follows:

1. Tumor mass is removed completely. The incomplete removal leads to recurrence and poor prognosis.
2. Efforts are made to prevent the intraoperative spread of the tumor to distal organs. Historically, application of metal tourniquets made up of iron, copper, zinc, and lead were used around the tumor to control the spread. The mass is then destroyed by cautery (*agni*), caustics (*kshara*), or surgically depending upon the depth and extent of the tumor.
3. Sushruta advocated a minimal invasive technique in inoperable tumors or tumors situated over vital areas (*marma*). In this case, a strong caustic thread (*ksharasutra*) is passed across the center of its base with the help of a needle. The ends of the thread should be tied firmly on either side, leading to avascular necrosis of the tumor mass.

These principles of treatment occupy an important place in surgical oncology even today. Application of tourniquets, the no-touch technique of excision, and the ligation of feeding vessels are some of the important operative techniques that are still in practice to prevent the spread of the tumor.

After surgical excision, the area is cauterized (*agni/kshara*) to achieve a complete cure. Cleansing (*shodhana karma*) of the wound should be undertaken after excision of the tumor. The wound has to be cleaned using the decoction of *aparajita* (*Clitorea teratea*), *jati* (*Jasminum grandiflorum*), and *karaveera* (*Neium odorum*). The oil prepared from *bharangi* (*Clerodendrum serratum*), *vidanga* (*Embelia ribes*), and the paste of *triphala* (*Terminalia chebula, Terminalia belerica, Emblica officinalis*) can enhance the healing of wounds. Suppurated wounds may be treated according to measures mentioned for the management of infected ulcers (*dushta vrana*).

The efficacy of the above-mentioned drugs in wound healing has been established by various experimental and clinical trials. Therefore, these drugs can be used safely in conjugation with conventional surgical treatment.

16.9.4.2 Conventional Medicine

There are three sets of goals in conventional management of cancer patients: therapeutic, human, and scientific.[1] Ayurvedic medicine has similar goals. The therapeutic goal is to

TABLE 16.8

Tumor Response to Chemotherapy in Conventional Medicine

Cure (>30%) of Advanced Disease	Significant Cures (5–30%)	Probably Increases Survival	Adjuvant Treatment Leading to Increased Cure
Choriocarcinoma, acute lymphocytic leukemia (childhood), malignant lymphoma (Hodgkin's disease)	Ovarian cancer	Breast cancer	Breast cancer
Hairy-cell leukemia	Bladder cancer	Multiple myeloma	Colon cancer
Testicular cancer	Small-cell lung cancer	Head and neck cancer	Osteogenic sarcoma
Childhood tumors (e.g., embryonal rhabdomyosarcoma, Ewing's sarcoma, Wilm's tumor)	Gastric cancer		Early stage of large-cell lymphoma
Acute myelocytic leukemia			
Acute lymphocytic leukemia (adult)			
Prtomyelocytic leukemia			

Source: From Goldman, L. and Bennett, J.C., *Cecil Text Book of Medicine,* Part XIV, W.B. Saunders, Philadelphia, 2000. With permission.

cure patients and return them to normal life. If this is not attainable, then the next step in this goal is to help patients achieve long, qualitatively satisfactory remission, or on a tertiary level, a remission of any kind and finally terminal comfort care. The human goal in oncology is that the needs of the patient, family, and social environment be understood and met. The scientific goal requires special methods in oncology provided by specialists to deliver optimal clinical care.

In conventional medicine, effective anticancer therapy has integrated medical management with surgery and radiation therapy. The development of new cytotoxic and endocrine agents and the introduction of biologic therapy based on recombinant synthesis of interferon and cytokines have helped expand medical management. Not all patients are candidates for cancer therapy because of limitations in available drugs or comorbidity from other medical problems. In addition, not all tumors are responsive to chemotherapy (Table 16.8). Although many of the tumors are manageable by various chemotherapeutic agents, they are associated with the causation of various toxicities (Table 16.9).[15]

Antitumor drugs fail to cure cancer because they cannot kill 100% of the cancer cells. Even if one cell survives the chemotherapy, that cell can grow very quickly into millions of cells. The result is a relapse of cancer because the body immunity defense does not recognize the remaining cancer cells as foreign cells and thus does not kill them. Cancer cells can hide behind the blood barriers for drugs, such as for blood-brain barrier, and therefore do not get killed. The other mechanisms responsible for the failure of chemotherapy are the metabolism of drugs to inactive form, removal of drugs by binding to plasma proteins, rapid urinary excretion, and the development of resistance in the tumor cells due to an increase in certain critical enzymes that are inhibited by the drug. For example, tumors resistant to methotrexate were found to have high levels of dihydrofolate reductase, a key enzyme.[16–22] Transport across the cell membrane is also an obstacle in reaching the agent to the malignant cell. This can sometimes present a formidable barrier

TABLE 16.9

Toxicity of Antitumor Drugs of Conventional Medicine

Type of Agent	Major Clinical Toxicities
Alylating agents	Cardiac, renal, hepatic, lungs, bone marrow, GI tract
Antifolates	Bone marrow depression, intestinal epithelium, interstitial pneumonitis, neurotoxicity
Pyrimidine analogs	GI toxicity, ulceration of GI mucosa, neurotoxicity, cardiotoxicity, myelosuppression, leucopenia
Purine analogs	Bone marrow suppression, GI tract toxicity, hepatic necrosis, immunosuppression
Vinca alkaloids	Leukopenia, neurotoxicity, GI tract toxicity
Paclitaxel	Neutropenia, bone marrow suppression, neurotoxicity, hypersensitivity reactions
Actinomycin D	GI tract toxicity, bone marrow suppression, hematopoetic suppression, ulceration of oral mucosa
Daunorubicin, doxorubicin, and idarubicin	Bone marrow suppression, GI tract toxicity, cardiac toxicity
Bleomycin	Myelosuppression, cutaneouss toxicity, pulmonary toxicity, hyperthermia, hypotension, exacerbations of rheumatoid arthritis
Plicamycin	Bone marrow depression, liver and kidney toxicity, GI tract toxicity and neurotoxicity
Platinum compounds	Nephrotoxicity, hearing loss, peripheral neuropathy, myelosuppression, hemolytic anemia, cardiotoxicity

Source: From Calabresi, P. and Chabner, B.A., *Goodman & Gillman's The Pharacological Basis of Therapeutics,* Sec. 10, McGraw-Hill, New York, 1996. With permission.

and may be one of the reasons why some tumors are insensitive to some of the chemotherapeutic agents.[23] Mechanisms of resistance to some common drugs are listed below.[1]

Methotrexate	Impaired transport or amplification of dihydrofolate reductase
Cytarabine	Decrease in deoxycytidine kinase or increase in cytidine deaminase
5-Fluorouracil	Increase in thymidylate synthetase enzyme
Cisplatin	Decreased uptake, increase in repair enzymes
Taxol-Vinca alkaloids	Multidrug resistance (MDR) expression, mutations in tubulin (decreased binding)
Doxorubicin	MDR expression, decrease or alterations in topoisomerase II
Irinotecan, topotecan	Decrease in topoisomerase I

Cancer chemotherapy research in conventional medicine is primarily focused on developing analogs of purines, pyrimidines, and various vitamins like folic acid, plant products, and biological products. Various approaches have also been tried to overcome tumor resistance to various drugs. For example, an attempt has been made to take advantage of an increase in the enzyme responsible for the drug resistance. This approach is called enzyme dependent lethal synthesis. It was speculated that tetrahydrohomofolic acid, an analog of natural tetrahydrofolic acid (an inhibitor of thymidylate sythetase), may inhibit DNA synthesis and overcome the resistance. Studies have shown that dihydrohomofolic acid, a good substrate of dihydrofolate reductase, produced selective tumor inhibition only in methotrexate-resistant tumors containing high levels of dihydrofolate reductase enzyme.[16–22] After administering dihydrohomofolic acid to tumor-bearing mice, several folds of higher levels of tetrahydrohomofolic acid were found only in resistant tumors containing high levels of dihydrofolate reductase enzyme than in the methotrexate sensitive tumors confirming the hypothesis. A similar approach can be used with other agents where an increase in a key enzyme is responsible for the drug resistance.

16.10 Scientific Basis

Giving due importance to the various drugs and formulations that have been mentioned for the management of various *arbuda*, the modern-day researchers have been trying these drugs in various animal models. The researchers' goal is to find the drug's mode of action, realizing the dream of generating a magical potion for the eradication of cancers.

Various herbs used in Ayurveda are being researched both experimentally and clinically in various institutions. Drugs and drug fractions with antitumor activity are summarized in Table 16.10. Clinical, animal, and *in vitro* studies on some of the Ayurvedic herbs are presented below.

16.10.1 Clinical Studies

There are only two clinical studies available on antitumor herbal formulations. In the first study,[24] an Ayuravedic formula containing *bhallataka* (*Semicarpus anacardium*), *rohitaka* (*Amoora rohitaka*), and *yastimadhu* (*Glyceriza glabra*) was studied on 100 patients with different types of malignancy, as an adjuvant therapy, in a dose of 1.5 g/day in two divided doses, given after food. The study concluded that this compound is effective in cancer patients as evidenced by increases in body weight, appetite status, and hemoglobin percentage. It also reduced the mortality rate in studied cases. It can be used along with conventional therapy to improve the general condition of the patient. This compound can be used in lymphoma patients along with chemotherapy and radiotherapy, as it reduces the lymphophenic effect of chemotherapy and improves the hemoglobin level of the patients.[25]

In the second study,[26] the efficacy and side effects of an Ayurvedic arsenic-compound formula were evaluated. This is in light of the fact that just over 100 years ago arsenic was recognized in the West as useful in the control of blood counts in patients with chronic myeloid leukemia.

16.10.2 *In Vitro* studies

In one *in vitro* study,[27] extracts of the flowers of *Calotropis procera* (asclepiadaceae) and the nuts of *Semecarpus anacardium* (anacardiaceae) displayed the strongest cytotoxic effect with 50% inhibitory dose (ID_{50}) values of 1.4 and 1.6 μg/ml, respectively.

16.10.3 Animal Studies

16.10.3.1 Ashwagandha (Withania somnifera)

Withaferin A, isolated from the roots of *W. somnifera*, was found effective in Ehrlich ascitis carcinoma when given at a dose of 30 mg/kg along with radiation therapy.[28,29] Antioxidant and detoxifying properties of *W. somnifera* may be responsible for chemopreventive activity.[30]

Administration of 75% methanolic extract of *W. somnifera* was found to significantly increase the total white blood cell (WBC) count in normal Balb/c mice and reduce the leucopenia induced by a sublethal dose of gamma radiation. Treatment with *W. somnifera* was found to significantly increase the bone marrow cellularity in mice. *W. somnifera*

TABLE 16.10

Herbs and Herbal Fractions with Antitumor Activity

Plant	Botanical Name	Parts Used	Dose	Action as Mentioned in Classics	Proven Actions	Ref.
Bhallataka	*Semicarpus anacardium*	Fruit	3–6 g	*Lekhana* (excises unhealthy tissues), *rasayana* (rejuvenator)	Has antitumor activity against experimental mammary carcinoma in animals	65,66
Ashwagandha	*Withania somnifera*	Root	3–6 g	*Shothahara* (reduces swellings), *rasayana* (rejuvenator)	Alcoholic extract of the root in doses of 400 mg/kg and above produces complete regression of two-stage skin carcinogenesis induced by DMBA and croton oil	35,67,68
Kumkuma	*Crocus sativa*	Stamens	$^1/_2$–1 g	*Shothahara* (reduces swellings), *rasayana* (rejuvenator)	Has antitumor activity toward sarcoma-180 and Ehrlich ascites carcinoma (EAC) solid tumors in mice	69
Bhunimba	*Andrographis paniculata*	All parts	1–3 g	*Raktashodhaka* (purifies vitiated blood), *shothahara* (reduces swellings)	Prevents chemotoxicity including carcinogenicity	70
Tulasi	*Ocimum sanctum*	Leaf, seed, root	1–3 g	*Vishaghna* (detoxifies), *shothahara* (reduces swellings), *raktashodhaka* (purifies vitiated blood)	Reduces 20-methylcholanthrene-induced tumor incidence and tumor volume	71
Manduka parni	*Centella asiatica*	All parts	Juice 10–20 ml	*Kaphahara* (cleanses vitiated *kapha*), *shothahara*, (reduces swellings), *rasayana* (rejuvenator)	Retards the development of solid and ascites tumors and increases the life span of these tumor-bearing mice	72
Arka	*Calotropis procera*	Root, latex, flower	0.5–1 g	*Kaphashamaka* (pacifies vitiated *kapha*), *shothahara* (reduces swellings), *raktashodhaka* (purifies *vitiated* blood), vishaghna (detoxifier)	Displays the strongest cytotoxic effect with ID_{50} values of 1.4 μg/ml	27
Chitraka	*Plumbago rosea*	Root bark	1–2 g	*Lekhana* (excises unhealthy tissue), *shothahara* (reduces swellings), *rasayana* (rejuvenator)	Used with radiation to enhance the tumor-killing effect	73
Bakuchi	*Psoralea coryfolia*	Seed, seed oil	1–3 g	*Kaphagna* (pacifies vitiated *kapha*), *shothahara* (reduces swellings), *vrana shodhana* (cleanses chronic wounds), *vrana ropana* (heals wounds)	100 mg/kg body weight (of the active fraction) inhibits the growth and delays the onset of papilloma formation in mice; the active fraction at the same dose, when administered orally inhibits the growth of subcutaneously injected 20-methylcholantherene-induced soft tissue fibrosarcoma significantly	74

Katuki	*Picrorhiza kurroa*	Root	½–1 g	*Kaphagna* (pacifies vitiated *kapha*), *shothahara* (reduces swellings), *raktashodhaka* (purifies vitiated blood), *lekhana* (excises unhealthy tissue)	Picroliv (100 and 200 mg/kg) inhibits the sarcoma development by 47 and 53%; it also delays the onset of first skin tumor in the group of animals treated with Picroliv; Picroliv administration increases the life span of transplanted Dalton's lymphoma ascites (DLA) and Ehrlich ascites carcinoma (EAC)-harboring mice and reduces the volume of transplanted solid tumors	75
Aragvadha	*Cassia fistula*	Fruit pulp, root bark	5–10 g	*Kaphashodhaka* (pacifies vitiated *kapha*), *shothahara* (reduces swellings)	Increases life span by decreasing the tumor volume and viable tumor cell count in the EAC tumor hosts; improves the hematological factors after methanolic extract treatment, like hemoglobin content, red blood cell count and bone marrow cell count of the tumor-bearing mice	76
Kumari	*Aloe vera*	Leaf	10–20 ml	Kaphahara (pacifies vitiated *kapha*), *shothahara* (reduces swellings), *vrana ropana* (heals wounds), *raktashodhaka* (purifies vitiated blood)	Detoxifies reactive metabolites including chemical carcinogens and drugs	77
Kalajaji	*Nigella sativa*	Seed	1–3 g	*Kaphashamaka* (pacifies vitiated *kapha*), *lekhana* (excises unhealthy tissue), *shothahara* (reduces swellings)	*In vivo* EAC tumor development is completely inhibited by the active principle at the dose of 2 mg/mouse/day $\times 10^{16}$	78
Vamsha	*Bambusa arundinacea*	Root, leaf, Shoot	50–100 ml	*Kaphashamaka* (pacifies vitiated *kapha*), *lekhana* (excises unhealthy tissue), *vishaghna* (detoxifier)	Antitumor activity against benzopyrene and 4-nitroquinolince-1-oxide-induced tumors is highest with 1% bamboo leaf extracts (0.71 mg/ml) and a direct action of bamboo leaf extracts on tumor cells is indicated	79
Hingu	*Ferula narthex*	Latex	Up to 0.5 g	*Kaphahara* (normalizes vitiated *kapha*)	Asafoetida is a potent antioxidant and can afford protection against free radical mediated diseases such as carcinogenesis	80
Methika	*Trigonella foenum-*Graecum	Seed	1–3 g	*Shothahara* (reduces swellings)	Has an anti-inflammatory and antineoplastic effect	81
Amala	*Emblica officinalis* Gaertn	Fruit	4–10 g	*Shothahara* (reduces swellings)	Antioxidant, antitumor, chemopreventive, prostate cancer, immunomodulator, anticlastogenic radiation protection	82–96

treatment of irradiated mice normalized the ratio of normochromatic erythrocytes and polychromatic erythrocytes. Major activity of *W. somnifera* seems to be in the stimulation of stem cell proliferation.[31]

The alcoholic extract of dried roots of *W. somnifera* and Withaferin A showed significant antitumor and radio-sensitizing effects in experimental tumors *in vivo* without any noticeable systemic toxicity. The mechanism of action, however, is not clear. The studies indicate that *W. somnifera* could prove to be a good natural source of a potent and relatively safe radio-sensitizer and chemotherapeutic agent. Further studies are needed to explore the clinical potential of the plant for cancer therapy.[32]

W. somnifera was injected at a dose of 500 mg/kg to tumor-bearing mice (tumor size: 50 $\pm$ 5 mm^3) for 10 days with one local exposure of radiation therapy followed by hyperthermia. It significantly increased the tumor cure rate, produced a delay in the growth of partially responding tumors, and increased animal survival. Study concluded that *W. somnifera*, in addition to having a tumor-inhibitory effect, also acts as a radio sensitizer.[33] *W. somnifera* extract also inhibited 20-methylcholanthrene-induced sarcoma development in mice at a dose of 20 mg/day.[34] *W. somnifera* extract was also found to reduce two-stage skin carcinogenesis induced by DMBA and croton oil.[35]

Withaferin A reduced survival of V79 cells in a dose-dependent manner. LD50 for survival was 16 μM. One-hour treatment with a non-toxic dose of 2.1 μM before irradiation significantly enhanced cell killing, giving a sensitizer enhancement ratio (SER) of 1.5 for 37% survival and 1.4 for 10% survival.[36] *W. somnifera* was found to significantly reduce leucopenia induced by cyclophosphamide (CTX) treatment. The total WBC count on the 12th day of the CTX-treated group was 3720 cells/mm^3; the WBC count in CTX-treated animals that were simultaneously treated with WS was 6120 cells/mm^3. Withania extract increased the number of alpha-esterase positive cells (1130/4000 cells) in the bone marrow of CTX plus *W. somnifera*-treated animals, compared with the CTX-treated group (687/4000 cells).[37]

W. somnifera was also found to enhance the levels of interferon gamma (IFN-gamma) (75.87 pg/ml), Interleukin-2 (IL-2) (14.16 pg/ml), and granulocyte macrophage colony-stimulating factor (GM-CSF) (49.22 pg/ml) in normal Balb/c mice. The lowered levels of IFN-gamma (30 pg/ml), IL-2 (4.5 pg/ml), and GM-CSF (19.12 pg/ml) after treatment with CTX was reversed by the administration of *W. somnifera* extract (IFN gamma = 74 pg/ml; IL-2 7.5 = pg/ml; GM-CSF = 35.47 pg/ml). *W. somnifera* extract lowered the levels of tumor necrosis factor alpha (TNF alpha) production. Administration of bone marrow cells from donor mice treated with WS extract increased the spleen nodular colonies in irradiated mice (8.33) compared with those treated with normal bonemarrow cells (3.03). The number of nodular colonies increased significantly after continuous treatment with WS. These results indicate the immunopotentiating and myeloprotective effects of *W. somnifera*.[38]

W. somnifera extract was also found effective as a chemopreventive agent. *W. somnifera* protected against 20-methylcholanthrene-induced fibrosarcoma tumors in Swiss albino mice. A single subcutaneous injection of 200 μg of 20-methylcholanthrene in 0.1 ml of dimethylsulphoxide into the thigh region of mice produced a high incidence (96%) of tumors. Oral treatment of animals with 400 mg/kg body weight of *W. somnifera* extract (1 week before injecting 20-methylcholanthrene and continuing until 15 weeks thereafter) significantly reduced the tumor incidence and tumor volume and enhanced the survival of the mice, compared with the untreated 20-methylcholanthrene-injected mice. The occurrence of tumors was also delayed in the treatment group. Liver biochemical parameters revealed a significant modulation of reduced glutathione, lipid peroxides, glutathione-S-transferase, catalase, and superoxide dismutase in extract-treated mice compared with 20-methylcholanthrene-injected mice. The authors suggested that the mechanism of chemopreventive activity of *Withania somnifera* extract may be due to its antioxidant and detoxifying properties.[39] *W. somnifera* was also found to increase the neutrophil count in mice with paclitaxel-induced neutropenia.[40]

16.10.3.2 Aloe vera Linn.

Di (2-ethylhexyl) phthalate (DEHP), an active principle isolated from *Aloe vera* Linn., has been shown to have antileukemic and antimutagenic effects *in vitro* in *Salmonella typhimurium* TA98 and TA 100 strains.[41] Aloes potentiated the antitumor effect of 5-fluorouracil and cyclophosphamide as components of combination chemotherapy.[42] Aloe-emodin, a hydroxyanthraquinone present in *Aloe vera* leaves, has been shown to have a specific *in vitro* and *in vivo* antineuroectodermal tumor activity.[43]

Aloe vera has been claimed to contain several important therapeutic properties, including anticancerous effects. The effect of this drug was studied on a pleural tumor in rat (Yoshida AH-130, ascite hematoma cells) and proved its therapeutic use in cancer.[44]

In one study, the antigenotoxic and chemopreventive effect of *Aloe barbadensis* Miller (polysaccharide fraction) on benzo[a]pyrene (B[a]P)-DNA adducts was investigated *in vitro* and *in vivo*. Aloe showed a time-course and dose-dependent inhibition of [3H]B[a]P-DNA adduct formation in primary rat hepatocytes (1×10^6 cells/ml) treated with [3H]B[a]P (4 nmol/ml).[45] The growth of human neuroectodermal tumors is inhibited in mice with severe combined immunodeficiency without any appreciable toxic effects on the animals. The compound does not inhibit the proliferation of normal fibroblasts nor that of hemopoietic progenitor cells. The cytotoxicity mechanism consists of the induction of apoptosis, whereas the selectivity against neuroectodermal tumor cells appear to depend upon a specific energy-dependent pathway of drug incorporation.[46]

Crude modified aloe polysaccharide (MAP) activated macrophage cells and stimulated fibroblast growth. Under the same conditions, native *Aloe barbadensis* gel had no effect on macrophage activation. MAP prevented ultraviolet B (UVB) irradiation-induced immune suppression as determined by contact hypersensitivity (CHS) response in C3H/HeN mice.[47] Aloin- or sennoside-enriched diets (0.03%) did not promote incidence and growth of adenomas and carcinomas after 20 weeks in a model of dimethylhydrazine-induced colorectal tumors in male mice. In addition, no significant changes in serum electrolytes and parameters of hepato- and nephrotoxicity were observed in the aloe-fed mice.[47]

A new immunostimulatory polysaccharide called Aloeride from commercial *Aloe vera* (*Aloe barbadensis*) juice has been isolated and characterized. It is between 4 and 7 million Da, and its glycosyl components include glucose (37.2%), galactose (23.9%), mannose (19.5%), and arabinose (10.3%). Although Aloeride comprises only 0.015% of the aloe juice dry weight, its potency for macrophage activation accounts fully for the activity of the crude juice.[48]

16.10.3.3 Coleus forskohlii

Forskolin, a diterpene from *C. forskohlii,* is a potent platelet aggregation inhibitor. It has been found to strongly inhibit the melanoma cell-induced human platelet aggregation and tumor colonization. The study suggests that forskolin could prove to be valuable in the clinic for the prevention of cancer metastasis.[49]

Roidex, a formulation of squalene, vitamin E, and *Aloe vera*, produced chemopreventive effect in chemically induced skin tumors in CD-1 mice. The tumors were induced by 7,12-dimethylbenz[*a*]-anthracene (DMBA) and promoted with 12-*O*-tetradecanoylphorbol-13-acetate (TPA). The mice were treated with either mineral oil, 5% squalene, or Roidex. There was a regression of 33.34% of the tumors in the Roidex-treated group (39 to 26 tumors) compared with the nontreated group, whose tumors regressed only 3.44% (29 to 28 tumors).[50] An immunomodulator fraction extracted from Aloe vahombe (Alva) was found to protect mice against bacterial, parasitic, and fungal infections. It also produced cures only in the case of the McC3-1 tumor; under different experimental conditions, the growth rate of tumors in animals treated was found to be slower than in those untreated.[51]

16.10.3.4 *Andrographis paniculata* Nees

The methanol extract of the aerial part of *Andrographis paniculata* Nees showed potent cell differentiation-inducing activity on mouse myeloid leukemia (M1) cells.[52]

16.10.3.5 *Santalum album*

The essential oil, emulsion, or paste of *S. album* has been used in India as an Ayurvedic medicinal agent for the treatment of inflammatory and eruptive skin diseases. Sandlewood-oil treatment showed chemopreventive effect in DMBA-initiated and TPA-promoted skin papillomas tumor model and TPA-induced ornithine decarboxylase (ODC) activity in CD-1 mice. Sandalwood-oil treatment significantly decreased papilloma incidence by 67%, multiplicity by 96%, and TPA-induced ODC activity by 70%. The study suggests that the oil could be an effective chemopreventive agent against skin cancers.[53]

16.10.3.6 *Picrorrhiza kurroa*

P. kurroa extract has been shown to have antitumor and anticarcinogenic activity in 20-methylcholanthrene (20 MC)-induced tumor model after oral administration. The extract also inhibited transplantable tumors.[54]

16.10.3.7 Cystone

Cystone, a polyherbal ayurvedic preparation, was found to protect tumor-bearing mice from cisplatin-induced nephrotoxicity when given intraperitoneal 1 h before cisplatin. Pretreatment with cystone did not reduce the antitumor activity of cisplatin. The study shows potential for use in protecting patients from nephrotoxicity of cisplatin.[55]

16.10.3.8 Sesame Oil

Sesame oil is extensively used as topical application in Ayurveda for skin health. In one study, it was found that sesame and safflower oils, both of which contain large amounts of linoleate in triglyceride form, selectively inhibited malignant melanoma growth over normal melanocytes; coconut, olive, and mineral oils, which contain little or no linoleate as triglyceride, did not. Further studies showed that only linoleic acid was selectively inhibitory, whereas palmitic and oleic acid were not. These fatty acids were tested in the range of 3 to 100 μg/ml. The study suggests that certain vegetable oils rich in linoleic acid, such as the sesame oil, recommended for topical use by Ayurveda, may actually contain selective antineoplastic properties.[56]

16.10.3.9 *Terminalia arjuna*

Methanol extract of *T. arjuna* was found to inhibit the growth of human normal fibroblasts (WI-38) *in vitro* without any effect on normal cells. A cyclin-dependent kinase inhibitor, p21WAF1, was induced in the transformed cell by *T. arjuna*. It is likely that *T. arjuna* has components that can inhibit of transformed cell by p53-dependent and independent pathways.[57]

16.11 Conclusions and Future Research

It is evident that early Ayurvedic physicians had a good understanding of etiology, clinical manifestations, symptoms, classification, malignant and benign nature of tumors, metastasis, recurrence diagnosis, prognosis, and treatment. It is remarkable that the basic information is fairly consistent with the current knowledge in these areas given the technology available 500 years ago. The physicians also recognized the fact that malignant tumors must be completely and extensively excised so that not a trace of tumor is left in the body for even a trace can grow back to a tumor. This is also consistent with the current knowledge about the nature of malignant tumors and their treatment. Various treatment methods, both local and systemic, and various herbal formulations found useful in many tumors are presented. The review has shown that Ayurvedic therapies are useful as an adjuvant to conventional chemotherapy. The following areas are identified for further research: (1) the use as an adjuvant to improve the well-being of the patient, (2) protection against the drug cytotoxicity (the major dose limiting side effect), (3) chemoprevention to reduce the cancer incidence, and (4) immunomodulation to help the body respond better to cancer chemotherapy.

References

1. Goldman, L. and Bennett, J.C., Eds., Oncology, in *Cecil Text Book of Medicine,* Part XIV, W.B. Saunders, Philadelphia, 2000.
2. Mishra, L.C., Criteria for Classifying Carcinogens in Consumer Products for Purpose of Labeling under the Federal Hazardous Substances Act. Labeling Requirements for Art Materials and Other Products; Final Rules. *16 CFR Part 1500, Federal Registe*r/Vol. 57. No. 197/Friday, October 8, Carcinogenicity, p. 46632–46637, 1992.
3. Parmar, R.K., Comparative Study of Ayurveda in Relation to Neoplastic Lesions and its Management by Indigenous Drugs, M.D. thesis (Ayurveda), Institute of Medical Sciences, Banaras Hindu University, Varanasi, India, 1983.
4. Singh, L., Response of Poorvakarma in Different Types of Cancer Treatment, M.D. thesis (Ayurveda), Department of Shalya Shalakya, Faculty of Ayurveda, Institute of Medical Sciences, Banaras Hindu University, Varanasi, India, 1989.
5. Mohanty, K.R., Study in Immunological Alteration in Cancer under the Influence of Indigenous Drugs, M.D. thesis (Shalya), Department of Shalya Shalakya, Faculty of Ayurveda, Institute of Medical Sciences, Banaras Hindu University, Varanasi, India, 1991.
6. Singh, R.K., Evaluation of an Ayurvedic Compound (Rohitaka, Bhallataka) in Hepatobiliary and Gastrointestinal Malignancy: A Comparative Study, M.S. thesis (Shalya), Department of Shalya Shalakya, Faculty of Ayurveda, Institute of Medical Sciences, Banaras Hindu University, Varanasi, India, 1998.
7. Chalapathi Rao, K.V., Studies on Combined Use of Rohitaka and Bhallataka as an Adjuvant Therapy in the Management of Squamous Cell Carcinoma, M.S. thesis (Shalya), Department of Shalya Shalakya, Faculty of Ayurveda, Institute of Medical Sciences, Banaras Hindu University, Varanasi, India, 1998.
8. Reddy, P.V.S. et al., 1992, Kavitha, S. K. et al., 1996, Dua, P.K.G. et al., 1997, M.S. thesis (Shalya), Department of Shalya Shalakya, Faculty of Ayurveda, Institute of Medical Sciences, Banaras Hindu University, Varanasi, India, 1998.
9. David, L. and Kuttan, G., Suppressive effect of cyclophosphamide-induced toxicity by Withania somnifera extract in mice, *J. Ethnopharmacol.*, 62(3), 209–214, 1998.

10. Davis, L. and Kuttan, G., Effect of Withania somnifera on cytokine production in normal and cyclophosphamide treated mice, *Immunopharmacol. Immunotoxicol.*, 21(4), 695–703, 1999.
11. Rao, M., Praveen Rao, P.N., Kamath, R., and Rao, M.N., Reduction of cisplatin-induced nephrotoxicity by Cystone, a polyherbal Ayurvedic preparation, in C57BL/6J mice bearing B16F1 melanoma without reducing its anti tumor activity, *J. Ethnopharmacol.*, 68(1–3), 77–81, 1999.
12. Smith, D.E. and Salerno, J.W., Selective growth inhibition of a human malignant melanoma cell line by sesame oil in vitro, *Prostaglandins Leukot Essent Fatty Acids*, 46(2), 145–150, 1992.
13. Sharma, P.V., Granthi Apachi *Arbuda* Galaganda chikitsa adhyaya in Sushruta Samhita by Acharya Sushruta, 2000, p. 18, verses 29–30.
14. Sharma, P.V., Granthi Apachi *Arbuda* Galaganda chikitsa adhyaya in Sushruta Samhita by Acharya Sushruta, 2000, p. 18, verse 31.
15. Calabresi, P. and Chabner, B.A., Chemotherapy of neoplastic diseases, in *Goodman & Gillman's The Pharacological Basis of Therapeutics,* Sec. 10, Hardman, J.G., Limbird, L.E., Molinoff, P.B., Ruddon, R.W., and Gillman, A.G., Eds., McGraw-Hill, New York, 1996.
16. Mishra, L.C., Parmar, A.S., and Mead, J. A.R., The anti-leukemic activity of dihydrohomofolate (H_2HF) and its reduction to tetrahydrohomofolate (H_4HF) in mice, *Proc. Am. Assn. Cancer Res.*, 11, 57, 1970.
17. Mishra, L.C., Parmar, A.S., and Mead, J.A.R., The effect of pretreatment with methotrexate on the reduction of dihydrohomofolic acid in mice, *Biochem. Pharmacol.*, 20, 2871, 1971.
18. Mishra, L.C., Parmar, A.S., and Mead, J.A.R., Chemical transformations of tetrahydrohomofolic acid in vitro and in vivo, *Chem.-Biol. Interact.*, 4, 97, 1971-1972.
19. Mishra, L.C. and Mead, J.A.R., On the biochemical mechanism of action of tetrahydrohomofolic acid, *Biochem. Pharmacol.*, 21, 579, 1972.
20. Mishra, L.C., Parmar, A.S., and Mead, J.A.R., Assessment of dihydrofolate reductase (H_2F-R) activity in vivo after administration of ^3H-dihydrofolate, *Pharmacologist,* 13, 208, 1971.
21. Mishra, L.C., Parmar, A.S., and Mead, J.A.R., A method to assess dihydrofolate-reductase inhibition in vivo, *Anal. Biochem.*, 48, 515, 1972.
22. Mishra, L.C., Parmar, A.S., and Mead, J.A.R., Regeneration of tetrahydrohomofolate in cells, *Biochem. Pharmacol.*, 23, 1827, 1974.
23. Double, J.A., Extra cellular factors affecting the response of tumors to chemotherapeutic agents in recent results in cancer research, *George's Math.*, 21, 24–25, 1969.
24. Sahu, M., Role of Certain Indigenous Drugs of an Adjuvant Therapy in the Management of Cancer, M.D. thesis (Shalya), Department of Shalya Shalakya, Faculty of Ayurveda, Institute of Medical Sciences, Banaras Hindu University, Varanasi, India, 1980.
25. Sahu, R.N., Role of Ayurvedic Compound as an Adjuvant in the Management of Lymphoma, M.D. thesis (Shalya), Department of Shalya Shalakya, Faculty of Ayurveda, Institute of Medical Sciences, Banaras Hindu University, Varanasi, India, 1998.
26. Treleaven, J., Meller, S., Farmer, P., Birchall, D., Goldman, J., and Piller, G., Arsenic and Ayurveda, *Leukemia Lymphoma*, 10, 343, 1993; comment in *Leukemia Lymphoma*, 16, 189, 1994.
27. Smit, H.F., Woerdenbag, H.J., and Singh, R.H., Ayurvedic herbal drugs with possible cytostatic activity, *J. Ethnopharmacol.*, 47(2), 75–84, 1995.
28. Devi, P.U., Sharada, A.C., and Solomon, F.E., In vivo growth inhibitory and radio sensitizing effects of Withaferin on mouse Ehrlich ascitis carcinoma, *Cancer Lett.*, 16, 95(1–2), 189–193, 1995.
29. Sharada, A.C., Solomon, F.E., Devi, P.U., Udupa, N., and Srinivasan, K.K., Anti tumor and radiosensitizing effects of Withaferin A on mouse Ehrlich ascites carcinoma in vivo, *Acta Oncol.*, 35(1), 95–100, 1996.
30. Prakash, J., Gupta, S.K., Kochupillai, V., Singh, N., Gupta, Y.K., and Joshi, S., Chemopreventive activity of *Withania somnifera* in experimentally induced fibrosarcoma tumors in Swiss albino mice, *Phytother. Res.*, 15(3), 240–244, 2001.
31. Kuttan, G., Use of Withania somnifera Dunal as an adjuvant during radiation therapy, *Indian J. Exp. Biol.*, 34(9), 854–856, 1996.
32. Devi, P.U., Withania somnifera Dunal (*Ashwagandha*) potential plant source of a promising drug for cancer chemotherapy and radio sensitization, *Indian J. Exp. Biol.*, 34(10), 927–932, 1996.

33. Devi, P.U., Sharada, A.C., and Solomon, F.E., Anti tumor and radiosensitizing effects of *Withania somnifera* (*Ashwagandha*) on a transplantable mouse tumor, Sarcoma-180, *Indian J. Exp. Biol.*, 31(7), 607–611, 1993.
34. Davis, L. and Kuttan, G., Effect of *Withania somnifera* on 20-methylcholanthrene induced fibrosarcoma, *J. Exp. Clin. Cancer Res.*, 19(2), 165–167, 2000.
35. Davis, L. and Kuttan, G., Effect of Withania somnifera on DMBA induced carcinogenesis, *J. Ethnopharmacol.*, 75(2–3), 165–168, 2001.
36. Devi, P.U., Akagi, K., Ostapenko, V., Tanaka, Y., and Sugahara, T., Withaferin A: a new radiosensitizer from the Indian medicinal plant Withania Somnifera, *Int. J. Radiat. Biol.*, 69, 193, 1996.
37. Davis, L. and Kuttan, G., Suppressive effect of cyclophosphamide-induced toxicity by Withania somnifera extract in mice, *J. Ethnopharmacol.*, 62, 209, 1998.
38. Davis, L. and Kuttan, G., Effect of Withania somnifera on cytokine production in normal and cyclophosphamide treated mice, *Immunopharmacol. Immunotoxicol.*, 21, 695, 1999.
39. Prakash, J., Gupta, S.K., Kochupillai, V., Singh, N., Gupta, Y.K., and Joshi, S., Chemopreventive activity of Withania somnifera in experimentally induced fibrosarcoma tumors in Swiss albino mice, *Phytother. Res.*, 15(3), 240-244, 2001.
40. Gupta, Y.K., Sharma, S.S., Rai, K., and Katiyar, C.K., Reversal of paclitaxel induced neutropenia by Withania somnifera in mice, *Indian J. Physiol. Pharmacol.*, 45, 253, 2001.
41. Lee, K.H., Kim, J.H., Lim, D.S., and Kim, C.H., Anti leukaemic and antimutagenic effects of di (2-ethylhexyl) phthalate isolated from *Aloe vera*, *J. Pharm. Pharmacol.*, 52(5), 593–598, 2000.
42. Gribel, N.V. and Pashinskii, V.G., Anti-metastatic properties of Aloe juice, *Vopr. Onkol.*, 32(12), 38–40, 1986.
43. Pecere, T., Gazzola, M.V., Mucignat, C., et al., *Aloe emodin* is a new type of anticancer agent with selective activity against neuroectodermal tumors, *Cancer Res.*, 60 (11), 2800–2804, 2000.
44. Corsi, M.M., Bertelli, A.A., Gaja, G., et al., The therapeutic potential of Aloe vera in tumor bearing rats, *Int. J. Tissue React.*, 20(4), 115–118, 1998.
45. Kim, H.S. and Lee, B.M., Inhibition of benz[a]pyrene-DNA adduct formation by Aloe barbendensis Miller, *Carcinogenesis*, 18, 771, 1997.
46. Pecere, T., Gazzola, M.V., Mucignat, C., Parolin, C., Vecchia, F.D., Cavaggioni, A., Basso, G., Diaspro, A., Salvato, B., Carli, M., and Palu, G., Aloe-emodine is a new type of anticancer agent with selective activity against neuroectodermal tumors, *Cancer Res.*, 60, 2800, 2000.
47. Qiu, Z., Jones, K., Wylie, M., Jia, Q., and Orndorff, S., Modified Aloe barbadensis polysaccharide with immunoregulatory activity, *Planta Medica*, 66, 152, 2000; Siegers, C.P., Siemers, J., and Baretton, G., Sennosides and aloin do not promote dimethylhydrazine-induced colorectal tumors in mice, *Pharmacology*, 47, 205, 1993.
48. Pugh, N., Ross, S.A., ElSohly, M.A., and Pasco, D.S., Characterization of aloeride, a new high-molecular-weight polysaccharide from Aloe vera, *J. Agric. Food Chem.*, 49, 1030, 2001.
49. Agarwal, K.C. and Parks, R., Jr., Forskolin: a potential antimetastatic agent, *Int. J. Cancer*, 32, 801, 1983.
50. Desai, K.N., Wei, H., and Lamartiniere, C.A., The preventive and therapeutic potential of the squalene-containing compound, Roidex, on tumor promotion and regression, *Cancer Lett.*, 101, 93, 1996.
51. Ralamboranto, L., Rakotovao, L.H., Le Deaut, J.Y., Chaussoux, D., Salomonm, J.C., Fournet, B., and Montreuil, J., Rakotonirina-Randriambeloma, P.J., Dulat, C., and Coulanges, P., Immunomodulating properties of an extract isolated and partially purified from Aloe vahombe. III. Study of antitumoral properties and contribution to the chemical nature and active principle, *Arch. Inst. Pasteur Madagascar*, 50, 227, 1982.
52. Matsuda, T., Kuroyanagi, M., Sugiyama, S., Umehara, K., Ueno, A., and Nishi, K., Cell differentiation-inducing diterpenes from Andrographis paniculata Nees, *Chem. Pharm. Bull.* (Tokyo), 42, 1216, 1994.
53. Dwivedi, C. and Abu-Ghazaleh, A., Chemopreventive effects of sandalwood oil on skin papillomas in mice, *Eur. J. Cancer Prev.*, 6, 399, 1997.

54. Joy, K.L., Rajeshkumar, N.V., Kuttan, G., and Kuttan, R., Effect of Picrorrhiza kurroa extract on transplanted tumours and chemical carcinogenesis in mice, *J. Ethnopharmacol.*, 71, 261, 2000.
55. Rao, M., Praveen Rao, P.N., Kamath, R., and Rao, M.N., Reduction of cisplatin-induced nephrotoxicity by cystone, a polyherbal ayurvedic preparation, in C57BL/6J mice bearing B16F1 melanoma without reducing its antitumor activity, *J. Ethnopharmacol.*, 68, 77, 1999.
56. Smith, D.E. and Salerno, J.W., Selective growth inhibition of a human malignant melanoma cell line by sesame oil in vitro, *Prostaglandins Leukot Essent Fatty Acids*, 46, 145, 1992.
57. Nagpal, A., Meena, L.S., Kaur, S., Grover, I.S., Wadhwa, R., and Kaul, S.C., Growth suppression of human transformed cells by treatment with bark extracts from a medicinal plant, Terminalia arjuna, in vitro, *Cell Dev. Biol. Anim.*, 36, 544, 2000.
58. Kaviraja Ambikadatta shastry, Galagandadi roga chikitsa prakarana in Bhaishajya ratanavali by Govindadasa, 2001, chap. 44, p. 583, verse 59.
59. Kaviraja Ambikadatta shastry, Pleehayakrut roga chikitsa prakarana in Bhaishajya Ratanavali by Govindadasa, 2001, chap. 41, p. 545, verse 90.
60. Mishra, S.N., Dhatu prakarana in Rasendra Chudamani by Acharya Somadeva, 1984, chap. 14, p. 247, verse 70.
61. Kulkarni, D.A., Maharasa in Ras Ratna Samucchaya by Acharya Vagbhata, 1998, chap. 2, p. 18, verse 2.
62. Mishra, S.N., Dhatu prakarana in Rasendra Chudamani, by Acharya Somadeva, 1984, chap. 14, pp. 234–235, verse 22–23.
63. Shastry, L.P., Arbuda chikitsa in Yogaratnakara, 1988, p. 156, verse 4-6.
64. Ganekar, B.G. and Vaidya, L.C., Samshodhana samshamaneeya Adhyaya in sutrasthana of Sushruta Samhita by Acharya Sushruta, 5th ed., 1994, chap. 40, p. 142, verse 7.
65. Sujatha, V. and Sachadanandam, P., Recuperative effect of Semicarpus anacardium Linn., nut milk extract on carbohydrate metabolizing enzymes in experimental mammary carcinoma bearing rats, *Phytother. Res.*, 16 (Suppl. 1), 14–18, 2002.
66. Premalatha, B., Sujatha, V., and Sachadanandam, P., Modulating effect of Semicarpus anacardium Linn., nut extract on glucose metabolizing enzymes in aflatoxin B induced experimental hepatocellular carcinoma, *Pharmacol. Res.*, 36(3), 187–192, 1997.
67. Mishra, L.C., Singh, B.B., and Dagenias, S., Scientific basis for the therapeutic use of Withania somnifera (ashwagandha), a review, *Altern. Med. Rev.*, 5(4), 334–346, 2000.
68. Devi, P.U., Sharada, A.C., Solomon, F.E., and Kamath, M.S., In vivo growth inhibitory effect of *Withania somnifera* (*Ashwagandha*) on a transplantable mouse tumor, Sarcoma 180, *Indian J. Exp. Biol.*, 30 (3), 169–72, 1992.
69. Nair, S.C., Salomi, M.J., et al., Effect of saffron on thymocye proliferation, intracellular glutathione levels and its anti tumor activity, *Biofactors*, 4(1), 51–54, 1992.
70. Singh, R.P., Banerjee, S., and Rao, A.R., Modulatory influence of Andrographis paniculata on mouse hepatic and extra hepatic carcinogen metabolizing enzymes and anti-oxidant status, *Phytother. Res.*, 15(5), 382–390, 2001.
71. Prakash, J. and Gupta, S.K., Chemo preventive activity of Ocimum sanctum seed oil, *J. Ethnopharmacol.*, 72(1–2), 29–34, 2000.
72. Babu, T.D., Kuttan, G., and Paddikala, J., Cytotoxic and anti-tumor properties of certain taxa of Umbelliferae with special reference to Centella asiatica (L) Urban, *J. Ethnopharmacol.*, 11, 48(1), 53–57, 1995.
73. Devi, P.U., Sharada, A.C., and Solomon, F.E., In vivo tumor inhibitory and radio sensitizing effects of an Indian medicinal plant, Plumbago rosea on experimental mouse tumor, *Indian J. Exp. Biol.*, 32(8), 523–528, 1994.
74. Latha, P.G. and Panikkar, K.R., Inhibition of chemical carcinogenesis by Psoralea corylifolia seeds, *J. Ethnopharmacol.*, 68(1–3), 295–298, 1999.
75. Rajesh Kumar, N.V. and Kuttan, R., Protective effect of Picroliv, the active constituent of *Picrorhiza kurroa*, against chemical carcinogenesis in mice, *Teratog. Carcinog. Mutagen*, 21(4), 303–313, 2001.
76. Gupta, M., Mazumdar, J.K., Rath, N., and Mukhopadhyay, D.K., Anti-tumor activity of methanolic extract of *Cassia fistula* L. seed against ehrlich ascites carcinoma, *J. Ethnopharmacol.*, 72(1–2), 151–156, 2000.

77. Singh, R.P., Dhanalakshmi, S., and Rao, A.R., Chemomodulatory action of *Aloe vera* on the profiles of enzymes associated with carcinogen metabolism and anti oxidant status regulation in mice, *Phytomedicine,* 7(3), 209–219, 2000.
78. Salomi, N.J., Nair, S.C., Jaywardhanan, K.K., et al., Anti-tumor principles from *Nigella sativa* seeds, *Cancer Lett.*, 63(1), 41–46, 1992.
79. Kuboyama, N., Fujii, A., and Tamura, T., Anti tumor activities of bamboo leaf extracts (BLE) and its lignin (BLL), *Nippon Yakurigaku Zasshi,* 77(6), 579–596, 1981.
80. Saleem, M., Alam, A., and Sultana, S., Asafoetida inhibits early events of carcinogenesis, a chemo preventive study, *Life Sci.*, 68(16), 1913–1921, 2001.
81. Sur, P., Das, M., et al., Trignonella foenum graecum (fenugreek) seed extract as an anti-neoplastic agent, *Phytother. Res.*, 15(3), 257–259, 2001.
82. Bhattacharya, A. et al., Antioxidant activity of active tannoid principles of Emblica officinalis (amla), *Indian J. Exp. Biol.*, 37, 676, 1999.
83. Biswas, S. et al., Protection against cytotoxic effects of arsenic by dietary supplementation with crude extract of Emblica officinalis fruit, *Phytother. Res.*, 13, 513, 1999.
84. Darzynkiewicz, Z., Traganos, F., Wu, J.M., and Chen, S., Chinese herbal mixture PC SPES in treatment of prostate cancer (review), *Int. J Oncol.*, 17(4), 729–736, Oct. 2000.
85. Dhir, H., Roy, A.K., et al., Relative efficiency of Phyllanthus emblica fruit extract and ascorbic acid in modifying lead and aluminium-induced sister-chromatid exchanges in mouse bone marrow, *Environ. Mol. Mutagenesis,* 21, 229, 1993.
86. Freedland, S.J., Pantuck, A.J., Weider, J., Zisman, A., and Belldegrun, A.S., Immunotherapy of prostate cancer, *Curr. Urol. Rep.*, 2, 242, 2001.
87. Ghosh, A., Sharma, A., et al., Comparison of the protection afforded by a crude extract of Phyllanthus emblica fruit and an equivalent amount of synthetic ascorbic acid against the cytotoxic effects of cesium chloride in mice, *Int. J. Pharmacognosy,* 31, 116, 1993.
88. Jeena, K.J. et al., Effect of Emblica officinalis, Phyllanthus amarus and Picrorrhiza kurroa on N-nitrosodiethylamine induced hepatocarcinogenesis, *Cancer Lett.*, 136, 11, 1999.
89. Jeena, K.J., Girija, K., and Kuttan, R., Antitumor activity of Emblica officinalis, *J. Ethnopharmacol.*, 75, 65, 2001.
90. Nandi, P. et al., Dietary chemoprevention of clastogenic effects of 3,4-benzo(a)pyrene by Emblica officinalis Gaertn. fruit extract, *Br. J. Cancer,* 76, 1279, 1997.
91. Rege, N.N. et al., Adaptogenic properties of six rasayana herbs used in Ayurvedic medicine, *Phytother. Res.*, 13, 275, 1999.
92. Roy, A.K., Dhir, H., Sharma, A., and Talukder, G., Modifying role of phyllanthus emblica and ascorbic acid against nickel clastogencity in mice, *Cancer Lett.*, 59, 9, 1991.
93. Sai Ram, M., Neetu, D., Yogesh, B., Anju, B., Dipti, P., Pauline, T., Sharma, S.K. et al., Cytoprotective and immunomodulating properties of Amla (Emblica officinalis) on lymphocytes: an in-vitro study, *J. Ethnopharmacol.*, 81, 5, 2002.
94. Smith, M.R., Complementary and alternative therapies for advanced prostate cancer, *Hematol. Oncol. Clin. North Am.*, 15, 559, 2001.
95. Suresh, K. and Vasudevan, D.M., Augmentation of murine natural killer cell and antibody dependent cellular cytotoxicity activities by Phyllanthus emblica, a new immunomodulator, *J. Ethnopharmacol.*, 44, 55, 1994.
96. Yadav, S.K., Protection against radiation-induced chromosome damage by Emblica officinalis fruit extract, *Cryology,* 40, 261, 1987.

17

Indigestion (Ajirna)

Shankar K. Mitra and Paramesh R. Rangesh

CONTENTS

0-8493-1366-X/04/$0.00+$1.50

17.1 Introduction

Gastrointestinal (GI) symptoms are among the most common and widespread of health complaints among the general populace. An alternative term is dyspepsia. Dyspepsia is often used to refer to upper abdominal pain or discomfort but may also encompass symptoms of early satiety, postprandial abdominal bloating or distension, nausea, and vomiting. Dyspepsia can be episodic or persistent and is often exacerbated by eating. Indigestion is a general term used to describe discomfort or pain in the upper abdomen or chest, usually after meals.

Ayurvedic treatment is focused on the correction of gastrointestinal pathology for most of the endogenous disorders ranging from indigestion to arthritis. Ayurvedic texts describe the anatomy and physiology of the digestive system at great lengths. Here is a brief insight into the concepts of digestion and indigestion.

17.2 Ayurvedic Concept

17.2.1 The Stomach and Digestion

The stomach is one of the vital organs of the body (*marma*). The other important organs are the heart, lungs, kidneys, and the brain. The stomach not only stores food during the process of digestion, but also makes it more permeable through the juices it produces. The stomach has minute glands from which gastric juice (*pachaka pitta*) is produced. The gastric juice helps break down food into smaller molecules. The moment food enters the stomach, the wall of the organ starts a churning action to mix the food with the gastric juice so that it becomes absorbable. Foods that are easy to digest (*laghu ahara*), such as fat-free or low-fat milk and fat-free cereals or fruits, take far less time to digest than heavier foods (*guru ahara*), such as fried substances, which are rich in fat.

The partially digested food from the stomach enters the intestine and is then exposed to the action of bile, pancreatic and intestinal juices, and bacteria. The food is broken down into various easily absorbable substances, which are vital for growth and development, because these form the building blocks of the body. It is only when food has been eliminated from the intestine that the process of digestion is complete and the process of absorption starts.

17.2.2 *Agni* and Disease

Ayurvedic literature has recognized 13 types of enzymes (*agni*); the most important is the digestive enzyme (*jatharagni*), the primary factor of digestion. The others are the seven intracellular enzymes (*dhatu agni*) and the five organic catalysts (*bhuta agni*). The digestive enzyme (also called *koshthagni*) contained in the gastric juice is the source of all the enzymes of the body. In addition to the digestive enzyme, there are six other factors that help digestion process. They are gastric juice, gut motility factor (*samana vata*), moisture and water, mucin (*kledaka kapha*), time, and a proper combination of the first five. The gut motility factor propels the food into the stomach, bringing it into contact with gastric juice, and supports the enzymes; moisture breaks down the compactness of the food and mucin softens the food. Time is required for completing the process of digestion, and a proper combination of all factors is vital for completion of the process. The food is digested with the help of the digestive enzyme. This process results in the separation of the nutrient factors from the food, which circulate in the body and help in tissue building through the help of intracellular enzymes.

As long as this enzyme is in homoeostasis, it results in a state of health. Disease is the result of a deviation from this state. The imbalance of the digestive enzyme (including the enzymes of the stomach and intestine) gives rise to most disorders of the stomach, particularly anorexia and dyspepsia. This enzyme occurs in four states: balanced (*samagni*), abnormal (*vishamagni*), increased (*tikshnagni*), and decreased (*mandagni*). Except the balanced state, others are pathological states. These pathological states of enzymes are due to the influence of three *dosas*: *vata*, *pitta*, and *kapha*, respectively.

Physiologically, food undergoes three stages of conversion in the GI tract. The first is a mucilaginous neutral stage (*madhurabhava*) under the influence of *kapha*. The second stage, due to the interference of *pitta*, is an acidic stage (*amlabhava*), and the final stage is a dry, pungent stage (*katubhava*) under the effect of *vata*. Due to etiological factors such as abnormal food habits, emotional disturbances, etc., a pathological state of enzyme results called *agnimandya*. *Agnimandya* is the principal cause for all metabolic disorders commencing with indigestion (*ajirna*).

17.2.3 Indigestion

Indigestion, a deviation in any of the steps described above, also known as upset stomach, dyspepsia, or gastric indigestion, is discomfort or a burning feeling in the upper abdomen. It is often accompanied by nausea, abdominal bloating, belching, and sometimes vomiting.[1] Dyspepsia, which means bad (dys) digestion (pepsia), is a term often used by doctors to describe a set of symptoms believed to have their cause somewhere in the upper part of the GI tract.

Ayurvedic physicians diagnose the disease with clinical interrogation about the state of digestive enzymes and digestion with certain clinical features such as absence of hunger, abdominal discomfort, and belching of undigested food. The physicians also examine the abdomen by palpation and percussion for the presence of flatulence.

To diagnose indigestion, the doctor of conventional medicine might perform tests for problems like ulcers. In the process of diagnosis, a person may have x-rays of the stomach and small intestine or undergo an endoscopy, in which the doctor uses an instrument to look at the inside of the upper GI tract.

17.3 Definition

According to classic Ayurveda, the word *ajirna* in Sanskrit means bad (a) digestion (*jirna*). It is defined as a pathological condition in which food is not digested easily and is the root cause for many internal diseases (metabolic). In conventional medicine, the term *dyspepsiais,* derived from the Greek words *dys* (bad) and *pepsis* (digestion), refers to symptoms thought to originate in the upper GI tract.

17.4 Clinical Description

Indigestion, lassitude, heaviness in the body, the retention of flatus and constipation, or loose motion are the common signs and symptoms of *ajirna*, as described in classic texts. In conventional medicine, dyspepsia is characterized by upper abdominal pain or discomfort. It may also encompass symptoms of early satiety, postprandial abdominal bloating or distension, nausea, and vomiting.

17.5 History and Epidemiology

Dyspepsia is common; surveys in Western societies have recorded a prevalence of between 23 and 41%. For many people, dyspeptic symptoms are an acceptable part of living. Why some sufferers (about 25% of the population) seek help from doctors is not clear, but concern about symptoms seems to be as important as the symptoms themselves. The minority of sufferers (5% of the population) who do consult doctors are the major consumers of resources. In the U.K., in 1994, more than 400 million pounds was spent on ulcer-healing drug prescriptions issued by general practitioners. About 4% of general practice consultations are for dyspepsia and 2% of the entire populations receive either an endoscopy or barium swallow (upper GI) each year. Time lost from work and interference with quality of life is more difficult to measure but are likely to be considerable.[2]

Only 10% of patients attending their general practitioner with dyspepsia will be referred for hospital consultation or investigation.

The prevalence of dyspepsia ranges from 26% in the U.S. to 41% in the U.K. Although only 20 to 25% of persons with dyspepsia seek medical care; the problem is responsible for 2 to 5% of visits to primary care physicians. Nonulcer dyspepsia results in substantial health-care costs.[2]

17.6 Etiology

According to Ayurveda, the chief causes that affect digestion are the following:

1. Drinking too much liquid or water
2. Irregular eating habits, which include erratic schedules and quantities (i.e., eating at abnormal intervals [between meals, middle of the night, etc.] or too large or too small a serving)
3. Food allergies
4. Iatrogenic indigestion due to improper application of *panchakarma* (the detoxification procedures)
5. Suppression of nature's call or urges like hunger, defecation, etc.
6. Sleep disturbances
7. Emotional disturbances (e.g., envy, phobia, fury, depression, vengeance)

8. Seasonal changes
9. Debilitating chronic illnesses

In general, food selection, frequency of intake, seasonal changes, and emotional disturbances affect digestion.

According to conventional medicine, the main causes of dyspepsia are overeating, eating wrong food combinations, eating too rapidly, and neglecting proper mastication and salivation of food. Causes also include overeating and making the stomach, liver, kidneys, and bowels harder. When the food putrefies, its poisons are absorbed into the blood and consequently the whole system is poisoned. Certain foods, if not properly cooked, can cause dyspepsia. Other causes are intake of fried, rich, and spicy foods; excessive smoking; intake of alcohol; constipation; insomnia; lack of exercise; and emotions such as jealousy, fear, and anger.

17.7 Pathogenesis and Pathology

Ayurvedic texts state that diminished digestive enzymes lead to a state in which the patient is unable to digest even wholesome (*satmya*) and easily digestible food taken in an orderly time frame. This condition is known as *ajirna*.

Etiological factors disturb the homoeostasis of the *dosas*, which in turn influence the digestive enzyme and result in three states dependent on the three *dosas*. They are the *vata*-dependent abnormal state (*vishamagni*), *pitta*-dependent increased state (*tikshnagni*) and *kapha*-dependent decreased state (*mandagni*). These three pathological states of enzyme bring about *dosa*-specific indigestion. They are static indigestion (*vishtabdha ajirna*), acid indigestion (*vidagdha ajirna*), and endotoxic indigestion (*ama ajirna*), which are caused by *vata, pitta,* and *kapha dosas*, respectively. Section 17.9 details the types indigestion as described in Ayurvedic texts.

17.8 Clinical Diagnosis

The following clinical features as described in classic Ayurveda help to diagnose the three pathological states of enzyme:

1. Abnormal state of enzyme (*vishamagni*) — In this state, the enzyme is antagonistic due to involvement of vitiated *vata*. Symptoms include a very unpredictable digestive capacity. Sometimes the food is digested well, whereas at other times even light food in small quantities cannot be tolerated. Gaseous distension is common.
2. Increased state of enzyme (*tikshnagni*) — In this circumstance, the appetite is good, but the food that is eaten is not assimilated in the body. At such times, eating more food does not help at all. In fact, the enzyme will become more disturbed and so will the digestion process. A typical feature of this condition is that whatever the food that is eaten (and digested) seems to disappear down a slightly overburdened gut.

3. Decreased state of enzyme (*mandagni*) — In this condition, simple meals are difficult to digest and there is an uneasy feeling of indigestion. Other symptoms are malaise and vomiting.

17.9 Classification of Indigestion

Ayurvedic literatures describe a total of six types of indigestion, of which three are pathological types. They are static indigestion (*vishtabdha ajirna*), acid indigestion (*vidagdha ajirna*), and endotoxic indigestion (*ama ajirna*). The other three are transient indigestion (*rasasesha ajirna*), diurnal indigestion (*dinapaki ajirna*), and successive indigestion (*prativasara ajirna*). Although the latter three are not pathological types, they are transitional and occur physiologically in between any two meals every day. Dislike for food intake until the earlier food is digested is known as transient indigestion. The feeling of abdominal heaviness and lethargy soon after food ingestion is a natural process called diurnal indigestion and successive indigestion. The three pathological types are described below.

1. Endotoxic indigestion (*ama ajirna*) — The clinical features, such as abdominal heaviness, hypersalivation, puffiness of face, and belching out undigested food particles help diagnose this type of indigestion.
2. Acid indigestion (*vidagdha ajirna*) — This condition is presented with clinical features such as giddiness, intense thirst, daze, acid reflux, increased sweating, and a burning sensation all over the body.
3. Static indigestion (*vishtabdha ajirna*) — Clinical features, such as pain in the abdomen, abdominal distension, obstruction to bowel and flatus movements, bewilderment, and myalgia, are presented in this type of indigestion.

In conventional medicine, the clinical diagnosis is based on several signs and symptoms. As dyspepsia is a group of symptoms, it alerts doctors to suspect diseases of the upper GI tract. It includes symptoms of upper abdominal discomfort, retrosternal pain, anorexia, nausea, vomiting, bloating, fullness, early satiety, and heartburn, among others. A firm clinical diagnosis can be difficult based on these symptoms, as few symptoms are discriminatory. Many diseases cause dyspepsia; these include peptic ulcers, esophagitis, cancer of the stomach or pancreas, and gallstones. In a large proportion of cases, no clear pathological cause for a patient's symptoms can be determined. Other symptoms include a foul taste in the mouth, coated tongue, and foul breath. At times, a sensation of tightness in the throat is experienced. In most cases of indigestion, the patients suffer from constipation.

An organic cause is found in 40% of patients with dyspeptic symptoms. The most common organic disorders causing dyspepsia are gastroduodenal ulcer, gastroesophageal reflux disease, and gastric cancer. In 50% of patients, no cause is apparent and the dyspepsia is considered idiopathic, meaning the diagnosis is essential, functional, or nonulcer dyspepsia.[2] The history and physical examination do not reliably differentiate organic from nonulcer dyspepsia.

Many people do not require invasive investigation. However, as persistent indigestion may suggest a more serious underlying complaint, the doctor of conventional medicine may decide to arrange the following:

1. An endoscopy to enable the doctor to look into the stomach
2. A barium swallow test to enable the outline of the stomach to show up on an x-ray
3. An ultrasound to scans the abdominal organs
4. A blood test to detect anemia or any other abnormality

Ayurvedic physicians currently also use these diagnostic procedures.

17.10 Clinical Course and Prognosis

Indigestion not treated in time may lead to the development of sequelae such as stupor (*murcha*), incoherent talk (*pralapa*), vomiting (*vamathu*), hypersalivation (*praseka*), severe myalgia (*sadana*), vertigo (*bhrama*), and even death (*marana*).[3] The GI disturbances that may be followed by metabolic imbalances, either due to toxic states (especially metabolic histotoxic anoxia) or malnutritional states (which are acute to begin with) may tend to become chronic.

The acute conditions are among others that are caused by the impairment of enzymes (*agni*) and the formation of endotoxin (*ama*). Among the subacute and chronic conditions, both GI and metabolic, that may occur in a kind of chain sequence, the following may be mentioned here: functional impairment of colon, liver damage, and hepatic diseases. In fact, according to Ayurveda, most of the diseases included under internal medicine may, from this point of view, be stated to be the outcome of this endotoxin and *dosa* combined with this, called *sama*.

There is increasing evidence that individuals with autoimmune diseases, like rheumatoid arthritis, have intestines that are more permeable to certain antigens, allowing these antigens to invade the body and stimulate the symptoms. These antigens may be akin with the Ayurvedic concept of *ama*.[4]

17.11 Management

17.11.1 Ayurvedic Therapy and Management of Indigestion

The management of indigestion begins with treating enzyme disturbance because it is considered the basic cause of this condition. *Agnimandya* is treated as follows[5]:

1. The abnormal state of enzyme is treated with food and drinks that have sour and salty tastes, along with some quantity of fat.
2. The increased state of enzyme is brought to equilibrium with dairy products such as curds, milk, and milk gruel (*payasam*).
3. The decreased state of enzyme is treated with food and drinks that have pungent, bitter, and astringent tastes, which stimulate enzymes.

Indigestion is generally treated with drugs that have digestive and carminative activities:

TABLE 17.1

Compound Formulas for Indigestion, Poor Digestion, and Dyspepsia

Name of Formulation	Activity	Dose	Adjuvant	Ref
Bhaskaralavana curna	Digestive, appetizer	1–3 g twice/day before meals	Warm water and lemon juice	10
Hingvastaka curna	Carminative, antiflatulent	1–2 g twice/day before or with meals	Warm water, buttermilk, and ghee	5
Panchakola curna	Digestive, carminative	1–2 g twice/day before or with meals	Warm water	10
Agnitudi vat	Carminative, antispasmodic	240–480 mg twice/day before meals	Warm water	10
Rasonadi vati	Digestive, antiflatulent	240–480 mg twice/day before meal	Warm water	10
Sankha vati	Digestive, antiflatulent	240–480 mg twice/day before meals	Lime water	6

1. In endotoxic indigestion, digestive drugs have to be used. If there is excess *kapha*, then *vamana* (emesis) is done under a physician's supervision followed by digestive drugs such as *panchakola curna, agnitudi vati,* and *rasonadi vati* (Table 17.1).
2. Acid indigestion is treated with light and easily digestible food. If there is excess *pitta, virecana* (purgation) is followed by using antacids, such as *sankha vati* (Table 17.1).
3. To control *vata* in static indigestion, *virecana* with castor oil or *Terminalia chebula* is used followed by *basti* (enema) treatment done under medical supervision. To relieve constipation and indigestion, compound herbal powders such as *bhaskaralavana curna* and *hingvastaka* curna are used (Table 17.1).
4. In any stage of indigestion, ginger (*Zingiber officinale*), cumin (*Cuminum cyminum*), asafetida (*Ferula foetida*), and rock salt are used as digestives and carminatives.[6]

Therapy for functional gastrointestinal disorders comes under phytotherapeutic treatment. From ancient times, phytotherapeutics played a very important role in patients with dyspeptic symptoms. Bitter herbal drugs stimulate at even very small concentrations, sensorially, the secretions of the stomach as well as the digestive glands, and also strengthen the smooth musculature of the digestive tract (via the gustatory system, vagus, and the enteric nervous system). At higher dosages, herbs and food articles with bitter tastes probably directly affect the mucous membranes of the stomach and the bowels as stimulants. Bitters often are combined with essential oils (some volatile oils such as aromatic bitters, drug combinations of a volatile oil with a bitter taste). Essential oils act primarily as spasmolytic, carminative, and local anesthetic. In the past few years, several controlled studies were carried out with phytotherapeutic combinations (e.g., with *Iberis amara*, caraway oil, peppermint oil, curcuma, and ginger extracts) in which the herbal drugs proved to be superior compared with placebo and were as effective as prokinetics (studies according to evidence-based medicine).[7]

17.11.2 Clinical Experiences

1. In case of abdominal pain, *shankha vati* is used at 250 to 500 mg twice daily with warm water.

2. To control and relieve *borborygmi*, 1 to 3 g of *hingvashtaka curna* is used with ½ tsp of cow's ghee along with the first morsel of cooked rice twice daily.
3. If there is constipation with indigestion, 1 to 3 g *bhaskaralavana curna* is used with warm water twice daily.

17.11.3 Lifestyle Changes

A person with an abnormal enzyme and indigestion should avoid stale, cold, and oily foodstuffs, cold drinks, and cold water. Onions, potatoes, sweet potatoes, eggplant, yogurts, bananas, pickles fried, hot and spicy foods, dairy products, liquor, and desserts should be avoided.

Items like ginger, garlic, cumin, coriander, coriander leaves, curry leaves, and lemon should be added to the diet. Vegetables such as radishes, yams, drumsticks, snake gourd, bitter gourd, and pumpkin or fruits (e.g., pomegranates) can be eaten freely. Whole wheat bread, whole cereals, and rice (harvested and stored for a long time) are also helpful.

To avoid indigestion, adhere to the following guidelines:

1. Eat meals at regular times.
2. Do not rush meals.
3. Enjoy eating and drinking, but do so in moderation.
4. Avoid those foods that are associated with symptoms.
5. Avoid nonsteroidal anti-inflammatory drugs (NSAIDs). If possible, consult a doctor before doing so.
6. Avoid stressful situations that cause emotional upset.
7. Stop smoking.[8]

17.11.4 Review of Ayurvedic Therapies

The provision of dosage information in this section does not constitute a recommendation or endorsement but rather indicates the range of doses commonly used in Ayurvedic practice. Doses are given for single herb use and must be adjusted when using herbs in combinations. Doses may also vary according to the type and severity of the condition treated and individual patient conditions.

17.11.4.1 Imbalanced States of Digestive Enzymes

1. 2 g of dried ginger (*Zingiber officinale*) powder taken, twice daily, with warm water stimulates enzymes and relieves indigestion.
2. 5 g of fresh ginger taken with salt or jaggery twice daily before meals.
3. 3 g of chebulic myrobalan (*Terminalia chebula*) powder taken twice daily before meals with salt or jaggery.
4. 7 to 14 ml of lemon juice taken three times daily after meals.
5. Heat 1 g each of long pepper (*Piper longum*) powder and salt on a half lemon fruit over blue flame. The juice of this cooked lemon is to be sucked two or three times daily with meals.

6. 1 g each of the powdered fruit of long pepper and salt to be taken with lemon juice twice daily with meals.
7. Take equal parts of fruit rind of chebulic myrobalan, dried ginger, and rock salt in powder form, and add to it jaggery (approximately one third of the total weight). This is to be taken in 1 to 3 g doses with warm water once daily before the first meal.[9]
8. Fennel is one of the ingredients in a compound pill called *rasonadi vati*. It is useful in low enzyme states.[10]
9. Distillate of peppermint leaves relieves nausea, stimulates enzyme secretion, and improves appetite and taste.[11]

17.11.4.2 Indigestion

Various Ayurvedic formulas commonly used for indigestion are commercially available (Table 17.1). Other simple home remedies consisting of single herbs or multiple herbs are listed below.

1. Dried ginger tea should be taken several times a day.
2. Take 1 to 3 g of the powdered fruit rind of black chebulic myrobalan (*Terminalia chebula*) with an equal quantity of raw unrefined sugar twice daily before meals.
3. 1 to 3 g powdered dried ginger taken three times daily with jaggery.
4. 3 to 6 g of a paste prepared from equal parts of chebulic myrobalan fruit rind, raw unrefined sugar, and raisins is to be taken with honey twice daily before meals.
5. 1 g of the powder of equal parts of rock salt, fruit rind of chebulic myrobalan, fruit of long pepper, and root of leadwort (*Plumbago zeylanica*) should be taken with warm water twice daily after meals.
6. 14 to 28 ml of a decoction prepared from equal parts of clove (*Syzygium aromaticum*), fruit rind of chebulic myrobalan, and rock salt should be taken twice daily before meals.
7. 14 to 28 ml of decoction of equal parts of fruit of coriander (*Coriandrum sativum*) and dried ginger should be taken twice daily before meals.[9]
8. The powder of the turmeric rhizome (3 g) is useful in distaste and indigestion.[11]

17.11.4.3 External Applications

1. A hot poultice prepared from equal parts of asafetida (*Ferula foetida*), rock salt, and hot water may be applied on the abdomen when it is warm to relieve abdominal discomfort.
2. A warm poultice prepared from equal parts of asafetida powder, black pepper (*Piper nigrum*), rock salt, and hot water may be applied on the abdomen to relieve abdominal discomfort.[9]

According to conventional medicine, the treatment of indigestion includes avoidance of the foods and situations that seem to cause indigestion; in some cases this is the most successful way to treat indgestion. Excess stomach acid does not usually cause or result from indigestion, so antacids are not an appropriate long-term treatment, although some people report that they do help. Smokers can help relieve their indigestion by quitting smoking, or at least not smoking right before eating. Exercising with a full stomach may cause indigestion, so scheduling exercise before a meal or at least an hour after might help.

To treat indigestion caused by a functional problem in the digestive tract, the doctor may prescribe medicine that affects stomach motility. Because indigestion can be a sign of or mimic a more serious disease, patients should see a doctor if they have vomiting; weight or appetite loss; black tarry stools or blood in the vomit; severe pain in the upper right abdomen; discomfort unrelated to eating; and indigestion accompanied by shortness of breath, sweating, or pain radiating to the jaw, neck, or arm.

17.12 Scientific Basis

17.12.1 *Zingiber officinale* (Ginger)

17.12.1.1 Antinausea and Antiemetic Effects

17.12.1.1.1 Animal Studies

In mice, ginger's effect in enhancing intestinal motility was similar to metoclopramide's.[12] In shrews, dogs, and rats, ginger extracts effectively reduced chemotherapy-associated vomiting.[13,14] Ginger also protected frogs against experimentally induced emesis.[15] An herbal combination including ginger and ginkgo was as effective as metoclopramide in another animal study of experimentally induced nausea.[16] Studies in rats and mice suggest that ginger produces its antiemetic effects by stimulating peripheral anticholinergic and antihistaminic receptors and by antagonizing 5-hydroxytryptamine (serotonin) receptors in the gut.[17,18]

17.12.1.1.2 Clinical Studies

Both during fasting and after a standard test meal, ginger extracts significantly enhanced gastroduodenal motility in 12 normal volunteers.[19] Several randomized controlled trials support ginger's use as an antiemetic for nausea secondary to several conditions: morning sickness, chemotherapy-associated nausea, postoperative nausea, and motion sickness. In a randomized, double-blind, placebo-controlled crossover trial of 30 women with hyperemesis gravidarum, ginger (250 mg four times daily) proved significantly more effective than placebo in preventing and reducing nausea.[20] Ginger also proved useful in treating chemotherapy-induced nausea in a small pilot study of 11 adult patients; their nausea scores fell from an average of 2 (out of maximum of 4) to 0.7 after taking 1.5 g of powdered ginger.[21] Another case series also supported ginger's use as an antiemetic in patients undergoing chemotherapy.[22]

Data on ginger's effectiveness in preventing postoperative nausea have been conflicting. In two randomized, double-blind studies of women undergoing gynecologic surgery, those treated with ginger had significantly less postoperative nausea and vomiting than those treated with placebo; ginger was as effective as metoclopramide in preventing postoperative GI symptoms.[23,24] Two other randomized, controlled trials failed to document any statistically significant benefits of preoperative ginger (500 to 2000 mg) on postoperative nausea or vomiting.[25,26] Several studies have evaluated ginger's effectiveness in preventing motion sickness or seasickness and the potential mechanisms for this effect. In an open study of 1741 tourists traveling by sea, ginger supplements (250 mg every 2 h) were as effective as both nonprescription and prescription medications in preventing sea sickness.[27]

In a randomized, crossover trial of eight healthy volunteers, ginger supplements were significantly more effective than placebo in alleviating vertigo associated with motion sickness.[28] In a randomized, controlled trial of naval cadets, ginger was significantly more effective than placebo in preventing seasickness, both vomiting and vertigo.[29] In an early trial involving 36 college students prone to motion sickness, ginger was as effective as a dimenhydrinate in preventing nausea.[30] In a randomized, controlled trial in healthy volunteers, ginger was an effective antiemetic, but its mechanism of action appeared not to rely on alterations in gastric emptying.[24] In a study evaluating potential mechanisms for ginger's ability to reduce motion sickness, ginger had no impact on experimentally induced nystagmus associated with motion sickness; the investigators concluded that ginger's primary effect was on the stomach rather than the central nervous system.[31] In one National Aeronautics and Space Administration (NASA)-sponsored study in healthy volunteers, ginger (500 to 1000 mg) had no apparent effect on gastric emptying.[32] Other studies have reported enhanced intestinal motility after oral administration of ginger.[12]

17.12.1.2 Carminative and Antiulcer Effect

17.12.1.2.1 Animal Studies

In mice, zingiberene and gingerol significantly reduced gastric ulceration experimentally induced by ethanol and hydrochloric acid.[33]

These results were confirmed in several subsequent studies using several of ginger's constituents, including beta-sesquiphellandrene, beta-bisabolene, gingesulfonic acid, curcumene, and 6-shogaol. The results showed a demonstration of antiulcer effects and protection of gastric mucosa against alcohol, NSAIDs, and hydrochloric acid.[34,35] Rats given ginger extracts (gingerols) had enhanced bile secretion.[36]

17.12.1.2.2 Clinical Studies

A Chinese case series reported that an herbal mixture containing ginger was effective in halting upper gastrointestinal hemorrhage.[37] There are no randomized, controlled trials in humans evaluating ginger's effect as a carminative or ulcer remedy.

17.12.1.2.3 Dose

There is disagreement on the optimal form and dose of ginger. A pediatric dose is not established. Reputable physicians and herbalists recommend a range of doses. A dose of dried ginger at 250 mg, four times daily taken orally,[38] is commonly used. Some German herbalists recommend up to four times this amount.[39] Chinese herbalists may use up to ten times this amount. The following methods for preparing ginger can be used:

1. Tea — 1 tsp of fresh ginger root boiled in 1 to 2 cups of water for 10 to 20 min. Cool for 5 minutes and sweeten as desired. May be mixed with peppermint or chamomile.
2. Ginger tincture — 1.5 to 3.0 ml/dose.[38]
3. Candied ginger — A 1-in. square piece is presumably equivalent to 500 to 1000 of dried ginger.[40,41]

Ginger is used worldwide as a cooking spice, condiment, and herbal remedy. Rhizomes of ginger have long been used in traditional medicine for alleviating symptoms of GI illness.[14] It is used as a carminative to enhance digestion and reduce intestinal gas and flatulence. In experimental studies, gingerol, an active constituent of ginger, had enhanced bile secretion.[36] Ginger in combination with long pepper and black pepper (the combination is called *trikatu* in Ayurvedic literature) promoted the secretion of digestive juices and an increased appetite; it is also reported useful in patients with gastric disorders accompanied with clinical symptoms of achlorhydria and hypochlorhydria.[42]

17.12.2 Foeniculum vulgare (Fennel)

Fennel is a promoter of normal GI motility and is an antispasmodic.[43] In experimental studies, fennel was reported to stimulate bile flow from the liver, which could help in relieving GI discomfort.[44]

17.12.3 Curcuma longa (Turmeric)

Experimental study with ethanolic extract of turmeric has proved its ability to inhibit gastric secretion and to protect gastroduodenal mucosa against the injuries caused by pyloric ligation; hypothermic-restraint stress; indomethacin; reserpine and cysteamine administration; and cytodestructive agents, including 80% ethanol, 0.6 *M* HCl, 0.2 *M* NaOH, and 25% NaCl. Turmeric extract has found to increase the gastric wall mucus and also restored the nonprotein sulfhydryl (NP-SH) content in the glandular stomachs of rats.[45]

A number of clinical trials on turmeric have proved it beneficial in the treatment of peptic ulcer and nonulcer dyspepsia and right upper abdominal pain that may often be caused by biliary dyskinesia.[46–50] Further acute and chronic oral toxicity studies on the turmeric rhizomes in mice, rats, guinea pigs, and monkeys found it to be safe.[51,52]

17.12.4 Mentha piperita (Peppermint Oil) and Carum carvi (Caraway Oil)

A combination of peppermint and caraway oils in the treatment of functional dyspepsia has been extensively studied in experimental models and in clinical conditions of dyspepsia.[53,54]

The peppermint and caraway oil combination was found to be a safe preparation that acted locally to cause GI smooth muscle relaxation.[55] The favorable risk-benefit ratio of a peppermint and caraway oil combination was demonstrated for the treatment of functional dyspepsia.[56] Peppermint oil was known to inhibit enterocyte glucose uptake via a direct action at the brush border membrane in the intestinal lumen.[57]

Acknowledgments

The authors acknowledge the data input provided by M.V. Venkatranganna and S. Gopumadhavan, Pre-Clinical Pharmacology Laboratory, R&D Center, The Himalaya Drug Company, Makali, Bangalore, India.

References

1. Anon., Indigestion, National Institute of Diabetes and Digestive and Kidney Diseases of NIH, NIH Publication No. 02-4549, National Institutes of Health, U.S.A, Feb. 2002, available at: http://www.niddk.nih.gov/health/digest/summary/ind/.
2. Drossman, D.A. et al., U.S. Householder survey of functional GI disorders: prevalence, sociodemography and health impact, *Dig. Dis. Sci.*, 38, 1569, 1993.
3. Dwarakanath, C., *Introduction to Kayachikitsa*, Chowkhambha Orientalia, Varanasi, U.P. India, 1996.
4. Madhava, *Madhavanidanam*, Vol. 1, Sastri, S. and Uapadhyaya, Y., Eds., Chaukhambha Sanskrit Sansthan, Varanasi, U.P. India, 1976, chap. 6, p. 198.
5. Bhavamishra, *Bhavaprakasha*, Vol. 2, Mishra, B.S., Ed., Chaukhambha Sanskrit Sansthan, Varanasi, U.P. India, 1972, chap. 6, p. 78.
6. Anon., *Yogaratnakara*, Part I, Shastri, B.B., Ed., Chaukhambha Sanskrit Sansthan, Varanasi, U.P. India, 1997, p. 310.
7. Saller, R. et al., Dyspeptic pain and phytotherapy: a review of traditional and modern herbal drugs, *Forsch. Komplementarmed. Klass Naturheilkd.*, 8(5), 263, 2001.
8. Anon., Dyspepsia Management Guidelines, British Society of Gastroenterology, London, 2002, available at: http://www.bsg.org.uk/clinical_prac/guidelines/dyspepisia.htm.
9. Anon., *Hand Book of Domestic Medicine and Common Ayurvedic Remedies*, Central Council for Research in Indian Medicine and Homoeopathy, New Delhi, India, 1978, chaps. 2 and 3, p. 43.
10. Das, G., *Bhaishajyaratnavali*, Chaukhambha Sanskrit Sansthan, Varanasi, U.P. India, 1997, chap. 10, p. 237.
11. Vaishya, S., *Shaligramanighantu Bhushana*, Vols. 7 and 8, Khemaraj Srikrishnadas Publications, Mumbai, Maharashtra, India, 1953, pp. 71 and 158.
12. Yamahara, J. et al., Gastrointestinal motility enhancing effect of ginger and its active constituents, *Chem. Pharm. Bull.* (Tokyo), 38, 430, 1990.
13. Yamahara, J. et al., Inhibition of cytotoxic drug-induced vomiting in suncus by a ginger constituent, *J. Ethnopharmacol.*, 27, 353, 1989.
14. Sharma, S.S. et al., Anti-emetic efficacy of ginger (Zingiber officinale) against cisplatin-induced emesis in dogs, *J. Ethnopharmacol.*, 57, 93, 1997.
15. Kawai, T. et al., Anti-emetic principles of Magnolia obovata bark and Zingiber officinale rhizome, *Planta Medica*, 60, 17, 1994.
16. Frisch, C. et al., Blockade of lithium chloride-induced conditioned place aversion as a test for antiemetic agents: comparison of metoclopramide with combined extracts of Zingiber officinale and Ginkgo biloba, *Pharmacol. Biochem. Behav.*, 52, 321, 1995.
17. Qian, D.S. and Liu, Z.S., Pharmacologic studies of antimotion sickness actions of ginger, *Chung Kuo Chung Hsi I Chieh Ho Tsa Chih*, 12, 95, 1992.
18. Huang, Q. et al., Anti-5-hydroxytryptamine effect of galanolactone, diterpenoid isolated from ginger, *Chem. Pharm. Bull.*, 39, 397, 1991.
19. Micklefield, G.H. et al., Effects of ginger on gastroduodenal motility, *Int. J. Clin. Pharmacol. Ther.*, 37, 341, 1999.
20. Fischer-Rasmussen, W. et al., Ginger treatment of hyperemesis gravidarum, *Eur. J. Obstet. Gynecol. Reprod. Biol.*, 38, 19, 1991.
21. Meyer, K. et al., Zingiber officinale (ginger) used to prevent 8-Mop associated nausea, *Dermatol. Nurs.*, 7, 242, 1995.
22. Pecoraro, A. et al., Efficacy of ginger as an adjunctive anti-emetic in acute chemotherapy-induced nausea and vomiting, *ASHP Midyear Clin. Meet.*, 33, 429E, 1998.
23. Bone, M.E. et al., Ginger root: a new antiemetic. The effect of ginger root on postoperative nausea and vomiting after major gynaecological surgery, *Anaesthesia*, 45, 669, 1990.
24. Phillips, S., Hutchinson, S., and Ruggier, R., Zingiber officinale does not affect gastric emptying rate. A randomised, placebo-controlled, crossover trial, *Anaesthesia*, 48, 393, 1993.

25. Arfeen, Z. et al., A double-blind randomized controlled trial of ginger for the prevention of postoperative nausea and vomiting, *Anaesth. Intensive Care*, 23, 449, 1995.
26. Visalyaputra, S. et al., The efficacy of ginger root in the prevention of postoperative nausea and vomiting after outpatient gynaecological laparoscopy, *Anaesthesia*, 53, 506, 1998.
27. Schmid, R. et al., Comparison of seven commonly used agents for prophylaxis of seasickness, *J. Travel Med.*, 1, 203, 1994.
28. Grontved, A. and Hentzer, E., Vertigo-reducing effect of ginger root: a controlled clinical study, ORL, *J. Otorhinolaryngol. Relat. Spec.*, 48, 282, 1986.
29. Grontved, A. et al., Ginger root against seasickness: a controlled trial on the open sea, *Acta Otolaryngol.* (Stockholm), 105, 45, 1988.
30. Mowrey, D.B. and Clayson, D.E., Motion sickness, ginger, and psychophysics, *Lancet*, 1, 655, 1982.
31. Holtmann, S. et al., The anti-motion sickness mechanism of ginger. A comparative study with placebo and dimenhydrinate, *Acta Otolaryngol.* (Stockholm), 108, 168, 1989.
32. Stewart, J.J. et al., Effects of ginger on motion sickness susceptibility and gastric function, *Pharmacology*, 42, 111, 1991.
33. Yamahara, J. et al., The anti-ulcer effect in rats of ginger constituents, *J. Ethnopharmacol.*, 23, 299, 1988.
34. Yamahara, J. et al., Stomachic principles in ginger. II. Pungent and anti-ulcer effects of low polar constituents isolated from ginger, the dried rhizoma of Zingiber officinale Roscoe cultivated in Taiwan: the absolute stereostructure of a new diarylheptanoid, *Yakugaku Zasshi*, 112, 645, 1992.
35. al-Yahya, M.A. et al., Gastroprotective activity of ginger Zingiber officinale rosc. in albino rats, *Am. J. Chin. Med.*, 17, 51, 1989.
36. Yamahara, J. et al., Cholagogic effect of ginger and its active constituents, *J. Ethnopharmacol.*, 13, 217, 1985.
37. Gong, Q.M., Wang, S.L., and Gan, C., A clinical study on the treatment of acute upper digestive tract hemorrhage with wen-she decoction, *Chung Hsi I Chieh Ho Tsa Chih*, 9, 272, 1989.
38. Newall, C.A., Anderson, L.A., and Phillipson, J.D., *Herbal medicines: A Guide for Health-Care Professionals*, Pharmaceutical Press, London, 1996, p. 296.
39. Blumenthal, M., *The Complete German Commission E Monographs: Therapeutic Guide to Herbal Medicine*, American Botanical Council, Austin, 1998.
40. Robbers, J.E. and Tyler, V.E., *Tyler's Herbs of Choice: The Therapeutic Use of Phytomedicinals*, Haworth Herbal Press, New York, 1999, p. 287.
41. Peirce, A., *The American Pharmaceutical Association Practical Guide to Natural Medicines*, William Morrow and Company, Inc., New York, 1999.
42. Johri, R.K. and Zutshi, U., An Ayurvedic formulation "trikatu" and its constituents, *J. Ethnopharmacol.*, 37, 85, 1992.
43. Westphal, J., Horning, M., and Leonhardt, K., Phytotherapy in functional upper abdominal complaints, *Phytomedicine*, 2, 285, 1996.
44. Kline, R.M. et al., Enteric-coated pH-dependent, peppermint oil capsules for the treatment of irritable bowel syndrome in children, *J. Pediatr.*, 138, 125, 2001.
45. Rafatullah, S. et al., Evaluation of turmeric (Curcuma longa) for gastric and duodenal antiulcer activity in rats, *J. Ethnopharmacol.*, 29(1), 25, 1990.
46. Prucksunand, C. et al., Phase II clinical trial on effect of the long turmeric (Curcuma longa Linn) on healing of peptic ulcer, *Southeast Asian J. Trop. Med. Public Health*, 32(1), 208, 2001.
47. Eigner, D. and Scholz, D., Ferula asafetida and Curcuma longa in traditional medical treatment and diet in Nepal, *J. Ethnopharmacol.*, 67(1), 1, 1999.
48. Niederau, C. and Gopfert, E., The effect of chelidonium- and turmeric root extract on upper abdominal pain due to functional disorders of the biliary system: results from a placebo-controlled double-blind study, *Med. Klin.*, 94(8), 425, 1999.
49. Kositchaiwat, C., Kositchaiwat, S., and Havanondha, J., Curcuma longa Linn. in the treatment of gastric ulcer comparison to liquid antacid: a controlled clinical trial, *J. Med. Assoc. Thailand*, 76(11), 601, 1993.

50. Thamlikitkul, V. et al., Randomized double blind study of *Curcuma domestica* Val. for dyspepsia, *J. Med. Assoc. Thailand*, 72(11), 613, 1989.
51. Qureshi, S., Shah, A.H., and Ageel, A.M., Toxicity studies on Alpinia galanga and Curcuma longa, *Planta Medica*, 58(2), 124, 1992.
52. Shankar, T.N. et al., Toxicity studies on turmeric (Curcuma longa): acute toxicity studies in rats, guineapigs and monkeys, *Indian J. Exp. Biol.*, 18(1), 73, 1980.
53. Freise, J. and Kohler, S., Peppermint oil-caraway oil fixed combination in non-ulcer dyspepsia: comparison of the effects of enteric preparations, *Pharmazie.*, 54(3), 210, 1999.
54. May, B. et al., Efficacy of a fixed peppermint oil/caraway oil combination in non-ulcer dyspepsia, *Arzneim. Forsch.*, 46(12), 1149, 1996.
55. Micklefield, G.H., Greving, I., and May, B., Effects of peppermint oil and caraway oil on gastroduodenal motility, *Phytother. Res.*, 14(1), 20, 2000.
56. May, B., Kohler, S., and Schneider, B., Efficacy and tolerability of a fixed combination of peppermint oil and caraway oil in patients suffering from functional dyspepsia, *Aliment Pharmacol. Ther.*, 14(12), 1671, 2000.
57. Beesley, A. et al., Influence of peppermint oil on absorptive and secretory processes in rat small intestine, *Gut*, 39(2), 214, 1996.

18

Constipation (Vibandha)

Shankar K. Mitra and Paramesh R. Rangesh

CONTENTS

0-8493-1366-X/04/$0.00+$1.50

18.1 Introduction

Constipation is the infrequent and difficult passage of stools. The frequency of bowel movements among healthy people varies greatly, ranging from three movements/day to three times/week. As a rule, if more than 3 days pass without a bowel movement, the intestinal contents may harden, and a person may have difficulty or even pain during elimination. Sometimes stools may harden and be painful to pass even after shorter intervals between bowel movements. Constipation is a common, often frustrating, and difficult to manage problem in the elderly. Approximately 25% of all Americans over 65 years old experience constipation.[1] Ayurvedic therapies are very effective treatments for constipation.

18.2 Ayurvedic Concept

Most people develop constipation after years of either an imbalanced lifestyle or diet. In general, there are some contributing factors. The most common is the suppression of natural urges resulting in the subsequent disappearance of the normal eliminative urges. For example, first thing in the morning (typically at or before dawn) there should be a natural urge to eliminate. We often find this natural urge inappropriate or inconvenient at certain times and force ourselves to suppress it. This habitual suppression can lead to a kind of psychosocial form of constipation whereby elimination may be regular but not complete. If elimination does not naturally conform to the Ayurvedic definition of normal (i.e., every morning), then the elimination cannot be complete and the colon is therefore constipated.

Normal elimination for one person may not be normal for someone else. In general, one is probably constipated if one passes hard stools fewer than three times/week.[2] In some cases, the person may also have a bloated feeling or abdominal cramping or pain.

A few commonsense lifestyle changes, including getting more exercise, eating high-fiber foods, and drinking plenty of fluids, especially water, can go a long way toward preventing and alleviating many cases of constipation.[3]

In Ayurveda, it is described that the normal stool has a definite consistency and hardness, which is called well-formed stool. During digestion, food undergoes an acidic state in which it is in semiliquid form in the small intestines. As it travels further in the large intestine, this digested food (called *ahara rasa*) is absorbed and the waste is left in the large intestine. The cecum, the first portion of this part of the gastrointestinal tract, has the dominance of *vata* and *pitta dosas* that helps in drying of waste and giving it a form. When these *dosas* are in a pathological state, it results in excess drying of the fecal matter. This stool becomes dry and hard and is expelled in small quantities with difficulty. In such situations, if an individual holds the urge to defecate for various reasons, there will be a possibility of collection of fecal matter that becomes very hard; this is a result of too much absorption of water from the stool. In many diseases, constipation occurs as a symptom. In order to avoid this, one has to drink large amounts of water.

18.3 Definition

In Ayurveda, constipation is called *vibandha*. The word *vibandha* is derived from "vi" prefixed to "bandh," meaning that which is especially bound (in the intestine) or obstructed. Its synonyms are *purishasanga, purishanaha* (both meaning the accumulation of feces), *vishtambha* (obstruction), *kricchravitka, alpavitka* (both meaning the passing of a small quantity of stool), and *anaha* (bloated abdomen due to accumulation of stools). Constipation is derived from Latin, "con" meaning together and "stipare," meaning to cram or pack.

18.4 Clinical Description

The clinical feature of the disease, described in conventional medicine as having a bowel movement not every day, does not necessarily mean one is constipated. A person is most likely constipated if he or she experiences the following:

1. Passes a hard stool fewer than three times/week
2. Strains more than one of four times
3. Has abdominal bloating or discomfort[3]

Ayurvedic literature describes the clinical features of the disease as the condition that is manifested with the following signs and symptoms:

1. Pain in the abdomen (left hypochondriac, iliac, and umbilical regions)
2. Reduced bowel movement
3. Painful defecation
4. Dry stools
5. Indigestion
6. Headache
7. Churning pain in rectum
8. Pain in the sacral region[4]

18.5 History and Epidemiology

This disease is referred to many times in *Caraka Samhita*.[5] Constipation is the most common gastrointestinal complaint in the U.S., resulting in about 2 million annual visits to the doctor.[6] Most people treat themselves without seeking medical help, as is evident from the $725 million Americans spend on laxatives each year.[7]

18.6 Etiology

According to Ayurveda, constipation is mainly caused by aggravation of *vata*, though it can sometimes be caused by aggravation of *pitta* and *kapha dosas*. Constipation is generally caused by wrong and untimely bowel habits, a controlled urge to defecate, improper eating habits and untimely food intake, eating food that is difficult to digest and dominated with astringent properties, and not eating enough vegetables or salads (dietary fiber). Frequent fasting is also considered as a cause of constipation. It is also caused by not sleeping well or sleeping very late at night, irritable colon, colitis, and negative emotions like stress, grief, fear, worry, etc.

The following are some of the most common causes of constipation, according to conventional medicine:

1. Improper diet — The most common cause of constipation may be a diet high in animal fats and refined sugar but low in fiber found in vegetables, fruits, and whole grains.
2. Not enough liquids — Liquids like water and juice add fluid to the colon and bulk to stools, making bowel movements softer and easier to pass. People who have problems with constipation should drink enough of these liquids every day, about eight 8-oz glasses. Other liquids that contain caffeine (e.g., coffee and cola) seem to have a dehydrating effect.
3. Lack of exercise — Lack of exercise can lead to constipation, although doctors do not know precisely why. For example, constipation often occurs after an accident or during an illness when one must take bed rest and cannot exercise.
4. Changes in life or routine — During pregnancy, women may be constipated because of hormonal changes or because the heavy uterus compresses the intestine. Aging may also affect bowel regularity, because a slower metabolism results in less intestinal activity and muscle tone.
5. Ignoring the urge to have a bowel movement — People who ignore the urge to have a bowel movement may eventually stop feeling the urge, which can lead to constipation.
6. Laxative abuse — People who habitually take laxatives become dependent upon them and may require increasing dosages until the intestine becomes insensitive and fails to work properly.
7. Travel — People often experience constipation when traveling long distances, which may relate to changes in lifestyle, schedule, diet, and drinking water.
8. Fissures and hemorrhoids — Painful conditions of the anus can produce a spasm of the anal sphincter muscle, which can delay a bowel movement.
9. Specific diseases — Diseases that cause constipation include neurological disorders, metabolic and endocrine disorders, and systemic conditions that affect organ systems. These disorders can slow the movement of stool through the colon, rectum, or anus.

10. Mechanical compression — Scarring, inflammation around diverticula, tumors, and cancer can produce mechanical compression of the intestine and result in constipation.
11. Irritable bowel syndrome (IBS) — Also known as spastic colon, IBS is one of the most common causes of constipation. Some people develop spasms of the colon that delay the speed with which the contents of the intestine move through the digestive tract, leading to constipation.
12. Nerve damage — Injuries to the spinal cord and tumors pressing on the spinal cord can produce constipation by affecting the nerves that lead to the intestine.
13. Medications — Many medications can cause constipation. These include pain medications (especially narcotics), antacids containing aluminum, antispasmodic drugs, antidepressant drugs, tranquilizers, iron supplements, anticonvulsants for epilepsy, antiparkinsonism drugs, and antihypertensive calcium channel blockers.
14. Problems with colon and rectum — The peristaltic activity of the intestine may be ineffective and result in colonic inertia or outlet obstruction. Intestinal obstruction, scar tissue (adhesions), diverticulosis, tumors, colorectal stricture, Hirschsprung's disease, or cancer can compress, squeeze, or narrow the intestine and rectum and cause constipation.

18.7 Pathogenesis and Pathology

Normally muscle contractions propel the waste products of digestion through the intestines. In the large intestine, reabsorption of up to 90% of the water and salt takes place because they are essential for many of our body's functions. If too much water is absorbed or if the waste moves too slowly, one may become constipated.[3]

According to Ayurveda, the *apana vata* affected (due to various etiological factors) dries up the stools, which obstructs the bowel movements and results in constipation. In short, the pathology of the disease is described as a result of the obstruction or reduced motility in the large intestine, the part of the excretory system, and due to the pathological changes in *apana vata* involving the fecal matter.

18.8 Clinical Features

The Ayurvedic literature describes two types of constipation:

1. Constipation due to *ama* (*amaja anaha*) — Constipation caused by *ama* presents with the following symptoms: thirst, burning sensation in the head, pain in the abdomen, and suppression of eructation and coryza.
2. Constipation due to feces (*purishaja anaha*) — In this type of constipation, retention of feces and urine, acute abdominal pain, and fainting are seen. Vomiting of undigested material and pedal edema may also occur in severe cases.

Current practitioners and information sources classify the types of constipation based on *dosa* dominance in a constitution.

18.8.1 *Vata* Constipation

In Ayurveda, excretory process is controlled by *vata*, the principle that governs all kinds of movement in the body. The particular *subdosa* of *vata* involved in constipation is called *apana vata*. *Apana vata* controls the movements in the pelvis and elimination and reproduction. Typically, when *apana vata* gets out of balance, it will first cause dryness in the colon where the stool can become hard and impacted.

18.8.2 *Pitta* Constipation

The dominance of *pitta*, whose property is heat, causes this form of constipation. An increased heat in the colon can also dry out the colon, aggravating *apana vata* and leading to constipation.

18.8.3 *Kapha* Constipation

When there is excess *vata* or dryness in the colon, the body will defend itself by producing more colonic mucus to combat dryness. When this happens in excess, the clogged colon with mucus causes a *kapha*-based constipation. This imbalance combined with a mucus-forming diet will result in a condition that could become chronic.[8]

18.9 Diagnosis

A diagnosis of constipation generally depends on the medical history and a physical examination. The doctor will first want to make sure there is no blockage (intestinal obstruction) in the small intestine or colon, an endocrine condition (e.g., hypothyroidism), or an electrolyte disturbance (e.g., excessive calcium in the blood [hypercalcemia]). The doctor may also check the medications in case they may be causing the constipation.

In some cases, the doctor may order a test for hidden (occult) blood in stools. Alternatively, one may have a barium enema. A sigmoidoscopy may help detect problems in the rectum and lower colon, in addition to routine blood, urine, and stool tests. One may also perform a proctosigmoidoscopy. In many cases, the doctor will be able to see the rectum and sigmoid colon more easily with this procedure than with a barium enema.[9]

18.9.1 Medical History

The doctor may ask a patient to describe the constipation, including duration of symptoms, frequency of bowel movements, consistency of stools, presence of blood in the stool, and toilet habits (frequency and place of bowel movements). Recording eating habits, medication, and level of physical activity or exercise under personal history also helps the doctor determine the cause of constipation.[10]

18.9.2 Physical Examination

A physical exam may include a digital rectal exam with a gloved, lubricated finger to evaluate the tone of the anal sphincter and to detect tenderness, obstruction, or blood.

18.9.3 Clinical Course and Prognosis

Constipation associated with intense thirst and weakness with severe abdominal pain is considered difficult to manage according to Ayurveda.

According to conventional medicine, medical intervention is necessary if one experiences a recent, unexplained onset of constipation or change in bowel habits or any of the following symptoms, which might indicate a more serious health condition:

1. Constipation that lasts longer than 7 days, despite changes in diet or exercise
2. Intense abdominal pain
3. Blood in the stool

Although constipation can be extremely bothersome, it usually is not serious. If it persists, and especially if straining results, one may develop complications such as hemorrhoids and cracks or tears in the anus called abrasions or fissures.

Very severe or chronic constipation can sometimes cause a fecal impaction, a mass of hardened stool not eliminated by a normal bowel movement. An impaction can be very dangerous, and one may need to have it manually removed by a nurse or doctor.

18.10 Therapy

Although treatment depends on the cause, severity, and duration, in most cases dietary and lifestyle changes will help relieve symptoms and help prevent constipation. As in all other gut problems, fasting is an important initial remedy. One should fast at least once a month so that the gut is clean and digestion is complete. This facilitates smooth passage of stools and a sense of complete evacuation. Along with oil, ghee (clarified butter), milk, and some roughage (i.e., green leafy vegetables) should be included in the diet.

If the staple diet consists of bread, boiled vegetables, vegetable or animal protein, salad or dry foodstuffs, the content of ghee in the diet should be increased. Paradoxical as this may sound, ghee in measured quantities does not increase bad cholesterol.[11] Ayurveda has instead attributed ghee to many useful effects, including the lubrication of blood vessels, which delays aging. One should pursue the habit of drinking milk before sleeping and add 1 tsp of ghee to it or use ghee with hot water; this is very beneficial in mild to moderate constipation. Administering a laxative will lubricate the walls and help elimination for the constipated patient and provides symptomatic relief at best. However, the goal of the Ayurvedic approach is to understand why and how the constipation manifested and to restore balance specifically while enlivening the body's natural ability to sustain normal elimination. With the proper diagnosis established, the treatment for constipation is relatively simple. The general line of treatment would include the following:

1. Application of oil massage (*abhyanga*) and sauna (*svedana*)

2. Intake of medicated fats (*snehapana*), purgation (*virecana*), and an enema (*anuvasana basti*) with honey, rock salt, and castor oil
3. Anal suppositories such as *phalavarti and snehavarti*

18.10.1 Purgation Therapy (*Virecana*)

Virecana, or purgation, is administered for cleansing of *pitta* and stools in the intestine. *Virecana* cleanses the small intestine and colon. Many herbs and other ingredients are used as laxatives or purgatives. These include senna, prunes, bran, flaxseed husk, psyllium husk, cow's milk, salt, castor oil, raisins, and mango juice. When taking these herbs, it is important to follow a restricted diet.

The dose and the selection of herbs also depend on the nature of one's bowel, called *koshta* in Ayurveda. The literature describes three types of bowels: extremely harsh, weak, and moderate. The extremely harsh bowel (*krura koshtha*) is controlled by more *vata* and *kapha*, and the person with this type fails to purge and needs drastic purgatives in higher doses. The extremely weak bowel (*mrudu koshtha*) is controlled by *pitta* and purges to the intake of milk and needs lower doses of purgatives. The moderate bowel (*madhya koshtha*), which is under the influence of balanced *dosas*, requires moderate doses of purgatives.

Among the Ayurvedic medicines available for treatment of constipation, the most common one is triphala powder (compound powder of fruit rinds of Indian gooseberry [*Emblica officinalis*], chebulic myrobalan [*Terminalia chebula*], and Belliric myrobalan [*Terminalia bellirica*]) to be taken with ghee. Otherwise, the mucosal lining becomes dry and leads to further constipation, setting a vicious cycle into motion. In keeping with the emphasis laid on individualization of treatment by Ayurveda, the doses of these medicines vary in different individuals.

Some of the laxatives that can be effectively used in constipation are the following:

1. *Bhagottara curna* — The powders of the following ingredients are mixed in increasing ratio: resin of asfetida (*Ferula foetida*), rhizome of sweet flag (*Acorus calamus*), blacksalt, rhizome of dried ginger (*Zingiber officinale*), cumin seeds (*Cuminum cyminum*), fruit rind of *chebulic myrobalan*, and root of inula (*Inula racemosa*). The mixture is taken twice/day at the dose of 3 to 6 g.
2. An equal quantity of powders of rhizome of sweet flag, fruit rind of chebulic myrobalan, root of leadwort (*Plumbago zeylanica*), salt of potassium and sodium (*yavakshara*), long pepper (*Piper longum*) fruit, atis root (*Aconitum heterophyllum*), and rhizome of costus (*Saussurea lappa*) is taken twice/day with warm water at a dose of 3 to 6 g.
3. 5 g of fruit pulp of Indian laburnum (*Cassia fistula*) is taken with 50 ml of water and 5 to 10 g of unrefined sugar once/day.
4. 5 g of fruit rind of small Chebulic myrobalan is to be taken with 0.5 g of salt at bed time.
5. A powder of purified and fried resin of *asafetida*, garcinia fruit (*Garcinia indica*), fruit of bishop's weed (*Ptychotis ajowan*), rock salt, and seed of fennel (*Foeniculum vulgare*) is taken in equal parts. A dose of 2 to 6 g of the powder can be taken with 5 ml of fresh lemon juice twice/day.

Commercially available Ayurvedic formulas commonly used to treat constipation are listed in Table 18.1.

TABLE 18.1

List of Ayurvedic Formulas Used for Constipation

Name of Formulation	Activity	Dose	Adjuvant	Ref.
Triphala Curna	Laxative, digestive	2–6 g two times/day	50 ml warm water and ghee	5
Hingvadi Curna	Carminative, antiflatulent, laxative	1–2 g two times/day before or with meals	Warm water, buttermilk and ghee	12
Yashtyadi Curna syn. Madhukadi curna or *Svadishta virecana*	Laxative	3–6 g at bedtime	Warm water	13
Pancasakara curna	Antiflatulent, laxative	3–6 g at bedtime	Warm water	13
Trivritadi leha	Laxative	6–12 g on an empty stomach in the morning	Warm water	5
Icchabhedi Rasa	Drastic purgative, contraindicated for regular use in constipation (for *virecana* therapy only)	120–240 mg on an empty stomach early morning	Cold water	12

Local applications:

1. Poultice of *asafetida* is applied around the umbilicus.
2. Poultice prepared from equal parts of salt petre, fruit rind of Indian gooseberry, ammonium chloride, and sesame seeds (*Sesamum indicum*) is applied around the umbilicus.

18.10.2 Enema (*Basti*)

The medication rectally administered to control *vata*, which is mainly located in the colon, is known as *basti* or medicated enema. In general, this treatment is used to flush out the loosened *dosas* (including stools) through the intestinal tract. This therapy is administered in chronic and extreme conditions of constipation. It is also administered to patients with habitual constipation and weak patients who cannot be subjected to purgation. This therapy is done under the supervision of a physician. There are over 100 specific enemas listed in Ayurveda to treat constipation and for other *panchakarma* procedures.

An enema involves introducing medicinal substances, such as sesame oil, cow's ghee, and other herbal decoctions, in a liquid medium into the rectum. This treatment is especially good for *vata* disorders and it alleviates constipation and abdominal distension.

The common type of enemas are the following:

1. Oil enema or *anuvasana basti* — $1/2$ to 1 cup of warm sesame oil or castor oil (for chronic constipation)
2. Decoction enema or *asthapana basti* (herbal enema) — $1/2$ cup of *gotukola* (*Centella asiatica*) decoction with $1/2$ cup of warm sesame oil or honey mixed with sesame oil and rock salt (for acute constipation)
3. Nutritional enema — 1 cup of warm milk, 1 cup of meat broth, or 1 cup of bone marrow soup[4] (for chronic constipation where general weakness is a problem)

Contraindications for the enema are people suffering from chronic indigestion, bleeding from the rectum, cough, breathlessness, diarrhea, diabetes, and severe anemia; the elderly; or children under 7 years old. People suffering from acute fever, diarrhea, cold, paralysis, heart pain, or severe pain in the abdomen are not given decoction enemas.

18.10.3 *Vata* Constipation

Oleation (*snehana*) and purgation (*virecana*) is the general line of treatment for all *vata*, *pitta*, and *kapha* constipations. A monthly oleation with ghee followed by castor oil purgation provides eliminative support and cumulatively reinstates a more unctuous environment in the colon. To ensure such an effect, moistening and *vata*-balancing herbs are administered between oleations and purgations. This kind of therapy should not be continued beyond 3 months, and the following procedure is helpful:

1. While eating light food for a week, one should start each day with progressively increasing amounts of liquid ghee (2–4–6 tsp) taken orally. (*Note*: Avoid this procedure if fat intolerant.)
2. On the eve of the 4th day, take a warm bath before retiring and drink 6 tsp of castor oil as a purgative.
3. If there is any sign of weakness or fatigue, avoid the procedure above and simply take 1/2 to 1 tsp of castor oil every night for 1 month. This should not produce a purgative effect. If it does, take less castor oil, because a continuous laxative effect can deplete body fluids and electrolytes.

For a proper diet, cold and dry foods should be avoided. Eat heavier warm foods with an emphasis on oily foods such as nuts, oils, and cooked grains.

18.10.4 *Pitta* Constipation

Purgation therapy provides a cooling, moistening, and eliminative effect, making it the treatment of choice for this type. Herb therapy includes the following:

1. Take 1 to 2 tsp of aloe gel (*Aloe vera*), three times/day.
2. Take 1 tsp of triphala with ghee to make a paste and take three times/day.
3. Take licorice (*Glycyrrhiza glabra*), *F. vulgare*, and coriander (*Coriandrum sativum*) tea three times/day.
4. Take 1 tsp of psyllium husk mixed well with 8 oz of warm water for 5 min before bedtime.
5. For severe cases, rhubarb root (*Rheum emodi*) and Indian senna (*Cassia angustifolia*) leaf can be taken individually or together as needed.

For a proper diet, one should favor foods that are slightly oily and cooked and avoid hot, spicy, and pungent foods.

18.10.5 *Kapha* Constipation

The aim of the treatment is to reduce *kapha* with dietary changes. Foods rich in hot and more pungent spices, such as ginger and black pepper, are recommended. Mucus-producing foods, including cheese, sugar, yogurt, bread, and pastries, should be especially avoided at night. The following herbal remedies are useful:

1. 1 to 2 tsp of psyllium husk (*Plantago ovata*) taken with 8 oz of water three times/day.
2. 8 to 10 glasses of warm honey water daily.
3. $^1/_2$ to 1 tsp of triphala taken with honey three times/day.
4. Aloe, rhubarb, and Indian senna are bitter laxatives that will combat the intestinal *kapha* and provide an eliminative effect.

Note: While treating for *vata*, *pitta*, or *kapha* constipation there should not be an excess of bowel movements. If there is such an effect, reduce the dose of recommended therapy. If there is no improvement in 2 weeks of treatment, the dosages should be increased.[8]

18.10.6 General Dietary Recommendation

A diet with enough fiber (20 to 35 g/day) helps form soft, bulky stools. A doctor or dietitian can help plan an appropriate diet. High-fiber foods include beans, whole grains, bran cereals, fresh fruits, and vegetables such as asparagus, sprouts, cabbage, and carrots. For people prone to constipation, limiting foods that have little or no fiber such as ice cream, cheese, meat, pizza, and processed foods are also important.

18.10.7 General Lifestyle Changes

Other changes that can help treat and prevent constipation include drinking enough water and other liquids (e.g., fruit and vegetable juices and clear soup), engaging in daily exercise, walking a mile, and reserving enough time to have a bowel movement. In addition, the urge to have a bowel movement should not be ignored. People who are dependent on laxatives need to gradually stop using the medications with the help of a physician.

18.10.8 Prevention of Constipation

It is well known that prevention is the best approach to constipation. Although there is no way to ensure never experiencing constipation, the following guidelines should help. It is important to eat a well-balanced diet that includes unprocessed bran, whole-wheat grains, fresh fruits, and vegetables. Drink plenty of fluids, exercise regularly, have a regular time for breakfast, lunch, dinner, and have undisturbed visits to the toilet. It is very important not to ignore the urge to defecate and avoid a dependence on laxatives. Improve the digestion with the use of light spices such as cumin seeds, coriander, turmeric powder, fennel, and asafetida. Drinking a glass of warm milk at bedtime helps in evacuation the next morning. Regulate your sleeping hours. Ayurveda advises the common saying, "early to bed and early to rise." In the morning after waking up, drink a glass or two of preferably warm water and then wait a few minutes before going for evacuation. Massaging the whole body with oil (*abhayanga*) once or twice a week and applying oil or ghee on the naval area daily helps in preventing constipation.

18.11 Scientific Basis

A review of pharmacological studies on various Ayurvedic plants used in the therapies of constipation are presented in this section.

18.11.1 *Aloe vera* (Aloe)

Barbaloin or aloin derived from the inner sheath cells of Aloe leaves is a laxative. *In vitro* studies have revealed the inhibitory effect on sodium and potassium pump and chloride channels at the colonic membrane.[14] Aloe anthroquinones were reported to enhance large-intestinal propulsion and water secretion in rats and mice.[15,16] Randomized controlled trials have documented its potency as a cathartic in chronically constipated adults.[17]

18.11.2 *Plantago ovata* (Psyllium)

The ground seeds or husks of psyllium are used in dietary supplements for increased fiber, cholesterol reduction, and laxative activity.[18] In a randomized double-blind placebo study,[19] psyllium was found to be effective for stool frequency and consistency in patients with chronic constipation. In an open study,[20,21] conducted in patients having manifestations of irritable bowel syndrome with constipation, psyllium showed good results.

18.11.3 *Cassia senna* (Senna)

Senna leaf contains 1.5 to 3% hydroxyanthracene glycosides, mainly sennosides A and B, which are rheindianthrones, and smaller amounts of sennosides C and D, which are rhein-aloe-emodin-heterodianthrones. Modern human studies have investigated the use of senna for the following:

1. Treating severe constipation[22,23]
2. Treating chronic constipation in long-stay elderly patients[24]
3. Managing morphine-induced constipation[25]
4. Improving colonoscopy preparation with lavage[26]
5. Managing constipation in the immediate postpartum period[27]
6. Managing postoperative constipation in anorectal surgery[28]
7. Treating disorders characterized by slow intestinal transit time or constipation[29]
8. Using as a laxative for terminal cancer patients treated with opiates[30]

18.11.4 *Rheum officinale* (Rhubarb)

The active chemical constituents of rhubarb are anthraquinone glycosides, aloe-emodin, and physcion.[31,32] Experimental studies[33] have revealed that the laxative effect is due to the inhibition of water and electrolyte reabsorption in the large colon and to a stimulant effect on intestinal motility. Clinically, it is used to soften stool in anal fissures and hemorrhoids and is used postoperatively for anorectal surgeries. It is also effective as a cathartic and therefore used for colonoscopy preparations.[34]

18.11.5 *Prunus persica* (Almond)

The leaf decoction of almond is used traditionally as anthelmintic and laxative. An experimental study[35] has revealed that the aqueous extract of leaves exhibits cholinomimetic activity, which may result in its laxative effect.

18.11.6 *Terminalia chebula* (Chebulic Myrobalan)

T. chebula is a commonly advocated agent in Ayurveda for improving gastrointestinal motility. Charles Foster rats were administered *T. chebula* (100 mg/kg/day for 15 days orally), metoclopramide, or atropine, which established prokinetic and antikinetic activities, respectively. *T. chebula* was found to increase the percent of gastric emptying. The enhancement of gastric emptying was comparable with that produced by metoclopramide. This indicates that *T. chebula* can be a useful alternative to the prokinetic drugs available today.[36,37]

18.11.7 *Cassia fistula* (Indian Laburnum)

The seeds and dried pulp in the pod of this fruit act as a purgative. The flowers soothe the eyes and the pods suppress acidity, making it useful in treating constipation associated with burning pain in the stomach (*pitta* type). The water extract is also used for treating constipation in pregnant women, children, and elderly persons. The pulp, prepared from its fruits, is a laxative used in the treatment of constipation.[38]

18.11.8 *Mallotus philippinensis* (Indian Kamala)

The *kampillaka* plant is excellent in treating constipation associated with worm infestation as it first kills worms and then, due to its purging effect, gets rid of them. A powder made of kampillaka is especially useful. Sometimes worm infestation causes itching of the skin. At such times, taking kampillaka powder at night in the dose of only 500 mg to 1 g is useful.[39]

18.11.9 *Ricinus communis* (Castor)

Castor seed oil is a harmless laxative in small doses. In large doses it is and can be safely used throughout the year.[40]

Acknowledgments

The authors acknowledge the data input provided by M.V. Venkatranganna and S. Gopumadhavan, Pre-Clinical Pharmacology Laboratory, R&D Center, The Himalaya Drug Company, Makali, Bangalore, India.

References

1. Harari, D., Gurwitz, J.H., and Minaker, K.L., Constipation in the elderly, *J. Am. Geriatr. Soc.*, 41, 1130, 1993.
2. Whitehead, W.E. et al., Constipation in the elderly living at home; definition, prevalence, and relationship to lifestyle and health status, *J. Am. Geriatr. Soc.*, 37, 423, 1989.
3. Anon., What is constipation? Mayo Clinic, http://www.mayoclinic.com.
4. Dhyani, S.C., *Kaya-Cikitsa*, 1st ed., Ayurvedic and Tibbi Academy, Lucknow, U.P. India, 1991, chap. 73, p. 257.
5. Agnivesa, *Caraka Samhita*, Part 2, Pande, G., Ed., Chowkhamba Sanskrit Series Office, Varanasi, U.P. India, 1970, chap. 26, p. 721.
6. Sonnenberg, A. and Koch, T.R., Physician visits in the United States for constipation: 1958 to 1986, *Dig. Dis. Sci.*, 34, 606, 1989.
7. Sweeney, M., Constipation: Diagnosis and Treatment, *Home Care Provider*, 2(5), 250, 1997.
8. John Douillard, D.C., Ayurvedic Specific Condition Review: Constipation, John Douillard's Life Spa, 6666 Gunpark Dr. East #102 Boulder, CO, http://www.lifespa.com/Ayurvedic%20Health%20Care%20Products/Life%20Spa%20Library/Constipation/constipation.htm.
9. Marshall, J.B., Chronic constipation in adults: how far should evaluation and treatment go?, *Postgrad. Med.*, 88(3), 49, 1990.
10. Manning, A.P., Wyman, J.B., and Heaton, K.W., How trustworthy are bowel histories? Comparison of recalled and recorded information, *Br. Med. J.*, 2, 213, 1976.
11. Tirtha, S.S., Ghee: Holy Food, *Ayurveda Health Center Newsletter*, http://www.ayurvedahc.com/Newsletter/Archive/Dec01/Ghee.htm.
12. Das, G., *Bhaishajyaratnavali*, Chaukhambha Sanskrit Sansthan, Varanasi, India, 1997, chap. 31, pp. 472, 476.
13. Acarya, Y.T., *Siddhayogasamgraha*, Shree Baidyanath Ayurveda Bhavan Ltd. Nagpur, Maharashtra, India, 1976, p. 55.
14. Honig, J., Geck, P., and Rauwald, H., Inhibition of Cl- channels as a possible base of laxative action of certain anthraquinones and anthrones, *Planta Med.*, 58, 586, 1992.
15. Ishii, Y. et al., Studies on Aloe VI-cathartic effect of isobarbaloin, *Biol. Pharm. Bull.*, 21(11), 1226, 1998.
16. Yagi, T., The synergistic purgative action of aloe-emodin anthrone and rhein anthrone in mice. Synergism in large intestinal propulsion and water secretion, *J. Pharm. Pharmacol.*, 49, 22, 1997.
17. Odes, H. and Madar, Z., A double-blind trial of a celandin, *Aloe vera* and psyllium laxative preparation in adult patients with constipation, *Digestion*, 49, 65, 1991.
18. Wichtl, M. and Bisset, N.G., *Herbal Drugs and Phytopharmaceuticals*, Medpharm Scientific Publishers, Stuttgart, Germany, 1994.
19. Thomas-Ridocci M. et al., The efficacy of *Plantago ovata* as a regulator of intestinal transit. A double-blind study compared to placebo, *Rev. Esp. Enferm. Dig.*, 82(1), 17, 1992.
20. Hotz, J. and Plein, K., Effectiveness of plantago seed husks in comparison with wheat bran on stool frequency and manifestations of irritable colon syndromes with constipation, *Med. Klin.*, 89(12), 645, 1994.
21. Marlett, J.A., Kajs, T.M., and Fischer, M.H., An unfermented gel component of psyllium seed husk promotes laxation as a lubricant in humans, *Am. J. Clin. Nutr.*, 72, 784, 2000.
22. Der Marderosian, A., *The Review of Natural Products, St. Louis: Facts and Comparisons*, Deutscher Apotheker Verlag, Stuttgart, Germany, 1999.
23. Pers, M. and Pers, B., A crossover comparative study with two bulk laxatives, *J. Int. Med. Res.*, 11(1), 51, 1983.
24. Passmore, A.P. et al., A comparison of agiolax and lactulose in elderly patients with chronic constipation, *Pharmacology*, 47(Suppl. 1), 249, 1993.
25. Ramesh, P.R. et al., Managing morphine-induced constipation: A controlled comparison of an Ayurvedic formulation and senna, *J. Pain Symptom Manage.*, 16(4), 240, 1998.

26. Ziegenhagen, D.J. et al., Addition of senna improves colonoscopy preparation with lavage: a prospective randomized trial, *Gastrointestinal Endoscopy*, 37(5), 547, 1991.
27. Shelton, M.G., Standardized senna in the management of constipation in the puerperium: a clinical trial, *South African Med. J.*, 57(3), 78, 1980.
28. Corman, M.L., Management of post-operative constipation in anorectal surgery, *Dis. Colon Rectum*, 22(3), 149, 1979.
29. Bossi, S. et al., Clinical study of a new preparation from plantago seeds and senna pods, *Acta Biomed. Atene. Parmense*, 57(5–6), 179, 1986.
30. Agra, Y. et al., Efficacy of senna versus lactulose in terminal cancer patients treated with opioids, *J. Pain Symptom Manage.*, 15(1), 1, 1998.
31. Peigen, X., Liyi, H., and Liwei, W., Ethnopharmacologic study of Chinese rhubarb, *J. Ethnopharmacol.*, 10, 275, 1984.
32. Chirikdjian, J.J., Kopp, B., and Beran, H., Laxative action of a new anthroquinone glycoside from rhubarb roots, *Planta Medica*, 48, 34, 1983.
33. Yamagishi, T. et al., New laxative constituents of rhubarb isolation and characterization of rheinosides A, B, C and D, *Chem. Pharm. Bull.*, 35, 3132, 1987.
34. Zhang, Y. et al., Tiao Wei Cheng Qi Tang decoction with liquid diet in bowel cleansing, *Bull. Hunan Medical Coll.*, 11, 299, 1986.
35. Gilani, A.H. et al., Pharmacological basis for the use of peach leaves in constipation, *J. Ethnopharmacol.*, 73, 87–93, 2000.
36. Tamhane, M.D. et al., Effect of oral administration of *Terminalia chebula* on gastric emptying: an experimental study, *J. Postgrad. Med.*, 43(1), 12, 1997.
37. Miglani, B.D., Sen, P., and Sanyal, R.K., Purgative action of an oil obtained from *Terminalia chebula*, *Indian J. Med. Res.*, 59(2), 281, 1971.
38. Iyengar, M.A., Pendse, G.S., and Narayana, N., Bioassay of *Cassia fistula*, *Planta Medica*, 14(3), 289, 1966.
39. Gupta, S.S., Verma, P., and Hishikar, K., Purgative and antihelmintic effects of *Mallotus philippinensis* in rats against tape worm, *Indian J. Physiol. Pharmacol.*, 28(1), 63, 1984.
40. Saez, L.R., Therapeutic proposals for the treatment of idiopathic constipation, *Ital. J. Gastroenterol.*, 23(8), 30, 1991.

19

Hyperacidity (Amlapitta)

Shankar K. Mitra and Paramesh R. Rangesh

CONTENTS

0-8493-1366-X/04/$0.00+$1.50

19.1 Introduction

Hyperacidity (*amlapitta*) is a disease caused by the excessive formation of acid in the stomach associated with the symptom of burning sensation in the throat and heart area. This condition appears in many diseases ranging from gastritis and peptic ulcer disease (PUD) to the currently named gastroesophageal reflux disease (GERD).

Gastritis includes myriad disorders that involve inflammatory changes in the gastric mucosa, including erosive gastritis caused by a noxious irritant, reflux gastritis from exposure to bile and pancreatic fluids, hemorrhagic gastritis, infectious gastritis, and gastric mucosal atrophy. PUD refers to a discrete mucosal defect in the portions of the gastrointestinal (GI) tract (gastric or duodenal) exposed to acid and pepsin secretion. Presentations of gastritis and PUD usually are indistinguishable, and the management is generally the same. GERD is a digestive disorder that affects the lower esophageal sphincter (LES), the muscle connecting the esophagus with the stomach. Many people, including pregnant women, suffer from heartburn or acid indigestion caused by GERD. Doctors believe that some people suffer from GERD due to a condition called hiatal hernia. In most cases, heartburn can be relieved through diet and lifestyle changes; some people may require medication or surgery.

Amlapitta is more generally classified as a GI disorder, which is due to imbalance in enzyme secretions. Caraka describes some of the common causes for such as deranged digestive enzymes. Fasting, overeating while having indigestion, practicing irregular eating habits, consuming unsuitable foods, eating in an unsupportive atmosphere or at the wrong time, or eating foods that have been improperly prepared will all produce acid indigestion.[1]

19.2 Definition

Amlapitta is defined as the digestive secretions (*pitta*) that have undergone an acidic and acrid state.[2]

Gastroesophageal refers to the stomach and esophagus and reflux means to flow back or return. Therefore, gastroesophageal reflux is the return of the stomach's contents into the esophagus.

19.3 Clinical Description

Hyperacidity is characterized by reflux of acid juice from the stomach, vomiting, a burning pain in the chest region, and headache.[2]

As described in conventional medicine, the most prevalent symptom is a burning pain in the area of the lower chest or upper abdomen. The pain of an ulcer can last anywhere from 30 min to a few hours. Additional symptoms that may be experienced are weight loss, a decrease in appetite, anemia, nausea, and vomiting. There may be times when the pain of an ulcer seems to be gone and then it suddenly returns. Pain associated with ulcers affect different people in different ways. Some people experience pain immediately after eating, whereas others may not be bothered for several hours. It is beneficial to figure out what may be responsible for producing excess stomach acid so these symptoms can be avoided.

19.4 History and Epidemiology

Hyperacidity is not described in detail in most of the ancient Ayurvedic literatures, including those of Caraka, Susruta, and Vagbhata that belong to the period *circa* 1500 B.C. to 600 A.D. However, Caraka has mentioned, while explaining irritable colon (*grahani*) disease, that this condition is the outcome of endotoxin, and the horsegram (*Dolicos biflorus*) seeds are known to be aggravating the disease.[1] For the first time, Kashyapa (*circa* 800 A.D.) has described this disease separately. Madhava (1000 A.D.) has given details about this disease.[3]

Looking back at the history of conventional medicine, PUD was a rare and generally unrecognized cause of symptoms and complications or death until the early 19th century. Despite sporadic case reports beginning in late 18th century, PUD did not become widely appreciated until early 20th century. The first 6 decades saw the dominance of surgery in the treatment of PUD. With the introduction of acid-suppressive drugs like histamine-2 blockers in the 1970s, the treatment of PUD was revolutionized. By the 1980s, the advent of *Helicobacter pylori* brought about a dramatic twist and possibly the cure.

Reflux disease is common. Approximately 15 to 20% of adults experience heartburn at least once a week. Obesity (body mass index [BMI] >30 kg/m^2), alcohol consumption (>7 standard drinks/week), and a first-degree relative with heartburn increase the risk of having reflux symptoms. Patients with connective tissue diseases, such as scleroderma, and chronic respiratory disease, such as asthma and cystic fibrosis, institutionalized and intellectually handicapped patients. Patients nursed in a supine position for prolonged periods are at increased risk of reflux disease.[4]

19.5 Etiology

According to Ayurvedic medicine, hyperacidity is caused by eating foods that are excessively sour, hot, and spicy; increasing the intake of alcohol; and eating oily, fried, or irritant foods. Violation of rules for eating and lifestyle changes, including overeating, having an incompatible diet, eating irritant and contaminated food, eating when suffering from indigestion, increasing the intake of horse gram, living in temperate climate, and experiencing factors that increase *pitta* (e.g., negative emotions and control of natural urges) are causes this disease.[1]

Dietary and lifestyle choices may contribute to GERD. Certain foods and beverages, including chocolate, peppermint, fried or fatty foods, coffee, or alcoholic beverages, may weaken the LES, causing reflux and heartburn. Studies show that cigarette smoking relaxes the LES. Obesity and pregnancy can also cause GERD.[4]

19.6 Pathogenesis and Pathology

In Ayurveda, hyperacidity may be an expression of excessive digestive enzymes (*pachaka pitta*) due to stimulation from *vata*. This excessive enzyme secretion will dry the mucous (*kaphadhara kala*) lining of the stomach, leading to irritation, hypersecretion, acidity, and eventually ulceration. There are two common causes of this type of *vata* stimulation:

1. *Samana vata* — This type of *vata* normally stimulates the digestive enzymes while eating. It is the controller of digestion and relates the state of mind. If one is stressed and hurried during a meal, skips a meal, or eats fast, nondigestible food, these stressors will affect the quality of digestion.
2. *Apana vata* — This type of *vata* is in the intestinal tract. It is often siphoned upward through the enteric cycle into the liver and digestive organs. This reversed flow of the *apana vata* can excessively stimulate the digestive enzyme in the stomach and irritate the stomach lining. Subsequently, *apana vata* can then be drawn upward from an already aggravated *pitta*. Also, *apana vata* may increase as a result of stress, wherein the nervous system is under such extreme influence that *apana vata* is drawn upward for nervous system support. Along the way, the *apana* would stimulate the digestive enzyme and leave the seat of *vata* in the intestines depleted.[2]

Pitta is at the root of such a disorder. This is typically seen in a *pitta* constitution with a *pitta* imbalance. *Pitta* constitution types are the ones who eat fast without awareness and have a very hectic lifestyle. *Pitta*, which increases by the etiological factors (especially with its acid state), results in hyperacidity. This state of *pitta* is burnt out to cause acid eructation.

Thus hyperacidity is a hypersecretory disorder of the stomach and duodenum. It involves the pathological state of *pitta* locally and blood systemically.

19.7 Diagnosis

The diagnosis of this condition is made by identifying a combination of signs and symptoms such as indigestion (*avipaka*), bitter and acid regurgitation (*tikta-amlodgara*), substernal burning (*hritkantha daha*), hypersalivation (*utklesha*), fatigue, and increased stress (*klama*).

19.7.1 Classification

Amlapitta is classified into two types: regurgitation through the mouth (*urdhvaga amlapitta*) and a similar type of movement in the lower GI tract (*adhoga amlapitta*). Based on the association of the *dosa* involvement, there are three types: *vata, kapha* and *vata kapha*.[2]

19.7.1.1 Hyperacidity Affecting the Upper GI Tract (Regurgitation through the Mouth)

Clinical features of this type are regurgitation of excessive sour, slimy, meat soup (with green, yellow, bluish, dark, blood-stained contents) and vomiting of bitter and sour contents despite having an empty or full stomach. Heartburn rising from the stomach or lower abdomen that continues to the chest and toward the neck, headache, a burning and hot feeling in the sole and palm, and distaste (usually associated with fever) are the other associated problems.

19.7.1.2 Hyperacidity Affecting the Lower GI Tract

This condition is characterized by the passing of loose stools with burning pain, excessive thirst, vertigo, stupor, hypersalivation, skin rashes, hypersweating, and horripilations.

19.7.1.3 Hyperacidity Due to Vata

This condition, in addition to the above symptoms, presents abdominal pain, tremors, horripilations, blackouts, delirious talk, stupor, and fatigue.

19.7.1.4 Hyperacidity Due to Kapha

This condition, in addition to the above symptoms, also has expectoration of sputum, heaviness of the body, loss of taste, vomiting, weakness, itching all over the body, and excessive sleep.[2]

19.7.2 Clinical Features of GERD

19.7.2.1 Heartburn

This is the hallmark symptom of reflux disease. It is characterized by a burning feeling below the sternum, rising from the stomach or lower chest toward the neck. It is typically provoked by meals, especially those containing fatty and highly spicy food; bending forward; straining; or lying down. It is usually eased or relieved by antacids.

19.7.2.2 Regurgitation

This is the other characteristic symptom of reflux disease. Regurgitated material is usually tasted and reswallowed but is sometimes so voluminous that it may be mistaken for "vomiting." Some patients may experience regurgitation as their predominant symptom.

19.7.2.3 Water Brash

Esophageal acidification may cause such sudden and brisk stimulation of salivation that the patient's mouth fills with saliva.

19.7.2.4 Atypical Symptoms

Reflux may cause a number of other symptoms not easily identified as being due to reflux. These include angina-like chest pain, excessive belching, dyspepsia and nonspecific queasiness, uneasiness, or nausea.

19.7.3 Complications of Reflux Disease

19.7.3.1 Respiratory Symptoms

Reflux has been incriminated as a cause of respiratory and laryngeal diseases such as asthma, chronic cough, laryngitis, and sinusitis. Coughing, wheezing, hoarseness, or a sore throat may occur and are occasionally the presenting symptoms. It is uncertain how important reflux is in causing these nonspecific symptoms, but this applies probably only in a minority.

19.7.3.2 Dysphagia

Dysphagia is common but is usually variable and due either to defective esophageal peristalsis or heightened esophageal sensitivity. Dysphagia that is associated with symptoms of bolus impaction is highly suggestive of a stricture.

19.7.3.3 Odynophagia (Painful Swallowing)

This may be a prominent symptom due to excessive sensitivity of the esophageal mucosa. It is usually associated with severe esophagitis.

19.7.3.4 Bleeding from Esophagitis

Hematemesis may be a presenting symptom but is rarely severe. Occasionally, iron deficiency may result.[5]

19.8 Clinical Course and Prognosis

Hyperacidity is amenable to treatment if treated early. It becomes palliative if delayed and is difficult to cure in patients not observing preventive follow-up.[2]

19.9 Therapy

In Ayurveda, the following procedures are used in treating hyperacidity:

1. Emesis therapy (vamana) with the water extracts of snakeguard (*Trichosanthes dioica*) and neem (*Azadirachta indica*) followed by purgation (*virecana*) with powders of trivrit (*Operculina turpethum*) or any one of the following: *avipattikara curna, amalakyadi curna, abhayarishta*, or *triphala curna*.
2. If the burning pain is intensive, the patient is advised to apply whole body massage with *candana taila* or *lakshadi taila*.
3. In conditions of regurgitation through the mouth, purgation is advised. In case of lower GI symptoms due to hyperacidity, emesis is the choice.[6]

19.9.1 Lifestyle Changes

Three factors are essential for good and balanced digestion. First, food must be fresh and grown locally, or at least seasonally, and prepared with a caring and loving attitude. Second, food must be eaten with attention and awareness. Our sense of taste both prepares and ignites the digestive process before food ever reaches the stomach, as does our sense of composure and calm. Being distracted with books, driving, computers, and phones during a meal negates any hope of a balanced digestive process. Third, eating is best done during *pitta* period, between 10 A.M. and 2 P.M.; this is when the enzymes are the strongest and digestion will be the most effective. Eating at other times will eventually compromise the body's ability to digest and assimilate nutrition and give energy over a long period.

19.9.2 Home Remedies for Hyperacidity

1. Take tender coconut (*Cocus nucifera*) water. A dose of 100 to 500 ml should be taken twice/day.
2. Take the powdered fruit rind of emblic myrobalan (*Emblica officinalis*). A dose of 3 to 6 g should be taken with 100 to 250 ml milk twice/day.
3. Mix a gruel of rice corn, raw sugar, and honey in equal quantity. A dose of 100 to 200 g should be taken twice/day.
4. Take powdered fruit rind of chebulic myrobalan (*Terminalia chebula*) and whole plant of thistles (*Eclipta alba*) in equal quantity. A dose of 3 to 6 g should be taken with 12 g of jaggery and warm water twice/day.
5. Take dried rhizome of turmeric (*Curcuma longa*), leaf of snakeguard (*Trichosanthes dioica*), and fruit rind of emblic myrobalan (*Emblica offcinalis*) in equal parts and make the powder. A dose of 3 to 6 g should be taken with the fresh juice of ginger and 30 drops of papaya latex twice/day.
6. Prepare a decoction from the equal parts of stem of tinospora (*Tinospora cordifolia*), fruit of neem, leaf of snakeguard, and *triphala*. A dose of 14 to 28 ml should be taken twice/day.
7. Prepare a decoction of equal parts of dried ginger, fruit of coriander, and leaf of snakeguard. A dose of 14 to 28 ml should be taken twice/day.
8. Prepare a decoction of equal parts of leaves of snakeguard and *vasaka*, dried ginger, stem of tinospora, and rhizome of katuki (*Picrorhiza curroa*). A dose of 14 to 28 ml should be taken with 4 to 6 g honey twice/day.
9. Prepare *mahasurdarshan churna*, containing triphala (*Emblica officinalis, Terminalia belerica, Terminalia chebula*), guduci (*Tinospora cordifolia*), katuka (*Picrorrhiza kurroa*), fumaria (*Fumaria officinalis*), lime juice, etc. A dose of 1/2 tsp three times/day after meals is recommended.
10. Prepare *avipattikara churna*, containing ginger, black pepper, triphala, nut grass (*Cyperus rotundus*), embelia fruits (*Embelia ribes*), cardamom (*Elettaria cardamomum*), clove (*Syzygium aromaticum*), cinnamon (*Cinnamomum cassia*), and sugar. This is the medicine of choice in treating hyperacidity. A dose of 1 tsp before meals three times/day with lemon juice is recommended.
11. Use aloe vera (*Aloe littoralis*). Prepare 1 tbsp of fresh gel from the plant and take three times/day.
12. Drink coriander (*Coriandrum sativum*) and cumin (*Cuminum cyminum*) tea.

TABLE 19.1

Common Ayurvedic Formulas Used To Treat Hyperacidity

Name of Formulation	Activity	Dose	Adjuvant	Ref.
Avipattikara curna	Digestive, pacifies *pitta*	3–6 g twice/day before meals	Warm water	6
Dhatri loha	Carminative, hemetinic	0.5–1 g twice/day	Ghee	8
Kamadudha rasa	Antacid	250–500 mg twice/day before meals	Honey and Water	8
Sankha bhasma, Kapardika bhasma, or Pravala bhasma	Antacid, antispasmodic	250–500 mg twice/day before meals	Honey and water	8
Sutasekhara rasa	Antacid, antispasmodic	250–500 mg twice/day before meals	Honey and water	8
Narikela khanda	Antacid, antiflatulent	6–12 g twice/day before meals	Milk	8

13. Take 1 tsp of psyllium (*Plantago ovata*) 1 h after meals with 8 oz of warm water.
14. Prepare a milk decoction of 1 tsp emblica myrobalan (*Emblica officinalis*), 1 tsp raw sugar, 1 cup of milk, and 1 cup of water. Boil to 1 cup. Drink as a tea with meals or anytime three times/day.
15. Prepare a decoction of fenugreek (*Trigonella foenum-graecum*), honey, ½ tsp of powder with ½ tsp of turmeric on an empty stomach with warm water or warm milk.
16. Prepare a licorice (*Glycyrrhiza glabra*) ghee. Make the decoction with 1 tsp of licorice in 2 cups of water. Boil to 1 cup. Add 1 cup ghee and 1 cup water. Boil off water. Take ½ tsp three times/day on an empty stomach with hot water. This ghee can be used in cooking.[7]

Compound formulas commonly used to treat hyperacidity are listed in Table 19.1.

19.10 Scientific Basis

The scientific studies relating to the treatment of GERD through natural products are diverse, which include not only the studies on gastric acidity, but also those which are suggestive of antiulcer activity. Some of the current studies on therapeutic procedures as well as the plants and herbomineral preparations are listed below.

19.10.1 Fat Preparations (*Snehapana*)

Various dehydrated butter (ghee) or oil preparations have been prescribed in Ayurveda for the management of *parinama sula*. Ghee in the duodenum inhibits gastric acid secretion; gastric inhibitory peptide (GIP) has been proposed as a candidate for this enterogastrone action. Moreover, extracts of various indigenous herbs are mixed in Ayurvedic ghee and oil preparations, making these preparations more useful. Utility of ghee and oil preparations in PUD is discussed below.

Snehapana of *dadimadya ghrta* (2 oz/day for 2 to 6 weeks) exhibited symptomatic relief in peptic ulcer syndrome. A significant reduction in gastric acidity was observed particularly in cases of nonulcer dyspepsia (NUD).[9]

Dadimadya ghrta or *accha ghrta* produced excellent results in 60% of cases with peptic ulcer syndrome (15-patient case study) when given in dose of 50 g/day for 2 to 3 weeks. Experimental studies[10] also confirmed the protective action of *ghrta* against histamine-induced ulcers.

In a control study, researchers have evaluated the efficacy of *panchakarma* (*snehana* and subsequent *virecana*) in 30 patients with *parinama sula*. A dose of 30 ml of *dadimadya ghrta* was given to the first group of 15 patients on the first day followed by a daily increase of 30 ml for 7 days. Thereafter, *virecana* with *avipattakara curna* was given. A control group of 15 patients was treated with *shankha vati* (6 tablets/day) for the same duration. Cases of both groups were followed for 3 months. Approximately 60% of the *snehana-virecana* group was completely cured from the disease for the whole period of follow-up along with radiological ulcer healing and reduction in gastric acidity. Other cases of this group had different degrees of relief. Patients of the control group were not completely cured. This cure probably works by virtue of elimination of *vata* and *pitta dosa* along with wound-healing effects.[10]

Tikta ghrta (*astangahrdaya*) was taken in doses of 40 ml/day. Results showed complete symptomatic relief in 82% of cases with *parinama sula* (38-patient case study). The study lacks laboratory or radiological evidence of improvement.[10]

Indukanta ghrta (*sahasrayoga*) was tested in 46 patients with *parinama sula* (28 with duodenal ulcer [DU], 10 with gastric ulcer, and 8 with hyperchlorhydria). *Snehapana* was given according to the *agnibala* of the patients for the first 7 days followed by *Svedana* (2 days). *Virecana* with castor oil (1 day) was followed by *samsarjana karma* for the next 3 days. During the *samana* period of 7 days, *indukanta ghrta* was given in doses of 30 ml/day. Complete symptomatic relief was observed in 84% of cases of this series. However, a gastric acid secretion augmented histamine test, barium meal, or endoscopial study has not been included in the evaluation of results.[10]

Kusadi ghrta has been studied in patients with peptic ulcers (18 with DU and 2 with gastric ulcer). A dose of 25 g of *ghrta* per day was given for 1 month. Apart from clinical improvement, *ghrta* reduced gastric acid secretion in the Fractional Test Meal test and caused complete ulcer healing confirmed radiologically in 65% of patients.[10]

Many single and combined herbs, herbominerals, and fat preparations have been found effective in treating PUD. *Amalaki, madhuyasthi, satavari,* and *bhringaraja* appear more useful among herbs. Real efficacy can be proved only by comparative and controlled study adopting endoscopic evaluation. These herbs have shown ulcer-healing property even on these parameters. Moreover, these herbs are cheap and nontoxic even with long-term use.[10]

19.10.2 Herbs, Herbal Preparations, *Rasas*, and *Bhasmas*

19.10.2.1 Emblica officinalis (Indian Gooseberry)

Dhatri lauha, frequently used in *amlapitta* and *parinama sula,* consists of two herbs (*amalaki* and *madhuyasthi*) and one mineral (iron). This preparation has been found to alleviate the common clinical complaints like epigastric pain, acid eructation, epigastric and retrosternal burning in the majority of patients with *amlapitta* along with an appreciable reduction in free and total acidity.[12] Fruits of *amalaki,* apart from having proven efficacy in experimental study, relieved the symptoms significantly in patients with *amlapitta* having hyperchlorhydria when given in doses of 3 g three times/day for 7 days. However, this study consisted of only a few patients.[10]

In a clinical trial on *amalaki* in a large series of patients with DU (27 cases) and NUD (12 cases), *amalaki* was given in a dose 9 to 13.5 g/day (in three divided doses) for an initial 2 weeks. This was followed by a dose of 6 to 9 g/day (two divided doses) for the rest of total duration of 3 months to the patients of both groups. Gastric acid secretion was measured by an AHT. Pepsin and mucin were also estimated in gastric juice. A significant decrease in acid and pepsin secretion was observed. Complete radiological healing was reported in peptic-ulcer patients. Marked symptomatic relief was found in most of the patients (78-patient case study) with the use of *amalaki*. Moreover, the drug exhibited prophylactic effect against the histamine-induced ulcer in albino rats. Furthermore, *amalaki* exhibited some anabolic activity evidenced by weight gain and also an increase in hemoglobin concentration.[13] Both the prophylactic and curative properties of *amalaki rasayana* have been observed in another study on experimental peptic ulcer.[14] *Amalaki* powder produced 66% symptomatic improvement, significant reduction in gastric acidity response (AHT), and endoscopic healing in 57% of cases with DU. However, there were only seven trial cases.[10]

19.10.2.2 *Glycyrrhiza glabra* (Licorice)

The second and important ingredient of *dhatri lauha* is *madhuyasthi* or licorice. The antiulcerogenic effect of *madhuyasthi* was observed against both the pyloric ligation and histamine-induced ulcers. The drug powder in doses of 18 g/day in three divided doses exhibited marked response in 80% of patients with DU (10-case study) within a week. Further clinical and experimental study was done on *madhuyasthi*.[15] The powder of the drug was given to 10 patients with NUD (6 g/day) and 15 patients with DU (6 g/day) for 1 to 3 months. Excellent response was reported in 30% of patients and good response was seen in 50% of patients with NUD. After 2 months of therapy in the duodenal ulcer group, pain was relieved completely in 56% of cases, whereas a burning sensation was reported in 78% of the cases. Complete radiological healing was observed in 50% of cases and partial in 40% of cases. No reduction in gastric acidity response was observed. Experimentally, *madhuyasthi* did not produce significant acid reduction. *Haridra* (*Curcuma longa*), *babula* (*Acacla arabica*), and *aparajita* (*Clitoria ternatia*) reduced acidity significantly in albino rats. Two herbs of *dhatri lauha*, *amalaki* and *madhuyasthi*, have been found quite effective for both types of patients, i.e., DU and NUD.[10]

19.10.2.3 *Asparagus racemosus* (Asparagus)

A clinical study has reported good response in 80% of patients with DU with the use of *satavari* (asparagus) powder in a dose of 20 g/day in three divided doses for 4 weeks. Free and total gastric acidity was reduced significantly in 15 patients with DU having hyperacidity. Workers also have observed a significant decline in free and total acidity of gastric juice of albino rats with *satavari*. In a double-blind, randomized drug trial, researchers have observed suppression of heartburn, nausea, or vomiting in 100% of cases and pain in 83% of cases with DU with the use of *satavari* powder (6 g/day for 6 weeks). Complete ulcer healing was observed in 50% of cases radiologically and in 62% of cases endoscopically. The drug also reduced hyperchlorhydria of these patients. Workers observed slightly better results with *satavari* in comparison with *amalaki*, but the study was conducted on only eight and seven patients, respectively.

A group of researchers have observed antiulcerogenic effect of *satavari* and *bhringaraja* in aspirin (200 mg/kg body weight for 4 days)-induced ulcers in albino rats. There was a decrease in ulcer score and severity in both the groups, along with reduction in gastric acidity and peptic activity and an increase in mucin activity. Continuity and thickness of gastric mucosa was maintained in comparison with aspirin-treated gastric mucosa. Histochemically, mucin content of gastric mucosa was increased in both the groups. Clinically, both the drugs (*satavari* and *bhringaraja*) exhibited radiological (in 83 and 67% of cases, respectively) as well as endoscopical healing (in 55 and 50% of patients, respectively) along with significant reduction in hyperacidity pattern. However, again the number of patients was fewer: only six in *satavari* group and nine in *bhringaraja* group.

Another group has observed significant symptomatic improvement in 26 patients with proved DU disease with the use of *satavari* root powder (12 g/day for 6 weeks). *Satavari* inhibited basal acid output by 32%, histamine-induced maximum output by 38%, and alcohol-induced output by only 32%. Approximately 75% of patients had radiologic and endoscopic evidence of ulcer healing. The drug was not found to possess antacid property *in vitro*. Direct healing effect was proposed probably by enhancement of mucosal barrier, prolongation of life span of mucosal cells, or cytoprotection.[10]

The antiulcerogenic activity of juice of fresh roots of asparagus has been reported against cold-restraint stress and pylorus ligation-induced gastric ulcers. The activity was reported to be due to both a decrease in offensive acid-pepsin secretion and an increase in defensive mucin secretion. Mucin secretion was quantified in terms of TC:P ratio in the gastric juice. The strengthening of the mucin barrier led to a further decrease in the dexoribonucleic acid (DNA) content of the gastric juice, indicating a decrease in cell shedding.[16] In continuation of earlier experimental work, a *satavari* containing Ayurvedic preparation, *satavari mandur,* has undergone clinical trails and shown promising results. It has been observed that when given *satavari mandur* at the dose of 1.5 g twice daily for a month, the preparation not only produced significant improvement in symptoms of peptic ulcer, but also healed endoscopically proved cases of ulcer dyspepsia by 75%. The biochemical estimations of offensive acid-pepsin and defensive mucin secretion and cell shedding before and after treatment with *satavari mandur* showed a tendency to decrease acid-pepsin secretion. The estimations also showed a significant decrease in cell shedding and an increase in mucin secretion indicating *satavari mandur's* predominant effect on mucosal defensive factors.[10]

19.10.2.4 Eclipta alba (Thistles)

Bhringaraja is used as a soaking agent for various Ayurvedic antiulcer preparations. As early as in 1968 researchers have reported the efficacy of *Eclipta alba* in treating hyperchlorhydria.[17] Later on, in a clinical trial done on 22 patients with NUD and 8 patients with DU, researchers observed a significant reduction in gastric acidity when *bhringaraja* (whole plant) was given in syrup form in a dose of 20 ml/day (20 g crude drug) in three divided doses for 6 weeks. Approximately 90% of dyspeptic patients were cured, whereas about 87% of ulcer patients improved. Seeing its efficacy, a team of scientists further evaluated its effectiveness in NUD and DU in a large series of 60 cases (35 of NUD and 25 of DU). The powder of whole herb was given in a daily dose of 30 g (in three divided doses) for 1 month to the NUD group and for 3 months to the DU group. The drug exhibited marked symptomatic relief in the majority of the patients and reduced gastric acidity significantly in both groups. Approximately 80% of patients with NUD responded well to this therapy. Radiological improvement was observed in 75% of cases out of 12 patients with DU who came for follow-up. Approximately 48% of patients of this series gained excellent relief with *bhringaraja*. Later another group further confirmed the effectivity of *bhringaraja* in 60% of cases (935-patient case study) with DU when given in dose of 30 g/day for 3 to 6 months.[10]

19.10.2.5 Trichosanthes dioica (Snakeguard)

Patoladi kasaya (prepeptone), consisting of *patola, haritaki, bibhitaka, amalaki, kutaki, cirayata, amrta, pittapapada, sunthi,* and *bhringaraja*, exhibited complete improvement in 50% of cases and partial improvement in 40% of cases with PUD (10-patient case study). The decoction was given in doses of 30 ml/day in three divided doses for 3 weeks. It decreased the acid response in hypersecretors and normalized the acid response in hyposecretors. Best results were observed in patients with *kaphaja parinama sula.*

Another *patoladi kasaya* consisting of only four herbs, *patola, sunthi, amrta,* and *kutaki,* was given in a follow-up study of 33 operated cases of DU. The drug kept the patients symptom- and complication-free when given in doses of 40 ml/day in two divided doses. It normalized both the hyper- and hypoacidity of these patients.

The efficacy of a single herb, *patola,* was studied in 20 patients with DU. Its decoction was given in doses of 150 ml/day (60 g crude drug) in three divided doses for three weeks. Drug exhibited marked clinical improvement and reduction in gastric hyperacidity. Excellent response with complete ulcer healing (radiological) was observed in 50% of patients, and good response in 35% of patients. Effectively of *patola* in DU (excellent response in 45% of 20 cases) has been further reported.[10]

19.10.2.6 Adhatoda vasica (Vasaka)

Vasaka in Ayurveda is indicated in bleeding disorders. PUD may cause hematemesis. Therefore, this drug was tried in 20 patients with DU. Approximately 60 ml of syrup (30 g crude drug) was given daily in four divided doses for 6 weeks. Clinical improvement along with reduction in gastric acidity was observed in 85% of patients in this series. Moreover, the drug also decreased gastric acid secretion in albino rats. The drug was not tried in patients with DU.[18,19]

19.10.2.7 Cocos nucifera (Coconut)

Coconut water has been reported to possess protective action against aspirin- and histamine-induced gastric mucosal damage. Its kernal reduced the gastric acidity and improved the clinical features in patients with DU. *Narikela khanda,* a famous preparation for *parinama sula,* was given in a dose 60 g/day in five divided doses for three weeks to eight patients of PUD. Approximately 62% of patients got complete relief, whereas the reamining cases got partial improvement. Best results were obtained in the *paittika* type of *parinama sula.*

Two researchers evaluated the effectivity of an Ayurvedic compound preparation consisting of *narikela lavana, trisankha bhasma,* and *avipittikara curna* in 60 cases of *amlapitta.* The compound clinically exhibited good response in 57% of cases and fair response in 26% of cases.[10]

19.10.2.8 Tamra bhasma (Copper Calx)

The use of herbomineral preparations in Ayurveda is well documented. *Tamra bhasma,* a traditional preparation of copper, has been suggested for its use in *amlapitta.* An earlier published study has given the composition of *tamra bhasma* as $CuO < 44.45\%$, $Fe_2O_3 < 6.03\%$, and $S < 2.75\%$.[20]

Extensive studies have been undertaken to unravel the antiulcerogenic activity of *tamrabhasma.* It has been shown to possess ulcer-protective activity against various gastric ulcers in 8-h immobilized, 4-h pylorous-ligated, and aspirin-induced rats and histamine-induced gastric and DUs in guinea pigs. The activity was due to both a decrease in offensive acid-pepsin and an increase in defensive mucin secretion.[21] Further evaluation of *tamra bhasma* from different sources were compared with pure compound and mixture of major ingredients of *tamra bhasma* for antiulcerogenic activity. Results revealed that *tamra bhasma* preparation was better than pure copper compound or a mixture of known ingredients.

Quantitative differences in *tamra bhasma* preparation also showed the importance of pharmaceutical processing in the therapeutic activity of *tamra bhasma*.[22] *Tamra bhasma* has an overall solubility in water of approximately 1% and 12 ng/ml of CuO forms a saturated solution at 50°C. This implies that when used orally it would have a local effect rather than being systemically absorbed, reducing the possibility of systemic toxicity with copper. Toxicity studies have shown that TMB was safe, and even 1000 times of the effective antiulcer dose was tolerable in rats.

Tamra bhasma was also found to have an antiulcerogenic effect against aspirin-induced ulcers without affecting the anti-inflammatory activity of aspirin. *Tamra bhasma* seemed to have prolonged effect, as the protective effect of *tamra bhasma* lasted up to 5 days after discontinuation of treatment. An aspirin–copper combination may reduce ulcerogenic activity of aspirin without affecting its anti-inflammatory effect. Researchers have reported the gastric protective effect of *tamra bhasma* against cold restraint stress-induced gastric ulcers in rats and guinea pigs and its healing effect against acetic acid-induced gastric ulcers in rats. *Tamra bhasma* was reported to increase prostaglandins (PGEs) and decrease leukotrine C4 (LTC4) in human gastric and colonic mucosal incubates. The mucosal protective effects of *tamra bhasma* and CuCl2 could be due to their effect on endogenous PGEs and LTs. *Tamra bhasma* showed better and potent effect when compared with CuCl2 on PGEs release both in gastric and colonic incubates, suggesting that other ingredients of TMB add to its effects. *Tamra bhasma* significantly protected rats against ethanol-induced ulcers, and the effect was ascribed to decrease in LTC4/D4 synthesis.[23]

Tamra bhasma has also been reported to increase the defensive mucopolysaccharides, including sialomucin and fucose. It has also been reported to decrease DNA in gastric juice, suggesting decrease in cell shedding and increase in life span of mucosal cells, with no change in mucosal DNA and incorporation of [^{3}H]-thymidine uptake in mucosal tissues, indicating absence of activity on cell proliferation. The effect of TMB on offensive acid-pepsin secretion and LTs and defensive mucus secretion, mucosal glycoproteins, prostaglandin, and cell shedding may contribute to its ulcer protective activity.[24]

Tamra bhasma (1 mg/kg) has shown antiulcerogenic effect in 8-h immobilized, 4-h pylorous ligated, aspirin-induced and histamine-induced gastric ulcers in albino rats and guinea pigs. The drug decreases total acid and pepsin output and increases carbohydrate protein ratio, indicating an increase in mucosal barrier. Acute and subacute toxicity of the drug was not observed.[25] *Tamra bhasma* has better and prolonged antiulcer effect than pure copper preparation. Moreover, it does not antagonize the anti-inflammatory effect of aspirin. It has been suggested to take it on alternate days or even twice a week only with all beneficial effects in PUD.[10]

19.10.2.9 Sutasekhara Rasa

Sutasekhara rasa, an herbomineral mercury preparation, is widely used for the treatment of *amlapitta* and *parinama sula*. It contains copper, aconite, datura, and certain other herbs like *bhringaraja*. Two types of *sutasekhara rasa,* those with gold and those without gold, are popular in treating DUs.

Two researchers evaluated the efficacy of modified *sutasekhara rasa* (devoid of gold and copper) in seven patients with NUD and three with DU. The drug was given in doses of 600 mg/day for 6 weeks. Excellent response was reported in 85% of patients with NUD and in 67% of patients with DU.

A team of researchers, in a comparative clinical trial done on 63 patients with *parinama sula* (DU), did not observe any significant difference in the effectivity of *sutasekhara rasa* with gold and without gold. Gold preparation (375 mg/day in three divided doses) exhibited relief in 70% of patients, whereas preparation without gold (750 mg/day in three divided doses) produced relief in 67% of patients in 45 days. Results were assessed only on symptomatic improvement and reduction in acid secretion (FTM) and not on radiological and endoscopical ulcer-healing criteria. They have recommended the use of *sutasekhara rasa* without gold because of the high cost and long-term toxicity of *sutasekhara rasa* with gold.[26] Another group has reported the relief in patients with DU after a course of *sutasekhara rasa* for 42 days. Workers believe that this preparation acts probably by modifying the homeostatic regulation of hormonal stimulation of Hy ion secretion.[27]

Recently, *sutasekhara rasa* (without gold, 600 mg/day) along with *ashvangandha* powder (*Withania somnifera*, 6 g/day) exhibited symptomatic radiological and endoscopical improvement. It also exhibited along with a reduction in gastric acidity (FTM) in all the four treated patients with DU in 6 weeks; *sutasekhara rasa* alone improved three out of four patients. Similarly, *sutasekhara rasa* and *asvangandha* separately exhibited good response in four out of five patients, whereas their combination showed response in all the five treated cases with NUD. The number of trial cases in each group was very low. A substantial inference cannot be drawn. Even then, this study highlights the utility of antianxiety indigenous herbs (medhya drugs) as an adjuvant in the management of PUD.[10]

There are many plants used in antiulcer herbal formulations that have not yet been individually investigated for their efficacy in this condition. A group of researchers has reported the antiulcer effect of an herbal formulation, UL-409, consisting of six medicinal plants: *Glycyrrhiza glabra* L. (root), *Saussurea lappa* C.B. Clarke (root), *Aegle marmelos* Corr. (fruit), *Foeniculum vulgare* Mill. (seed), *Rosa damascena* Mill. (flower petals), and *Santalum album* L. (stem). This herbal formulation was found to increase the stomach mucus and decrease the acid volume, free and total acid content, in rats. Moreover, this formulation significantly prevented the occurrence of stress-induced ulceration and significantly inhibited gastric ulceration induced by ethanol, aspirin, pylorus-ligation, histamine, and indomethacin in rats and guinea pigs. It was found to have antiulcer activity due to a modulation of defensive factors, thereby improving gastric cytoprotection.[28,29]

A clinical trial was conducted in 56 patients with peptic ulcers, as confirmed by endoscopy, with UL-409. Results showed the formulation's beneficial effect in patients with PUD without any side effects in any of the patients.[30]

In another clinical trail,[31] patients with *H. pylori* infection (UL-409) showed clinical improvements without any side effects.

19.11 Future Ayurvedic Formulas

A variety of botanical products have been reported to possess antiulcer activity (especially from ethnopharmacological studies), but the documented literature has centered primarily on pharmacological action in experimental animals. Except for a few phytogenic compounds (i.e., liquorice and chilli), limited clinical data are available to support the use of herbs as gastroprotective agents and, thus, the data on efficacy and safety are limited. Despite this, there are several botanical products with potential therapeutic applications because of their high efficacy and low toxicity. Finally, it should be noted that substances, such as flavonoids, aescin, aloe gel, and many others, that possess both anti-inflammatory and antiulcer activity are of particular therapeutic importance. This is because most of the anti-inflammatory drugs used in modern medicine are ulcerogenic.

Several plants and herbs are used in folk medicine to treat gastrointestinal disorders, including peptic ulcers. Recently, there has been a growing interest in identifying new antiulcer agents from plant sources.

References

1. Caraka, *Caraka Samhita*, Part II, Pande, G., Ed., Chowkhamba Sanskrit Series Office, Varanasi, U.P. India, 1970, chap. 15, p. 386.
2. Madhava, *Madhavanidanam*, Part II, Upadhyaya, Y., Ed., Chowkhamba Sanskrit Series Office, Varanasi, U.P. India, 1973, chap. 51, p. 171.
3. Dhyani, S.C., *Kaya Chikitsa*, 1st ed., Ayurvedic & Tibbi Academy, Lucknow, U.P. India, 1991, chap. 67, p. 213.
4. Spechler, S.J., Epidemiology and natural history of gastro-oesophageal reflux disease, *Digestion*, 51(Suppl. 1), 24–29, 1992.
5. Fennerty, M.B. and Sampliner, R.E., Gastroesophageal reflux disease, *Hosp. Med.*, 29(4), 28–40, 1993.
6. Anon., *Yogaratnakara*, Part II, Sastri, B., Ed., Chowkhamba Sanskrit Series Office, Varanasi, U.P. India, 1973, p. 237.
7. Anon., *Hand Book of Domestic & Common Ayurvedic Remedies*, 1st ed., Central Council for Research in Indian Medicine and Homoeopathy, New Delhi, India, 1978, chap 9, p. 63.
8. Das, G., *Bhaishajyaratnavali*, Chaukhambha Sanskrit Sansthan, Varanasi, U.P. India, 1997, chap. 56, p. 643.
9. Singh, R.H. and Chaturvedi, G.N., Studies on pancha karma therapy. VII. Therapeutic value of Snehapan in the management of peptic ulcer syndrome, *Nagarjuna*, 10(11), 572, 1967.
10. Singh, K.P. and Singh, R.H., Recent advances in the management of *amlapitta-parinama sula* (non-ulcer dyspepsia and peptic ulcer disease), *J. Res. Ayurveda Siddha*, 6, 132, 1985.
11. Sarda Amma, L. and Narayan Sharma, K.P., Efficacy of dadimadighrita (*snehapana*) subsequent virechana in the treatment of parinamasula (duodenal ulcer), *J. Res. Educ. Ind. Med.*, 1(4), 27, 1982.
12. Das, S. and Shaw, B.P., Effect of dhatri lauha on gastric acidity of the patients of *amlapitta*, *J. Ayur. Yoga*, 4, 7, 1983.
13. Varma, M.D. et al., *Amalaki rasayana* in the treatment of peptic ulcer, *J. Res. Ind. Med. Yoga Homoeo.*, 12(4), 19, 1977.
14. Banu, N. et al., Role of *amalaki* (Emblica officinalis Linn.) *rasayana* in experimental peptic ulcer, *J. Res. Educ. Ind. Med.*, 1(1), 29, 1982.
15. Chaturvedi, G.N. et al., Some clinical and experimental studies on whole root of *Glycyrrhiza glabra* Linn. (Yashtimadhu) in peptic ulcer, *Ind. Med. Gaz.*, 113(6), 200, 1979.
16. De, B. et. al., Effect of some sitavirya drugs on gastric secretion and ulceration, *Indian J. Exp. Biol.*, 35, 1084, 1997.
17. Chaturvedi, G.N. and Singh, R.N., Treatment of hyperchlorhydria with an indigenous drug *Eclipta alba*, *Curr. Med. Pract.*, 8, 283, 1968.
18. Chaturvedi, G.N., Krishan Mohan, and Ariyawansa, H.A.S., Clinical correlation of amalapitta and its treatment with indigenous drug vasa (*Adhatoda vasica* Nees.), *Nagarjuna*, 24(8), 170, 1981.
19. Chaturvedi, G.N. et al., Clinical trial of *Adhatoda vasica* syrup (vasa) in the patients of non-ulcer dyspepsia (*amlapitta*), *Ancient Sci. Life*, 3(1), 19, 1983.
20. Raghunathan, K., *Pharmacopoeial Standards for Ayurvedic Formulations*, Central Council for Research in Indian Medicine and Homeopathy, New Delhi, India, 1976, p. 363.
21. Sanyal, A.K., Pandey, B.L., and Goel, R.K., The effect of a traditional preparation of copper, *tamrabhasma*, on experimental ulcers and gastric secretion, *J. Ethnopharmacol.*, 5, 78, 1982.

22. Pandey, B.L., Goel, R.K., and Das, P.K., A study of the effects of *tamrabhasma*, and indigenous preparation of copper on experimental gastric ulcers and secretion, *Ind. J. Exp. Biol.*, 21, 258, 1983.
23. Goel, R.K., Tavares, I.A., and Bennett, A., Effects of cupric chloride and *tamrabhasma*, a traditional Indian preparation of copper, on eicosanoid production by human gastric and colonic mucosa, *J. Pharm. Pharmacol.*, 44(10), 862, 1992.
24. Goel, R.K., Maiti, R.N., and Mukhopadhyaya, K., Effect of *tamrabhasma*, an Indian indigenous preparation of copper, on rat gastric mucosal resistance, *Indian J. Exp Biol.*, 32(8), 559, 1994.
25. Sanyal, A.K., Pandey, B.L., and Goel, R.K., The effect of a traditional preparation of copper, *tamrabhasma*, on experimental ulcers and gastric secretion, *J. Ethnopharmacol.*, 5(1), 79, 1982.
26. Kishore, P. et al., Clinical study on parinama sulacomparative clinical evaluation of swarna sutasekhar rasa and suta sekhara rasa, *J. Res. Ayu. Siddh.*, 2(3), 200, 1981.
27. Vaidya, A.B., Investigative gastroenterology and clinical pharmacology — a brief review and reminiscences, *J. Res. Educ. Ind. Med.*, 1(4), 1, 1982.
28. Mitra, S.K. et al., Protective effect of UL-409, a herbal formulation against physical and chemical factor induced gastric and duodenal ulcers in experimental animals, *J. Ethnopharmacol.*, 52, 165, 1996.
29. Kulkarni, S.K. and Goel, R.K., Gastric antiulcer activity of UL-409 in rats, *Indian J. Exp. Biol.*, 34, 683, 1996.
30. Rajasambandam, P., Peptic ulcer disease and cytoprotection: a possible herbal therapy, *Indian Pract.*, 54(8), 577, 2001.
31. Chandrashekar, N. and Vijaya, D., Ulcitum in gastroduodenal disease, *Indian J. Clin. Pract.*, 12(11), 49, 2001.

20

Irritable Colon (Grahani)

Shankar K. Mitra and Paramesh R. Rangesh

CONTENTS

0-8493-1366-X/04/$0.00+$1.50

20.1 Introduction

Irritable colon is also known as Irritable Bowel Syndrome (IBS). It is a gastrointestinal (GI) motility disorder for which there is no organic or structural cause. Because the symptoms of IBS can mimic other disorders, such as hypothyroidism, it is diagnosed when all other local and systemic conditions have been ruled out.

In Ayurvedic literature, the symptom of a disease called *grahani* resembles most of IBS symptoms. According to Ayurveda, grahani can be due to a number of factors such as improper diet, heavy foods, overeating, constipation, hemorrhoids, drinking too much fluid (especially cold water when hungry), exercising too soon after eating, forcing or straining natural urges, and taking chemical drugs.

20.2 Definition

The disease condition is called *grahani,* which indicates the pathological state of function and integrity of the intestinal tract (mostly small intestine), a particular part of the GI system known as *grahani* in Sanskrit.[1] *Grahani* is the seat of enzymes (agni). Normally, it holds up the food (until it is digested) and releases it from the side after it is digested. But when it is deranged due to weak digestive enzymes, it releases the ingested material even in undigested conditions.[1]

A disorder characterized by abnormally increased motility of the small and large intestines, producing abdominal pain, constipation, or diarrhea, is also known as irritable colon, spastic colon, or mucous colitis.

20.3 Clinical Description

Ayurvedic literature characterizes the disease by the passage of stools alternated with constipation or diarrhea and with undigested food particles. This disease is also associated with thirst, distaste, blackouts, pedal edema, pain in the bone, fever, and vomiting.[2] It is a motility disorder involving the entire GI tract, causing recurring upper and lower GI symptoms, including variable degrees of abdominal pain, constipation and diarrhea, and abdominal bloating.

20.4 History and Epidemiology

IBS has been a problem for people for thousands of years, as it is mentioned in the earlier literatures of Ayurveda. IBS, also known as spastic colon, is a common disorder affecting as many as 20% of the population, more so among women than men. Because it is a clinical diagnosis, the prevalence figures vary depending upon the definition of IBS used. Although only about 10% of IBS patients actually seek medical attention, it accounts for about 3 million physician visits and over 2 million prescriptions in the U.S. annually. It is the seventh leading diagnosis among all physicians, and these patients utilize an additional $300 per year of health-care costs than do their non-IBS counterparts.[3]

20.5 Etiology

Although no specific causes are mentioned in Ayurvedic literatures, most of them focus on the dietary injudiciousness as the foremost cause of IBS. Examples include the quality of food, such as extremely dry, astringent, spicy, and heavy to digest (protein rich) foods; the quantity of intake (e.g., overeating); and the improper frequency of intake (e.g., untimely eating habits). Certain lifestyles including excessive traveling and controlling various natural urges (e.g., defecation and urination) are described to be the foremost causes that affect the function and integrity of digestive system.[4]

In conventional medicine, the cause of IBS is unknown. No anatomical cause can be found. Emotional factors, diet, drugs, or hormones may precipitate or aggravate heightened GI motility. Some patients have anxiety disorders (particularly panic disorders), major depressive disorders, and somatization disorders. Stress and emotional conflict do not always coincide with symptom onset and recurrence. Some patients with IBS appear to have a learned aberrant illness behavior (i.e., they tend to express emotional conflict as a GI complaint, usually abdominal pain). The physician evaluating patients with IBS, particularly those with refractory symptoms, should investigate for unresolved psychological issues, including the possibility of sexual or physical abuse.[3]

20.5.1 Food Intolerance

True food allergy is mediated by the immune system and is associated with hives, asthma, eczema, nasal discharge, and positive skin-prick radioallergosorbent test (RAST) scores or other allergy tests.[5] However, food intolerance, rather than true food allergy, is believed to be more significant in IBS.[6] Between 33 and 66% of IBS patients report having one or more food intolerances.[5] The most common culprits are dairy (40 to 44%) and grains (40 to 60%); the resulting GI bloating, flatulence, and pain caused by this reaction appears to be mediated by inflammatory prostaglandin synthesis.[6]

20.5.2 Neurochemical Imbalance

Interaction between the brain and the gut occurs via nerves that send neurotransmitter signals. An imbalance between two of these neurotransmitters, serotonin and norepinephrine, are implicated in IBS. Constipation may result when levels of norepinephrine increase, causing a reduction in serotonin levels and inhibition of another neurotransmitter called acetylcholine. Conversely, diarrhea can occur when increased serotonin inhibits norepinephrine and causes levels of acetylcholine to increase. For IBS patients, such an imbalance in the nervous system can lead to the fluctuating bowel symptoms of constipation and diarrhea.[7]

20.5.3 History of Analgesic Use

The use of acetaminophen, a common pain-relieving medication, is associated with diarrhea-predominant IBS. Its action may be due to an imbalance in the neurotransmitter serotonin. Because acetaminophen can cause elevated levels of the serotonin by-product 5-hydroxy-indole-acetic acid (HIAA) in the urine, it is possible that acetaminophen somehow interferes with serotonin metabolism. Plasma serotonin levels have indeed been shown to be elevated after eating by patients with diarrhea-predominant IBS. Clinically, a drug that blocks the 5- HT3 serotonin receptor (5-HT3 receptor antagonist) is effective for women with diarrhea-predominant IBS. It is interesting to note that asthma, another condition associated with disordered smooth muscle function, was recently found to be associated with acetaminophen.[8]

20.5.4 Reproductive Hormones

IBS occurs more than twice as frequently in women than in men and tends to follow a cyclic pattern, with aggravation during the postovulatory (progesterone predominant) and premenstrual phases of the menstrual cycle.[9] Progesterone is known to delay gastric emptying and cause constipation; constipation with straining and the frequent passage of hard stools is a more prevalent IBS manifestation in women, especially during the postovulatory phase.[10] At the end of the postovulatory phase, the sudden withdrawal of progesterone that occurs with the start of the premenstrual phase may trigger increased bowel activity. Women frequently report loose stools and diarrhea before or with the onset of menstruation. In contrast to progesterone, estrogen has not been associated with exacerbations of IBS symptoms.[11]

Along with progesterone levels in women, prostaglandins E2 and F2 alpha also increase in the premenstrual phase. Because they are powerful stimulants of bowel contractions, it is possible that women with IBS may have an exaggerated response to these prostaglandins.[9]

20.5.5 Mood

Anxiety, hostile feelings, sadness, depression, and sleep disturbance are associated with IBS. Adverse life events such as family death, marital stress, financial difficulties, and especially physical and sexual abuse have also been reported more frequently in IBS patients than in the general population. However, it is possible that IBS patients with this social or psychological background may be more likely to seek medical treatment or participate in research studies.[5]

The impact of stress on bowel motility and pain were explored in one study[5] by administering corticotrophin-releasing factor (CRF), a hormone released in the body during stress. CRF increases motility of the descending colon and can induce abdominal pain. The researchers found that IBS patients had greater colonic motility and more abdominal pain after receiving CRF.

20.5.6 Small Intestine Bacterial Overgrowth

Excess bacteria in the small intestine, an area that is normally relatively bacteria free, is being recognized as important in the development of IBS. When these bacteria are present in the small intestine, excessive gas, bloating, abdominal distension and pain, and altered gut motility can result.[5]

20.6 Pathogenesis and Pathology

According to Ayurveda, there is a certain pathogenesis of this disorder. Due to the above causative factors, the enzyme secretion gets disturbed by the dominant *dosa*, which results in the production of enterotoxin. This toxin causes the food to undergo acidification, which damages the mucous membrane of the intestines; the result is a decrease of intestinal transit time, causing early evacuation of bowel contents or alternated with a state of constipation, which is influenced by *apana vata*.[2]

In IBS, the circular and longitudinal muscles of the small bowel and sigmoid are particularly susceptible to motor abnormalities. The proximal small bowel appears to be hyperreactive to food or parasympathomimetic drugs. Small-bowel transit is variable in patients with IBS, and changes in bowel transit time often do not correlate with symptoms. Intraluminal pressure studies of the sigmoid show that functional constipation can occur when austral segmentation becomes hyperreactive (i.e., increased frequency and amplitude of contractions); in contrast, diarrhea is associated with diminished motor function.

Excess mucus production, which often occurs in IBS, is not related to mucosal injury. Its cause is unclear, but it may be related to cholinergic hyperactivity. Hypersensitivity to normal amounts of intraluminal distention exists, as does a heightened perception of pain in the presence of normal quantity and quality of intestinal gas. The pain of IBS seems to be caused by an abnormally strong contraction of the intestinal smooth muscle or by an increased sensitivity of the intestine to distention. Hypersensitivity to the hormones gastrin and cholecystokinin may also be present. However, hormonal fluctuations do not correlate with clinical symptoms. The caloric density of food intake may increase the magnitude and frequency of myoelectrical activity and gastric motility. Fat ingestion may cause a delayed peak of motor activity, which can be exaggerated in IBS. The first few days of menstruation can lead to transiently elevated prostaglandin E2, resulting in increased pain and diarrhea. This is not caused by estrogen or progesterone but by the release of prostaglandins.[3]

20.7 Diagnosis

Ayurvedic literature indicates that there are four different types of IBS. They are constipation-predominant IBS (*vata grahani*), diarrhea-predominant IBS (*pitta grahani*), dysentery-predominant IBS (*kapha grahani*), and complex IBS (*tridosha grahani*). All three *dosas* are involved (*vata*, *pitta*, and *kapha*). Other literature also describes two chronic types of IBS: accrual IBS (*samgraha grahani*) and an incurable type called tympanitis predominant IBS (*ghatiyanthra grahani*).[2] The clinical features of all types of IBS are described below.

1. Constipation-predominant IBS — This type of IBS presents the clinical features of dryness in skin, mouth, or throat; more constipation or alternating constipation and diarrhea; thirst; bloating; flatulence; and a cold feeling. It is also associated with back or groin pain, weight loss, debility, anal fissures, insomnia, and anxiety.
2. Diarrhea-predominant IBS — This type of IBS clinically shows the presence of heartburn, thirst, feeling hot, irritable or angry, inflammation, sweating and fever, fluid, and foul smelling stools and eructation.

3. Dysentery-predominant IBS — This type of IBS exhibits the presence of nausea, indigestion, and excess sputum in the pharyngeal region, heaviness in the chest and abdomen, bad-smelling eructation, lethargy, sluggish bowels, and mucus in the stools.
4. Complex IBS — This type reveals the combined signs and symptoms of all the above types.
5. Accrual IBS — This type of IBS presents the combined features of all the *tridosas* and is more chronic. It is specially diagnosed with clinical features of *borborygmi*, diurnal changes that the bowel movements are increased in the daytime and stop at night. The nature of the stool will be pastier and slimy, have undigested food particles, and be eliminated with pain. The pattern of the bowel movement will be accumulation of stools for some days followed by passage of loose stools for several days.
6. Tympanites-predominant IBS — In this type of IBS, the clinical symptoms are rumbling sounds heard in abdomen and increased bowel movements with lots of undigested food particles.[2]

Conventional medicine states that IBS tends to begin in the second and third decades of life, causing bouts of symptoms that recur at irregular periods. Onset in late adult life is rare. Symptoms usually occur in the awake patient and rarely rouse the sleeping patient. Symptoms can be triggered by stress or the ingestion of food.

The features of IBS are pain relieved by defecation, an alternating pattern of bowel habits, abdominal distention, mucus in the stool, and sensation of incomplete evacuation after defecation. The more symptoms that are present, the likelier it is that the patient has IBS. In general, the character and location of pain, precipitating factors, and defecatory pattern are distinct for each patient. Variations or deviations from the usual symptoms may suggest intercurrent organic disease and should be thoroughly investigated. Patients with IBS may also have extra intestinal symptoms (e.g., fibromyalgia, headaches, dyspareunia, temporomandibular joint [TMJ] syndrome).

Two major clinical types of IBS have been described. In *constipation-predominant IBS*, constipation is common, but bowel habits vary. Most patients have pain over at least one area of the colon, associated with periodic constipation alternating with a more normal stool frequency. Stool often contains clear or white mucus. The pain is either colicky, comes in bouts, or has a continuous dull ache; it may be relieved by a bowel movement. Eating commonly triggers symptoms. Bloating, flatulence, nausea, dyspepsia, and pyrosis can also occur.

Diarrhea-predominant IBS is characterized by precipitous diarrhea that occurs immediately on rising or during or immediately after eating. Nocturnal diarrhea is unusual. Pain, bloating, and rectal urgency are common, and incontinence may occur. Painless diarrhea is not typical and should lead the physician to consider other diagnostic possibilities (e.g., malabsorption, osmotic diarrhea).[3]

Diagnosis of IBS is based on characteristic bowel patterns, time and character of pain, and exclusion of other disease processes through physical examination and routine diagnostic tests. Standardized criteria have been developed for IBS. The Rome criteria for IBS include abdominal pain relieved with defecation and a varying pattern of altered stool frequency or form, bloating, or mucus. The key to diagnosis is effective history taking. This requires attention to directed (but not controlled), elaboration of the presenting symptoms, history of present illness, past medical history, family history, familial interrelationships, and drug and dietary histories. The patient's interpretation of personal problems and overall emotional state are equally important. The quality of patient–physician interaction is key to diagnostic and therapeutic efficacy.

On *physical examination*, patients with IBS generally appear to be healthy. Palpation of the abdomen may reveal tenderness, particularly in the left lower quadrant, at times associated with a palpable, tender sigmoid. A routine digital rectal examination should be performed on all patients, and a pelvic examination should be performed on women. Stool examination for occult blood (preferably a 3-day series) should be performed. Routine testing for ova and parasites or a stool culture is rarely indicated without a supporting travel history or supporting symptoms (e.g., fever, bloody diarrhea, acute onset of severe diarrhea).

Proctosigmoidoscopy with a flexible fiber-optic instrument should be performed. Introduction of the sigmoidoscope and air insufflation frequently trigger bowel spasm and pain. The mucosal and vascular pattern in IBS usually appears normal. In patients with chronic diarrhea, particularly older women, mucosal biopsy can rule out possible microscopic colitis, which has two variants: collagenous colitis, seen on trichrome stain as increased submucosal collagen deposition, and lymphocytic colitis, characterized by increased numbers of mucosal lymphocytes. The mean age of presentation for these disorders is 60 to 65 years old, with a female predominance. Similar to IBS, presentation involves nonbloody, watery diarrhea. Diagnosis can be made via rectal mucosal biopsy.

Laboratory examination should include a complete blood count (CBC); erythrocyte sedimentation rate; 6- and 12-channel biochemical profile (sequential multiple analyses 6 and 12), including serum amylase; urinalysis; and thyroid-stimulating hormone. An abdominal sonogram, barium enema x-ray, and upper GI esophagogastroduodenoscopy or colonoscopy may be selectively used, based on the patient's history, physical examination, age, and follow-up evaluations. These studies should be undertaken only when less invasive and less expensive studies reveal objective abnormalities.

Diagnosis of IBS should never preclude suspicion of intercurrent disease. Changes in symptoms may signal another disease process. For example, a change in the location, type, or intensity of pain; a change in bowel habits; constipation and diarrhea; and new symptoms or complaints (e.g., nocturnal diarrhea) may be clinically significant. Other symptoms that require investigation include fresh blood in the stool, weight loss, very severe abdominal pain or unusual abdominal distention, steatorrhea or noticeably foul-smelling stools, fever or chills, persistent vomiting, hematemesis, symptoms that wake the patient from sleep (e.g., pain, the urge to defecate), or a steady progressive worsening of symptoms. Patients more than 40 years old are more likely than younger patients to have an intercurrent organic illness.[3]

Characteristic symptoms of IBS include recurrent abdominal pain; abdominal pain relieved by defecation; disordered bowel habit, including constipation, diarrhea, or an alternation between the two; and abdominal distension and bloating.[12]

IBS is also associated with nongastrointestinal conditions such as headache, low back pain, arthritis, noncardiac chest pain, difficult urination, and fibromyalgia.[13]

20.8 Clinical Course and Prognosis

According to Ayurvedic literature, IBS is curable in children, difficult to treat in middle age, and incurable in older patients. The chronic accrual IBS is difficult to cure whereas tympanites-predominant IBS is incurable.

20.9 Therapy

The Ayurvedic principle of the involvement of *dosas* is very helpful because it provides an understanding of the symptoms and how they vary from one type to another. It also provides a system of treatment specific to that particular *dosa* imbalance. Ayurveda utilizes not only diet and herbs, but also lifestyle advice so that treatment of IBS can be more specific and more successful.

Generally, Ayurveda suggests drinking warm water at first, when morbidity and enterotoxin is located in IBS and is flared up with the improperly digested food. Appetizers, a light diet (e.g., liquid gruel) followed by ghee mixed with appetizers, *vata*-alleviating drugs, and an enema are then advised as a line of treatment. Ayurvedic treatment is based on the nature of the stool with (*sama*) or without (*nirama*) enterotoxin stool. The therapy process is highlighted as follows:

1. According to Ayurveda, dyspepsia and enterotoxin in IBS are important pathological processes that have to be treated effectively along with consideration of bowel movements with respect of stools with or without mucus discharge. When enterotoxin dominates this stage, it is treated with fasting and administration of digestives and carminatives. Use of warm water is highly recommended.
2. In constipation-predominant IBS, the first line of treatment is administration of digestives like *chitrakadi vati* and *shankha vati* to eliminate enterotoxin. It is recommended to follow the digestive with an administration of medicinal ghee preparations such as *dashmuladi ghrita* and *thryushanadi ghrita*.
3. Emesis (*vamana*) is the first line of treatment in diarrhea-predominant IBS, followed by the herbal bitters.
4. The first line of treatment for dysentery-predominant IBS is laxatives (*virechana*) followed by the administration of herbs with spicy and sour tastes.
5. Complex IBS is treated with the *panchakarma* line of treatment and supported by digestives and carminative preparations.
6. Generally, in the treatment of IBS, the use of buttermilk (*takra*) is emphasized. The patient has to be kept on the diet of buttermilk, which is the treatment and nutrition in IBS. Buttermilk is digestive, astringent, and light to digest and helps in improving the consistency of the stool. Buttermilk is given along with asafetida, cumin, and rock-salt powder to control the bowel movements. It contains a good amount of lactobacillus bacteria, which helps restore the normal flora of the intestines.[14]

When treating IBS, a light diet is advised. Indigestible foods such as bread; cheese; red meat; and cold, hard, and raw foods should be avoided. A light fast can be helpful taking only vegetable soups and a little basmati rice and green gram beans. Herbs like ginger, fennel, and cumin that stimulate enzyme secretions will improve digestion, absorption, and clear *ama* from the digestive tract.

20.9.1 Common Herbs Used in IBS

20.9.1.1 Constipation-Predominant IBS

The following herbs are used in this type of IBS for their respective benefits:

1. Ginger, clove, fennel, cumin, cardamom, and a little cinnamon will all stimulate digestive enzymes.
2. Chebulic myrobalan (*Terminalia chebula*) clears excess *vata* from the bowel. *Triphala*, a mixture of chebulic myrobalan, Indian gooseberry (*Emblica Officinalis*), and belliric myrobalan (*Terminalia belerica*), is a gentle bowel tonic excellent for chronic constipation and IBS and for clearing toxins from the bowel. It can be taken in powder or capsule form at bedtime.
3. Asparagus (*Asparagus racemosus*), *ashwagandha* (*Withania somnifera*), and sesame oil all calm *vata*. This is often given as an enema but can also be massaged over the body, particularly over the abdomen 5 min before soaking in a warm bath. Sweet, sour, and salty foods are best.

20.9.1.2 Diarrhea-Predominant IBS

The following herbs are used in this type of IBS for their respective benefits:

1. Indian gooseberry (*Emblica officinalis*) is a rejuvenative tonic and renowned remedy for *pita* problems, which balances *dosas*.
2. Coriander water cools *pita*, as does sandalwood powder prepared in ghee, which is often mixed with fennel, long pepper, black pepper, and cloves.
3. Nutgrass (*Cyperus rotundus*) improves intestinal absorption and stops diarrhea.
4. Aloe vera juice, turmeric, Indian madder (*Rubia cordifolia*), guduchi (*Tinospora cordifolia*) and Indian asparagus (*Asparagus racemosus*) are all excellent for balancing *pitta*. Sweet, bitter, and astringent foods are best.

20.9.1.3 Dysentery-Predominant IBS

The following herbs are used in this type of IBS for their respective benefits:

1. Ginger, lime juice, and honey are excellent to control *kapha*.
2. *Trikatu*, a compound containing black pepper, long pepper, and ginger, is specific for low enzyme and high enterotoxin.
3. Turmeric, cardamom, cinnamon, cloves, sandalwood, cumin, nutmeg, rock salt, and long pepper raise digestive enzyme and clear *kapha*.
4. $^1/_2$ tsp of *Hingvastaka*, a mixture of asafetida, ginger, black pepper, rock salt, etc. taken in a little warm water 1 to 2 h before lunch and supper, increases enzymes and clears enterotoxin. Pungent, bitter, and astringent tasting foods are best.[14]

20.9.2 Lifestyle Changes

The following changes in lifestyle help to control IBS:

1. Identify and remove food intolerances — A trained practitioner can supervise an elimination diet. Many foods are removed from the diet for a brief period and then reintroduced sequentially to isolate the body's reaction to the offending foods. Because grains are a common culprit, it is important to remember that carbohydrate digestion begins in the mouth and that chewing grains thoroughly allows amylase, the digestive enzyme present in saliva, to digest the grains.
2. Improve gut motility — Soluble fiber increases bowel transit, stools, and relieves constipation. Wheat bran has been used in some research studies, but it is not recommended for people who may have intolerances to wheat. Psyllium is a good source of soluble fiber and is readily available. Sufficient water should be taken or fiber can have the opposite effect and result in greater constipation. Flaxseed (*Linum usitatissimum*) also acts as a gentle laxative. It is useful for chronic constipation, damage to the colon wall from laxative abuse, irritable colon, and soothing GI inflammation.
3. Restore a healthy balance of bacteria in the gut — *Lactobacillus acidophilus* and *Bifidobacterium bifidum* can help restore a healthy balance of bacteria in the gut. They can decrease the amount of bacteria with gas-producing abilities and relieve IBS symptoms such as abdominal distension and flatulence. Bifidobacterium acts as a barrier against colonization of the gastrointestinal tract by pathogenic bacteria, and lactobacillus inhibits the attachment of pathogens onto the intestinal mucous lining.[5]

   Low fiber intake is associated with an overgrowth of toxin-producing bacteria and a lower percentage of lactobacillus bacteria. A diet high in dietary fiber increases the formation of short-chain fatty acids, such as butyrate, which is the preferred energy source of the cells that line the colon.[15]
4. Pancreatic enzymes — These enzymes help inhibit the growth of bacteria in the small intestine. They help improve protein digestion. Goldenseal (*Hydrastis canadensis*) also inhibits bacteria and prevents the conversion of proteins to vasoactive amines.[6]
5. Mind–body therapy — Brief psychotherapy was found to be helpful in improving IBS symptoms of pain and diarrhea. Relaxation training to induce whole-body relaxation and stress management, hypnosis, and biofeedback have all been helpful in treating IBS.[16] Antidepressants have been shown to be very effective for treating bowel motility and visceral nerve responses, in addition to addressing the emotional component of IBS.

Therapy is supportive and palliative. A physician's sympathetic understanding and guidance are of overriding importance. The physician must explain the nature of the underlying condition and convincingly demonstrate to the patient that no organic disease is present. This requires time for listening and explaining normal bowel physiology and the bowel's hypersensitivity to stress, food, or drugs. These explanations form the foundation for attempting to reestablish a regular bowel routine and individualize therapy. The prevalence, chronicity, and need for continuing care of IBS should be emphasized. Psychological stress and anxiety or mood disorders should be sought, evaluated, and treated. Regular physical activity helps relieve stress and assists in bowel function, particularly in patients who present with constipation.

In general, a normal diet should be followed. Patients with abdominal distention and increased flatulence may benefit from dietary reduction or elimination of beans, cabbage, and other foods containing fermentable carbohydrates. Reduced intake of apple and grape juice, bananas, nuts, and raisins may also lessen the incidence of flatulence. Patients with evidence of lactose intolerance should reduce their intake of milk and dairy products. Bowel function may also be disturbed by the ingestion of sorbitol, mannitol, fructose, or combinations of sorbitol and fructose. Sorbitol and mannitol are artificial sweeteners used in dietetic foods and as drug vehicles, whereas fructose is a common constituent of fruits, berries, and plants. Patients with postprandial abdominal pain may try a low-fat diet supplemented with increased protein.

Increasing dietary fiber can help many patients with IBS, particularly those with constipation. A bland bulk-producing agent may be used (e.g., raw bran, starting with 15 ml [1 Tbsp] with each meal, supplemented with increased fluid intake). Alternatively, psyllium hydrophilic mucilloid with two glasses of water tends to stabilize the water content of the bowel and provide bulk. These agents help retain water in the bowel and prevent constipation. They also can reduce colonic transit time and act as a shock absorber to prevent spasm of the bowel walls against each other. Fiber added in small amounts may also help reduce IBS-induced diarrhea by absorbing water and solidifying stool. Excessive use of fiber can lead to bloating and diarrhea. Fiber doses must therefore be adjusted to individual patient needs.

Anticholinergic (antispasmodic) drugs (e.g., hyoscyamine [0.125 mg 30 to 60 min before meals]) may be used in combination with fiber agents. The use of narcotics, sedative hypnotics, and other drugs that produce dependency is discouraged. In patients with diarrhea, 2.5 to 5 mg of diphenoxylate (1 to 2 tablets) or 2 to 4 mg of loperamide (1 to 2 capsules) may be given before meals. Chronic use of antidiarrheals is discouraged because tolerance to the antidiarrheal effect may occur. Antidepressants (e.g., desipramine, imipramine, and amitriptyline [50 to 150 mg/day]) help many patients with both constipation- and diarrhea-predominant IBS. In addition to constipation and diarrhea, abdominal pain and bloating are relieved by antidepressants. These drugs can also reduce pain by down regulating the activity of spinal cord and cortical afferent pathways arriving from the intestine. Finally, certain aromatic oils (carminatives) can relax smooth muscles and relieve pain caused by cramps in some patients. Peppermint oil is the most commonly used agent in this class.[3]

Available information and indications on some of the treatments are given below.

1. Peppermint oil (*Mentha piperita*) — Abdominal pain, the most frequent and disabling symptom of IBS, improves when the intestinal smooth muscles are relaxed. Peppermint oil can reduce abdominal pain and distension of IBS, possibly by blocking the influx of calcium into muscle cells and inhibiting the excess contraction of intestinal smooth muscles.[19] It is a carminative, which means it helps eliminate intestinal gas. Peppermint oil should be used only in enteric-coated capsules to ensure that it reaches the intestines intact; otherwise, the oil can relax the lower esophageal sphincter and cause heartburn.

   In a randomized, double-blind controlled trial,[20] in children with irritable bowel syndrome (IBS), enteric-coated peppermint oil capsules proved to be effective by reducing the severity of pain associated with IBS.

TABLE 20.1

Ayurvedic Formulas Commonly Used in the Treatment of IBS

Name of Formulation	Activity	Dose	Adjuvant	Ref.
Brhat gangadhara curna	Astringent	1–3 g three times/ day before meals	Warm water	14
Dadimastaka curna	Carminative, hemetinic	1–3 g three times/ day before meals	Warm water	17
Jatiphaladi curna	Antacid	1–3 g three times/ day before meals	Warm water	17
Bilvadi lehyam	Antacid, antispasmodic	3–6 g ½ h before meals	3–6 g butter three times/day	17
Chitrakadi vati	Relieves enterotoxin, carminative	250–500 mg two times/day	Warm water	18
Shankha vati	Digestive, antispasmodic	250–500 mg two times/day	Warm water	14
Dashmuladi ghrita	Carminative, nutritive	1–2 tsp two times/day	Warm water	1
Pancamrta parpati	Antacid, antispasmodic	120–360 mg three times/day	Honey and water	17
Rasa-parpati	Antacid, antiflatulent	120–360 mg three times/day	Honey	17

2. Fennel seed (*Foeniculum vulgare*) — Fennel is another herb that is used to relieve spasm of the gastrointestinal tract, feelings of fullness, and flatulence.[21]
3. Psyllium (*Plantago ovata*) — An herbal product derived from seeds of the plantago plant, psyllium is a source of dietary fiber that may aid constipation and diarrhea by absorbing water and adding bulk to the stool. (Be sure to drink one to two glasses of water when you take psyllium, and drink plenty of extra water throughout the day.) If psyllium aggravates symptoms instead of relieving them, discontinue using it.
4. Acidophilus — This form of beneficial bacteria normally inhabits the digestive tract, helps digest food, and also fortifies the body against digestive disorders by stopping the harmful bacteria that cause disease from growing uncurbed. It is especially important to take after a round of antibiotics. (Obtain pills containing 1 to 2 billion "live" organisms per pill.) You can enhance the effect of the acidophilus by taking it in combination with fructo-oligosaccharides (FOS), a supplement containing indigestible carbohydrates that feed the friendly bacteria.
5. Gammaoryzanol — This is a natural substance isolated from rice-bran oil. Studies have shown that it protects the mucous lining of the GI tract by regulating nervous system control and exerting antioxidant activity. Clinically, gammaoryzanol has been found to be effective in a broad range of GI complaints, including IBS. Earlier studies suggested that gammaoryzanol may act on the hypothalamus and pituitary glands of the brain, resulting in an inhibition of leutinizing hormone; further research has not supported this finding.[15]

Compound formulations commonly used for the treatment of IBS are given in Table 20.1.

20.10 Scientific Basis

20.10.1 Review of Clinical Trials

20.10.1.1 Holarrhena antidysenterica, Beans of Acacia arabica, Fruit Pulp of Aegle marmelos, and Seeds of Cuminum cyminum

In a study on 60 cases of IBS diagnosed according to Ayurvedic guidelines, patients were separated into two equal groups. The first group received a herbal combination of equal quantities of the powders of the stem bark of *Holarrhena antidysenterica*, beans of *Acacia arabica*, fruit pulp of *Aegle marmelos*, and seeds of *Cuminum cyminum* in the dose of 1 g three times/day with water and showed better response in the character of the stools within a week of treatment. The second group received *kutaja ghanavati* (dry extract of the bark of *Holarrhena antidysenterica*) in the dose of 1 g three times/day with two drops *shankha drava* (dissolved in ½ oz of water). This group showed marked relief with more than 75% of the signs and symptoms of the disease being controlled along with significant improvement in body weight, hemoglobin and fat, and undigested food particles in the stool. The duration of the treatment was 3 weeks.[22]

20.10.1.2 Zingiber officinale

Powder of the rhizome of *Zingiber officinale* at the dose of 3 g three times/day with warm water was given to 30 patients with *grahani* for 4 weeks. The results showed a definite effect on the bowel movement by way of controlling the number of motions and changes in the consistency of the stool within 7 days of the treatment. It also has shown improvement in hemoglobin and body weight. Observation of clearance of giardia and entamebic cyst in the stool was also made.[23] Further, it was reconfirmed on 111 cases of *grahani* that the administration of powder of the rhizome of *Zingiber officinale* is effective in controlling frequency of bowel movements, consistency, improvement in general health and anemia, and the relief of associated symptoms in most of the patients. The effect of this powder on the elimination of amoebiasis and giardiasis is also significantly observed, though it does not have any effect on ascaris.[24]

20.10.1.3 Acorus calamus Rhizome, Aegle marmelos Fruit, Withania somnifera Roots, Sesame Oil, and Common Salt Powder

A randomized, placebo-controlled trial[25] studied the effect of *vasti* (medicated enema comprising of extracts of *Acorus calamus* rhizome, *Aegle marmelos* fruit, *Withania somnifera* roots, sesame oil, common salt powder) on 53 patients with IBS. Results showed a significant reduction in abdominal distention and pain and increased retention time and D-xylose excretion when compared with a control group. It is concluded that *vasti* alters the visceral pain perception, acting via the regulation of the enteric nervous system, and brings about anxiolytic and antidepressant effects.

20.10.1.4 Aegle marmelos and Bacopa monniere

Among 169 patients with IBS, standard therapy (with clidinium bromide, chlordiazepoxide, and isaphaghulla) and a compound Ayurvedic preparation (with *Aegle marmelos* correa and *Bacopa monniere* Linn.), along with a matching placebo were given in a double-blind, randomized trial for 6 weeks. The Ayurvedic preparation in 57 patients was found effective in 64.9%, whereas standard therapy (60 patients) was useful in 78.3%. Patients on placebo (52 patients) showed improvement in only 32.7%. Ayurvedic therapy was particularly beneficial in the diarrhea-predominant form as compared with the placebo. The standard therapy was more useful in the painful form of IBS as compared with the placebo and Ayurvedic preparation. In the gas-predominant form, the effects of standard and Ayurvedic therapy were similar to the placebo. Long-term follow-up (greater than 6 months) showed that both forms of therapy were no better than the placebo in limiting the relapse.[26]

Acknowledgments

The authors acknowledge the data input provided by M.V. Venkataranganna S. Gopumadhavan, Pre-Clinical Pharmacology Laboratory, R&D Center, The Himalaya Drug Company, Makali, Bangalore, India.

References

1. Caraka, *Caraka Samhita*, Part II, Pande, G., Ed., Chowkhamba Sanskrit Series Office, Varanasi, U.P. India, 1970, chap. 15, p. 452.
2. Madhava, *Madhavanidanam*, Part I, Upadhyaya, Y., Ed., Chowkhamba Sanskrit Series Office, Varanasi, U.P. India, 1973, chap. 4, p. 162.
3. Beers, M.H. and Berkow, R., Eds., *The Merck Manual of Diagnosis and Therapy*, 17th ed., Section 3, Chapter 32, Merck and Co., Whitehouse Station, NJ, http://www.merck.com/pubs/mmanual/section3/chapter32/32a.htm
4. Dhyani, S.C., *Kaya Chikitsa*, 1st ed., Ayurvedic & Tibbi Academy, Lucknow, U.P. India, 1991, chap. 69, p. 223.
5. Jones, J. et al., British Society of Gastroenterology guidelines for the management of irritable bowel syndrome, *Gut*, 47(Suppl. 2), 1, 2000.
6. Murray, M. and Pizzorno, J., *Textbook of Natural Medicine*, Vols. 1 and 2, Harcourt Publishers, Edinburgh, 1999.
7. Talley, N.J., Serotoninergic neuroenteric modulators, *Lancet*, 358(9298), 2061, 2001.
8. Shaheen, S.O. et al., Frequent paracetamol use and asthma in adults, *Thorax*, 55, 266, 2000.
9. Case, A.M. and Reid, R.L., Effects of the menstrual cycle on medical disorders, *Arch. Intern. Med.*, 158, 1405, 1998.
10. Whitehead, W.E. et al., Evidence for exacerbation of irritable bowel syndrome during menses, *Gastroenterology*, 98, 1485, 1990.
11. Eliakim, R., Abulafia, O., and Shere, D.M., Estrogen, progesterone, and the gastrointestinal tract, *J. Reproduc. Med.*, 45(10), 781, 2000.
12. Gilbody, J.S., Fletcher, C.P., Hughes, I.W., and Kidman, S.P., Comparison of two different formulations of mebeverine hydrochloride in irritable bowel syndrome, *Intern. J. Clin. Pract.*, 54(7), 461, 2000.

13. Azpiroz, F. et al., Nongastrointestinal disorders in the irritable bowel syndrome, *Digestion*, 62, 66, 2000.
14. Anon., *Yogaratnakara*, Part I, Sastri, B., Ed., Chowkhamba Sanskrit Series Office, Varanasi, U.P. India, 1973, p. 278.
15. Murray, M., *Encyclopedia of Nutritional Supplements*, Prima Publishing, Rocklin, CA, 1996.
16. Coleman, D. and Gurin, J., *Mind Body Medicine: How to Use Your Mind for Better Health*, Consumer Reports Books, Yonkers, NY, 1993.
17. Das, G., *Bhaishajyaratnavali*, Chaukhambha Sanskrit Sansthan, Varanasi, U.P. India, 1997, chap. 8, p. 166.
18. Bhavamishra, *Bhavaprakasha*, Part II, Misra, B., Ed., Chowkhamba Sanskrit Sansthan, Varanasi, U.P. India, 1968, chaps. 4, 30.
19. Liu, J. et al. Enteric-coated peppermint capsules in the treatment of irritable bowel syndrome: a prospective, randomized trial, *J. Gastroenterol.*, 32, 765, 1997.
20. Kline, R.M. et al., Enteric coated, pH-dependent, peppermint oil capsules for the treatment of irritable bowel syndrome in children, *J. Pediat.*, 138, 125, 2001.
21. Blumental, M., Goldberg, A., and Brinckman, J., Herbal Medicine Expanded Commission E Monographs, 1st ed., American Botanical Council with Integrative Medicine Communications, Newton, MA, 2000.
22. Kumar, N. and Kumar, A., A comparison of different drug schedules under different groups of *Grahani* Roga, *J. Res. Ayurveda Siddha*, 18(3–4), 79, 1997.
23. Nanda, G.C., Tewari, N.S., and Kishore, P., Clinical studies on the role of Sunthi in the treatment of *Grahani* Roga, *J. Res. Ayurveda Siddha*, 6(1, 3, 4), 78, 1985.
24. Nanda, G.C., Tewari, N.S., and Kishore, P., Clinical evaluation of Sunthi (*Zingiber officinale*) in the treatment of *Grahani* Roga, *J. Res. Ayurveda Siddha*, 14(1, 2), 34, 1993.
25. Shastry, M.K., Yadava, R.K., and Singh, R.H., Effect of *vasti* therapy in the management of irritable bowel syndrome (Pakwasayagata *Vata* Vyadhi), *J. Res. Ayurveda Siddha*, 17(1, 2), 16, 1996.
26. Yadav, S.K. et al. Irritable bowel syndrome: therapeutic evaluation of indigenous drugs, *Indian J. Med. Res.*, 90, 496, 1989.

21

Diarrhea (Atisara) and Dysentery (Pravahika)

Shankar K. Mitra and Paramesh R. Rangesh

CONTENTS

0-8493-1366-X/04/$0.00+$1.50

21.1 Diarrhea

21.1.1 Introduction

Diarrhea, a condition of loose, watery stools that occur more than three times in a day, is a common problem that usually lasts a day or two and goes away on its own without any special treatment. Prolonged diarrhea can be a sign of other problems. Diarrhea can cause dehydration, which is particularly dangerous in children and the elderly, and it must be treated promptly to avoid serious health problems. People of all ages can get diarrhea. The average adult has a bout of diarrhea about four times a year.

Diarrhea is called *atisara* in Ayurveda. Frequent passing of watery stools is the cardinal feature. According to Ayurveda, diarrhea results from the excess mass of stools and endotoxins (*ama*) in the gastrointestinal (GI) tract, and this excess is eliminated through the nearest outlet (rectum) as diarrhea. Digestive and excretory systems, the two parts of the GI tract called *mahasrotas*, influence each other. The common etiological factors in the diseases of these systems are dyspepsia and endotoxin.[1]

21.1.2 Definition

Atisara in Sanskrit means frequent passing of excessively watery, unformed stool. Other descriptions include watery stools, frequent bowel movements, and loose bowel movements.

TABLE 21.1

Clinical Features of Different Types of Diarrhea

Nature	*Vata*	*Pitta*	*Kapha*	*Tridosa*	Emotional
Color of stool	Bluish	Yellow, reddish	Whitish	Fatty and meat-soup like	Blood red
Nature of stool	Frothy	Watery, foul smell	Mucus, foul smell	Watery	Watery, with or without smell
Frequency	Frequently with sound	Not frequently	Less, without sound, incompletely	Alternate	Frequently
Quantity	Less	More	Less	Sometimes more or less	More
Associated symptoms	Pain in abdomen and pelvis	Fever, thirst, sweating	Drowsy, nausea, horripulation	Combination	Headache, burning sensation
Complication	Rectum prolapse	Inflammation of rectum	Painful rectum	Combination of all	Rectum prolapse

21.1.3 Clinical Description

Clinical features of different types of diarrhea are listed in Table 21.1. The major clinical features of diarrhea are increased fluidity in stools, increased frequency of bowel movement, and increased stool volume.

Although diarrhea is not considered a disease or disorder on its own in conventional medicine, Ayurvedic literature records it as both a symptom and an independent disease.

The World Health Organization (WHO) defines diarrhea as the passage of loose or watery stools, at least thrice in a 24-h period. However, it is the consistency of the stools rather than the frequency that is most important. Frequent passing of formed stools is not diarrhea.[2]

21.1.4 History and Epidemiology

Diarrhea dates back to history of human life. According to Indian mythology, the disease was said to exist in the first age (*sathya yuga*) and was observed to be the outcome of abnormal food habits and emotional disturbance.[3]

More than 1 billion people worldwide suffer one or more episodes of acute diarrhea each year. Because of poor sanitation and more limited access to health care, acute infectious diarrhea remains one of the most common causes of mortality in developing countries, particularly among children younger than 3 years old. It accounts for 5 to 8 million deaths every year.

On average, children in developing countries experience three episodes of diarrhea each year. In 1993, an estimated 3.2 million children under 5 years old died from diarrheal disorders. Eight of 10 of these deaths occur in the first 2 years of life. In many countries, diarrheal disorders, including cholera, are also an important cause of morbidity among older children and adults.[2]

21.1.5 Etiology

According to Ayurveda, diarrhea is caused mainly by the consumption of excessive food that is hard to digest (e.g., protein-rich and fatty foods). In addition, eating foods that are too dry, too hot, or too cold; drinking contaminated water and alcoholic beverages; eating foods with contradictory properties (*viruddhasana*); eating frequently (*adhyasana*); eating improperly cooked foods (*aparipakvasana*); and eating incompatible foods (*asathmya bhojana*) also result in diarrhea. Certain behaviors and lifestyles may also lead to diarrhea. Examples include emotional stress, fear, or grief and controlling natural urges such as urination and defecation (*vega dharana*). Disorders such as indigestion (*ajirna*), irritable colon (*grahani*), hemorrhoids (*arshas*), helminthiasis (including microbial infection [*krimi*] also result in diarrhea.[1]

Conventional medicine indicates that diarrhea may be caused by an infection or an intestinal disease. A few of the more common causes of diarrhea are bacterial or viral infections from consuming contaminated food or water. The common bacteria known to cause diarrhea are campylobacter, salmonella, shigella, *Escherichia coli,* and viral infections (e.g., rotavirus, Norwalk virus, cytomegalovirus, herpes simplex virus, viral hepatitis, etc.). Certain food intolerances such as lactose (sugar found in milk) and parasites that can enter the body through food or water (e.g., *Giardia lamblia, Entamoeba histolytica,* and *Cryptosporidium*) can cause diarrhea. Reaction to medicines, such as antibiotics, blood pressure medications, and antacids containing magnesium; intestinal diseases, such as inflammatory bowel disease and celiac disease; functional bowel disorders, such as irritable bowel syndrome (IBS); poststomach surgery; and gallbladder removal can result in diarrhea.

Certain people who travel to foreign countries are at risk for traveler's diarrhea due to consuming food or drinking water contaminated with bacteria, viruses, or parasites. Traveler's diarrhea is a particular problem for people visiting developing countries.[2] Children can have acute (short-term) or chronic (long-term) forms of diarrhea. Causes include bacteria, viruses, parasites, medications, functional disorders, and food sensitivities. Infection with the rotavirus is the most common cause of acute childhood diarrhea. Rotavirus diarrhea usually resolves in 5 to 8 days.

21.1.6 Pathogenesis and Pathology

Ayurveda describes the pathogenesis of diarrhea as caused by various etiological factors discussed above. The fluid content of the intestines increase, slowing down the activity of digestive enzymes. This fluid that mixes with the stool in the intestine increases the bulk and is propelled by the force of *vata*; as a result, the contents of the intestine are thrown out in the form of diarrhea.[1]

In conventional medicine, the pathology of this disease is due to infections, generally short lived and self-limiting. Common forms of diarrhea are grouped under terms such as gastroenteritis. These conditions may include vomiting and often appear in mini-epidemics in schools, neighborhoods, or families. Most cases of diarrhea will stop without treatment in a few days.

Diarrhea broadly has infectious, drug-induced, food-related, postsurgical, inflammatory, transit-related, and psychological causes. These causes produce diarrhea by four distinct mechanisms: increased osmotic load, inflammation, fluid secretion, and decreased absorption time.

21.1.7 Diagnosis

21.1.7.1 Prodromal Features of Diarrhea

According to Ayurveda, the clinical manifestation of diarrhea is preceded with the following signs and symptoms: pricking pain in the epigastric, umbilical, anal, and general abdominal regions; general body malaise; constipation and obstruction in flatus movement; abdominal bloating; and indigestion.[4]

21.1.7.2 Main Types of Diarrhea

There are broadly six types of diarrhea:

1. Diarrhea due to the imbalance of *vata* (*vata atisara*)
2. Diarrhea due to the imbalance of *pitta* (*pitta atisara*)
3. Diarrhea due to the imbalance of *kapha* (*kapha atisara*)
4. Diarrhea due to imbalance of *tridosa* (*sannipata atisara*)
5. Diarrhea due to emotional disturbances (*sokaja* including *bhayaja*)
6. Diarrhea due to the imbalance of and due to enterotoxin (*ama atisara*)

Table 21.1 shows the details of their presenting features.[1]

21.1.7.2.1 Enterotoxic Diarrhea (Ama Atisara)

To aid treatment, enterotoxic diarrhea is classified into two kinds: with enterotoxin (*sama*) and without enterotoxin (*nirama* or *pakva*). The characteristic features of the stool with enterotoxin are described as improperly digested stool with a distinct foul smell that is slimy or incompacted and is associated with flatulence, abdominal pain, and salivation. The nonenterotoxic diarrhea is devoid of the above features and it also sinks in water.[4] The diarrhea could be mild, moderate, or intense.

21.1.7.3 Other Types of Diarrhea

21.1.7.3.1 Hemorrhagic Diarrhea (Rakta Atisara)

Hemorrhagic diarrhea is an exacerbated variant or latter stage of *pitta-atisara*. If a patient is suffering from *pittaja* diarrhea, then ventures into excessive use of spicy foods, salt, or alcohol may result in hemorrhagic diarrhea, which is characterized by the passage of blood along with the stools.[1]

21.1.7.3.2 Infective Diarrhea (Jvara Atisara)

Etiology of infective diarrhea is the result of etiological factors of fever and diarrhea, with the symptoms of diarrhea associated with fever.[1]

21.1.7.3.3 Clincial Types of Diarrhea

In conventional medicine, four clinical types of diarrhea are recognized:

1. Acute bloody diarrhea (also known as dysentery) — The main dangers are intestinal damage, sepsis, and malnutrition. Other complications, including dehydration, may also occur.
2. Acute watery diarrhea (including cholera) — This type of diarrhea lasts several hours or days. The main danger is dehydration, and weight loss also occurs if feeding is not continued.
3. Persistent diarrhea — This type of diarrhea lasts 14 days or longer. The main danger is malnutrition and serious nonintestinal infection. Dehydration may also occur.

4. Diarrhea with severe malnutrition (marasmus or *kwashiorkor*) — The main dangers of this type of diarrhea are severe systemic infection, dehydration, heart failure, and vitamin and mineral deficiency.

The management of each type of diarrhea should prevent or treat the main cause that each one presents.[2]

Diagnostic tests to find the cause of diarrhea include the following:

1. Medical history and physical examination
2. Stool culture to determine the bacterial infection
3. Blood tests
4. Fasting tests
5. Sigmoidoscopy
6. Colonoscopy (similar to sigmoidoscopy, but the doctor looks at the entire colon)

21.1.8 Clinical Course and Prognosis

According to Ayurveda, diarrhea is difficult to cure if the stool is purple (ripe jamun fruit) or liver brown; amount of stool elimination is small; the consistency resembles dehydrated butter (*ghee*), oil, fat, or meat soup; embedded with shiny particles; and has a very fishy odor. Patients with severe thirst, generalized burning sensation, unconsciousness, dyspnea, relaxed rectal sphincters, rectal prolapse, loss of strength, muscular wasting, loss of blood, and severe arthritic pain along with diarrhea will be very difficult to cure.

The diarrhea due to the involvement of all three *dosas* and emotional types are also difficult to treat successfully.[4]

Diarrhea can be either acute or chronic. The acute form, which lasts less than 3 weeks, is usually related to a bacterial, viral, or parasitic infection. Chronic diarrhea lasts more than 3 weeks and is usually related to functional disorders like IBS or diseases like celiac disease or inflammatory bowel disease.

21.1.8.1 Complications

Common complications of diarrhea are pain in the abdomen, dysentery, tymphanitis, rectal prolapse, anuria, edema, severe infection, and loss of consciousness.[1]

According to conventional medicine, fluid loss with consequent dehydration, electrolyte loss (Na, K, Mg, Cl), and even vascular collapse may occur. Patients who are very young, old, or debilitated may collapse rapidly or have severe diarrhea (such as those with cholera). HCO_3 loss may cause metabolic acidosis. Serum sodium concentrations vary according to the composition of diarrheal losses relative to plasma. Hypokalemia may occur in severe or chronic diarrhea or if the stools contain excess mucus. Hypomagnesemia after prolonged diarrhea may cause tetany.

21.1.9 Therapy

The fundamental principle of treatment in diarrhea is to keep away from the causative factors as previously described. Treatment has to be undertaken based on the nature of the stool — with endotoxin (of recent origin) or without endotoxin (chronic).

21.1.9.1 Enterotoxic Diarrhea

In case of a mild degree of toxin, advice on diet and carminatives are used. While in moderate degree, digestives are administered. In case of an intense degree, the patient is subjected to detoxification (*shodhana–virecana, basti*), using herbs to eliminate toxins.[2]

The use of antimotility drugs is contraindicated in the beginning of enterotoxic diarrhea, in order to prevent the enterotoxin from remaining in the gut. The reduction of bowel movement results in convulsive disorders, abdominal distension, irritable colon, hemorrhoids, anal fissures, edema, anemia, and splenomegaly. Antimotility drugs are used in cases of infants, the elderly, dehydrated conditions, infective diarrhea, and excess diarrhea.[5]

The diet should be restricted to light food like soup of *mudga* (green gram) with ginger or cooked rice (100 to 250 g with 1 to 6 g of ghee). Depending upon the desire and taste, using buttermilk, rice gruel, or rice corn soaked in water is advised. These will be more nourishing and act as a digestive aid.

The following herbal mixtures are recommended (see Section 21.1.10 for the names of the herbs):

1. Chebulic myrobalan (*Terminalia chebula*) fruit powder at a dose of 1 to 3 g with 250 mg of long pepper (*Piper longum*) fruit powder are advised along with warm water. Care should be taken, as large doses of this will result in more bowel movements. This formula helps eliminate toxins.
2. A tea made of rhizomes of calamus (*Acorus calamus*), aconitum species, nutgrass (*Cyperus rotundus*), aerial parts of fumaria (*Fumaria officinalis*), root of pavonia (*Pavonia odorata*), and rhizome of ginger taken at a dose of 50 ml two to three times/day is given to improve digestion.[3]
3. Powder of fried cumin (*Cuminum cyminum*), rhizome of nutgrass, long pepper, or ginger at a dose of 5 g is mixed with 1 l of buttermilk and divided into four parts. Each dose should be taken at 6-h intervals.
4. Ginger powder (1 to 3 g) taken with an equal quantity of sugar two times/day is useful in relieving the symptoms of enterotoxin.
5. Powder of kurchi seed (*Holarrhena antidysenterica*), bark of cinnamomum (*Cinnamomum zeylanicum*), root of vetiver (*Vetivera zizanioides*), seed of jambul (*Syzygium cumini*), and fruit pulp of bael (*Aegle marmelos*) are mixed in equal quantities. A dose of 3 to 6 g of this mixture is taken with buttermilk three times/day.
6. Equal quantities of the powder of pop of old paddy (*laja*), fruit of coriander (*Coriandrum sativum*), and resin of silk cotton tree (*Bombax ceiba*) are mixed with double-quantity fennel seeds (*Foeniculum vulgare*). A dose of 3 to 6 g of this mixture is taken with warm water two times/day.
7. Powder of nutmeg (*Myristica fragrans*), cumin seeds, and fruit pulp of bael are mixed in equal quantity and triturated with lime water to make pills each weighing 800 mg. One pill is taken in the morning with rice water in the case of *pitta* diarrhea and with 25 to 75 ml camphor water for *kapha* diarrhea.[6]

A few compound formulations used in the treatment of enterotoxic diarrhea are given below:

Name of Formulation	Activity	Dose	Adjuvant	Ref.
Gangadhara curna	Digestive, appetizer, antidiarrheal	1–3 g three times/day	Jaggery, buttermilk and honey	7
Jatiphaladi curna	Carminative, antidiarrheal	1–2 g three times/day	Honey, buttermilk and water	7
Lai curna	Antiflatulent, antidiarrheal	1–3 g three times/day	Buttermilk	5
Jatiphaladi vati	Antimotility, antispasmodic	60–120 mg three times/day	Buttermilk and water	8
Karpura vati	Antimotility, antispasmodic	120–240 mg two times/day	Honey	8
Kutajarishta[8]	Digestive, antidysenteric	15–30 ml two times/day	Equal quantity of water	8

21.1.9.2 Nonenterotoxic Diarrhea

This condition is treated with carminatives and antimotility herbs. The following herbal mixtures are recommended:

1. A dose of 3 to 6 g of a mixture of equal quantity of powders of the bark of kurchi and rhizome of aconitum species is taken three to four times/day with honey.[5]
2. A dose of 3 to 6 g of powder of fruit pulp of bael mixed with 100 to 250 ml buttermilk is taken three to four times/day.
3. A dose of 3 to 6 g of powder of bark or seeds of kurchi is taken with 100 to 250 ml buttermilk three to four times/day.
4. A decoction of equal parts of fruit pulp of bael, rhizomes of pavonia and aconite species, rhizomes of nutgrass, and sida root (*Sida cordifolia*) and bark of kurchi is taken at the dose of 14 to 28 ml three times/day.[7]

21.1.9.3 Vata Diarrhea

Vata diarrhea is treated with herbs that improves digestion, followed by antidiarrheal herbal formulas. A decoction of rhizomes of calamus, aconitum, and nutgrass, and seed of kurchi is given.[9]

21.1.9.4 Pitta Diarrhea

Pitta diarrhea is treated with a light diet, carminatives, fluids, and mineral supplements such as rice gruels and fruit juice. If this fails, resort to palliatives and antimotility agents and medicated enema. A mixture of equal quantity of powders of dry extract of berberis (*Berberis aristata*), rhizome of aconite, bark of kurchi, flowers of woodfordia (*Woodfordia fruitcosa*), and ginger is given at a dose of 3 to 6 g with rice water two to three times/day. For a medicated decoction enema (asthapana basti), the paste of the fennel seeds (*Foeniculum vulgare*), roots of asperagus (*Asparagus racemosus*), cow's milk, roots of licorice (*Glycyrrhiza glabra*), sesame oil, cow's ghee, and fruit pulp of bael are used.[3] This herbal combination helps to decrease the motility of intestine. The diet includes goat milk and meat soup with rice.[9]

21.1.9.5 *Kapha* Diarrhea

Kapha diarrhea is treated best with fasting and by improving digestion because it occurs due to excessive eating. A decoction of chaba (*Piper chaba*), aconite, nutgrass, bael, ginger, kurchi seed and bark, and chebulic myrobalan in equal quantities are given at a dose of 15 to 30 ml.[9]

A few compound formulations used in the treatment of *vata* and *kapha* diarrheas are given here:

Name Formulation	Activity	Dose	Adjuvant	Ref.
Kutajavaleha	Antidiarrheal	5–10 g three times/day	Water	10
Agasthisutaraja rasa	Antidiarrheal	60–120 mg three times/day	Cumin, nutmeg, powders	5
Kanakasundara rasa	Antidiarrheal	60–120 mg three times/day	Buttermilk	8

21.1.9.6 Hemorrhagic Diarrhea

The bleeding in hemorrhagic diarrhea has to be stopped immediately. Analgesics (*vadanasthapana*) and styptics (*rakthasthambhaka*) as well as antidiarrheals have to be used. The following herbal mixtures are recommended:

1. A dose of 3 to 6 g of the powder of asparagus (*Asparagus racemosus*) root mixed with 120 ml of goat's milk, three to four times/day, is taken while following a strict rice-milk diet.[3]
2. A dose of 3 to 6 g of white sandalwood (*Santalum album*) powder is mixed with an equal quantity of honey and 5 to 10 g of sugar. It is taken two or three times/day along with rice water and relieves thirst, burning, and bleeding.
3. A dose of 5 to 10 g of cow's milk butter mixed with honey and candy sugar in equal quantities helps stop bleeding.[9]
4. A dose of 3 to 6 g of powder of the fruit pulp of bael is taken with an equal quantity of jaggery.
5. A dose of 3 to 6 g of banyan shoot (*Ficus bengalensis*) paste is taken with 100 to 250 ml of rice water three times/day.
6. A dose of 28 ml of the fresh juice of the leaves of jambul, Indian gooseberry, and mango in equal quantity is mixed with 14 g of honey and 100 ml of goat's milk. The solution is taken three times/day.
7. A dose of 2 to 6 g of red sandalwood (*Pterocarpus santalinus*) powder with 6 g of sugar and 6 g of honey, followed by a potion of 100 to 250 ml of rice water, is taken two times/day.[5]

Goat's milk is given with honey and sugar as a drink and even as a rectal douche.[3]

A few compound formulations used in the treatment of hemorrhagic diarrhea are given below:

Name of Formulation	Activity	Dose	Adjuvant	Ref.
Dadimashtaka curna	Antidysenteric	3–6 g three times/day	Water	5
Dadimavaleha	Antidysenteric	6–12 g three times/day	Honey and water	11
Ushirasava	Hemostatic	15–30 ml two times/day	Equal water	8
Bola parpati	Hemostatic	120–240 mg three times/day	Sugar, honey, buttermilk	5

21.1.9.7 Emotional Diarrhea

Treatment in emotional diarrhea is similar to *vata* diarrhea. In addition, entertainment and counseling is advised.

21.1.9.8 Infective Diarrhea

The line of treatment in this condition involves fasting or taking light and easily digestible food and digestive agents along with antipyretic drugs. A dose of 15 to 30 ml of a decoction of the equal parts of fruit pulp of bael, rhizomes of ginger and musk, fruit of coriander, and roots of sida should be taken once daily early in the morning. A 15- to 30-ml dose of the following decoction is given two times/day: equal quantities of aerial parts of velvet leaf (*Cissampelos pareira*), andrographis, fumaria, rhizomes of nutgrass, ginger, seeds of kurchi, and tinospora stem in water.[7]

The compound formulations used in the treatment of infective diarrhea are listedbelow:

Name of Formulation	Activity	Dose	Adjuvant	Ref.
Karpura rasa	Digestive, antipyretic, antidiarrheal	60–120 mg three times/day	Water	8
Lakshminarayana rasa	Antipyretic and antidiarrheal	120–240 mg three times/day	Ginger juice and honey	5
Mritasanjivini rasa	Antidiarrheal	360 mg two times/day	Honey	5

21.1.9.9 Rectal Prolapse

If the anal region is inflamed, a sitz bath with cold extract of snakeguard leaves (*Trichosanthes dioica*) and licorice is given. If it is associated with a burning sensation, goat's milk mixed with honey and sugar is douched or applied as a wash locally and is also taken internally. A poultice of Woodfordia flower, Lodh bark (*Symplocos racemosa*), and blackgram seeds helps reduce inflammation and bleeding and is applied on the end part. A cotton swab soaked in a medicated ghee (*shatadhoutha ghrita*) is also applied or plugged locally.[9,12]

The compound formulations for all types of diarrheas are listed as follows:

Name of Formulation	Activity	Dose	Adjuvant	Ref.
Rasa parpati	Intestinal antiseptic	125 mg two times/day	Honey	13
Panchamrita parpati	Antidysenteric	125–250 mg two times/day	Honey, curd, and buttermilk	8
Svarna parpati	Antidysenteric, tonic	125 mg two times/day	Honey	5
Vijaya parpati	Antidysenteric, tonic	125–375 mg two times/day	Water and honey	8

21.1.9.10 Lifestyle Changes

Old rice, mung beans, asafetida, garlic, Indian gooseberry, a liquid diet, and raw bananas are all advised in treating diarrhea. Sleeping immediately after a meal also helps control diarrhea and helps in recovery. As one improves, soft and bland foods, raw bananas, guava fruit, plain rice, baked potatoes or dioscorea tubers, toast, crackers, cooked carrots, and baked chicken without the skin or fat are recommended. For children, the bananas, rice, apple sauce, and toast diet is recommened.[14]

Fatty foods (which are heavy for digestion); excess of meat; milk products; and foods that are greasy, high fiber, or very sweet are contraindicated. Negative emotions like fear, grief, and anger, and suppression of the urges of defecation and urination should also be avoided.

The treatment of any type of diarrhea is considered complete when urination and passage of flatus without the appearance of stool, increased appetite, and a feeling of lightness in the abdomen are observed.[4]

21.1.10 Scientific Basis

The inhibitory effect of ayurvedic plants on enteropathogenic bacterias is presented in Table 21.2. Other studies on ayurvedic herbs are summarized below.

21.1.10.1 Holarrhena antidysenterica (Kurchi)

This herb has been indicated in many diseases apart from dysentery in all the forms described in Ayurveda.[15] The total alkaloids of the bark has shown antibacterial activity on the intestinal bacteria, *E. coli*.[16] Kurchamine, an alkaloidal fraction from the bark, effectively reduced the intestinal amoebic infection in rats and hepatic amoebiasis in hamsters. The activity was comparable with emetine hydrochloride.[17] Clinical tests with conessine from the bark on patients with intestinal and hepatic amebiasis have been given results comparable with those obtained with emetine.[18]

21.1.10.2 Myristica fragrans (Nutmeg)

The seed or nutmeg of *Myristica fragrans* is considered a folk remedy for diarrhea. Experimental studies with petroleum ether, chloroform, and ethanol extract showed a reduction in fecal output, inhibition of castor oil-induced diarrhea, and enteropooling in rats. The protective effect of nutmeg in castor oil-induced diarrhea indicates the action could be due to the inhibition of prostaglandin biosynthesis.[19]

TABLE 21.2

Inhibitory Effect of Ayurvedic Plants on Enteropathogenic Bacterias

Name	Part	Solvent	A[a]	B[a]	C[a]	D[a]	MICD/IC_{50} (mg or mg/ml, or μg or μg/ml)	Ref.
Ocimum basilicum	Leaf	Ethanol	6	6	6	NT	*S. typhi* (>10 mg)	49
Psidium guajava	Leaf	Methanol	9	8	13	NT	*S. flexneri* (>10 mg)	49
Punica granatum	Fruit	Methanol	N/A	N/A	NT	NT	12 mg/ml	50
Bergenia ciliata	Rhizome	Methanol	15	NT	NT	12	1.0 mg	51
Caesalpinia bonducella	Seeds	Methanol	20	19	15	NT	*E. coli* (10 mg/ml), *S. typhi* (0.62 mg/ml), *S. flexneri* (2.5 mg/ml)	52
Ficus racemosa	Leaf	Petroleum ether	19	NT	NT	NT	25 mg/ml	53
Capsicum annum	Fruit	Ethanol	N/A	NT	NT	NT	100 mg/ml	54
Holarrhena antidysenterica	Stem bark	Aqueous	>25	>25	>20	>30	200 mg/ml	55
Murraya koenigii	Leaf	Chloroform	8	NT	10	NT	500 μg	56
Syzygium cumini	Stem bark	Ethanol	N/A	N/A	NT	NT	128 μg/ml	57
Astercantha longifolia	Whole plant	Chloroform	15	NT	NT	NT	100 mg/ml	58
Leptadenia arborca	Whole plant	Methanol	16	NT	NT	NT	100 mg/ml	58
Tephrosia purpurea	Whole plant	Methanol	17	NT	NT	NT	100 mg/ml	58
Withania somnifera	Whole plant	Methanol	15	NT	NT	NT	100 mg/ml	58
Evolvulus alsinoides	Leaf	Methanol	17	NT	NT	NT	100 mg/ml	59
		Chloroform	17	NT	NT	NT	100 mg/ml	59
Abrus precatorius	Stem	Methanol	18	NT	NT	NT	100 mg/ml	59
Clitoria ternatea	Whole plant	Methanol	15	NT	NT	NT	100 mg/ml	59
Plumbago zeylanica	Stem and leaf	Methanol	19	NT	NT	NT	100 mg/ml	59
Calotropis procera	Root	Ethanol	15	NT	NT	NT	10 mg/ml	60
Trigonella foenum graecum	Seeds	Ethanol	20	NT	NT	NT	100 mg/ml	61
Allium sativum	Cloves	Water	12	18	30	32	30 μg	62
Cassia occidentalis	Flower	Ethanol	8	NT	NT	NT	10 μg	63
	Callus	Ethanol	8	NT	NT	NT	10 μg	63
Tachyspermum ammi	Fruit	Ethanol	N/A	NT	NT	NT	6.25 mg/ml	64
Hemidesmus indicus	Root	Ethanol	N/A	NT	NT	NT	25 mg/ml	64
Cassia fistula	Seed	Ethanol	N/A	NT	NT	NT	12.5 mg/ml	64
Terminalia bellerica	Exocarp	Ethanol	N/A	NT	NT	NT	12.5 mg/ml	64
Phylanthus emblica	Fruit	Ethanol	N/A	NT	NT	NT	12.5 mg/ml	64
Oxalis corniculata	Leaf	Ethanol	N/A	NT	NT	NT	12.5 mg/ml	64
Plumbago indica	Leaf	Ethanol	N/A	NT	NT	NT	12.5 mg/ml	64
Aegle marmelos	Leaf	Methanol	5	8	5	NT	50 μg/ml	65
Terminalia chebula	Fruit	Alcoholic	>20	>20	NT	NT	200 mg/ml	66
Emblica officinalis	Fruit	Alcoholic	>20	>20	NT	NT	200 mg/ml	66

[a] A = *Escherichia coli*; B = *Salmonella typhi*; C = *Shigella flexneri*; D = *Vibrio cholerae*.

Note: Values indicate bacterial inhibition zone (mm); MICD = minimal inhibitory concentration in disk.

21.1.10.3 *Dioscorea oppositifolia* (Chinese Wild Yam)

The tuber extract is known to have antidiarrheal activity in infantile diarrhea.[20]

21.1.10.4 *Psidium guajava* (Guava)

In fruits with therapeutic properties for antidiarrheal and laxative uses, the presence of lectins may be the bioactive properties that interfere with bacterial adhesion, which are thought to be competing for glycoside signal sites in the attachment. Guava has a galactose-specific lectin that prevents adhesion of *E. coli* O157:H7 to red cells; this lectin is mediated by galactose. Prevention could also be due to their capacity of agglutinating *E. coli* by guava.[21] The antidiarrheal properties of the water and methanolic extracts of *Psidium guajava* leaves have been demonstrated with anteriority; their spasmolytic effect was attributed to quercetin, a flavonoid contained in this plant.[22] The spasmolytic effects of *Psidium guajava* leaf methanol, hexane, and water extracts were demonstrated in the guinea pig isolated ileum-perfused model suggesting the existence of two different types of active components.[23]

21.1.10.5 *Musa paradisica* (Banana)

Banana flakes can be used as a safe, cost-effective treatment for diarrhea in critically ill tube-fed patients. Banana flakes can be given concurrently with a workup for *Clostridium difficile* colitis, expediting the treatment of diarrhea.[24]

21.1.10.6 *Nelumbo nucifera* (Sacred Lotus)

Extract of *Nelumbo nucifera* rhizome reduced not only the frequency of defecation, wetness of fecal dropping and prostaglandin-2 (PGE_2)-induced enteropooling, but also significantly reduced the propulsive movements of charcoal meal significantly in experimental rats. [25,26]

21.1.10.7 *Ficus bengalensis* (Banyan Tree) and *Syzygium cumini* (Jamun)

Ethanol extracts of *Ficus bengalensis* Linn. (hanging roots) and *Syzygium cumini* Linn. (bark) showed significant inhibitory activity against castor oil-induced diarrhea and PGE_2-induced enteropooling in rats. These extracts also showed a significant reduction in GI motility in charcoal meal tests in rats. The results obtained establish the efficacy of all these plant materials as antidiarrheal agents.[27]

21.1.10.8 *Acorus calamus* (Sweet Flag) and *Aegle marmelos* (Bael)

A study was conducted on the effect of aqueous and methanolic plant extracts of *Acorus calamus* rhizome, *Pongamia glabra* leaves, *Aegle marmelos* unripe fruit, and *Strychnos nux-vomica* root bark for their antidiarrheal potential against castor oil-induced diarrhea in mice. Results showed that methanolic extracts were more effective than were aqueous plant extracts. The methanolic extracts significantly reduced induction time of diarrhea and total weight of the feces. The result establishes the efficacy of these plant extracts as antidiarrheal agents.[28]

21.1.10.9 *Clerodendrum phlomidis* (Clerodendrum)

The methanolic extract from the leaves of *Clerodendrum phlomidis* Linn. (*Agnimantha*) (MECP) was examined for its antidiarrheal potential against several experimental models of diarrhea in Wistar albino rats. MECP showed significant inhibitory activity against castor oil-induced diarrhea and PGE_2-induced enteropooling in rats. The extract also showed a significant reduction in GI motility in charcoal meal test in rats. The results obtained establish the efficacy and substantiated the folklore claim as an antidiarrheal agent.[29]

21.1.10.10 *Piper nigrum* (Black Pepper)

Antidiarrheal activity of piperine (*Piper nigrum*) against castor oil, magnesium sulphate, and arachidonic acid was studied in mice. It significantly inhibited diarrhea produced by these cathartics at an oral dose of 8 and 32 mg/kg. Inhibition of castor oil-induced enteropooling by piperine suggests its inhibitory effect on prostaglandins.[30]

21.1.10.11 *Berberis aristata* (Indian Barberry)

Berberine was effective in reducing water and electrolyte secretions induced by *E. coli* heat-stable enterotoxin. These findings indicate that berberine may be an effective antidiarrheal agent in *E. coli* heat-stable enterotoxin-mediated secretory diarrhea. The results also provided a basis for the frequent empirical use of berberine alkaloid and berberine-containing plants in gastroenteritis and infectious diarrhea in Asian and other countries.[31]

21.1.10.12 *Punica granatum* (Pomegranate)

Experimental studies[32] on methanolic extract of *Punica granatum* fruit rind have reported antidiarrheal and antibacterial activity against *Staphylococcus aureus, E. coli, Kleibsella pneumoniae, Proteus vulgaris,* and *Salmonella typhi.*

21.1.10.13 *Tinospora cordifolia* (Tinospora gulancha)

Tinospora cordifolia was reported to be active against *Entamoeba histolytica*.[33]

21.1.10.14 Clinical Trials

21.1.10.14.1 Diarex

Diarex is a polyherbal formulation containing *Holarrhena antidysenterica, Tinospora cordifolia, Aegle marmelos, Punica granatum,* and *Cyperus rotundus* as its constituents. *Holarrhena antidysenterica* is reported to be more effective in treating amoebic dysentery.[34] *Aegle marmelos* is reported to be a very effective remedy in controlling acute diarrhea.[35] A combination of *Aegle marmelos, Punica granatum,* and *Tinospora cordifolia* along with other herbs is known to have potential antispasmodic activity.[36] Clinical trials of diarex have showed to be effective in acute chronic and infectious diarrhea.[37]

21.1.10.14.2 *Calotropis procera* (Indian Madder)

A pilot study was conducted on the effect of the root bark of *Calatropis procera* (arka) in 73 patients of diarrhea. The powder was administered at 250 mg three times/day with buttermilk for 7 days. The consistency of the stools was achieved on the first day of the treatment. There were 49 patients (67.1%) who had complete relief and 18 patients (24.7%) who had marked relief.[38]

21.1.10.14.3 Compound herbal powder (Solanum torvum, Murraya koenigii, Mangifera indica, Carum roxburghianum, Emblica officinalis, Punica granatum, and Trigonella foenum-graecum)

An open clinical trial[39] examined the role of a compound herbal powder (consisting of *Solanum torvum, Murraya koenigii, Mangifera indica, Carum roxburghianum, Emblica officinalis, Punica granatum,* and *Trigonella foenum-graecum*) in the management of nonspecific diarrhea in 25 subjects. Results showed marked relief in loose stools (76%), tenasmus (85%), acid belching (69.5%), borborygmus (66.6%), and bloating of abdomen (62.5%). During the study no adverse reactions were noted.

21.1.10.14.4 Valeriana officinalis (Valerian)

In a clinical observation and experimental study,[40] *Valeriana officinalis* was found to be an effective medicine in controlling infantile rota viral diarrhea.

21.1.10.14.5 Green bananas

In a double-blind trial,[41] green bananas and pectin were shown to be useful in the dietary management of persistent diarrhea in hospitalized patients. The plantain flour-based solution proved effective for the treatment of dehydration due to acute diarrheal diseases and should be considered as an alternative when standard WHO oral rehydration solution (WHO-ORS) is not available.[42]

21.1.10.14.6 Soy fiber

A randomized, blind clinical trial[43] was conducted on soy fiber and rice-based oral rehydration solutions. Results showed that these solutions reduced the duration of watery stools during acute diarrhea caused by bacterial and viral pathogens.

21.2 Dysentery

21.2.1 Introduction

Dysentery is a term used for diarrhea when there is evidence that organisms have invaded the intestinal wall and caused pus, mucus, and blood to appear in the stool. There is often fever and abdominal cramps as well. Although the term dysentery conjures up more emotion, there is no clear-cut line between diarrhea and dysentery, and treatments are often the same.

In its classic form, dysentery leads to symptoms of cramping abdominal pain, diarrhea, and blood and mucus in the feces. Initially, the diarrhea may be copious but soon becomes frequent and of small volume; the patient often complains of painful defecation. It is sometimes accompanied by other symptoms such as vomiting and fever. The *shigella* infection (Sd1) rarely involves other parts of the body. However, more severe forms of infection can occur, particularly in travellers abroad. In these cases, the patient may become very ill and dehydrated, and in the absence of medical treatment, dysentery can be fatal.[44]

Some authors of Ayurvedic literature consider this disease as an advanced stage of *kapha* diarrhea as well as enterotoxic diarrhea.[3] Others consider it an individual disease.[4]

21.2.2 Definition

In Ayurvedic medicine *pravahika* is the term used to indicate dysentery, which means moving with force. It is synonymous with *visramsa, antargranthi, annagranthi, niscaraka,* or *nissaraka.* Dysentery is an acute disease in which the stools and mucus secretion causes a delay in evacuation due to *kapha* and *vata dosas* resulting in straining down the stools.[1] The word *dysentery* is derived from the Greek *dusenteria,* meaning bad intestine.

21.2.3 Clinical Description

Passage of stool with mucus and tenesmus and a feeling of incomplete evacuation characterize the disease.[1] Dysentery is a disease in which the patient passes a small quantity of mucoid, slimy, or bloodstained stool with considerable tenesmus, gripping abdominal pain, and burning sensation.[14] More or less fever, loss of appetite, sleeplessness, and restlessness at night also are noticed. Sometimes the abdomen is distended.

Severe symptoms include having a high fever, being very thirsty and having a red tongue; the abdomen may appear sunken in some cases, straining ceases, and the bowels become relaxed and may prolapse. The passage of urine is infrequent and is accompanied by a burning sensation. The pulse becomes slow, breathing becomes rapid, and generally, the patient looks pale and emaciated. This condition should not be allowed to continue.[1]

21.2.4 History and Epidemiology

Man has known dysentery in its severe form since ancient times, but most cases acquired in the developed world today are mild. The earliest literature in Ayurveda describes this disease in the chapter on diarrhea, whereas the latest authors have recorded this disease as an individual entity.

Shigella infection has caused epidemics of dysentery throughout the world. It caused a 4-year epidemic in Central America beginning in 1968 that resulted in more than 500,000 cases and at least 20,000 deaths.[44]

21.2.5 Etiology

Accoring to Ayurveda, the main causes for this disease are similar to diarrhea. These causes especially include foods that are incompatible (*Ahita*), extremely spicy, and heavy to digest (e.g., protein-rich foods). Drinking contaminated water is also another important cause.[1]

In conventional medicine, bacterial or viral infection, infestation of protozoa or parasitic worms, and chemical irritants are described as major causes of the disease. Some of these causes include the following:

1. Inflammation of the rectum and large intestine
2. Eating insufficient foods
3. Having an improper diet
4. Drinking too much liquid with meals

5. Overeating
6. Eating the wrong combinations of foods
7. Being in unhygienic surroundings
8. Eating fruits or vegetables that have started decomposing
9. Eating foods that have been in pantries that are not well ventilated
10. Eating improperly refrigerated, contaminated foods

Irritated bowels, habitual constipation, and taking certain types of medicine (e.g., laxatives) may also be the cause.

21.2.6 Pathogenesis

This disease can occur in two stages. The primary stage is due to food and other factors, whereas the secondary stage is due to *kapha* diarrhea.

21.2.6.1 Transmission

In conventional medicine, few studies have been done to determine how dysentery is spread. The most likely modes of transmission are person-to-person contact and contaminated water and food. Epidemics of Sd1 usually occur in impoverished areas. They affect people of all ages, with the highest age-specific incidence occurring among adults and the highest case-fatality rates occurring among children.[44]

21.2.7 Diagnosis

According to Ayurveda, dysentery is diagnosed into four types. These categories are based on the nature of signs and symptoms and are diagnosed into the following four types:

1. *Vata* dysentery — Defecation with tenesmus and abdominal pain
2. *Pitta* dysentery — Defecation with a burning sensation
3. *Kapha* dysentery — Defecation with mucus
4. *Rakta* dysentery — Defecation with blood

The enterotoxic and nonenterotoxic stages of this disease are diagnosed based on the tests described in diarrhea.[1]

The types of dysentery, such as amebic, bacillary, balantidial, malignant, and viral, are determined based on microscopic examination of the stool.[44]

21.2.8 Clinical Course and Prognosis

Dysentery is a curable disease. If it is left untreated, it leads to irritable colon disease.[1]

21.2.9 Therapy

The treatment of dysentery is aimed at eliminating the offending and toxic matter from the intestines, alleviating painful symptoms, stopping the virulence of the bacteria, and promoting the healing of any ulcers in the intestine. Antimotility agents should not be used in the early stages of dysentery because of the presence of enterotoxin. In such conditions, mild laxatives are recommended. Using herbal formulas to improve digestion and produce a carminative effect is preferred to achieve a long-lasting effect.

The bark of kurchi (*Holaarhena antidysenterica*) and the raw, tender fruit pulp of bael (*Aegle marmelos*) are the most important herbal ingredients in dysentery. Bastard saffron (*Mesua ferrea*) flower bud, lodh bark (*Symplocos racemosa*), and silk cotton-tree resin (*Bombax malabarica*) are the styptic plants to be used. All prescriptions for diarrhea are also useful for dysentery.[12]

Among specific herbal remedies, bael fruit is, perhaps, the most efficacious in the treatment of dysentery of both the varieties. The pulp of this fruit is mixed with jaggery and should be given three times/day. To deal with a chronic case of dysentery, unripe bael fruit is roasted over a fire and the pulp is mixed with water. Large quantities of the infusion are administered with jaggery. The pulp of the unripe fruit mixed with an equal quantity of dried ginger can also be given with buttermilk.

The use of pomegranate rind is another effective remedy for dysentery. About 60 g of the rind is boiled in 250 g of milk until half of the milk has evaporated. It is administered to the patient in three equal doses at suitable intervals.[45]

21.2.9.1 Food and Lifestyle

Adequate bedrest; a light diet; the use of potassium broth, soybean milk, or oatmeal milk; and drinking at least 1 pt/day of ginger or barley water are highly recommended. Chewing the food thoroughly before swallowing is most important.

Fasting is the best corrective remedy for dysentery. The patient should fast as long as acute symptoms are present. During the period of fasting, only fruit juice (orange) and water should be taken. In the alternative, the patient should subsist on buttermilk until the acute symptoms are over. Buttermilk combats offending bacteria and helps establish helpful microorganisms in the intestines.

The following foods are useful for patients with dysentery:

1. Old rice
2. Gruel prepared from pop of paddy
3. Soup prepared from phaseolus bean or lentil
4. Milk and butter from a goat or cow
5. Fresh or dried ginger
6. Leaves of wood sorrel
7. Fruits of jamun (*Eugenia jambulana*), pomegranate, and bael (*Aegle marmelos*)
8. Flower and fruit of banana

In addition, dysentery patients should avoid the following:

1. Uncherished food (*asatmya bjojana*)
2. Spicy and sour food
3. Incompatible articles of food (*viruddha ahara*)
4. Food that is difficult to digest
5. Products of sugarcane, wheat, black phaseolus bean, barley, and leaves of a variety of chenopodium

Excessive water intake and bathing, staying awake late in the night, and irregular hours of sleep should also be avoided.[7]

Compound formulations used in the treatment of dysentery are listed below:

Name of Formulation	Activity	Dose	Adjuvant	Ref.
Gangadhara curna	Digestive, appetiser, antidiarrheal	1–3 g three times/day	Jaggery, buttermilk and honey	6
Hingvashtaka curna	Carminative, digestive, antidysenteric	1–2 g two times/day	Warm water before meals	5
Agnimukha curna	Carminative, digestive, antidysenteric	1–3 g two times/day	Buttermilk	5
Bilvadi curna	Carminative, digestive, antidysenteric	2–6 g two times/day	Buttermilk (50–100 ml)	8
Kutajaghana vati	Antidysenteric	250–500 mg two times/day	Buttermilk (50–100 ml)	11
Jatiphaladi vati	Antimotility, Antispasmodic	60–120 mg three times/day	Buttermilk and water	8
Karpura vati	Antimotility, Antispasmodic	120–240 mg two times/day	Honey	8
Kutajarishta	Digestive, antidysenteric	15–30 ml two times/day	Equal quantity of water	8
Kutajavaleha	Antidysenteric	5–10 g three times/day	Water	8
Sankha bhasma, Kapardika bhasma, or *Pravala bhasma*	Antiflatulent, digestive, and intestinal adsorbant	0.25–0.5 g two times/day	Lemon juice before meals	46
Agasthisutaraja rasa	Antidiarrheal	60–120 mg three times/day	Cumin, nutmeg powders	5
Kanakasundara rasa	Antidiarrheal	60–120 mg three times/day	Buttermilk	8

21.2.10 Scientific Basis

21.2.10.1 Punica granatum (Pomegranate)

A decoction or tea infusion of *Punica granatum* peel was used in the *in vitro* experiments against *Vibrio cholerae*. Results showed the best bactericidal effect, and it is suggested to use them to stop cholera spreading.[14]

21.2.10.2 Berberis aristata (Indian Barberry)

Berberine, an alkaloid from the plant *Berberis aristata*, inhibited by approximately 70% of the secretory responses of the heat-labile enterotoxins of *V. cholerae* and *E. coli* in the rabbit-ligated intestinal loop model. The drug was effective when given either before or after enterotoxin binding and when given either intraluminally or parenterally; it did not inhibit the stimulation of adenylate cyclase by cholera enterotoxin and caused no histological damage to intestinal mucosa. Berberine also markedly inhibited the secretory response of *E. coli* heat-stable enterotoxin in the infant mouse model. Although the mechanism of action of the drug is not yet known, these data provide a rationale for its apparent clinical usefulness in treating acute diarrheal disease.[47]

21.2.10.3 Medicinal Herbs (*Boerhaavia diffusa, Berberis aristata, Tinospora cordifolia, Terminalia chebula,* and *Zingiber officinale*)

The antiamoebic effect of a crude drug formulation against *Entamoeba histolytica* was studied. The formula is composed of five medicinal herbs: *Boerhaavia diffusa, Berberis aristata, Tinospora cordifolia, Terminalia chebula,* and *Zingiber officinale*. The dried and pulverized plants were extracted in ethanol together and individually. *In vitro* amebicidal activity was studied to determine the minimal inhibitory concentration (MIC) values of all the constituent extracts as well as the whole formulation. The formulation had an MIC of 1000 μg/ml as compared with 10 μg/ml of metronidazole. In experimental cecal amebiasis in rats, the formulation had a curative rate of 89%; with the average degree of infection (ADI) reduced to 0.4 in a group dosed with 500 mg/kg/day as compared with an ADI of 3.8 for the sham-treated control group of rats. Metronidazole had a cure rate of 89% (ADI = 0.4) at a dose of 100 mg/kg/day and cured the infection completely (ADI = 0) when the dosage was doubled to 200 mg/kg/day. There were varying degrees of inhibition of the following enzyme activities of crude extracts of axenically cultured amoebae: deoxyribonuclease, ribonuclease, aldolase, alkaline phosphatase, acid phosphatase, alpha-amylase, and protease.[48]

Ayurvedic plants having inhibitory activity on enteropathogenic bacteria are shown in Table 21.2.

References

1. Madhava, *Madhavanidanam*, Part I, Upadhyaya, Y., Ed., Chowkhamba Sanskrit Series Office, Varanasi, U.P. India, 1973, chap. 3, p. 141.
2. Anon., *The Treatment of Diarrhea: A Manual for Physicians and Other Senior Health Workers*, WHO/CDR/95.3 10/95 World Health Organization, Geneva, 1990.
3. Agnivesha, *Caraka Samhita*, Part II, Pande, G., Ed., Chowkhamba Sanskrit Series Office, Varanasi, U.P. India, 1970, chap. 19, p. 556.
4. Susruta, *Susruta Samhita*, Acharya, Y.T., Ed., Chaukhambha Orientalia, Varanasi, U.P. India, 1997, chap. 40, p. 210.
5. Anon., *Yogaratnakara*, Part I, Sastri, B., Ed., Chowkhamba Sanskrit Series Office, Varanasi, U.P. India, 1973, p. 254.
6. Anon., *Hand Book of Domestic & Common Ayurvedic Remedies*, 1st ed., Central Council for Research in Indian Medicine and Homoeopathy, New Delhi, India, 1978, chap. 4, p. 49.
7. Sharngadhara, *Sharngadhara Samhita*, Parashara, R.K., Ed., Shree Baidyanath Ayurved Bhavan Ltd., Nagpur, Maharashtra, India, 1974, p. 314.
8. Das, G., *Bhaishajyaratnavali*, Chaukhambha Sanskrit Sansthan, Varanasi, U.P. India, 1997, chap. 7, p. 149.
9. Bhavamishra, *Bhavaprakasha*, Part II, Misra, B., Ed., Chowkhamba Sanskrit Sansthan, Varanasi, U.P. India, 1968, chap. 2, p. 1.
10. Cakrapani, *Cakradatta*, Sharma, P.V., Ed., Chaukhambha Orientalia, Varanasi, U.P. India, 1994, chap. 3, p. 47.
11. Anon., *Ayurveda Sarasamgraha*, Shree Baidyanath Ayurved Bhavan Ltd., Nagpur, Maharashtra, India, 1986, p. 547.
12. Dhyani, S.C., *Kaya Chikitsa*, 1st ed., Ayurvedic & Tibbi Academy, Lucknow, U.P. India, 1991, chap. 70, p. 236.

13. Acharya, Y.T., *Siddhayoga Samgraha*, Shree Baidyanath Ayurved Bhavan Ltd., Nagpur, Maharashtra, India, 1976, p. 23.
14. Guevara, J.M., Chumpitaz, J., and Valencia, E., The in vitro action of plants on Vibrio cholerae, *Rev. Gastroenterol. Peru*, 14(1), 27, 1994.
15. Singh, K.P. and Chaturvedi, G.N., Traditional research potentialities of Kutaja (Kurchi) (Holarrhena antidysenterica Wall), *J. Res. Ayurveda Siddha*, 4(1–4), 6, 1983.
16. Chakraborty, A. and Brantner, A.H., Antibacterial steroid alkaloids from the stem bark of Holarrhena pubescens, *J. Ethnopharmacol.*, 68(1–3), 339, 1999.
17. Bertho, A., Pharmakologische Prufung der extrakte und alkaloiden aus Holarrhena antidysenterica, *Archiven der Experimentellen Pathologie und Pharmakologie*, 203, 1323, 1944.
18. Crosnier, R. et al., Traitement de la dysenterie amibienne par les extraits d' Holarrhena floribunda, *Bull. Acad. Med.*, 132, 336, 1948.
19. Pillai, N.R. and Lillykutty, L., Anti-diarrhoeal potential of Myristica fragrans seed extracts, *Ancient Sci. Life*, 11(1 and 2), 74, 1991.
20. Vaishya, S., *Saligramanighantubhushana*, Vols. 7 and 8, Khemaraj Shrikrishnadas Prakashan, Bombay, Maharashtra, India, 1953, p. 420.
21. Coutino-Rodriguez, R., Hernandez-Cruz, P., and Giles-Rios, H., Lectins in fruits having gastrointestinal activity: their participation in the hemagglutinating property of *Escherichia coli* O157:H7, *Arch. Med. Res.*, 32(4), 251, 2001.
22. Morales, M.A. et al., Calcium-antagonist effect of quercetin and its relation with the spasmolytic properties of Psidium guajava L., *Arch. Med. Res.*, 25(1), 17, 1994.
23. Lozoya, X., Becerril, G., and Martinez, M., Model of intraluminal perfusion of the guinea pig ileum *in vitro* in the study of the antidiarrheal properties of the guava (Psidium guajava), *Arch. Invest. Med.* (Mexico), 21(2), 155, 1990.
24. Emery, E.A. et al., Banana flakes control diarrhea in enterally fed patients, *Nutr. Clin. Pract.*, 12(2), 72, 1997.
25. Talukder, M.J. and Nessa, J., Effect of Nelumbo nucifera rhizome extract on the gastrointestinal tract of rat, *Bangladesh Med. Res. Counc. Bull.*, 24(1), 6, 1998.
26. Mukherjee, P.K. et al., Antidiarrheal evaluation of Nelumbo nucifera rhizome extract, *Indian J. Pharmacol.*, 27, 262, 1995.
27. Mukherjee, P.K. et al., Screening of anti-diarrhoeal profile of some plant extracts of a specific region of West Bengal, India, *J. Ethnopharmacol.*, 60(1), 85, 1998.
28. Shoba, F.G. and Thomas, M., Study of antidiarrhoeal activity of four medicinal plants in castor-oil induced diarrhea, *J. Ethnopharmacol.*, 76(1), 73, 2001.
29. Rani, S. et al., Anti-diarrhoeal evaluation of Clerodendrum phlomidis Linn. leaf extract in rats, *J. Ethnopharmacol.*, 68(1–3), 315, 1999.
30. Bajad, S. et al., Antidiarrheal activity of piperine in mice, *Planta Medica*, 67(3), 284, 2001.
31. Zhu, B. and Ahrens, F.A., Effect of berberine on intestinal secretion mediated by *Escherichia coli* heat-stable enterotoxin in jejunum of pigs, *Am. J. Vet. Res.*, 43(9), 1594, 1982.
32. Das, A.K. et al., Studies on antidiarrheal activity of *Punica granatum* seed extract in rats, *J. Ethnopharmacol.*, 68, 205, 1999.
33. Sohni, Y.R. and Bhatt, R.M., Activity of crude extract formulation in experimental hepatic amoebiasis and in immunomodulation studies, *J. Ethnopharmacol.*, 54, 119, 1996.
34. Kumar, A. and Ali, M., A new steroidal alkaloid from the seeds of Holarrhena antidysenterica, *Fitoterapia*, 7, 101, 2000.
35. Singh, A.K., Abhimanyu Kumar, and Sharma, K.K., Shriphal powder: antidysenteric action, *Sachitra Ayurveda*, 46(8), 574, 1993.
36. Srivastava, D.N. and Bhatt, K.R., Effect of Neblon on transit time of ingesta in and gut of albino rats, *Indian J. Indigenous Med.*, 10(1), 23, 1993.
37. Kulkarni, K.S. and Joshi, V.K., New diarex in diarrhea, *Indian J. Clin. Pract.*, 12(10), 37, 2002.
38. Jain, P.K. et al., Clinical trial of arka mula tvaka bark of *Calotropis procera*, on atisar and pravahika – a preliminary study, *J. Res. Ayurveda Siddha*, (1, 3, and 4), 88, 1985.
39. Saroja, P.R., Sivaprakasam, K., and Veluchamy, G., Role of Chundaivattral Churnam in the management of (non-specific diarrhoea) Athisaram, *J. Res. Ayurveda Siddha*, 3-4, 128, 1998.

40. Jing, M. et al., Study on the mechanism of *Valeriana officinalis* for infantile viral diarrhea, *Yunnan J. Traditional Chin. Med.*, 8(4), 1, 1987.
41. Rabbani, G.H. et al., Clinical studies in persistent diarrhea: dietary management with green banana or pectin in Bangladeshi children, *Gastroenterology*, 121(3), 554, 2001.
42. Arias, M.M. et al., Oral rehydration with a plantain flour-based solution in children dehydrated by acute diarrhea: a clinical trial, *Acta Paediatr.*, 86(10), 1047, 1997.
43. Vanderhoof, J.A. et al., Use of soy fiber in acute diarrhea in infants and toddlers, *Clin. Pediatr.* (Philadelphia), 36(3), 135, 1997.
44. Anon., Epidemic Dysentery Fact Sheet No. 108, Division of Emerging and other Communicable Diseases Surveillance and Control WHO, Geneva, revised Oct. 1996, http://www.who.int/inf-fs/en/fact108.html.
45. Anon., Dysentery in *A Complete Handbook of Nature Care*, Healthlibrary.com, 2002, http://www.healthlibrary.com/reading/ncure/chap44.htm.
46. Anon., *The Ayurvedic Formulary of India*, Vol. 1, Part 1, Ministry of Health and family Welfare, Government of India, New Delhi, 1978.
47. Sack, R.B. and Froehlich, J.L., Berberine inhibits intestinal secretory response of Vibrio cholerae and *Escherichia coli* enterotoxins, *Infect. Immun.*, 35(2), 471, 1982.
48. Sohni, Y.R., Kaimal, P., and Bhatt, R.M., The antiamoebic effect of a crude drug formulation of herbal extracts against Entamoeba histolytica in vitro and in vivo, *J. Ethnopharmacol.*, 45(1), 43, 1995.
49. Caceres, A. et al., Plants used in Guatemala for the treatment of gastrointestinal disorders. III. Confirmation of activity against enterobacteria of 16 plants, *J. Ethnopharmacol.*, 38, 31, 1993.
50. Prashanth, D., Asha, M.K., and Amit, A., Antibacterial activity of Punica granatum, *Fitoterapia*, 72, 171, 2001.
51. Sinha, S. et al. Antibacterial activity of Bergenia ciliata rhizome, *Fitoterapia*, 72, 550, 2001.
52. Saeed, A.M. and Sabir, A.W., Antibacterial activity of Caesalpinia bonducella seeds, *Fitoterapia*, 72, 807, 2001.
53. Mandal, S.C., Saha, B.P., and Pal, M., Studies on antibacterial activity of Ficus racemosa Linn. Leaf extract, *Phytother. Res.*, 14, 278, 2000.
54. De, M., De, A.K., and Banerjee, A.B., Antimicrobial screening of some Indian spices, *Phytother. Res.*, 13, 616, 1999.
55. Ballal, M. et al., Antibacterial activity of Holarrhena antidysenterica (Kurchi) against the enteric pathogens, *Indian J. Pharmacol.*, 32(6), 392, 2000.
56. Nutan, M.T.H., Hasnat, A., and Rashid, M.A., Antibacterial and cytotoxic activities of Murraya koenigii, *Fitoterapia*, 69(2), 173, 1998.
57. Chattopadhyay, D., Sinha, B.K., and Vaid, L.K., Antibacterial activity of Syzigium species, *Fitoterapia*, 69(4), 365, 1998.
58. El Egani, A.A. et al., Sudanese plants used in folkloric medicine. VIII. Screening for antibacterial activity, *Fitoterapia*, 69(4), 369, 1998.
59. El Fatih, M. et al., Sudanese plants used in folk-loric medicine. VII. Screening for antibacterial activity, *Fitoterapia*, 68(6), 549, 1997.
60. Jain, S.C. et al., Antimicrobial activity of Calotropis procera, *Fitoterapia*, 68(3), 275, 1996.
61. Bhatti, M.A. et al., Antibacterial activity of Trigonella foenum-graecum, *Fitoterapia*, 67(4), 372, 1996.
62. Ahsan, M. and Islam, S.N., Garlic: a broad-spectrum antibacterial agent effective against common pathogenic bacteria, *Fitoterapia*, 67(4), 374, 1996.
63. Jain, S.C. et al., Antibacterial screening of Cassia occidentalis L. in vivo and in vitro, *Phytother. Res.*, 12, 200, 1998.
64. Valsaraj, R. et al., Antimicrobial screening of selected medicinal plants from India, *J. Ethnopharmacol.*, 58, 75, 1997.
65. Vijayalakshmi, K. et al., Activity of leaf extract of Aegle marmelos (L.) correa against some pathogenic bacteria, *Amruth*, 6(3), 17, 2002.
66. Ahmad, I., Mehmood, Z., and Mohammed, F., Screening of some Indian medicinal plants for their antimicrobial properties, *J. Ethnopharmacol.*, 62, 183, 1998.

22

Gastroduodenal Ulcers

Krishnamurthy Sairam and Sailaja Vani Batchu

CONTENTS

0-8493-1366-X/04/$0.00+$1.50

22.1 Introduction

In Ayurveda, peptic ulcers or gastroduodenal ulcers generally refer to *parinamasula*. It is the disease of the gastrointestinal tract, especially the stomach. Abdominal pain during digestion is the main symptom in these diseases. Earlier Ayurvedic classics like *Charaka Samhita* and *Sushrut Samhita* mentioned abdominal pain as relating to digestion but not as a separate clinical entity.[1,2] For the first time, in 7th century A.D., Madhavakar described this disease separately with the name *parinamashula* in his famous treatise, *Madhava Nidana,* which mainly deals with the etiology and pathology of different diseases. He has given a precise description of *parinamasula*, but *Vijayarakshita*, the commentary of *Madhava Nidana,* later elaborated it. This disease has been mentioned in all the later books like *Bhavaprakash*, *Yogaratnakar*, *Sharangadhara Samhita*, and *Chakradatta*.[3–5] Apart from the stress placed on food habits and personal hygiene, some herbal drugs have also been mentioned in the treatment of this disease. The gastric ulcer (GU) remains a major global health problem, eluding satisfactory therapeutic regimen. Modern medicine has not adequately evaluated the usefulness of natural drugs in ulcer therapy, although studies have been reported.

It is now assumed that the antiulcer drugs ultimately balance the aggressive factors (acid, pepsin, *H. pylori*, bile salts) and defensive factors (mucin secretion, cellular mucus, bicarbonate secretion, mucosal blood flow, cell turnover, etc.).[6] New etiological factors, such as involvement of free radicals[7] and *H. pylori*,[8,9] have gained attention. Resistance of *H. pylori* to antimicrobials[10] and poor patient compliance due to multiple doses[11] are reported to be major causes for the failure of antiulcer therapy. This necessitates using newer antibacterials and reducing doses during therapy. Antiulcer drugs with antioxidant and antibacterial effects would be superior to combined therapies.[12] These attributes are found with herbal drugs.

In this chapter, literature on Ayurvedic therapies of GUs and duodenal ulcers (DUs) is reviewed and compared with therapies in conventional medicine. Many similarities between the two systems are noted.

22.2 Clinical Description, History, and Epidemiology

According to Ayurveda, abdominal pain that is aggravated during digestion is known as *parinamashula*. Various synonyms of *parinamashula* mentioned in the texts (i.e., *annadravashula, paktishula, annavidahajashula,* etc.) are related to food and digestive factors. According to Ayurveda, the word *parinama* implies digestion. It actually starts after the emptying of the stomach. The word *shula* refers to pain. Hence the pain that occurs during the digestion period is called *parinamashula*.

Similarly, in conventional medicine, peptic ulcer disease (PUD) is described to be associated with epigastric pain exacerbated by fasting and improvement with food. The patient has a history of alterations in bowel habits, especially diarrhea or constipation.[13]

As discussed earlier, the GU or DU has not been recognized as a separate clinical entity, making information on history and epidemiology limited.

22.3 Etiology

When we compare and contrast GUs and DUs, both seem to be very much similar. PUD, according to the modern concept, is a multifactorial disease.[13] The causes include genetic, dietetic, psychological (stress and emotional factors), endocrine, and drug-induced infections. The common result of all these initiating factors is a breakage in mucous membrane of either the stomach or duodenum (common sites). There may be a difference in incidence, placement of ulcer, symptomatology, or prognosis of DUs and GUs, but the presence or absence of an ulcer is determined by a delicate interplay between the aggressive factors (acid and pepsin) and defensive factors (mucosal resistance).[1]

The defense mechanism of the gastrointestinal mucosa against aggressive factors, such as hydrochloric acid, bile acid, free radicals, *H. pylori* colonization, nonsteroidal anti-inflammatory drugs (NSAIDs), etc., mainly consists of functional, humoral, and neuronal factors.[14] These coincide with the Ayurvedic concept of PUDs, where it is believed to be an imbalance between *kapha* and *pitta*. The important factors responsible for ulcerogenesis are described below.

22.3.1 Offensive Factors

Pitta represents the aggressive factors such as acid and pepsin. *Vata* is the main factor in production of pain and represents the neuronal part of acid secretion. The symptomatology of *parinamashula* and PUD have similar symptoms such as pain in the epigastrium and other sites, nausea, vomiting, and pain relieving with intake of food (in DUs) or after digestion (i.e., in an empty stomach or with vomiting [in GUs], heartburn, abdominal pain, etc.)

22.3.1.1 Acid and Pepsin Secretion

The role of hydrochloric acid in the pathogenesis of gastric ulcer is well established.[15] Many commonly used antiulcer agents heal ulcers by blocking acid secretion.

22.3.1.2 H. pylori colonization

H. pylori, a gram-negative bacterium, is found in more than 90% of DU cases and 75% of GU cases.[16] Clinical outcomes associated with *H. pylori* infection include GU, DU, gastric adrenocarcinoma, and gastric-mucosa–associated lymphoid tissue lymphoma. The pathogenicity of *H. pylori* depends on bacterial and host factors.[16] Even though there have been advances in eradication of *H. pylori* in peptic ulcer patients by using multiple therapies, there are several reports on the limitations of such treatments, such as resistance to *H. pylori*[11] and poor patient compliance due to multiple doses.[12] Further treatment can be accompanied by nausea, diarrhea, abdominal pain, and pseudomembraneous colitis.[17] These adverse effects contribute to patient noncompliance and reduce the efficacy of therapy.

22.3.1.3 Histamine

Histamine has been found in the gastric wall and is a powerful stimulant for gastric secretion. Histamine blockers such as ranitidine have been reported to prevent even psychological stress-induced gastric ulceration.[18]

22.3.1.4 Drugs (NSAIDs)

NSAIDs are widely prescribed for treating many conditions. The risk of ulcer complications, such as bleeding, perforation, and death, is increased approximately fourfold in NSAID users. NSAIDs disrupt the GI mucosal-protective and acid-limiting properties of prostaglandins (PGs) and also have a direct topical irritant effect. NSAIDs induce gastric damage through generation of reactive oxygen species.[19] Adverse side effects may be significantly reduced through the use of cyclooxgenase-2 (COX-2)–specific inhibitors.[20]

22.3.1.5 Free Radicals

Free radicals are defined as chemical species possessing unpaired electrons. The role of oxygen-derived free radicals has been demonstrated in acute and chronic ulceration.[21] Several natural drugs have been reported to have antioxidant activity, which contributes to their activity.[22–24]

22.3.2 Gastric Mucosal Defense Mechanisms

The role of *kapha* is that of mucosal defensive mechanism and was clearly mentioned in the pathogenesis of *parinamashula* in 7th century A.D. According to modern medicine, the malfunctioning of certain defensive (protective) mechanisms of the GI tract mucosa are the important determinants in the development of ulcers. These mechanisms are presented here.

22.3.2.1 Mucus-Bicarbonate Barrier

The entire surface of the gastric mucosa is covered by a continuous layer of mucus gel, which has a variable thickness of less than 500 μm.[25] Mucus is made up of glycoprotein and contains sulfhydryl groups (-SH), which protect the mucosa from free-radical–induced injury.[26] Mucus provides a mixing barrier at the mucosal surface and also prevents the activation of pepsinogen to pepsin apart from providing a microenvironment for repair and restitution.[27]

22.3.2.2 Gastric Mucosal Renewal and Restitution

The rapid proliferation of gastric mucosa plays an important role in mucosal protection during normal state and after mucosal damage.[28]

22.3.2.3 Gastric Motility

Gastric motility changes have been reported to cause both gastric and duodenal ulceration.[29] Incompetence of the pyloric sphincter and delayed gastric emptying may lead to stasis and delayed clearing of refluxed duodenal contents; these actions can lead to increase gastric release and a subsequently higher rate of acid secretion.

22.3.2.4 Mucosal and Submucosal Blood Flow

Constituents of mucosal blood flow are important in mucosal defense. They play a vital role in protecting the mucosa by delivering oxygen, nutrients, and bicarbonate to the cells. They also remove hydrogen ions that have penetrated the mucus-bicarbonate and epithelial barrier.[30]

22.3.2.5 Prostaglandins

PGs, namely, prostaglandin E and prostaglandin I (PGE and PGI), have been shown to protect against experimental necrotic damage. PGs increase gastric mucosal blood flow, mucus, and bicarbonate secretion and strengthen the mucus bicarbonate barrier. Thus, inhibition of the production predisposes the stomach to injury. The beneficial effects of COX-2 inhibitors are still controversial.[31]

22.3.2.6 Antioxidants

Antioxidants are stated to be any substance, even present at low concentrations compared with those of an oxidizable substrate, that significantly delays or prevents oxidation of that substrate. Uncontrolled oxidation in aerobic organisms produces oxidative stress, cell damage, and eventually cell death. An array of cellular defense systems exists to counterbalance reactive oxygen species (ROS).[32] Antioxidants neutralize free radicals, thus protecting essential micro- and macromolecules in the body from the oxidative damage.

22.3.3 Other Causative Factors

Other causative factors can be broadly divided into three types: diet (*ahara*), lifestyle (*vihara*), and seasonal (*kala*) factors.

22.3.3.1 Dietetic Factors (Ahara)

Excessive use of sour, salty, pungent, spicy, astringent, and dry foods; alcohol intake; oil; mustard; pulses (e.g., peas, beans); and a nonvegetarian diet may all lead to ulcer development. Consuming food before digesting a previous meal, eating incompatible food, and being gluttonous may also cause peptic ulcers.

There are also recent reports from modern medicine on the influence of food on the genesis of GUs and DUs.[34–36] Factors such as being a male, having a family history of ulcers, having an O-blood type, skipping breakfast or more than one meal, drinking excessive amount of coffee, and smoking cigarettes were reported to be associated with increased incidences of DUs.[37]

22.3.3.2 Lifestyle Factors (Vihara)

Lifestyle factors include the following:

1. Physical factors — Examples include excessive exercise, hard work, excessive sexual indulgence, excessive exposure to sun or fire, waking up at night, and suppressing natural urges.

2. Mental factors — Examples include anger, grief, anxiety, and depression.
3. Psychological factors — Lifestyle factors can be equated with psychological factors. Although there has not been much information on patterns of life on ulcers in conventional medicine, there are reports on the psychological changes, which are an immediate fallout of these physical factors.
4. Stressful life events — According to modern medicine, these events have been associated with the onset or symptom exacerbation of some of the most common chronic disorders of the digestive system, including functional GI disorders, inflammatory bowel disease, gastroesophageal reflux disease, and PUD.[38] There is considerable evidence that supports the role of stressful life events in the etiology of PUD. These mechanisms involve both the cortical and subcortical levels.[39] Many investigators have suggested the role of ROS in stress-induced ulcers.[40]
5. Cigarette smoking — This is a major lifestyle risk factor for the development and recurrence of peptic ulcers. The association between ulcerative disease and smoking cannot be explained on the basis of an effect on gastric secretion of acid or pepsin, blood flow, or pancreatic secretion.
6. Seasonal factors (*kala*) — Seasonal factors, including rainy season, autumn, spring, cold weather, evening time, midday, midnight, and sunrise, may trigger ulcer development.

22.4 Pathogenesis

According to Ayurveda, in his description of the gastroduodenal ulcers, Madhavakar has not mentioned the specific etiological factors. However, he did state that all the exogenous and endogenous factors that cause the vitiation of *vata* are responsible for the initiation of pathogenesis of ulcers; *kapha* and *pitta* are also involved.[33] Hence the provocating factors mentioned in reference to *shularoga* were found to be relevant for gastrodudenal ulcers. Because of the indulgence in specific etiological factors, the *dosas* may start accumulating at their own sites followed by vitiation. The vitiation of any one of these *dosas* may disturb other *dosas*. Even when one of the three *dosas* is in a state of vitiation, the biofire (i.e., *agni*) tends to be deranged, hindering the process of digestion and leading to the formation of defective juices from inadequate digestion of food (*ahara rasa*).

The stomach (*amashaya*) is the site of specific *kaphas* (*kledakakapha*, *pachakapitta*, and *samanavata*). According to Ayurveda, *kledakakapha* protects the stomach from the ill effects of *pachakapitta*. The role of *samana vata* is to stimulate the *pachakapitta*. So, the eroding effect of *pitta* is counteracted by *kledakakapha* and *vata* maintains the motility and movements of the stomach. Because of indulgence in etiological factors, the displaced *kapha* from its site admixtures with the *pitta* and is inactivated with the help of *vata*, which produces the pain during the period of digestion. *Parinamashula* is a *tridoshik* disease, but *pitta* is the predomint *dosa*, as it plays important role during the period of digestion (i.e., *parinamakala*).

22.5 Clinical Examination

The cardinal feature of this disease, according to Ayurveda, is pain in the abdomen during the process of food digestion. Important sites of the pain are the epigastrium (*kukshi*), flanks (*jathara parshwe*), umbilical region (*nabhau*), retrosternal region (*stanantare*), and back (*prishtamoola pradesha*); the pain sometimes occurs in all the above mentioned sites simultaneously (*sarveshu*). There are seven clinical types mentioned, but basically they are derived from the permutations and combinations of three dosic states. Pain may be aggravated through the consumption of a specific variety rice (*raktashali*) and may be relieved by taking a meal and vomiting. As in modern medicine, the food habits and other personal clinical history features (e.g., previous drug intake) are taken into consideration, and modern techniques such as radiological and histological examinations are routinely done.

22.6 Clinical Course and Prognosis

The characters of pain are burning (*daha*), dull aching (*swalpa ruk*), flatulence (*borborygmi*), trembling (*vepana*), and acute continuous pain (*dirgha santata ruk*). *Borborygmi* is due to *vata* with systemic features of flatulence, constipation, and restlessness. These symptoms can be relieved by a hot and fatty diet. Burning sensation due to *pitta* with systemic features of thirst, restlessness, and excessive perspiration can be aggravated (*shula vriddhi*) by sour and salty food intake. Dull aching and continuous acute pain due to *kapha* with systemic features including nausea, drowsiness, and vomiting can be vitiated by pungent and bitter food.

The dual (*dwandaja*) type and triple (*tridoshaja*) type are clinical mixtures of above-mentioned three types of *parinamashula*. The *tridoshaja* variety is associated with excessive weakness and markedly diminished digestive capacity; it is considered incurable.

22.7 Therapy

In Ayurveda, the whole armamentarium of treatment of any disease has been broadly divided into two types: biopurificatory (*samshodhana*) and palliative (*samshamana*), along with avoidance of causative factors (*nidana parivarjana*):

1. *Samshodhan* therapy[41,42] — This type of treatment is used in strong and suitable persons who can bear the impact of various procedures like *langhan, vaman, virechan, anuvasan,* and *niruha vasti.*
2. *Samshamana* — Limited drugs have been mentioned[41,42] for this type of treatment (see Tables 22.1 and 22.2).
3. *Nidana parivarjana* — Also known as the withdrawal from the etiological factors, *nidana parivarjana* is considered to be crucial in the treatment of this disease.

TABLE 22.1

Single Herbal Drugs

Drug	Form of Drug	Dosage
Patola	Ghee prepared with fruits	25 ml twice daily with milk
Shatavari	Root powder	3-4 g three times with milk
	Ghee prepared with roots	25 ml twice daily with milk or hot water
Yashtimadhu	Root powder	4–5 g three times daily
Aswagandha	Root powder	4–5 g three times daily
Bhringaraja	Powder of whole plant	4–5 g four times daily
Amalaki	Powder of fruit pulp	1 g twice daily
Aparajita	Root paste	4–5 g twice daily

TABLE 22.2

Compound Ayurvedic Formulas Used in the Treatment of Gastroduodenal Ulcers

Preparation Type	Name of Preparation
Churna [powder]	*Avipattikara churna*
	Amalaki Rasayan
Avaleha	*Kushmandavaleha*
	Dadimavaleha
Gutika [pill]	*Shankha vati*
	Mahashankha vati
Bhasma [ash]	*Shankha bhasma*
	Varata bhasma
	Shambooka bhasma
Lauha [iron preparations]	*Saptamrita lauha*
	Dhatri lauha
Mandur	*Shatavari mandur*
Rasaushadhi	*Sutashekhara ras*
	Kamadudha ras
	Pravala panchamrit
Khanda	*Narikelakhanda*

The main principle of treatment of *parinamashula* is aimed at the following: (1) alleviation of excited *vata*, (2) controlling or reducing the hyperactivity of *pitta*, and (3) repairing and maintaining the integrity of the *rasavaha srotas* situated at the site of lesion by increasing the *kapha*.

22.7.1 Diet and Regularized Lifestyle (*Pathya ahara* and *Vihara*)

Bajra, wheat, Indian gooseberry (*amalaki*), milk, buttermilk, and all bitter and sweet foods are compatible. Mental and physical rest are also helpful to control the symptoms of the disease. Anger, grief, waking up at night, and excessive exposure to sun, cereals (e.g., blackgram, sesame), excessive sour and salty foods, alcohol, and foods that are heavy for digestion are all considered incompatible for a proper lifestyle and diet.

22.7.2 Conventional Therapies

Conventional drugs are reviewed here to understand their mechanism of action, which can be correlated with Ayurvedic drugs discussed later. This section also highlights their balance of therapeutic efficiency to adverse effects, drug interactions, and the need for alternative strategies.

22.7.2.1 Antacids

The effect of antacids on the stomach is due to partial neutralization of gastric HCl and inhibition of pepsin. Although adverse effects with antacids are minimal, significant adverse reactions can occur with long-term use.[43]

22.7.2.2 Histamine H_2-Receptor Antagonists

Histamine H_2-receptor antagonists (H_2RAs) competitively inhibit histamine action at all H_2 receptors. Their main clinical use is as inhibitors of gastric-acid secretion. There are reports suggesting non–acid-related effects contributing to the activity of H_2RAs defying the previously held view as only antisecretory drugs.[44] Reports suggest that the central nervous system (CNS) may be partially responsible for antiulcerogenic activities of H_2RAs.[45] This correlates well with the Ayurvedic view of influence of psychological factors and the use of adaptogens (*rasayanas*) for ulcer therapy. Human gastric carcinoid was detected during the development of tolerance and rebound acid secretion during the long-term treatment with H_2RAs.[46]

22.7.2.3 Proton Pump Inhibitors (PPIs)

Proton pump inhibitors (PPIs) act by irreversible interaction with the SH group of the H^+-K^+adenosine triphosphatase (ATPase), forming a disulphide bond. Reported side effects include headache, diarrhea, skin rash, and reversible abnormalities in biochemical liver function tests. Long-term inhibition has been reported to produce gastric carcinoma,[47] achlorhydria, and hypergastrenemia.[48] Omeprazole has been reported to reduce the secretion, synthesis, and gene expression of pepsinogen, which may create problems in the protein digestion and result in diarrhea.[49] There are reports of potential CNS side effects after PPI treatment, which need further evaluation.[50] PPIs have also been reported to have some drug interactions. Recently, lansaprasole has been reported to potentiate vecuronium-induced paralysis in patients.[51]

22.8 Preventive Measures

Preventive measures essentially include dietary intervention and lifestyle changes based on the factors as suggested in Ayurveda (see Sections 22.4 and Section 22.7).

22.9 Scientific Basis of Ayurvedic Therapies

Because the etiological factors for gastroduodenal ulcers in Ayurveda and conventional medicine are similar (e.g., imbalance of offensive [*vata*] and defensive factors [*kapha*]), animal models used to evaluate modern medicine are often used to evaluate Ayurvedic therapies.

The upcoming review of some selected drugs gives an elaborate and clear view of how modern evaluation models are suitably used for screening natural drugs. The success of Ayurvedic drugs in the commercial market depends on stringent evaluation followed closely in line with modern experimentation and clinical evaluation. One of the major hurdles is to clearly define the composition of Ayurvedic drugs and the identification of active ingredients. Without the knowledge of active ingredients, the product cannot be standardized or the amount of active ingredient cannot be quantified and would fall short of drug enforcement standards. Investigations not taken to this level will be of academic interest only and not of any practical value. This review gives major trust for drugs that have been actively quantified or have been standardized for active ingredients.

22.9.1 Animal Studies

22.9.1.1 *Musa sapientum var. paradisiaca (Unripe Plantain Banana)*

Plantain banana has been subjected to extensive experimental and clinical studies. Dried powder of banana pulp (DRBP) was effective against experimental ulcers.[52] The antiulcer activity of DRBP was reported to be due to its predominant effect on mucosal defensive factors rather than on the offensive acid-pepsin secretion.[53–55]

Ethanolic extract of banana was reported to increase the accumulation of eicosonoids like PGE, prostaglandin I_2 (PGI_2), and leukotrienes B_4 and C_4/D_4 (LTB_4, C_4/D_4) in the human gastric and colonic mucosal incubates.[56] Many active principles such as steryl-aclyglycosides, and sitoindosides I-IV were isolated and characterized from many vegetables and bananas and were reported to have antiulcerogenic activity both in animal and human models.[57–59] Methanolic extract of banana was reported to have an antioxidant effect but was devoid of anti-*H. pylori* activity *in vitro*.[24]

22.9.1.2 *Tambrabhasma*

Herbomineral preparations have been widely mentioned in Ayurveda.[60] *Tambrabhasma* (TMB), a traditional preparation of copper (containing CuO $\geq$ 44.45% $\leq$ 66.13%, Fe_2O_3 < 6.03%, and S < 2.75%) has been advocated for use in *amlapitta*. *Tambrabhasma* showed antiulcer activity against experimental GUs and DUs. The activity of *tambrabhasma* was ascribed due to a decrease in offensive acid-pepsin secretion and an increase in defensive factors; the effect was also free from toxicity.[61,62]

22.9.1.3 *Mahakasya Drugs*

A water decoction of ginger, which makes up one of the constituents of *mahakasyaya* drugs, along with a water decoction of *Piper longum* and a colloidal solution of *Ferula foetida,* has been reported to protect against cold-restraint stress, aspirin, and pyloric-ligation–induced GUs in rats. Although increase in offensive acid-pepsin secretion was observed in this study, the increase in defensive mucin secretion was sufficient enough to protect against experimental ulcers.[63]

22.9.1.4 *Bacopa monniera (Bramhi)*

Bacopa monniera Wettst. (syn. *Herpestis monniera* L.; scrophulariaceae) is classified as a *medhya rasayana,* a class of plant drugs used to promote mental health and improve memory and intellect.[64] It is a classic example where an adaptogenic drug has antiulcer activity. It is intriguing that *Bacopa monniera* has shown both anxiolytic and antidepressant activity.[65–67] *Bacopa monniera* contains active chemicals, such as bacoside A, which have been reported to be responsible for facilitation of memory[68] and the antiulcerogenic effect.[69]

Fresh juice of *Bacopa monniera* and its standardized methanolic extract, containing 35% of bacoside A,[23] has been reported to have an antiulcerogenic effect. *Bacopa monniera* extract (20 mg/kg) showed no effect on offensive factors, but it increased the defensive factors. *Bacopa monniera* showed significant antioxidant effect *per se* in stressed animals. *In vitro* studies with *H. pylori* showed significant inhibition at the concentration of 1000 (μg/ml of *Bacopa monniera* extract.[70] Even though effective antimicrobial therapy is available to eradicate *H. pylori* infection, current therapies require patients to ingest multiple agents several times a day for at least 1 week, leading to noncompliance of treatment schedules. An antiulcer agent having anti-*H. pylori* activity can have better compliance among patients and can also decrease incidences of drug interactions. *Bacopa monniera* extract also increased *in vitro* accumulation of PGs on human colonic mucosa cells.[70]

22.9.2 Clinical Studies

22.9.2.1 DRBP

The clinical effectiveness of DRBP was confirmed by radiological and endoscopic studies in the several clinical trials. DRBP was found to decrease or delay the relapse of peptic ulcer for 6 to 12 months after a 3-month continuous treatment at the dose level of 1 g four times/day. It became commercially available as Musapep® after phase IV clinical trials. A double-blind study[71] done at multiple centers has shown that about 40 to 70% of endoscopically proved DUs healed after 12 weeks of treatment with DRBP, as compared with about 16% with placebo. In another clinical study[72] with Musapep in nonulcer dyspepsia (NUD), there was a reported 75% relief in symptoms after 8 weeks of treatment compared with 20% in the control. The authors advocated that the therapeutic trials with this dose justified the use of DRBP on clinical grounds to be safe and effective in the treatment of NUD.

22.9.2.2 Satavari mandur

Effect of *Satavari mandur* was studied in 40 cases of *parinamashula*, including 10 cases of peptic ulcer, 15 cases of erosive mucosal disorder, and 15 cases of NUD. The improvement was assessed by clinical and radiological or endoscopic findings, together with the biochemical study of gastric juice in eight patients. The drug was given in a dose of 3 g/day in two divided doses with ghee for 2 months in NUD cases and 3 months in peptic ulcer cases. A significant improvement was observed in all the groups, but it was more prominent in ulcer dyspepsia than NUD. *Satavari mandur* showed significant improvement in healing ulcers (marked healing of 50%, partial healing of 30% in ulcer group) as well as significant improvement in symptoms. The biochemical study of gastric juice in eight patients showed a significant increase in mucosal defensive factors such as decreased cell shedding, increased individual carbohydrates, and increased total carbohydrate to protein ratio. These findings indicate the drug was promoting the mucosal defensive mechanism rather than affecting the acid and pepsin secretion.[41]

22.9.2.3 Eclipta alba (Bhringaraja)

In a clinical trial (n = 55), *Eclipta alba* showed marked symptomatic relief in NUD and peptic ulcer patients. Total response in NUD was excellent in 62.9%, good in 17.1%, poor

TABLE 22.3

Antiulcerogenic Activity of Some Medicinal Plants

Drugs (Common/Ayurvedic Name)	Experimental Models	Mechanism of Action	Ref.
Abies pindrow Royle, Fam. Pinaceae (*Talisapatra*) Petroleum ether (PE), acetone (AE), chloroform (CE), and ethanolic (EE) extracts of leaves	CRS- induced GU in rats	Antistress activity	74
Benincasa hispida, Fam. Cucurbitaceae (*Petha* or *Golkaddu*) Fresh juice, supernatant and residue fraction of centrifuged juice, PE and EE	Aspirin (ASP) + restraint, swimming stress, indomethacin plus histamine- and serotonin-induced ulcers in rats and mice	—	75
Camellia sinensis, Fam. Ternstroemiaceae (green tea) Hot water extract	Cold + restraint–stress-induced ulcers in rats		76
Centella asiatica, Fam. Umbelliferae (*Brahma-manduki*) Fresh juice of whole plant	CRS-, EtOH-, ASP-, and PL-induced GU in rats	No effect on acid-pepsin secretion, increase in mucin secretion and life span of mucosal cells	77
Convolvulus pluricaulis, Fam. Convolvulaceae (*Shankupuspi*) Fresh juice of whole plant	CRS-, EtOH-, ASP-, and PL-induced GU in rats	No effect on acid-pepsin secretion, increase in mucin secretion and life span of mucosal cells	78
Emblica officinalis Gaertn. Fam. Euphorbiaceae (*Amla*) Fresh juice of fruit plup	CRS-, EtOH-, ASP-, and PL-induced GU in rats and acetic-acid–induced healing model	Decreased the acid and pepsin secretion and increased mucus secretion	79
Garcinia cambogia, Fam. Guttiferae (*Kukum*) Fruit extract	Indomethacin	Decrease in acid-pepsin secretion and promotion of mucosal defensive	80
Honey	Ethanol-induced increased vascular permeability changes in the rat stomach	Free-radical scavenger	81
Pongamia pinnata, Leguminosae (*Karanj* or *Karanja*)		—	82, 83
PE, AE, CE, and EE extracts of seeds	RS-induced GU in mice	Decrease in acid pepsin	
PE, AE, CE, and EE extracts of roots	RS- and PL- induced GU in rats		
Satavari Mandur	PL- and CRS-induced GU in rats	No effect on acid-pepsin secretion and promotes mucosal defensive factors by enhancing mucin secretion and life span of mucosal cells	84
Shilajit *per se* effect	PL-, IS-, and ASP-induced GU in rats and CYS- and HIST-induced DU in rats and GP, respectively	Tendency to decrease acid-pepsin secretion and significant increase in mucin secretion	85

TABLE 22.3 (continued)

Antiulcerogenic Activity of Some Medicinal Plants

Drugs (Common/Ayurvedic Name)	Experimental Models	Mechanism of Action	Ref.
Sitavirya drugs a. Asparagus racemosus, Fam. Liliaceae (*Satawari*) Fresh juice of roots b. *Glycyrrhiza glabra*, Fam. Leguminosae (*Mulhatti*) Water decoction of roots c. *Holarrhene antidysenterica* Wall., Fam. Apocynaceae (*Kurachi*) water decoction of barks d. *Ficus religiosa*, Fam. Urticaceae (*Peepalbanti*) Water decoction of barks	 PL- and CRS-induced GU in rats PL- and CRS-induced GU in rats PL- and CRS-induced GU, CYS-induced DU in rats PL- and CRS-induced GU and CYS-induced DU in rats	No effect on acid-pepsin secretion and promotes mucosal defensive factors by enhancing mucin secretion and life span of mucosal cells	86
Tectona grandis L. Fam. Verbenaceae (Sagwan) Ethanolic fraction of trunk bark and wood chips	Pylorus ligation (PL) restraint stress (RS)- and prendnisolone-induced GU in rats Histamine (HIST)-induced GU and DU in guinea pigs (GP)	No effect on acid-pepsin secretion but caused an increase in mucin secretion	87
Withania somnifera, Fam. Solanaceae (*Aswagandha*) (Roots) SG-1 [total Me OH-H_2O (1:1)] SG-2 (sitoindosides VII, VIII, and withaferin-A)	RS-induced GU in rats	Antistress activity	88

in 5.7%, and 14.3% patients dropped out of the study. Radiological assessment confirmed the symptomatic improvement. Of 25 DU cases, 48% were under excellent response, 24% were under good response, and 16% showed poor response; 12% did not show any response to the treatment. The was drug given in the form of powder (30 g) in three divided doses/day for 1 month in NUD cases and for 3 months in DU cases. The drug also showed significant reduction in free HCL and total acidity in both the groups (NUD and UD).[73]

Various other herbal drugs have been reported to have antiulcerogenic activity. These are summarized in Table 22.3. Some of these drugs have been chemically characterized and the entities involved in the activity have been isolated. These are summarized in Tables 22.3 and 22.4.

22.10 Summary

Ayurveda has a clear description of etiology, pathology, and treatment for gastroduodenal ulcers. Scientific evidence was also found in the literature in support of use of the following Ayurvedic herbs: *Abies pindrow, Benincasa hispida, Camellia sinensis, Centella asiatica, Convolvulus pluricaulis, Emblica officinalis, Tambra bhasma, unripe plantain banana, Piper longum,*

TABLE 22.4

Ulcer Protective Effect of Some Active Constituents Isolated From Herbal Drugs

Plants	Active Constituents	Models	Mode of Action	Ref.
Aegle marmelos Correa, Fam. rutaceae (Bael (seeds)	Luvangetin	-do-	—	89
Asparagus racemosus, Fam. Liliaceae (*Satawari*)	Standardized extract to active saponins	CRS-, EtOH-, ASP- and PL-induced GU in rats	No effect on acid pepsin secretion, increase in mucin secretion and life span of mucosal cells	90
Azadhiracta indica, Fam. Meliaceae (Neem)	Nimbidin	ASP-, prednisolone, indomethacin-, serotonin stress-, and acetic acid-induced GU in rats; HIST-induced DU in GP CYS-induced DU in rats	—	91
Emblica officinalis Gaertn., Fam. Euphorbiaceae (Amla) methanolic extract	Standardized to the tannoids, emblicanin A and B	CRS-, EtOH-, ASP-, and PL-induced GU in rats and acetic-acid–induced healing model	Decreased the acid and pepsin secretion and increased mucus secretion	22
Garcinia indica, Fam. Guttiferae (*Kumkum*) Fruit rind	Garcinol	Water-immersion stress	Free-radical scavenger	92
Ocimum basilum, Fam. Leguminosae (*Tulsi*)	Fixed oil	ASP-, indomethacin-, EtOH-, Hist-, reserpine, Serotonin-, PL-, and stress-induced GU in rats	Antisecretory	93
Shilajit	Fulvic acid, 4′- methoxy 6 carbomethoxybi-phenyl	PL-, PL+ASP-, and RS–induced GU and CYS-induced DU in rats	*Per se* decrease in acid-pepsin secretion and cell shedding, tendency to increase mucin secretion, but reversed the increase in cell shedding and decrease in mucin secretion induced by ASP	94
Tectona grandis L., Fam. Verbenaceae (Sagwan) (Trunk bark and wood chips)	Lapachol	Immobilization stress (IS)- and ASP-induced GU in rats; CYS-and HIST-induced DU in rats and GP, respectively	*Per se* no significant effect on both offensive and defensive factors but reversed the ASP-induced increase in peptic activity and decrease in sialic acid and mucin secretion	95
Zingiber officinale Roscoe. (Ginger) (Adrak)	6-Gingesulphonic acid, 6-shogaol, and ar-curcumene	—	Gastric motility	76, 77, 96

Ferula foetida, Bacopa monniera, Eclipta alba, Garcinia cambogia, Pongamia pinnata, Tectona grandis, Withania somnifera, and *Satavari mandur.* These therapies are relatively safe and effective.

References

1. Goel, R.K. and Bhattacharya, S.K., Gastroduodenal mucosal defense and mucosal protective agents, *Indian J. Exp. Biol.*, 29, 701, 1991.
2. Borrelli, F. and Izzo, A.A., The plant kingdom as a source of antiulcer remedies, *Phytother. Res.*, 14, 581, 2000.
3. Sharma, P.V., Cititsastana to Siddhistana, in *Caraka Samhita,* Vol. 4, Sharma, P.V., Ed., Chaukhamba Orientalia, Delhi, India, 1994, p. 3.
4. Sharma, P.V., Sutrastana, in *Susruta Samhita,* Vol. 1, Sharma, P.V., Ed., Chaukhambha Visva Bharati, Varanasi, India, 1999, p. 519.
5. Tewari, P.V., Kumar, N., Sharma, R.D., and Kumar, A., Treatment of *amlapitta* (khila sthana), in *Kasyapa Samhita,* Tewari, P.V., Ed., Chaukhambha Visva Bharati, Varanasi, 1996, p. 630.
6. Translated by a board of scholars, Sutrastana, in *Astanga Hrdaya of Vagbada,* Vol. 1, Sri Satguru Publications, Delhi, India, 1999, p. 125.
7. Sharma, P.V., Treatment of *parinamasula,* in *Cakradatta, A Treatise on Principles and Practices of Ayurvedic Medicine,* Sharma, P.V., Ed., Chaukhambha Orientalia, Varanasi, India, 1994, p. 249.
8. Perry, M.A. et al., Role of oxygen radicals in ischemia induced lesions in the cat stomach, *Gastroenterology,* 90, 362, 1986.
9. Blaser, M.J., Hypothesis. The changing relationships of helicobacter pylori infection and humans: implications for health and disease, *J. Infect. Dis.*, 179, 1523, 1999.
10. Kuruta, S.H. and Nogawa, A.N., Meta-analysis of risk factors for peptic ulcer. Nonsteroidal antiinflammatory drugs, *Helicobacter pylori* and smoking, *J. Clin. Gastroenterol.*, 24, 2, 1997.
11. Megraud, F., Resistance of *Helicobacter pylori* to antibiotics, the main limitation of current proton-pump inhibitor triple therapy, *Eur. J. Gastroenterol. Hepatol.,* 11(Suppl. 2), S35, 1999.
12. Buring, S.M. et al., Discontinuation rates of *Helicobacter pylori* treatment regimens: a meta analysis, *Pharmacotherapy,* 19, 324, 1999.
13. McGuigan, J.E., Peptic ulcer and gastritis, in *Harrison's Principles of Internal Medicine,* 12th ed., Wilson, J.D. et al., Eds., McGraw,Hill, New York, 1991, p. 1229.
14. Tsukimi, Y. and Okabe, S., Recent advances in gastrointestinal pathophysiology, role of heat shock proteins in mucosal defense and ulcer healing, *Biol. Pharm. Bull.*, 24, 1, 2001.
15. Morris, G.P. and Wallace, J.L., The roles of ethanol and acid in the production of gastric mucosal erosions in rats, *Virchows Arch.*, 46, 239, 1981.
16. Marshall, B.J. and Warren, J.R., Spiral bacteria in the human stomach a common finding in patients with gastritis and duodenal ulcer, in *Campylobacter II,* Pearson, A.D. et al., Eds., Public Health Laboratory Service, London, 1983, p. 11.
17. Rauws, E.A.J., Reasons for failure of Helicobacter pylori treatment, *Eur. J. Gastroenterol. Hepatol.* 5(Suppl. 2), S92, 1993.
18. Black, J.W. et al., Definition and antagonism of histamine H_2-receptors, *Nature,* 236, 385, 1972.
19. Yoshikawa, T. et al., Role of active oxygen, lipid peroxidation and antioxidants in the pathogenesis of gastric mucosal injury induced by indomethacin in rats, *Gut,* 34, 732, 1993.
20. Ballinger, A. and Smith, G., COX-2 inhibitors vs. NSAIDs in gastrointestinal damage and prevention, *Expert Opin. Pharmacother.* 2, 31, 2001.
21. Bast, A., Haenen, G.R.M.M., and Doelman, C.J.A., Oxidants and antioxidants: state of the art, *Am. J. Med.*, 91, 2S, 1991.
22. Sairam, K. et al., Antiulcerogenic effect of methanolic extract of Emblica officinalis: an experimental study, *J. Ethnopharmacol.*, 82(1), 1, 2002.
23. Sairam, K. et al., Prophylactic and curative effects of *Bacopa monniera* in gastric ulcer models, *Phytomedicine,* 8, 423, 2001.

24. Goel, R.K. et al., Role of gastric antioxidant and anti-Helicobacter pylori activities in the antiulcerogenic activity of plantain banana (*Musa sapientum* var. paradisiaca), *Indian J. Exp. Biol.*, 39, 719, 2001.
25. Allen, A. et al., Gastroduodenal mucosal protection, *Physiol. Rev.*, 73, 823, 1993.
26. Williams, S.E. and Turnberg, L.A., Studies of the protective properties of gastric mucus: evidence for a mucus, bicarbonate barrier, *Gut*, 22, 94, 1981.
27. Lacy, E.R., Rapid restitution of the superficially damaged gastric mucosa, in *Advances in Peptic Ulcer Pathogenesis*, Ress, W.D.W., Ed., Lancaster, U.K., 1988, p. 163.
28. Mangla, J.C. et al., Effect of duodenal ulcerogens cysteamine, Meprizole and MPTP on duodenal myoelectric activity in rats, *Dig. Dis. Sci.*, 34, 537, 1989.
29. Sato, N. et al., Gastric blood flow in ulcer disease, *Scand. J. Gastroenterol.*, 30, 14, 1995.
30. Wallace, J.L., Mechanisms of protection and healing, current knowledge and future research, *Am. J. Med.*, 8(Suppl. 1), S19, 2001.
31. Jackson, L.M. et al., Cyclooxygenase (COX) 1 and 2 in normal, inflamed, and ulcerated human gastric mucosa, *Gut*, 47, 762, 2000.
32. Buettner, G.R., The packing order of free radicals and antioxidants, lipid peroxidation, a-tocopheral, and ascorbate, *Arch. Biochem. Biophys.*, p. 300, 1993.
33. *Madhava Nidanam*, Madhukosha commentary by Vijaya rakshita and Srikantadatta, Vidyotani Commentary by Sri Sudharshan Shastry, 15th ed., Chaukambha Sanskrit Sansthan, Varanasi, India, 1985, p. 472
34. Misciagna, G., Cisternino, A.M., and Freudenheim, J., Diet and duodenal ulcer, *Dig. Liver Dis.*, 32, 468, 2000.
35. Alarcon de la Lastra, C. et al., Mediterranean diet and health, biological importance of olive oil, *Curr. Pharm. Dis.*, 7, 933, 2001.
36. Jayaraj, A.P. et al., Dietary factors in relation to the distribution of duodenal ulcer in India as assessed by studies in rats, *J. Gastroenterol. Hepatol.*, 16, 501, 2001.
37. Villegas, I., Alarcon de la Lastra, C., La Casa, C., Motilva, V., and Martin, M.J., Effects of food intake and oxidative stress on intestinal lesions caused by meloxicam and piroxicam in rats, *Eur. J. Pharmacol.*, 414, 79, 2001.
38. Gwee, K.A., The role of psychological and biological factors in postinfective gut dysfunction, *Gut*, 44, 400–406, 1999.
39. McEwen, B.S., Protective and damaging effects of damaging effects of stress meditors, *N. Engl. J. Med.*, 338, 171, 1998.
40. Das, D. and Banerjee, R.F., Effect of stress on the antioxidant enzymes and gastric ulceration, *Mol. Cell. Biochem.*, 125, 115, 1993.
41. Sailaja, V., Further Studies on the Effect of Shatavari Mandur in Cases of *Parinamashula* vis-a-vis Acid Peptic Disorders, M.D. (Ayurveda) thesis, I.M.S., Banaras Hindu University, Varanasi, India, 2000.
42. Goel, R.K. and Sairam, K., Antiulcer drugs from indigenous sources with emphasis on *Musa sapientum, tamrabasma, Asparagus racemosus* and *Zingiber officinale*, *Indian J. Pharmacol.*, 34, 100, 2001.
43. Maton, P.N. and Burton, M.E., Antacids revisited: a review of their clinical pharmacology and recommended therapeutic use, *Drugs*, 57, 855, 1999.
44. Ichikawa, T. et al., Lafutidine-induced stimulation of mucin biosynthesis mediated by nitric oxide is limited to surface mucous cells of rat gastric oxyntic mucosa, *Life Sci.*, 62, PL259, 1998.
45. Chang, M., Saito, H., and Abe, K., Cimetidine inhibits the induction of long-term potentiation in the dentate gyrus of rats *in vivo*, *Jpn. J. Pharmacol.*, 74, 281, 1997.
46. Sandvik, A.K., Brenna, E., and Waldum, H.L., Review article, the pharmacological inhibition of gastric acid secretion: tolerance and rebound, *Aliment. Pharmacol. Ther.*, 11, 1013, 1997.
47. Larsson, H. et al., Plasma gastrin concentration and gastric enterochromaffin like cell activation and proliferation studies with omeprazole and ranitidine in intact and antrectomatized rats, *Gastroenterology*, 90, 391–399, 1986.
48. Wetscher, G.J. et al., Gastric acid blockade with omeprazole promotes gastric carcinogenesis induced by duodenogastric reflux, *Dig. Dis. Sci.*, 44, 1132, 1999.

49. Kakei, N. et al., Omeprazole a proton pump inhibitor, reduces the secretion, synthesis and gene expression of pepsinogen in the rat stomach, *Biochem. Biophys. Res. Commun.*, 195, 997, 1993.
50. Fireman, Z., Kopelman, Y., and Strenberg, A., Central nervous system side effects after proton pump inhibitor treatment, *J. Clin Gastroenterol.*, 25, 718, 1997.
51. Ahmed, S.M. et al., Lansoprasole potentiates vecuronium paralysis, *J. Indian Med. Assoc.*, 95, 422, 1997.
52. Sanyal, A.K., Banerjee, C.R., and Das, P.K., Studies on peptic ulceration. II. Role of banana in restraint and prednisolone-induced ulcer in albino rats, *Arch. Int. Pharmacodynamics*, 155, 244, 1965.
53. Goel, R.K., Chakrabarthy, A., and Sanyal, A.K., The effect of biological variables on the anti-ulcerogenic effect of vegetable plantain banana, *Planta Med.*, 2, 85, 1985.
54. Goel, R.K. et al., Antiulcerogenic effect of banana powder (*Musa sapientum* var. *Paradisiaca*) and its effect on mucosal resistance, *J. Ethnopharmacol.*, 18, 33, 1986.
55. Mukhopadhyay, K. et al., Effect of banana powder (*Musa sapientum* var. paradisiaca) on gastric mucosal shedding, *J. Ethnopharmacol.*, 21, 11, 1987.
56. Tavares, I.A. and Benntt, A., Stimulation of gastric and colonic mucosal eicosanoid synthesis of plantain banana, *J. Pharm. Pharmacol.*, 41, 747, 1989.
57. Ghosal, S., Steryl glycosides and acylsteryl glycosides from *Musa paradisiaca*, *Phytochemistry*, 241, 807, 1985.
58. Chattopadhyay, S., Chaudhuri, S., and Ghosal, S., Activation of peritoneal macrophages by sitoindoside-IV, an anti-ulcerogenic acylsteryl glycoside from *Musa paradisiaca*, *Planta Med.*, 53, 16, 1987.
59. Lewis, D.A., Fields, W.N., and Shaw, G.P., A natural flavanoid present in unripe banana plup (*Musa sapientum* L. var. *paradisiaca*) protects the gastric mucosa from aspirin-induced erosions, *J. Ethnopharmacol.*, 65, 283, 1999.
60. Varga, D., Misra, B.S., and Vaisya, R.L., Eds., 5th ed., *Bhavaprakash Nighantu of Shri Bhava Misra (1500–1600 A.D.)*, Chaukhambha Sanskrit Santhan, Varanasi, India, 1969, p. 605.
61. Goel, R.K., Tavares, I.A., and Bennett, A., Effects of cupric chloride and tamrabhasma: a traditional Indian preparation of copper, on eicosanoid production by human gastric and colonic mucosa, *J. Pharm. Pharmacol.*, 44, 862, 1992.
62. Goel, R.K., Maiti, R.N., and Mukhopadhyaya, K., Effect of Tamrabhasma, an Indian indigenous preparation of copper on rat gastric mucosal resistance, *Indian J. Exp. Biol.*, 32, 559, 1994.
63. Agrawal, A.K. et al., Effect of *Piper longum, Zingiber officinale* Linn and *Ferula* species on gastric ulceration and secretion in rats, *Indian J. Exp. Biol.*, 38, 994, 2000.
64. Udupa, K.N. and Singh, R.H., *Clinical and Experimental Studies on Rasayana drugs and Panchkarma Therapy*, Central Council for Research in Ayurveda and Siddha, New Delhi, India, 1995.
65. Bhattacharya, S.K. and Ghosal, S., Anxiolytic activity of a standardized extract of *Bacopa monniera*, an experimental study, *Phytomedicine*, 5, 77, 1998.
66. Sairam, K. et al., Antidepressant activity of standardized extract of *Bacopa monniera* in experimental models of depression in rats. *Phytomedicine*, 9, 207, 2002.
67. Bhattacharya, S.K. et al., Anxiolytic-antidepressant activity of Withania somnifera glycowithanolides, an experimental study, *Phytomedicine*, 7, 463, 2000.
68. Rastogi, R.P., Pal, R., and Kulshreshtha, D.K., Bacoside A_3, a triterpinoid saponin from *Bacopa monniera*, *Phytochemistry*, 36, 133, 1994.
69. Rao, Ch.V., Sairam, K., and Goel, R.K., Experimental evaluation of *Bacopa monniera* on rat gastric ulceration and secretion, *Indian J. Physiol. Pharmacol.*, 44, 35, 2000.
70. Goel, R.K. et al., *In vitro* evaluation of *Bacopa monniera* on accumulation of prostaglandins and anti-*Helicobacter pylori* activity, *Phytomedicine*, accepted.
71. Goel, R.K., Effect of Vegetable Banana on Gastric Secretion and Ulceration: An Experimental and Clinical Study, Ph.D. thesis, submitted to Banaras Hindu University, Varanasi, India, 1983.
72. Arora, A. and Sharma, M.P., Use of banana in non-ulcer dyspepsia, *Lancet*, 435, 612, 1990.

73. Tiwari, S.K., Chaturvedi, G.N., and Gupta, J.P., Comparative Studies on Gastroduodenal Diseases (*Amlapitta* and *Parinamashula*) in Ayurveda and Modern Medicine with Therapeutic Evaluation of *Bhringaraja* (Eclipta alba) in Peptic Ulcer and Nonulcer Dyspepsia, Ph.D. thesis, I.M.S., Banaras Hindu University, Varanasi, India, 1979.
74. Singh, R.K. et al., Pharmacological actions of *Abies Pindrow* Royle leaf, *Indian. J. Exp. Biol.*, 36, 187, 1998.
75. Grover, J.K. et al., Extracts of *Benincasa hispida* prevent development of experimental ulcers, *J. Ethnopharmacol.*, 78, 159, 2001.
76. Maity, S., Vedasiromani, J.R., and Ganguly, D.K., Anti-ulcer effect of the hot water extract of black tea (*Camellia sinesis*), *J. Ethnopharmacol.*, 46, 167, 1995.
77. Sairam, K., Rao, Ch.V., and Goel, R.K., Effect of *Centella asiatica* Linn on physical and chemical factors induced gastric ulceration and secretion, *Indian J. Exp. Biol.*, 39, 137, 2001.
78. Sairam, K., Rao, Ch.V., and Goel, R.K., Effect of *Convolvulus pluricaulis* Chois on gastric ulceration and secretion in rats, *Indian J. Exp. Biol.*, 39, 350, 2001.
79. Rao, Ch.V., Sairam, K., and Goel, R.K., Effect of E*mblica officinalis* fruit in gastric ulceration and secretion, *Acta Pharmaceutica Turcica,* in press.
80. Mahendran, P., Vanisree, A.J., and Shyamala Devi, C.S., The antiulcer activity of *Garcinia cambogia* extract against indomethacin-induced gastric ulcer in rats, *Phytother. Res.*, 16, 80, 2002.
81. Mobarok Ali, A.T. and al-Swayeh, O.A., Natural honey prevents ethanol-induced increased vascular permeability changes in the rat stomach, *J. Ethnopharmacol.*, 55, 231, 1997.
82. Singh, R.K. et al., Pharmacological action of *Pongamia pinnata* seeds: a preliminary study, *Indian J. Exp. Biol.*, 34, 1204, 1996.
83. Singh, R.K. et al., Pharmacological actions of *Pongamia pinnata* roots in albino rats, *Indian J. Exp. Biol.*, 35, 831, 1997.
84. Datla, G.K. et al., Anti-ulcerogenic activity of *Satavari mandur* — an Ayurvedic herbo-mineral preparation, *Indian J. Exp. Biol.*, accepted.
85. Goel, R.K., Banerjee, R.S., and Acharya, S.B., Antiulcerogenic and antiinflammatory studies with *shilajit*, *J. Ethnopharmacol.*, 29,95, 1990.
86. De, B. et al., Effect of some Sitavirya drugs on gastric secretion and ulceration, *Indian J. Exp. Biol.*, 35, 1084, 1997.
87. Pandey, B.L. et al., Effect of *Tectonia grandis* Linn. (common teak tree) on experimental ulcers and gastric secretion, *Indian J. Med. Res.*, 76, 224, 1982.
88. Bhattacharya, S.K. et al., Activity of sitoindosides VII and VIII, new acylsterylglcosides from *Withania somnifera*, *Phytother. Res.*, 1, 32, 1987.
89. Goel, R.K. et al., Antiulcer activity of naturally occurring pyranocoumarin and isocoumarin and their effect on prostanoids synthesis using human colonic mucosa, *Indian J. Exp. Biol.*, 35, 1080, 1997.
90. Sairam, K. et al., Anti-gastroduodenal ulcerogenic activity of *Asparagus racemosus* — an experimental, biochemical and histological study, *J. Ethnopharmacol.*, accepted.
91. Pillai, N.R. and Santha Kumari, G., Toxicity studies on nimbidin, a potential antiulcer drug, *Planta Med.*, 46, 143, 1984.
92. Yamaguchi, F. et al., Free radical scavenging activity and antiulcer activity of garcinol from *Garcinia indica* fruit rind, *J. Agric. Food Chem.*, 48, 2320, 2000.
93. Singh, S., Evaluation of gastric antiulcer activity of fixed oil of *Ocimum basilicum* Linn. and its possible mechanism of action, *Indian J. Exp. Biol.*, 36, 253, 1999.
94. Ghosal, S. et al., Antiulcerogenic activity of fulvic acids and 4-metoxy-6-carbomethyl biphenyl isolated from shilajit, *Phytother. Res.*, 2, 187, 1988.
95. Goel, R.K. et al., Effect of *lapachol,* a naphthaquinone isolated from *Tectona grandis*, on experimental peptic ulcer and gastric secretion, *J. Pharm. Pharmacol.*, 39, 138, 1987.
96. Yoshikawa, M. et al., 6-Gingesulfonic acid, a new antiulcer principle and gingerglycolipids A, B and C, three new monoacyldigalactosyt glycerols, from *Zingiberis rhizoma* originating in Taiwan, *Chem. Pharm. Bull.*, 40, 2239, 1992.

23

Alzheimer's Disease

Divya Shangari Vohora and Lakshmi Chandra Mishra

CONTENTS

23.1 Introduction

Mental diseases and mental temperaments have been extensively described in Ayurveda (e.g., nervous disorders [*vata vyadhi*], epilepsy [*Apasmara*], insanity, psychosis [*unmada*], loss of consciousness, fainting [*murccha, moha, tamaka*], impairment in functioning of mind [*Pramoha*], amnesia [*Vismriti*], etc.)[1,2] Alzheimer's disease (AD) is a neurodegenerative disorder associated with the progressively worsening of cognitive functions and behavioral disturbances; it is the most common form of primary dementia and mortality in the geriatric population. Although there is no precise equivalent for AD in Ayurveda, cognitive dysfunction has been described in convulsive disorders[1,3] and with the aging process, which is known to be associated with physical and mental disability.[4,5] Thus it can be seen

0-8493-1366-X/04/$0.00+$1.50

that in spite of the terminological differences between the Ayurvedic and the modern systems of medicine, there are areas of similarity between the two. It is necessary to bridge the terminology gap between the Eastern and Western concepts and management for a better understanding and control of cognitive disorders. The present review is aimed toward this objective.

23.2 Clinical Description

The major clinical manifestations of AD are memory disturbances, spatial and temporal disorientation, and getting lost in familiar surroundings. As the disease progresses, aphasia, apraxia, acalculia, and sleepwalking may develop.[6]

23.3 Epidemiology

AD is a worldwide problem that affects 5 million people in the U.S.[7] As the life span is increasing, AD is becoming a more common disorder. Approximately 10% of the population older than 65 years are affected.[6] In a recent report, AD was listed as the eighth cause of death in the U.S. in 2000.[8]

23.4 Etiology and Pathophysiology

In Ayurveda, AD is considered age related with no specific etiology except that the *vata dosa* is involved. Conventional medicine is using several working hypotheses to find an effective treatment for AD and develop prevention strategies. These hypotheses include defective beta-amyloid (Abeta) protein metabolism; abnormalities of glutamatergic, adrenergic, serotonergic, dopaminergic, and cholinergic neurotransmission; and the potential involvement of inflammatory, oxidative, and hormonal pathways.[9–12] Another suggested possible cause is a diet containing excessive intake of sugar, refined carbohydrates (with high glycemic index), and animal products (with high content of saturated fats), and a decrease intake of unrefined seeds (cereals, legumes, and oleaginous seeds), vegetables (with high fibrous content, vitamins, polyphenols, and other antioxidant substances [e.g., phytoestrogens]), and seafood (rich in omega-3 fatty acids).[13] The other causative factors hypothesized are insulin resistance, decreased endothelial production of nitric oxide, free-radical excess, inflammatory metabolites, homocysteine deficiency, and estrogen deficiency.[13]

In a prospective analysis of risk factors, increasing age, lack of education, and the apolipoprotein E epsilon4 allele were found to be significantly associated with increased risk of AD. On the other hand, use of nonsteroidal anti-inflammatory drugs (NSAIDs), wine, and regular physical activity were found to be significantly associated with reduced risk of AD.[14] Some evidence suggests that oxidative damage of brain tissue may be involved in pathogenesis, which precedes the occurrence of symptoms and the formation of amyloid-containing plaques and neurofibrillary tangles.[15]

Genetic factors may also be involved, but they do not explain in full the etiopathogensis of AD, implying a role for environmental factors.[16] The discovery of pathogenic mutations in the beta-amyloid peptide (beta-APP) and the presenilin genes provides strong support for the genetic hypothesis because Abeta production and deposition contribute to the etiology of AD.[17]

There is some evidence that alterations in the lysosomal system may have a role in the pathogenesis of AD.[18] The lysosomal system contributes to protein deposits associated with different types of age-related neurodegeneration. Lysosomes are highly susceptible to free-radical oxidative stress in the aging brain and leads to the gradual loss of metabolic activity over the life span of an individual.[19]

23.5 Clinical Examination and Diagnosis

Ayurvedic examination primarily consists of an eight-point examination to determine the vitiated *dosas,* body constitution, and manifestations of the disease to determine appropriate treatment (Chapter 2). Patients are examined for memory disturbances, difficulty in learning, spatial and temporal disorientation, and decline in daily living activities (e.g., eating and difficulty in grooming, dressing, and undressing). Patients generally begin to feel spatially lost in familiar surroundings. It is important to rule out the other causes of dementia such as metabolic causes (e.g., diabetes, medication-induced psychiatric illness) before treating the patient with cholinesterase inhibitors. Because many causes of dementia are rare and can be excluded by careful historical information, serial examination, and some structural examination, an accurate diagnosis can be made by using clinical criteria.[6]

23.6 Clinical Course and Prognosis

AD is a uniformly progressive disease. It ultimately results in irreversible debilitating cognitive impairment in patients. Although some medications appear to produce transient improvement, there is no medication available that can halt the progression of AD.[19]

23.7 Management

Ayurveda uses natural products (drugs of plant, animal, and mineral origin) for the treatment of all physical and mental ailments, including cognitive dysfunction. There are two approaches: one is aimed at general or total well-being, including mental exercises (memory games, reading, card games) and meditation, whereas the other specifically targets intellect (*medha*) and memory (*smriti*). Ayurvedic *rasayana tantra*, which describes these approaches, was defined by the Ayurvedic physician Susruta (500 B.C.) as the measure that prolongs longevity, develops positive health and mental faculties, and imparts resistance and immunity against disease.[4] These measures do not appear to differ from the adaptogenic,[20] immunomodulatory,[21] and antioxidant[22] therapeutic approaches used in modern medicine. The host-oriented approach of *rasayana* drugs is believed to vitalize the digestion and metabolism and improve microcirculation and tissue perfusion[5] to elicit the desired therapeutic effects.

23.7.1 Brain Tonics (*Medhya Rasayana*)

Abhang[23] reviewed the past, present, and future of *medhya rasayana* drugs: a special class of *rasayana* agents that rejuvenate mental faculties, intellect, and memory. In ancient India most of the education was imparted by oral instructions. The students retained and recalled this knowledge by repeated recitation. Therefore, intelligence was considered synonymous with memory, and drugs that helped reduce time for learning (memorizing) the lesson were developed from natural sources. Many such products, particularly of plant origin, have been described in Ayurvedic texts. Some of these are particularly reputed for *medhya rasayana* properties since ancient times of great Ayurvedic physicians Charaka (400 B.C.) and Susruta (500 B.C.). The following brain vitalizers have been mentioned in *Charak Samhita*[24]:

1. Expressed juice of Indian pennywort (*Centella asiatica*)
2. Powder of licorice (*Glycyrrhiza glabra*) with milk
3. Juice of *guduchi* (*Tinospora cordifolia*)
4. Paste made from small leaves of *shankhpushpi* (*Convolvulus pluricaulis*) mixed with its roots and flowers

A large number of Indian medicinal plants are attributed with brain tonic and memory-enhancing effects. These plants are rarely used singly and are mostly incorporated in polyherbal formulations containing 4 to 20 ingredients. The latter may occasionally include mineral-origin drugs in addition to medicinal plants. Polypharmacy appears to be the rule (rather than exception) in Ayurveda as in other traditional systems of medicine practiced in India (e.g., Unani-Tibb and Siddha). It is claimed that such combinations enhance activity and mitigate side effects of individual components.

Some plant ingredients are common to many formulations. A look at the composition of 6 polyherbal formulations, marketed in India for memory enhancing effects, revealed the presence of 32 medicinal plant ingredients (Table 23.1).

In conventional medicine, the only drugs currently approved for the treatment of AD are cholinomimetics, such as tacrine, which have the pharmacologic profile of acetylcholinesterase (AChE) inhibitors.[12,25,26] Tacrine has been shown to affect some measures of memory performance, but the magnitude of improvement was very modest.[27] The side effects of tacrine, such as abdominal cramping, nausea, vomiting, and diarrhea, may be significant and dose limiting. Considerable research is being conducted in other areas, such as using selective anti-inflammatory drugs (selective cyclooxgenase-2 [COX-2] inhib-

TABLE 23.1

Plant Ingredients of Six Polyherbal Formulations Marketed in India for Memory-Improving Effects

No.	Latin Name (Vernacular Name)
1	*Acorus calamus (vacha)*
2	*Amomum subulatum (badi ilaichi)*
3	*Asparagus racemosus (shatawar)*[a]
4	*Bacopa monniera (brahmi)*[a]
5	*Butea frondosa (dhak, palash)*
6	*Canscora decussata (sankha holi)*
7	*Cinnamomum zeylanicum (dalchini)*
8	*Convolvulus pluricaulis (shankhpushpi)*[a]
9	*Delphinium denudatum (jadwar shireen)*
10	*Elettaria cardamomum (choti elaichi)*
11	*Emblica officinalis (amla)*
12	*Embelia ribes (vayu vidang)*
13	*Eugenia caryophyllus (laung)*
14	*Foeniculum vulgare (bari saunf)*
15	*Ipomea paniculata (vidari kand)*
16	*Nardostachys jatamansi (jatamansi)*
17	*Operculum tarpethum (nishoth)*
18	*Paenia emodi (uood saleeb)*
19	*Pandanus odoratissimus (keora)*
20	*Pimpinella anisum (saunf)*
21	*Piper aurantiacum (renuka)*
22	*Piper longum (peepal, pippali)*
23	*Prunus amygdalis (badam)*
24	*Rosa damascena (gulab)*
25	*Sassurea lappa (kuth)*
26	*Terminalia belerica (bahera)*
27	*Terminalia chebula (harar, hareetaki)*
28	*Tinospora card folia (giloe)*
29	*Valerian walachia (tagar)*
30	*Vetiverica zizinoides (khas)*
31	*Withania somnifera (ashwagandha)*[a]
32	*Zingiber officinalis (adrakh)*

[a]Top four most frequently occurring plant ingredients in commercial polyherbal formulations used in the management of AD.

itors) to reduce inflammatory activity in the brain and antioxidants.[7,11,15] Other areas of research are antiamyloid strategies (e.g., immunization, aggregation inhibitors, secretase inhibitors), transition metal chelators (e.g., clioquinol), lipid-lowering agents, antihypertensives, vitamins, and neurotransmitter receptors.[9]

Studies on herbal materials with AChE inhibitory properties have shown some promise.[28,29] Ayurveda has many formulations and herbomineral drugs discussed below that are used to improve cognitive functions. The precise biochemical mechanism of action of these herbs is not clear. It is likely that antioxidant and anti-inflammatory properties of these herbs may be responsible for their beneficial effect in the treatment of AD.

23.8 Scientific Basis

23.8.1 Nootropic Plants

This findings of experimental studies on Indian medicinal plants with nootropic actions (activating or stimulating mental activity or causing cerebral or intellectual activity) are given below.

23.8.1.1 Pharmacological Studies on Single Herbs

23.8.1.1.1 Bacopa monniera Linn. (Herpestis monniera Linn.) (Brahmi)[30–35]

This plant has been extensively investigated at the Central Drug Research Institute, Lucknow, India, for memory-enhancing effects and is a component of Mentat (commercially marketed polyherbal preparation). Ethanolic extract of *B. monniera* was demonstrated to facilitate acquisition, consolidation, and retention of memory in animal models of the following cognitive functions: (1) active conditioned avoidance response, (2) Sidman's continuous avoidance response, and (3) foot shock-motivated brightness discrimination. Bacosides A and B (Saponins) were identified as active principles. Administration of bacosides attenuated the retrograde amnesia produced by immobilization induced stress, electroconvulsive shock, and scopolamine. Protein kinase activity and protein content of the hippocampus were increased. Improvement was observed in learning capacity and correction of epilepsy-associated abnormal behavior to some extent. Maze learning by albino rats was facilitated and brain glutamic acid and gamma-aminobutyric acid (GABA) concentrations were elevated.

The protective action of *B. monniera* was recently demonstrated against phenytoin-induced cognitive deficit. Phenytoin (25 mg/kg orally for 14 days) adversely affected the passive avoidance task in mice. An extract of this plant (Memory Plus, 40 mg/kg orally for 7 days along with phenytoin in the second week of the 2-week regimen) significantly reversed phenytoin-induced impairment without affecting its anticonvulsant efficacy. The observed cognitive effects of phenytoin and the plant extract were found to be independent of motor stimulation.

23.8.1.1.2 Centella asiatica (Mandookparni, Brahmi)[36]

Aqueous extract of this plant was shown to improve learning and memory in shuttle box, stepdown paradigm, and elevated plus maze in rats. When tested on oxidative stress parameters, it decreased brain levels of malondialdehyde (MDA) with a simultaneous increase in the level of glutathione. The drug also increased catalase levels. As a result, antioxidant mechanism in the cognition-enhancing effect of the drug was suggested.

23.8.1.1.3 Convolvulus pluricaulis Chois (Shankhpushpi)[37]

Ethanolic extract of the drug was made alcohol free and suspended in water to study the effect on brain neurotransmitter content in normal and stressed rats. The drug decreased the acetylcholine (ACh) content of the whole brain homogenate, but markedly increased ACh content in the cortex. The catecholamine and 5-hydroxytryptamine (5-HT) contents were also raised in treated rats. The histamine content was lowered in the whole brain homogenate but raised in the cortex. The changes were more pronounced in rats subjected to swimming stress. These changes suggest tranquilizing action and improvement of mental function.

23.8.1.1.4 Eugenia caryophyllus spl. (Laung)[38]

The aqueous extract of *E. caryophyllus* reduced hydrolysis of ACh by AChE, indicating the presence of water-soluble substances with anti-AChE activity in the plant.

23.8.1.1.5 Glycyrrhiza glabra Linn. (Yastimadhu, Mulethi)[37]

The alcoholic extract of *G. glabra* reduced ACh content in the whole brain but increased it in the cortex.

23.8.1.1.6 Hydrocotyl asiatica Linn. (Syn. Centella asiatica Linn. [Mandookparni])[37]

The effects of this plant are similar to *G. glabra* described above.

23.8.1.1.7 Lawsonia inermis Linn. (Mehndi)[39]

Significant nootropic effect was observed in acetone soluble fraction of petroleum ether extract of leaves on elevated plus maze and passive avoidance paradigms. It affected 5-HT and noradrenaline-mediated behavior in experimental animals.

23.8.1.1.8 Nardostachys jatamansi DC (Jatamansi)[40–42]

This plant has been demonstrated to reduce brain serotonin content, reaction time of trained animals for passage through tunnel in a Columbia obstruction box, and conditioned-avoidance response. It has also impaired biosynthesis and metabolism of 5-HT in rabbit brain. It is a constituent of Mentat, a polyherbal formulation with cognition facilitatory effects.

23.8.1.1.9 Paeonia emodi Wall (Uood Saleb)[43]

This plant is an ingredient of *shimotsu-to,* a traditional Chinese medicine shown to improve spatial-working memory in rats.

23.8.1.1.10 Pongamia pinnata (Karanj)[44]

Petroleum ether extract was tested in experimental models of AD (ibotenic-acid induced lesioning of nuclear basalis magnocellularis). It reversed both the cognitive deficits and reduction in cholinergic markers after 2 weeks of treatment. Reversal of perturbed cholinergic function was suggested as a possible mechanism of action.

23.8.1.1.11 Tinospora cordifolia F.Vill (Giloe, Guduchi)[37]

Ethanolic extract of this plant reduced ACh content in the whole brain but increased it in the cortex.

23.8.1.1.12 Withania somnifera Dunal (Ashwagandha)[45–47]

Active principles (equimolar amounts of sitoindosides VII-X and withoferin A) of *W. somnifera* were investigated in animal model of AD (ibotenic-acid–induced lesioning of nucleus basalis magnocellularis) in rats. The lesions caused marked cognitive deficit as evidenced by (1) severe reduction in learned task, (2) significant decrease in ACh levels in the frontal cortex and hippocampus, (3) reduction in choline acetyl transferase activity, and (4) muscarinic cholinergic binding. The drug (50 mg/kg) significantly reversed these alterations after 2 weeks of treatment.

W. somnifera induced depletion of ACh and catecholamines and increased serotonin and histamine concentrations in the whole brain tissue. It also elicited differential effect on AChE activity in basal forebrain nuclei by producing a slight enhancement in the lateral septum and globus pallidus and a reduction in vertical diagonal band. The changes were accompanied by enhanced M1-muscarinic cholinergic receptor binding in lateral and medium septum and frontal cortex. GABA and benzodiazepine receptor binding and n-methyl-d-aspartate (NMDA) and α-amino 3-hydroxy 5-methyl 4-isoxazole propionic acid (AMPA) glutamate receptor subtypes were not affected after treatment with *W. somnifera* principles, suggesting preferential effect of the drug on events in the cortical and basal forebrain cholinergic signal transduction cascade. The drug induced an increase in cortical muscarinic ACh-receptor capacity. This finding partly explains the nootropic action of the *W. somnifera*.

23.8.1.2 Clinical Studies on Nootropic Plants

The gist of information on clinical studies on Indian medicinal plants for nootropic effects is presented below.

23.8.1.2.1 *Bacopa monniera Linn.* (*Syn. Herpestis monniera Linn. [Brahmi]*)[48–49]

A significant increase in intelligent quotient (IQ) scores was observed after treatment of 110 males aged 10 to 13 years for 9 months with a *suksma* (micro) medicine derived from *B. monniera*. Memory (direct) and arithmatic tests were used. The drug was well tolerated in single (20 to 300 mg) and multiple (100 and 200 mg for 4 weeks) doses in a double-blind placebo-controlled and non-crossover phase I clinical trial in human volunteers.

23.8.1.2.2 *Centella asiatica Linn. (Syn: Hydrocotyle asiatica Linn. [Mandookparni, Brahm mandooki])*[50–52]

Double-blind studies with this herb revealed no change of the height, weight, and intelligence of mentally normal children but showed favorable action in mentally retarded children (free from epilepsy). A significant increase in general ability and behavioral pattern was noted even when the drug was administered only for 12 weeks. Another double-blind study, carried out on 30 mentally retarded children (9 to 13 years old) with an IQ range of 55 to 90, revealed better intelligence scores and psychological and biochemical parameters after treatment with the test drug for 9 months. The Binet test and Senguin Form Board test were used for assessing intelligence and performance of children.

23.8.1.3 Pharmacological and Clinical Studies on Nootropic Plant Formulations

23.8.1.3.1 *Mentat*

The preparation for Mentat (*Himalaya*) was developed at the Central Drug Research Institute, Lucknow, India. The formula (50 to 500 mg/kg) was found to improve the acquisition and retention of passive-avoidance task in a stepdown paradigm in mice. It reversed scopolamine-induced amnesia and attenuated amnesia produced by electroconvulsive shock (ECS) immediately after training. Chronic treatment with ECS for 6 successive days at 24-h intervals disrupted memory consolidation on day 7. Daily administration of Mentat (50 and 100 mg/kg for 6 days) significantly improved memory consolidation in mice. Administration of drug on day 7 also attenuated ECS-induced disruption of memory. Scopolamine-induced delay in transfer latency was reversed on day 1. Physostigmine enhanced the efficacy of Mentat against scopolamine-induced amnesia. When administered in combination with GABA and Aniracetam, the test drug improved learning and memory retrieval. The results suggest nootropic action in naive and amnesic mice and involvement of cholinergic and GABA-ergic modulation as possible mechanisms of action.[41,53]

The drug was shown to augment acquisition and retention of learning in normal rats and in states of cognitive deficits induced by undernutrition, environmental impoverishment, sodium nitrite hypoxia, aluminum, aging, and ECS-induced anterograde and retrograde amnesia. The parameters included active avoidance learning, food motivational behavior (Hebb Willam maze), and avoidance learning during endurance performance (Runimex circular runway).[54–56]

23.8.1.3.2 Trasina (Deys Pharmaceuticals)

Treatment with Trasina for 21 days exhibited significant nootropic effects in two experimental models of AD: (1) intracerebroventricular injection of colchicine (15 μg/rat) and (2) lesioning of nucleus basalis magnocellularis by ibotenic acid (10 μg/rat). The drug improved both memory and cholinergic markers (e.g., ACh concentration, choline acetyl transferase activity) and muscarinic cholinergic receptor binding in frontal cortex and hippocampus of rat brain. Nootropic action was attributed to correction of cholinergic dysfunction.[57]

23.8.1.3.3 Memorin (Phytopharma)

Pretreatment with this drug (200 mg/kg/day) attenuated ECS-induced retrograde amnesia in rats. The method used was a passive-avoidance test in a shuttle box.[57]

23.8.1.3.4 Syrup Shankhpushpi (Baidyanath)

This drug exhibited nootropic action in various experimental models of cognitive function such as active-avoidance learning in young and old rats, passive-avoidance learning in normal and scopolamine-amnesic mice, transfer latency using elevated plus maze in mice, and food and thirst motivational behavior in rats. It caused significant reduction in brain AChE activity but elicited no significant effects on L-glutamate, L-aspartate, and GABA content of whole brain tissue. The maximum tolerated dose was found to be >40 ml/kg orally, indicating it to be quite safe. Nootropic activity appears to be mediated through cholinergic mechanism.[30]

23.8.1.3.5 Saraswatarisht (Baidyanath)

This formulation (20 ml two times/day for 1 year) showed good antiepileptic activity in 25 patients; there was a significant reduction in the frequency and severity of convulsions and even complete absence of fits in some cases. The drug was found to be free from side effects.[58,59]

The drug showed cognition facilitatary effects against various experimental models of learning and memory in rats and mice. The effects were duly noted in normal animals, and no activity was discernible against amnesia induced by scopolamine and ECS. The activity appeared to be mediated through cholinergic mechanisms.[30]

23.8.1.3.6 Vidyarthi Amrit (Maharishi Ayurved)

Vidyarthi amrit exhibited nootropic activity in active-avoidance learning in aged rats, passive-avoidance learning in normal mice, and food and thirst motivational behavior in rats. No activity was discernible on transfer latency and against scopolamine- and ECS-amnesic mice. The drug caused a decrease in AChE and L-glutamate and an increase in

L-aspartate and GABA levels of whole brain tissue. The nootropic effects appear to be mediated through cholinergic mechanisms.[30]

23.8.1.3.7 Dimagh Pushtak Rasayan (Baidyanath)

This drug exhibited nootropic effects in active- and passive-avoidance paradigms in both normal and scopolamine-amnesic animals, transfer latency test, and thirst-motivational behavior. No effects were observed against food motivational behavior in the Hebb William maze, possibly because this test involved a single dose schedule which may not be adequate for effective drug concentrations. At least three of its ingredients, *Centella asiatica, Convolvulus pluricaulis,* and *siddh makardhwaja*, are reported to have nootropic effects. The memory-enhancing effects of the formulation were attributed to cholinergic mechanisms.[30]

23.8.1.3.8 Geriforte (Himalaya)

Clinical psychobiological studies on apparently normal-aged subjects 45 to 50 years were treated for 3 months with the test formulation. Results showed an increasing feeling of well-being, physical efficiency, and improvement in mental functions. The therapy reduced anxiety and helped in better nitrogen retention. The drug appears to be a rational combination of herbal components for arresting rapid onset of mental and physical disability in aged persons. The effects were attributed to its constituent drugs (e.g., *chyavanprasha* [chief ingredient *Emblica officinalis*]), *Bacopa monniera, Withania somnifera,* etc.).[60]

23.8.1.3.9 Combination of Four Plants: Convolvulus pluricaulis, Bacopa monniera, Withania somnifera, and Acorus calamas

The combination exhibited encouraging effects in patients of *unmada* (psychosis).[61]

23.8.1.4 Herbs with Allied Activities

The following is a summary of studies on Indian medicinal plants with properties considered allied to general well-being and nootropic action such as adaptogenic, immunomodulatory, anxiolytic, antioxidant, and antiaging effects.

23.8.1.4.1 Asparagus racemosus Wild (Shatawari)

Aqueous extract exhibited adaptogenic activity as evidenced by protection against a variety of biological, physical, and chemical stressors in experimental animals. It also normalized cisplatin-induced intestinal hypermotility.[62]

23.8.1.4.2 Bacopa monniera Linn. (Brahmi)

With this herb, significant anxiolytic effects in experimental animals have been reported.[63]

23.8.1.4.3 Boerhavia diffusa Linn. (Punarnava)

Milk fortified with this plant extract revealed growth-promoting and hematinic effects in children. The plant did not elicit appreciable effect on body weight, total proteins, and hematological parameters of normal adults (45 to 50 years).[64,65]

23.8.1.4.4 Centella asiatica Linn. (Mandookparni)

Aqueous extract of this plant, which is claimed to be a brain tonic, was given at 25 mg/kg i.p. Results showed decreased spontaneous motor activity and delayed pentylenetetrazol-induced convulsions in mice. The activity was comparable with diazepam (4 mg/kg i.p.). The extract potentiated pentobarbitone-induced sleep but did not affect immobility time in the swimming test. The results suggest an anxiolytic effect but no action on behavioral despair. Another report found antidepressant activity with 50% of ethanolic extract as evidenced by the reduction of immobility time in the forced swimming test. The effect appears to be mediated through D_2 receptor.[66,67]

Results of a double blind trial in 43 normal adults (45 to 50 years old) after 6 months revealed that the drug caused an increase in erythrocyte count, hemoglobin, blood sugar and serum cholesterol levels, vital capacity, and total proteins. It decreased mean blood urea and serum phosphatase concentrations.[65]

23.8.1.4.5 Syrup Shankhpushpi (Chief Ingredient: Convolvulus pluricaulis)

One month treatment with syrup *Shankhpushpi* formulation (10 ml three times/day) elicited beneficial action in 30 cases of anxiety neurosis. The symptoms and levels of plasma cortisol and urinary catecholamines were reduced.[68]

23.8.1.4.6 Embelia ribes (Amla)

The protection of *E. ribes* observed against a variety of stressors (biological, chemical, and physical), indicating adaptogenic action. The drug strengthened the defense against free-radical–induced damage during stress.[62]

23.8.1.4.7 Piper longum Linn. (Pippali)

This plant drug exhibited adaptogenic effects similar to *E. ribes* described above. [62]

23.8.1.4.8 Terminalia Chebula Retz (Harar)

This plant drug exhibited adaptogenic effects similar to *E. ribes* described above.[62]

23.8.1.4.9 Tinospora cordifolia F.Vill (Giloe, Guduchi)

Besides adaptogenic activity against different stressors, *T. cordifolia* normalized phagocytic function irrespective of the direction of change. The protection against stress-induced mucosal damage was lost when macrophage activity was blocked.[62]

23.8.1.4.10 Withania somnifera Dunal (Ashwagandha)

This reputed nootropic plant has been extensively investigated by many workers. It showed antistress, anxiolytic, rejuvenating, anticonvulsant, free-radical scavenging, adaptogenic, and antiaging properties in experimental and clinical studies.[43,46,69–74]

23.8.2 Nootropic Mineral Preparations

Although the majority of the preparations used in Ayurveda as a whole and for memory-enhancing effects are of plant origin, some reports on mineral prepartions are also available. The mineral-origin drugs are used mostly in calcined forms. Ayurvedic physicians use even those metals for therapeutic purposes, which are considered toxic and not used for internal administration in modern medicine (e.g., mercury and arsenic). It is believed that the specialized techniques used during preparation of the oxides (*Bhasmas*) (ash) "purify" the metal and make it therapeutically effective and safe for internal use. These techniques involve (1) incorporation of some herbal juices during the calcination process and (2) repeated calcination and trituration to fine powder forms. The mineral preparations, in contrast to herbal drugs, have not received much attention by researchers. The Department of Medical Elementology and Toxicology of Hamdard University, New Delhi, India, ventured into this neglected field and found encouraging results. Some interesting findings for effects of calcined metal preparations on animal models of learning and memory are summarized below.

23.8.2.1 Siddh Makardhwaja (Mercury)

The preparation helped in total development (physical and mental) of experimental animals. It revealed growth-promoting, memory-improving, and carbohydrate-sparing properties without affecting other central nervous system (CNS) parameters (e.g., pentobarbitone-induced sleeping time, activity index in traction test, activity counts in water wheel, rectal temperature, behavioral despair in forced swimming test, acetic acid-induced writhing episodes, and amphetamine aggregate toxicity) in rats and mice. Facilitation of cognition was shown by marked increase in acquisition, (control = 81.25%, treated = 100%), retention (control = 69.23%, treated = 80%), and learning scores (control = 4.00, treated = 5.26) in the active-avoidance learning test. The drug restored exercise-depleted liver and muscle glycogen concentrations, suggesting antifatigue action. Incorporation of this mineral in the diet (0.01% w/w) of young rat pups (45 to 70 g) for 6 weeks exhibited better growth rate vs. control pups.[74]

23.8.2.2 Swarna Bhasma (Gold)

The preparation (25 mg/kg orally for 7 to 10 days) exhibited a nootropic effect in active- and passive-avoidance learning in rats and mice. It caused significant increase in acquisition, retention, and learning scores in treated rats vs. the control group. The results compared well with panax ginseng tea (350 mg/kg orally for 10 days). Significant reduction in latency to reach shock free-zone and stepdown errors was observed in treated mice. Brain acetyl cholinestrase was significantly decreased in the frontal cortex, hypothalamus, hippocampus, midbrain, cerebellum, brain stem, and corpus striatum after the 10-day treatment in rats. Decreased AChE activity possibly led to increased ACh levels in brain with an improvement in cognitive function. The drug also exhibited glycogen-sparing, adaptogenic, and immunomodulatory activities. The drug showed a wide therapeutic index (effective dose = 25 mg/kg orally, maximum tolerated dose = >2 g/kg orally) and lack of gross behavioral effects, weight loss, or adverse effects on hematological parameters.[75–79]

23.9 Summary and Discussion

The revival of Ayurvedic medicine with special emphasis for research on medicinal plants has received considerable attention in India during the past 4 to 5 decades.[80] Research effort on medicinal plants and nootropic drugs that act on CNS gained momentum during the past 5 to 10 years. This has generated substantial data, giving a rational basis to ancient Ayurvedic remedies for deficits in learning and memory. Experimental and clinical data presented earlier provide support for the use of these herbs for the management of AD. However, further research need to be conducted to better utilize these herbs.

In conventional medicine, the drugs currently approved for the treatment of AD are cholinomimetics, such as tacrine, which has the pharmacologic profile of AChE inhibitors.[12,25,26] Modern drugs used for ameliorating intellectual impairment, confusion, behavioral disorders of senility, mental retardation, and learning problems in children include CNS stimulants and activators such as pyritinol (Encephabol) and nootropic agents such as Piracetam (Cerecetam, neurocetam, Nootropil, Normobarin, and Pirtam). Some of the adverse effects associated with these drugs include anorexia, epigastric distress, nausea, vomiting, headache, fatigue, excitement, restlessness, sleep disturbances, and skin rash. In addition, special care is required if these drugs are used for patients with hepatic, renal, or cardiac diseases. Ayurvedic herbal preparations have not been shown to produce adverse side effects. They offer a safe alternative in the management of AD.

In a recent study, leisure activities such as reading, playing board games, musical instruments, and dancing are associated with a reduced risk of dementia. This is consistent with the Ayurvedic concept of regular physical and mental exercise, and meditation as a part of disease prevention and treatment strategy.[81]

References

1. Dash, B. and Kashyap, L., *Diagnosis and Treatment of Diseases in Ayurveda,* Part 3, Concept Publishing Company, New Delhi, India, 1984, p. 124.
2. Frawley, D., *Ayurvedic Healing,* Motilal Banarsidass Publishers, Delhi, India, 1989, p. 247.
3. Dwivedi, K.K. and Singh, R.H., A clinical study of medhya rasayana therapy in the management of convulsive disorder, *J. Res. Ayurveda Siddha,* 13, 97, 1978.
4. Singh, R.H. and Sinha, B.N., Clinical and pharmacological studies on the effect of indigenous compound Rasayana drug in apparently normal and aged persons, *J. Res. Indian Med. Yoga Homeopathy,* 13, 8, 1978.
5. Singh, R.H. and Sinha, B.N., Further studies on the effect of an indigenous compound Rasayana drug on physical and mental disability in aged persons, *J. Res. Indian Yoga Homeopathy,* 14, 45, 1979.
6. Nakawastase, T.V. and Cummings, J.L., Alzheimers' disease and related dementias in *Cecil Text Book of Medicine*, Goldman, L. and Bennett, J.C., Eds., W.B. Saunders, New York, 2000, chap. 25.
7. Aisen, P.S., Evaluation of selective COX-2 inhibitors for the treatment of Alzheimer's disease, *J. Pain Symptom Manage.*, 23, S35, 2002.
8. Anderson, R.N., Deaths: leading causes for 2000, *Natl. Vital. Stat. Rep.*, 50, 1, 2002.
9. Doraiswamy, P.M., Non-cholinergic strategies for treating and preventing Alzheimer's disease, *CNS Drugs*, 16, 24, 2002.
10. Lemstra, A.W., Eikelenboom, P., and Van Gool, W.A., The cholinergic deficiency syndrome and its therapeutic implications, *Gerontology*, 49, 55, 2003.
11. Pasinetti, G.M., From epidemiology to therapeutic trials with anti-inflammatory drugs in Alzheimer's disease: the role of NSAIDs and cyclooxygenase in beta-amyloidosis and clinical dementia, *J. Alzheimers Dis.*, 4, 435, 2002.
12. Spiegel, R., Rivastigmine: a review of its clinical effectiveness, *Rev. Neurol.*, 35, 859, 2002; Clegg, B.J., Nicholson, T., McIntyre, L., De Broe, S., Gerard, K., and Waugh, N., Clinical and cost-effectiveness of donepezil, rivastigmine, and galantamine for Alzheimer's disease: a systematic review, *Int. J. Technol. Assess Health Care*, 18, 497, 2002.
13. Berrino, F., Western diet and Alzheimer's disease, *Epidemiol. Prev.*, 26, 107, 2002.
14. Lindsay, J., Laurin, D., Verreault, R., Hebert, R., Helliwell, B., Hill, G.B., and McDowell, I., Risk factors for Alzheimer's disease: a prospective analysis from the Canadian Study of Health and Aging, *Am. J. Epidemiol.*, 156, 445, 2002; Aisen, P.S., Anti-inflammatory agents in Alzheimer's disease, *Curr. Neurol. Neurosci. Rep.*, 2, 405, 2002.

15. Rutten, B.P., Steinbusch, H.W., Korr, H., and Schmitz, C., Antioxidants and Alzheimer's disease: from bench to bedside (and back again), *Curr. Opin. Clin. Nutr. Metab. Care,* 5, 645, 2002.
16. Cacabelos, R., Pharmacogenomics for the treatment of dementia, *Ann. Med.*, 34, 357, 2002.
17. Roberts, S.B., Gamma-secretase inhibitors and Alzheimer's disease, *Adv. Drug Deliv. Rev.*, 54, 1579, 2002.
18. Bahr, B.A. and Bendiske, J., The neuropathogenic contributions of lysosomal dysfunction, *J. Neurochem.*, 83, 481, 2002.
19. Gelb, D.J., Measurement of progression in Alzheimer's disease: a clinician perspective, *Stat. Med.*, 19, 1390, 2000.
20. Brekman, I.I. and Dardymov, I.V., New substances of plant origin which increase non-specific resistance, *Ann. Rev. Pharmacol.*, 9, 419, 1969.
21. Hashimotto, K. and Whilemist, C.E., Immunomodulatory effects of therapeutic gold compounds, *Am. Soc. Clin. Invest. Inc.*, 89, 1839, 1992.
22. Tolonen, M., Sarna, S., Westermarck, T., Nordberg, U.R., Halme, M., Tuominen, S.E.J., Keionen, M., and Schrijver, J., Antioxidant supplementation decreases TBA reactants in the serum of the elderly: a double blind clinical trial, in *Metabolism of Minerals and Trace Elements in Human Disease,* Abdulla, M. et al., Eds., Smith-Gordon, Nishimura, India, 1989.
23. Abhang, R.Y., Medhya rasayana: past, present and future, *Deerghayu Int.*, 4, 8, 1987.
24. Anon., *Caraka Samhita*, Shree Gulabkunverba Ayurvedic Society, Jamnagar, India, 5, 490, 1949.
25. Camps, P. and Munoz-Torrer, D., Cholinergic drugs in pharmacotherapy of Alzheimer's disease, *Mini Rev. Med. Chem.*, 2, 11, 2002.
26. Clegg, A., Bryant, J., Nicholson, T., McIntyre, L., De Broe, S., Gerard, K., and Waugh, N., Clinical and cost-effectiveness of donepezil, rivastigmine, and galantamine for Alzheimer's disease: a systematic review, *Int. J. Technol. Assessment Health Care,* 18, 497, Summer 2002.
27. Chatellier, G. and Lacomblez, L., Tacrine (teterahydroaminoacridine; THA) and lecithine in senile dementia of the Alzheimer type: a multicenter trial, *Br. J. Med.*, 300, 495, 1990.
28. Chung, Y.K., Heo, H.J., Kim, E.K., Kim, H.K., Huh, T.L., Lim, Y., Kim, S.K., and Shin, D.H., Inhibitory effect of ursolic acid purified from Origanum majorana L on the acetylcholinesterase, *Mol. Cells,* 137, 43, 2001.
29. Perry, E.K., Pickering, A.T., Wang, W.W., Houghton, P.J., and Perry, N.S., Medicinal plants and Alzheimer's disease: from ethnobotany to phytotherapy, *J. Pharm. Pharmacol.*, 51, 527, 1999.
30. Sivaraman, R., Nootropic Effects of Some Herbal Formulations Available in India, Ph.D. thesis, Department of Medical Elementology and Toxicology, Faculty of Science, Jamia Hamdard, New Delhi, India, 2002.
31. Dhawan, B.N., Centrally acting agents from Indian plants, in *Decade of the Brain India/USA Research on Mental Health and Neuroscience,* Koslow, S.H., Murthy, R.S., and Coelho, G.V., Eds., National Institute of Mental Health, Rockville, MD, 1995.
32. Shukla, B., Khanna, N.K., and Godhwani, J.L., Effect of brahmi rasayan on central nervous system, *J. Ethnopharmacol.,* 21, 65, 1987.
33. Singh, H.K. and Dhawan, B.N., Drugs affecting learning and memory, in *Lectures in Neurobiology,* Tandon, P.N., Bijlani, V., and Wadhwa, S., Eds., Wiley Eastern Ltd., New Delhi, 1992.
34. Vaidya, A.B., The status and scope of Indian medicinal plants acting on the central nervous system, *Indian J. Pharmacol.*, 29, S 340, 1997.
35. Vohora, D., Pal, S.N., and Pillai, K.K., Protection from phenytoin-induced cognitive deficit by *Bacopa monniera*, a reputed Indian nootropic plant, *J. Ethnopharmacol.*, 71, 383, 2000.
36. Veerender Kumar, M.H. and Gupta, Y.K., Effect of different extracts of *Centella asiatica* on cognition and makers of oxidative stress in rats, *J. Ethnopharmacol.,* 79, 253, 2002.
37. Singh, R.H., Sinha, B.N., Sarkar, F.H., and Udupa, K.N., Comparative biochemical studies on the effect of four Medhya Rasayana drugs described by Caraka on some central neurotransmitters in normal and stressed rats, *J. Indian Med. Yoga Homeopathy,* 14, 7, 1979.
38. Akinrimisi, E.D. and Akinwande, A.I., Effect of aqueous extract of *Eugenia caryophyllus* on brain acetylcholine estrase in rats, *West Afr. J. Pharmacol. Drug Res.*, 2, 127, 1975.
39. Iyer, M.R., Pal, S.C., Kasture, V.S., and Kasture, S.B., Effect of *Lawsonia inermis* on memory and behaviour mediated via monoamine oxidase neurotransmitters, *Indian J. Pharmacol.,* 30, 181, 1998.

40. Satyavati, G.V., Gupta, A.K., Tandon, N., and Seth, S.D., *Medicinal Plants of India*, Vol. 2, Indian Council of Medical Research, New Delhi, India, 1987.
41. Kulkarni, S.K. and Verma, A., Evidence for nootropic effect of BR-16A (Mentat): a polyherbal psychotropic preparation in mice, *Indian J. Physiol. Pharmacol.*, 36, 29, 1992.
42. Kulkarni, S.K. and Verma, A., BR-16A (Mentat) a herbal preparation improves learning and memory performance in mice, *Indian Drugs*, 30, 97, 1993.
43. Watanabe, H., Candidates for cognitive enhances extracted from medicinal plants: paenifloarin and tetramethyl pyrazine, *Behav. Brain Res.*, 83, 135, 1997.
44. Dahanukar, S.A., Kulkarni, R.A., and Rege, N.N., Pharmacology of medicinal plants and natural products, *Indian J. Pharmacol.*, 32, S 81, 2000.
45. Bhattacharya, S.K. and Kumar, A., Effect of glycowithanolides from *Withania somnifera* on an animal model of Alzheimers disease and perturbed central cholinergic markers of cognition in rats, *Phytother. Res.*, 9, 110, 1995.
46. Singh, R.H., Malviya, P.C., Sarkar, F.H., and Udupa, K.N., Studies on the psychotropic effect of Indian indigenous drug: ashwagandha (*Withania somnifera* Dural), *J. Res Indian Med. Yoga Homeopathy*, 14, 49, 1979.
47. Schiloers, R., Liermann, A., Bhattacharya, S.K., Kumar, A., Ghoshal, S., and Rich, V., Systemic administration of defined extracts from Withania somnifera (Indian ginseng) and shilajit differentially affects cholinergic but not glutaminergic and gabaergic markers in rat brain, *Neurochem. Int.*, 30, 181, 1997.
48. Abhang, R., Study to evaluate the effect of a micro (suksma) medicine derived from brahmi (*Herpestis monniera*) on students of average intelligence, *J. Res. Ayurveda Siddha*, 14, 10, 1993.
49. Singh, H.K. and Dhawan, B.N., Neuropsycho-pharmacological effects of Ayurvedic nootropic *Bacopa monniera* Linn (Brahmi), *Indian J. Physiol. Pharmacol.*, 20, S359, 1997.
50. Kuppurajan, K., Srinivasan, K., and Janki, K., A double blind study on the effect of Mandookparni on the general mental ability of normal children, *J. Res. Indian Med. Yoga Homeopathy*, 13, 37, 1978.
51. Apparao, M.V.R., Srinivasan, K., and Koteswara Rao, T., The effect of Mandookparni (*Centella asiatica*) on the general mental ability (Medhya) of mentally retarded children, *J. Res. Indian Med.*, 8, 9, 1973.
52. Abhang, R.Y., A study to evaluate the effect of a micro (suksma) medicine from a Medhya Rasayana on intelligence of mentally retarded children using psychological and biochemical parameters, *J. Res. Ayurveda Siddha*, 13, 35, 1992.
53. Kulkarni, S.K. and Verma, A., BR 16-A (Mentat): a herbal preparation improves learning and memory performance in mice, *Probe*, 33, 222, 1994.
54. Faruqi, S., Andrade, C., and Ramteke, S., Herbal pharmacotherapy for the attenuation of electroconvulsive shock-induced anterograde and retrograde amnesic deficits, *Convuls. Ther.*, 11, 241, 1995.
55. Bhardwaj, S.K. and Srivastava, K.K., Effect of a composite Indian herbal preparation CIHP (III) on avoidance learning during endurance performance in rats, *Indian J. Exp. Biol.*, 33, 580, 1995.
56. Handa, S.S. and Bhargava, V.K., Effect of BR 16-A (Mentat) on cognitive deficits in aluminum treated and aged rats, *Indian J. Pharmacol.*, 28, 258, 1997.
57. Dahanukar, S.A., Kulkarni, R.A., and Rege, N.N., Pharmacology of medicinal plants and natural products, *Indian J. Pharmacol.*, 32, S 81, 2000.
58. Singh, R.H. and Murthy, A.R.V., Medhya rasayana therapy in the management of apasmara vis-à-vis epilepsies, *J. Res Educ. Indian Med.*, 8, 13, 1989.
59. Dwivedi, K.K. and Singh, R.H., A clinical study of Medhya Rasayana therapy in the management of convulsive disorders, *J. Res Ayurveda Siddha*, 13, 97, 1992.
60. Singh, R.H. and Sinha, B.N., Clinical and psychobiological studies on the effect of an indigenous compound Rasayana drug on apparently normal aged persons, *J. Res. Indian Med. Yoga Homeopathy*, 13, 8, 1978.
61. Dash, S.C., Tripathi, S.N., and Singh, R.H., Clinical assessment of medhya drugs in the management of psychosis (unmada), *Ancient Sci. Life*, 3, 77, 1983.

62. Rege, N.N., Thatte, U.M., and Dahanukar, A., Adaptogenic properties of six rasayana herbs used in Ayurvedic medicine, *Phytotherapy Res.*, 9, 275, 1998.
63. Singh, R.H., Singh, L., and Sen, S.P., Studies on antianxiety effect of the medhya rasayana drug brahmi (*Bacopa monniera* Linn). II. Experimental studies, *J. Res. Indian Med. Yoga Homeopathy*, 14, 1, 1979.
64. Venkataraghvan, S., Seshadri, C., Sundaresan, T.P., Revathi, R., Rajgopalan, V., and Janki, K., The comparative effect of milk fortified with Ashwagandha and Punarnava in children: a double blind study, *J. Res. Ayurveda Siddha*, 1, 370, 1980.
65. Apparao, M.V.R., Usha, S.P., Rajgopalan, S.S., and Sarangan, R., Six months results of a double-blind trial to study the effect of Mandookparni and Punarnava on normal adults, *J. Res. Indian Med.*, 2, 79, 1967.
66. Diwan, P.V., Karwande, I., and Singh, A.K., Anti-anxiety profile of mandukparni (*Centella asiatica*) in animals, *Fitoterapia*, 57, 253, 1991.
67. Sakina, M.R. and Dandiya, P.C., A psycho-neuro pharmacological profile of *Centella asiatica* extract, *Fitoterapia*, 56, 291, 1990.
68. Singh, R.H. and Mehta, A.K., Studies on psychotropic effect of medhya rasayana drug shankhpushpi (*Convolvulus pluricaulis*). I. Clinical studies, *J. Res. Indian Med. Yoga Homeopathy*, 12, 18, 1977.
69. Singh, R.H. and Malviya, P.C., Studies on the psychotropic effect of an indigenous Rasayana drug Ashwagandha (*Withania somnifera*). I. Clinical studies, *J. Res Indian Med. Yoga Homeopathy*, 13, 15, 1978.
70. Sharma, K. and Dandiya, P.C., *Withania somnifera* Dunal: present status, *Indian Drugs*, 29, 247, 1992.
71. Kulkarni, S.K., Sharma, A., Verma, A., and Ticku, M.K., GABA receptor-mediated anti convulsant action of *Withania somnifera* root extract, *Indian Drugs*, 30, 305, 1993.
72. Kulkarni, S.K., George, B., and Nayar, U., Amygdaloid kindling in rats: protective effect of *Withania somnifera* (ashwagandha) root extract, *Indian Drugs*, 32, 37, 1994.
73. Panda, S. and Kar, A., Evidence of free radical scavenging activity of ashwagandha rood powder in mice, *Indian J. Physiol. Pharmacol.*, 41, 424, 1997.
74. Vohora, S.B., Kim, H.S., Shah, S.A., Khanna, T., and Dandiya, P.C., CNS and adaptogenic effects of Siddh Makardhwaja: an Ayurvedic mercury preparation, in *Trace Elements in Nutrition and Health*, Abdulla, M., Vohora, S.B., and Athar, M., Jamia Hamdard and Wiley Eastern Ltd., New Delhi, India, 1995.
75. Bajaj, S., Neuropsychopharmacological and Immunomodulatory Studies on Gold Preparations Used in Indian Systems of Medicine, Ph.D. thesis (Toxicology), Hamdard University, New Delhi, India, 1999.
76. Bajaj, S., Ahamad, I., Fatima, M., Raisuddin, S., and Vohora, S.B., Immunomadulatory activity of a Unani gold preparation used in Indian system of medicine, *Immunopharmacol. Immunotoxicol.*, 21, 151, 1999.
77. Bajaj, S. and Vohora, S.B., Anticataleptic, anti-anxiety and anti-depressant activity of gold preparation used in Indian systems of medicine, *Indian J. Pharmacol.*, 32, 339, 2000.
78. Bajaj, S., Ahmad, I., Raisuddin, S., and Vohora, S.B., Augmentation of non-specifc immunity in mice by gold preparations used in Indian systems of medicine, *Indian J. Med. Res.*, 113, 192, 2001.
79. Bajaj, S. and Vohora, S.B., Nootropic Effects of Korean Ginseng Tea and Calcined Gold Preparations Used in Ayurveda and Unani-Tibb, International Colloquium on Brain Research, Indian National Science Academy, New Delhi, India, 1999.
80. Vohora, S.B., Research on medicinal plants in India: a review of reviews, *Curare*, 12, 16, 1989.
81. Verghese, J., Lipton, R.B., Katz, M.J., Hall, C.B., Derby, C.A., Kuslansky, G., Ambrose, A.F., Sliwinski, M., and Buschke, H., Leisure activities and the risk of dementia in the elderly, *N. Engl. J. Med.*, 348, 2508, 2003.

24

Epilepsy

Heena A. Bhatt, Nithya J. Gogtay, Sudeshna S. Dalvi, and Nilima A. Kshirsagar

CONTENTS

24.1 Introduction

Epilepsy is one of the most common neurological disorders and afflicts more than 50 million people worldwide.[1] Data from the World Health Organization (WHO) suggest that as many as 1 in 20 people at some point in their lives have an epileptic seizure and that at least 1 in 200 people have epilepsy.[2] Over four fifths of the 50 million people with epilepsy are thought to be in developing countries, and 90% of these people do not receive appropriate treatment.[3] In India, it was estimated that by the end of the year 2001, the number of patients afflicted with epilepsy would be 5.5 million and the number of new cases each year would be close to half a million.[4] In India, over 70% of the population is rural, whereas 70% of the medical manpower, and nearly 100% of neurologists, are urban based.[5]

Facilities for neurological investigations such as the computered tomography (CT) scan, magnetic resonance imaging (MRI), and electroencephalogram (EEG), as well as most first-line and second-line antiepileptic drugs, are beyond the reach of a vast majority of patients. Against this backdrop, the Ayurvedic management of epilepsy, which is sometimes the only form of treatment available to the rural population, assumes great importance. Epilepsy was first documented in the ancient Ayurvedic literature as *apasmaara* in

0-8493-1366-X/04/$0.00+$1.50

Sanskrit. This review provides a comparative study of modern and Ayurvedic medicine in hopes of providing the scientific basis for the use of Ayurvedic therapies in epilepsy. In addition, our own experiences in the management of epilepsy with the use of therapeutic drug monitoring, and the identification of interactions of allopathic and Ayurvedic antiepileptic drugs are also discussed.

24.2 Definition

Apasmaara, or epilepsy, in Ayurveda has been described as one of the earliest eight diseases known (diagnosed) and can be controlled only with medical therapies that can sometimes be incurable and remain uncontrolled.[6] The parallels can be found in allopathic medicine where, despite the best available treatment, 10 to 12% of the patients still have uncontrolled seizures.[7] Epilepsy as per Ayurveda is defined as the transient derangement of memory, intelligence, and the mind, resulting in a temporary blackout of vision, loathsome activities, and unconsciousness. *Vagbhata* defines it as loss or destruction (*apaya*) of memory (*smriti*).[8] Modern medicine defines a seizure as a transient alteration of behavior due to the disordered, synchronous, and rhythmic firing of populations of neurons. Epilepsy per se is defined as a disorder of brain function characterized by the periodic and unpredictable occurrence of seizures.[7] Whereas the Ayurvedic definition describes the effect, the modern definition describes the cause of epilepsy.

24.3 Clinical Description

The clinical description as mentioned in Ayurvedic texts is classified as prodromal signs and symptoms (*purvarupa*) and clinical manifestations (*rupa*). The prodromal signs and symptoms include raising of eyebrows, frequent abnormal movements of eyes, hearing of sounds not perceived by others, excessive oozing of saliva and nasal mucus, aversion to food, anorexia, indigestion, distension of abdomen, debility, body ache, transient blackout, giddiness, profuse sweating, increased thirst, fainting, hallucinations, delusions, falling, aura, and insomnia.[6] This description is very similar to the description in modern medicine of generalized tonic clonic (GTC) seizures. These seizures are characterized by an abrupt onset, sometimes with premonitory symptoms, loud cry, excessive salivation, postictal unresponsiveness, headache, muscle ache, fatigue, and an increase in heart rate and pupillary size.[9] The loss of memory as described by *Vagbhata* is similar to the description of absence seizures, which are characterized by loss of consciousness for a longer duration and are less abrupt in onset and cessation.

In Ayurveda, epilepsy is divided into four types according to the dominant *dosa* involved in the disease pathogenesis: *vataja, pittaja, kaphaja,* and *sannipataja*; signs and symptoms manifest accordingly. The *vataja* type involves *vata* as the dominating *dosa* and is characterized by having frequent fits; regaining consciousness in the shortest time interval, bulging eyes, excessive crying, frothing at the mouth, irregularly contracted fingers, reddish, rough, and blackish nails, eyes, face, and skin, hallucinations, trembling, and visions of unstable, coarse, and rough objects. *Pitta* is the leading *dosa* in *pittaja* type with distinctive features of regaining consciousness in shorter periods, scratching the ground, greenish-yellowish and coppery nails, eyes, face, and skin, and visions of bloody, agitated, irritated, frightful, and burning objects. The *kaphaja* type denotes *kapha dosa* as the principal *dosa* including features such as delayed fits, delayed recovery, increased frothing at mouth, white nails, eyes, face, and skin, and visions of white, heavy, unctuous, smooth objects. *Sannipataja* means all the three *dosas* are in conjunction with each other. It is their simultaneous vitiation that gives rise to the combination of signs and symptoms.

Vataja and *kaphaja* types match the description of GTC seizures, *pittaja* matches complex partial seizures, and *sannipataja* matches the characteristics of a mixed-seizure profile.

24.4 Etiology (*Vyaadhi hetu*)

As per the classical texts, the basic etiology is threefold for epilepsy. Endogenous factors (*nija*) include genetic, congenital, constitutional (*prakriti*), enzymatic disturbance (*agni vikruti*), and idiopathic. Exogenous factors (*agantuka*) include habitual intake of unwholesome and unhygienic foods and drinks that have mutually contradictory properties (*apathya aahar*), especially those with properties similar to *vata dosa* causing its aggravation and trauma; this aggravation is due to worms (*krimijanya*) and environmental and idiopathic factors. Psychological trigger factors (*manasika*) include excessive worry, grief, fear, passion, anger, anxiety, attachment, and excitement. Modern medicine describes the etiology of epilepsy in a similar manner while giving an agewise classification of the causes. In neonates, genetic disorders, metabolic disturbances, and acute central nervous system (CNS) infection are the common causes. Infants and children have genetic disorders, febrile seizures, traumas, and CNS infections as common causes. Etiology for adults includes trauma, infection, tumor, and metabolic disorders in the case of older adults.[9] The relationship between the mind and the somatic response is well established.[10]

24.5 Pathogenesis

Of the three *dosas*, *vata* is the rudimentary element responsible for all the beneficial and harmful effects in the body in its normal and abnormal states, respectively, as mentioned in the authentic text, *Charak Samhita*. In epilepsy, *vata* is predominately vitiated and is the fundamental cause in the pathology of the disease. Neurological disorders, as understood in Ayurveda, are considered to be due to imbalance of *vata*.[11]

All the three etiological factors contribute in the accumulation and vitiation of the psychosomatic *dosa*, specifically *vata* affecting consciousness and all the sense organs. After it is aggravated, the *dosa* spreads throughout the body and through the nerves (*dhamanis*), leading to a manifestation of the epileptic episode. The agitated *vata dosa* abruptly proceeds through the nerves of the body, shaking it in a quick succession (shaking jerks) called "*akshepaka*," which means convulsion.[12] Another term for this condition is *apatanaka* where the patient falls on the ground without spasm at intervals that could be correlated with absence-seizure type of epilepsy.

According to modern medicine, epilepsy results from a focus of hyperexcitable neurons in the cortex. During seizures, the permeability of the cytoplasmic membrane of the neurons changes. This results in increased levels of intracellular calcium and extracellular potassium, which contributes to overall excitability of the epileptic neuronal aggregate. The neurons become susceptible to hypoglycemia, hyponatremia, hypocalcemia, sleep deprivation, and photic stimulation.[7,9] An epileptic seizure has two phases: initiation phase and seizure propagation phase. The initiation phase is characterized by two concurrent events: high frequency bursts of action potentials and hypersynchronization. In epileptogenesis, a normal neuronal network transforms into one that is chronically hyperexcitable. Ayurveda also has the concept of seizure propagation where the *vata dosa* spreads rapidly throughout the body.

24.6 Clinical Examination and Diagnosis

Following the principles of an Ayurvedic diagnosis, a comprehensive examination of the patient (*rogi pariksha*) precedes the disease diagnosis (*roga pariksha*). As in the modern approach of history taking, Ayurveda also emphasizes on the detailed history of the patient as well as features of the case definition of the disease. The type of epilepsy is diagnosed as explained under clinical description. Today, even Ayurvedic physicians establish their diagnosis utilizing modern techniques such as the EEG, CT scan, and MRI. As per Brodie,[13] the choice of treatment in newly diagnosed epilepsy should take into consideration the patient's age, general health, coexisting disabilities, concomitant medication, and lifestyle that is consistent with the Ayurvedic principles of treatment.

24.7 Clinical Course and Prognosis

According to Ayurveda, because epilepsy arises from the aggravation of the *dosas* of the body and mind together and is localized in an important vital organ (*mahamarma*), the brain (*shiromarma*), it is difficult to treat and cure. Sannipatika-type epilepsy, where all three *dosas* are vitiated, is incurable. Chronic epilepsy and the presence of concomitant diseases compound the problem. The case is worsened if the underlying *dosa* and the constitution (*prakriti*) of the patient are similar. For example, if the patient is of *vata pitta* constitution, his or her epilepsy is more difficult to treat than that patient with a different constitution.[6] Modern medicine determines the prognosis of epilepsy by the epilepsy syndrome type; these are classified into four groups: excellent, good, uncertain, and poor prognosis.[14] Interestingly, the terms are strikingly similar to the Ayurvedic concept of prognosis terms of *sukhsadhya, kashtasadhya, yapya,* and *pratyakheya,* respectively.

24.8 Management

All the three streams of Ayurvedic therapy are used in treatment of epilepsy: divine therapy (*deva vyapashraya*), rational therapy (*yukti vyapashraya*), and psychotherapy (*satvavajaya*). Divine therapy is often practiced with the principles of astrology, stones, religious scriptures, and auspicious rites. Rational therapy mainly includes purification and evacuatory (*samshodhana and panchakarma*) and curative and pacificatory (*samshamana*) with diet, drug, and lifestyle modification followed by restorative therapy (*rasayana*). Psychotherapy is practiced by incorporating the philosophy of assurance therapy (*aashvasana*) and the substitute of passions from negative to positive. Psychoneuroimmunology is a well-known concept in modern medicine where interaction between the brain and immune system is studied and used to treat patients. Consulting to produce positive emotions is an important aspect of the therapy.[15] The potential for behavioral interventions to affect psychological adaptations and the course of immune-related diseases should be investigated. Physicians should first restore the activities of the heart, mind, and channels (*srotas*) occluded by the *dosa* by using *samshodhana chikitsa. Vataja* should be treated with enema therapy (*basti*), *pittaja* with purgation therapy (*virechana*), and *kaphaja* with emesis therapy (*vamana*). This is followed by medicinal recipes. *Samshamana* therapy does not work well if purification is not made a priority.[6] A study by Nagashayana et al.[16] establishes the necessity of *panchakarma* therapy in Ayurveda medication before palliative therapy.

Primary therapy described in epilepsy is oleation (*snehana*) where *narayan tail* is commonly used followed by fomentation (*swedana*). These are also the preparatory measures for the *panchakarma* described in Chapter 4. Keeping in mind the particular patient, a physician may use emesis therapy in epilepsy where drugs are suitably prepared; a common vehicle is honey and rock salt followed by a postemesis regimen. Nasal insufflation (*nasya*) is also an important treatment wherein herbal powders and medicated oils are administered in the nostrils as per the case; *vacha* powder and oil, *anu tail, panchendriya vardhan tail,* and fresh juice of *nirgundi* are commonly used formulations.[17] *Shirodhara* is another part of the treatment (*shiro* = head and *dhara* = slow uniform dripping of a liquid substance). This is basically the pacificatory therapy wherein liquid medicaments like medicated oil, *ghrita* (clarified butter made out of cow's milk), decoctions of various suitable herbs, and buttermilk are allowed to trickle slowly on the forehead of the patient in a supine posture.

Formulations used in the treatment are as follows:

1. *Brahmi ghruta* containing *vacha, brahmi, kushtha, shankhpushpi*, and *ghruta*
2. *Kushmanda ghruta* made by cooking *ghruta* with 18 times its quantity of *kushmanda* juice and paste of *yashtimadhu*
3. *Kalyanaka churna* containing 17 herbs
4. *Sarasvata churna* containing 12 ingredients having *vacha* as the main constituent

The treatment of chronic epilepsy includes garlic with oil, *brahmi* juice with honey or *vacha* powder with honey, and *shatavari* with milk.

Strong emetics cannot be given in an acute attack of epilepsy but could be beneficial after the patient is stable and suitable to receive the therapy following the guidelines of authentic texts. In the current practice, Ayurvedic physicians use conventional medicines in the acute phase and subsequently *panchakarma* therapy followed by *rasayana* therapy to get the optimum benefit for the patient. It is shown that the blood histamine level decreased from 0.9 to 0.37 μg/ml by *vamana,* and the same is emitted in vomitus. This indicates elimination of toxic materials (*sukshma malas*) from the cellular level.[18]

The management of elderly patients is also an important issue.[19] The elderly may have many disorders, take multiple concomitant medications, and have different metabolic features; they are also more sensitive to the adverse effects of drugs. The incidence of epilepsy in the elderly is rising; an ideal anticonvulsant for use in an elderly patient in modern medicine is not currently available.[20] Furthermore, febrile seizures are the most common convulsive events in childhood, occurring in 2 to 5% of children. Approximately 20 to 30% of these children may have recurrence during a subsequent febrile infection. These could be nonepileptic. Because the side effects of the antiepileptic drugs outweigh their benefits, their continuous use is no longer recommended.[21] In both these circumstances, Ayurveda as an individualized therapy could be of great value.

The dos and don'ts (*pathyapathya*) for an epileptic patient have been mentioned in classical texts. The beneficial regime (*pathya*) includes a hot-water shower, consuming an ample amount of clarified butter (*ghruta*) as per the digestive capacity, massaging the soles in the evenings with *narayan tail* followed by hot water, fomentation, and living in a pleasant atmosphere. Furthermore, the patient should never go out alone and never be around a lake or fireplace or ride a horse. Patients should not be told any good or bad news suddenly so that they get emotionally disturbed. Products and regimes causing aggravation of *vata dosa* should be strictly avoided. The parallels in allopathy can be seen in the use of prophylactic therapy, a ketogenic diet, and mono- and polytherapy based on an individual patient's response.

24.9 Cost of Epilepsy Management

The costs of Ayurvedic medicines and conventional therapy for epilepsy are more or less similar in India contrary to the West.[22] However, in epilepsy treatment due to milder and fewer adverse effects and toxicities than modern medicine, the ultimate expenses would be certainly less than the conventional therapy. In many countries the vast majority of sufferers remain untreated.[23] The use of Ayurvedic therapies could help solve this problem worldwide. The Ayurvedic formulations used in the treatment of epilepsy available in the Indian market are given in Table 24.1[24] and the conventional medicines are given in Table 24.2.[25]

24.10 Scientific Basis

Conventional drugs for epilepsy should be further investigated for a safe and effective drug because none is available at this time. Carbamazepine treatment has potential risks that should be weighed against its benefits before initiating the therapy.[26] Weight gain in patients on antiepileptic drugs disturbs the general health. It causes cosmetic adverse effects and can have serious psychological effects that may lead to withdrawal of the drug.[27] Hepatotoxicity and teratogenecity of antiepileptic drugs like valproate are rare, but severe adverse effects have been reported.[28] Hepatoprotective Ayurvedic therapies may be used as an adjuvant to protect from hepatotoxicity of conventional drugs. All conventional antiepileptic drugs may provoke positive or negative psychiatric reactions in individual patients, and these reactions depend on the strength of the drugs and genetic and biographic psychiatric predisposition of the patient.[29] These adverse side effects can be prevented using Ayurvedic therapies where the concept of *prakriti* plays a vital role in the treatment.

Although they provide a scientific basis with modern parameters for Ayurvedic antiepileptic drugs, the majority of the herbs are investigated only in animal models. Rats and

TABLE 24.1

Ayurvedic Medicines for Epilepsy Available in the Indian Market

Formulation	Dose	Manufacturers[a]	Ref.[b]
Asvagandhadyarishta	12–24 ml twice/day	2–6, 8–10, 13	BR
Bala tail	For *snehana* and *abhyanga* (local application)	4, 9, 10	AH
Brahmi ghruta	12 g/day	3, 6, 7, 9, 10, 12, 13	AH
Chandanadi tail	For *snehana* and *abhyanga* (local application)	3, 4, 9–11, 13	YR
Chaturmukha rasa	125 mg twice/day	2, 6, 13	BR
Haratala bhasma	125–250 mg/day	2, 6	AP
Kalyanaka ghruta	12 g/day	4, 9–11	AH
Kumaryasava	12–24 ml twice/day	2, 4–6, 8–10, 13	YR
Mahakalyanaka ghruta	12 g /day	9, 10	AH
Mahamrutyunjaya rasa	125 mg twice/day	2, 3, 6, 9	ASS
Rajata bhasma	125 mg twice/day	2, 7, 8, 11, 13	Rasamrita
Saarasvatarishta	12–24 ml twice/day	2–6, 8–11, 13	BR
Sarpagandha vati	2–3 pills twice/day	2, 6, 11, 13	ASS
Svarna bhasma	15.5–62.5 mg/day	6, 7, 9, 11, 13	Rasamrita
Svarnamakshika bhasma	125–250 mg/day	2, 6–8	RSS
Vaatakulantaka rasa	125–250 mg/day	3, 6, 8, 12	BR
Yogendra rasa	125–250 mg/day	6–8, 11	BR

[a] Numbers denote the manufacturer in the Table. (1) Arya Vaidya Sala, Kottakkal, 676 503, Kerala; (2) Dabur Research Foundation, Ghaziabad, 201 010, Uttar Pradesh; (3) IMIS Pharmaceuticals Pvt. Ltd., Dubagunta nivas, Kari Marx Road, Vijayawada, 520 002; (4) Kerala Ayurveda Pharmacy Ltd., Athani Post Office, 683 585, Aluva, Kerala; (5) Sandu Brothers Pvt. ltd., Sandu Nagar, DK Sandu Marg, Chembur, Mumbai, 400 071; (6) Shree Baidyanath Ayurveda Bhawan Pvt. Ltd., Bamgani, Gopalgunj, M.P.; (7) Shree Bhuvaneshwari, Aushadhashhram, Gondal, 360 311, Gujarat; (8) Shree Dhootapapeshwar Ltd., 135, Nanubhai Deasai Road, Khetwadi, Mumbai, 400 004; (9) The Arya Vaidya Pharmacy (Coimbatore) Ltd., 326, Perumal Koli Street, Ramanathapuram, Coimbatore, 641 045; (10) Vaidyaratnam Oushadhasala, Ollur, Thaikkattussery, Thrissur, 680 322; (11) Venkateswara Ayurveda Nilayam Pvt. Ltd., Chintalru, 533 232 A.P.; (12) Vyas Pharmaceuticals, 98-C, Sanver Road, Sector-E, Indore; (13) Zandu Pharmaceutical Works Ltd., 70 Gokhale Road (South), Dadar, Mumbai, 400 025.

[b] BR = *Bhaishajya ratnavali*; AH = *Ashtang hridiya*; YR = *Yoga ratnakar*; RSS = *Rasendra sara sangraha*; AP = Ayurveda *prakash*; ASS = Ayurveda *sara sangraha*.

mice are subjected to kindling, which involves periodic administration of low-intensity electrical stimuli. Systemic administration of convulsant chemical agents, such as pentylenetetrazole and pilocarpine, are also used for animal models to study the antiepileptic activity of the drugs.

In one study, the first ultrastructural evidence of neuroprotective properties in *Semecarpus anacardium* and *Withania somnifera* has been reported.[30] Today's molecular pharmacology has made it possible to understand the mechanism of the action of Ayurvedic drugs. *Ashwagandha* (*W. somnifera*) is gamma-aminobutyric acid-A (GABA-A) receptor agonist, and *katuka* (*P. kurroa*) has antioxidant action equal to alfa-tocopherol, which has an effect on glutathion metabolism in the liver and brain.[31] It is believed to maintain the levels of cellular endogenous antioxidants in liver and brain. Subacute toxicity studies of drugs like *W. somnifera* did not reveal any toxicity.[32] A methanolic extract of *W. somnifera* root contains an ingredient that has a GABA-mimetic activity.[33]

A clinical trial of rejuvenating drugs for the nervous system (*medhya rasayana*) on epilepsy suggested that these medicines reduce the frequency, duration, and severity of

TABLE 24.2

Allopathic Antiepileptic Drugs

Generic Name	Dose (mg/day)
Phenytoin sodium (100 mg)	100–600
Carbamazepine (200 mg)	200–1200
Phenobarbitone (30 mg)	30–210
Sodium valproate (200 mg)	600–2500
Lamotrigine (25 mg)	25–150
Primidone (250 mg)	125–500
Oxcarbazepine (300 mg)	600–1200
Topiramate (25 mg)	25–800

seizures and have not shown any side effects.[34] *Brahmi rasayan*, an Ayurvedic preparation, was studied in mice and rats for its effects on the CNS at oral doses ranging between 1 and 30 g/kg. The study suggests an involvement of the GABA-ergic system in the mediation of the CNS effects of *brahmi rasayan*.[35] Piperine, an active alkaloid of *Piper longum* and *Piper nigrum*, exerted a significant protection against tertbutyl hydroperoxide and carbon tetrachloride hepatotoxicity by reducing both *in vitro* and *in vivo* lipid peroxidation, reducing enzymatic leakage of glutamate pyruvate transaminase (GPT) and alkaline phosphatase (AP), and preventing the depletion of reduced glutathione (GSH) and total thiols in the intoxicated mice.[36] Piperine and its derivatives are effective anticonvulsant drugs that antagonize convulsions induced by physical and chemical methods. They also have sedative, tranquilizing, and muscle-relaxing effects.[37]

The effects of piperine on convulsions induced in mice by agonists at different excitatory amino acid receptor subtypes were studied. Piperine significantly blocked convulsions induced by intracerebroventricular injection of threshold doses of kinate.[38] Toxicity evaluation of potassium embelate from *Embelia ribes* Burm. did not indicate adverse effects.[39] Vohora et al.[40] screened the ethanol extract of *Acorus calamus* rhizomes for CNS effects and found that it exhibited a large number of actions similar to alpha-asarone (an active principle of *A. calamus*). The effect of acute and subchronic administration of an alcoholic extract of *Nardostachys jatamansi* roots on norepinephrine (NE), dopamine (DA), serotonin (5-HT), and GABA were studied in male albino Wistar rats. A 15-day treatment resulted in a significant increase in the levels of NE, DA, 5-HT, and GABA, which indicates that the extract causes an overall increase in the levels of central monoamines and inhibitory amino acids.[41]

The anticonvulsant activity of *Myristica fragrance* was studied against seizures induced by maximum electric shock (MES), pentylene tetrazole (PTZ), lithium sulphate-pilocarpine nitrate (Li-pilo), and picrotoxin. Results showed that *M. fragrans* inhibited seizures induced by MES, PTZ, and Li-pilo, but not by picrotoxin.[42] An animal study with *Sesbania grandiflora* (*Agastya*) showed a wide spectrum of anticonvulsant profile and anxiolytic activity.[43] *Brahmi rasayan* offered a graded protection against audiogenic seizures in mice and antagonized the mescaline-scratch response in mice, indicating its tranquilizing properties.[44]

The therapeutic efficacy of an Ayurvedic formulation is due to actions of various components of the plant and their interactions. Studies on the efficacy of the whole plant cannot be confirmed by fragmented research using the plant extracts or isolated phytochemicals.

24.11 Drug Interactions in Epilepsy Management

In India, Ayurvedic medicines have been used for thousands of years, and adverse drug reactions are also fewer in frequency and severity.[45,46] These facts lead to the concomitant use of both Ayurvedic and modern medicine by the patient without the physician's knowledge. This can ultimately lead to drug interactions, which could be useful or harmful for the patient. At our therapeutic drug-monitoring clinic, we observed two patients who had well-controlled seizures who presented with sudden loss of seizure control. A detailed history taking revealed that they had started taking *shankhapushpi,* a purported memory enhancer. Animal studies with rats were carried out with single and multiple doses of the two drugs given alone and in combination. It was seen that on chronic administration, both the antiepileptic effect and plasma levels of phenytoin were reduced by *shankhapushpi.* Single-dose administration of the drugs did not lead to any change in phenytoin levels but decreased its antiepileptic effect. The interaction was found to be pharmacokinetic and pharmacodynamic.[47,48]

Another marketed memory enhancer, Mentat, has been shown to increase phenytoin levels in rabbits.[49] Likewise, studies on the possible interactions between traditional Chinese medicines and antiepileptic drugs are in progress.[50] Honey, a substance widely used as a good vehicle for a given Ayurvedic medicine, has shown to decrease the bioavailability of carbamazepine.[51]

24.12 The Future

Instead of using single-drug or various formulations mentioned in the authentic texts, the principle of threefold therapy should be validated where yoga can be practiced under divine therapy. Several parameters have been proposed to monitor the level of *tridosa,* where *vata* can be monitored in terms of membrane-bound signal transduction.[52] With reference to epilepsy, a *vata*-dominant disease, such a hypothesis should be validated. Allopathic and Ayurvedic practitioners and researchers should also plan effective healthcare delivery systems for epilepsy to improve the overall quality of life. Traditional systems of medicine like Ayurveda in India are here to stay. It is also inevitable that they will be used concomitantly with the allopathic system of medicine in the years to come. The worldwide herbal medicine market has grown by leaps and bounds. In the light of this, an understanding of the scientific basis of Ayurvedic therapies based on systematic studies of principles and practices and using current scientific principles and technology would certainly help contribute toward better patient care.

References

1. Porter, R.J., Therapy of epilepsy, *Curr. Opinions Neurol. Neurosurg.*, 1, 206, 1988.
2. Shorvon, S.D., Epidemiology, classification, natural history and genetics of epilepsy, *Lancet*, 366, 93, 1990.

3. Scott, R.A., Lhatoo, S.D., and Sander, J.W.A.S., The treatment of epilepsy in developing countries: where do we go from here?, *Bull. World Health Org.*, 79, 344, 2001.
4. Sridharan, R. and Murthy, B.N., Prevalence and pattern of epilepsy in India, *Epilepsia*, 40, 631, 1999.
5. Mani, K.S. et al., Epilepsy control with Phenobarbital or phenytoin in rural south India — the Yelandur study, *Lancet*, 357, 1316, 2001.
6. Sharma, R.K. and Dash, B., *Charaka Samhita*, 6th ed., Chaukhamba Sanskrit studies, Varanasi, India, 1999.
7. McNamara, J.O., Drugs effective in the therapy of the Epilepsies, in *Goodman & Gilman's The Pharmacological Basis of Therapeutics*, 10th ed., McGraw-Hill Medical Publishing Division, New York, 2001, p. 521.
8. Shrikanthamurthy, K.R., *Ashtanga Samgraha of Vagbhata*, 5th ed., Vol. 1, Chaukhambha Orientalia, Varanasi, India, 2002.
9. Lowenstein, D.H., Seizures and epilepsy, in *Harrison's Principles of Internal Medicine*, 15th ed.,Vol. 2, McGraw-Hill Medical Publishing Division, New York, 2001, p. 2354.
10. Singh, N.B. and Singh, R.K.L., Mental health: the journey ahead, *J. Med. Sci.*, 16, 1, 2002.
11. Gourie-Devi, M. and Venkataram, B.S., Concept of disorders of muscles in Indian medical treatise — relevance to modern mycology, *Neurol. India*, 31, 13, 1983.
12. Bhishagaratna, K.K., *Sushruta Samhita*, 1st ed., Vol. 1, Chowkhamba Sanskrit series Office, Varanasi, India, 1998.
13. Brodie, M.J., Monostars: an aid to choosing an antiepileptic drug as monotherapy, *Epilepsia*, 40, S17, 1999.
14. Mukherjee, A. and Chakravarty, A., Prognosis of Epilepsy, *Neurosci. Today*, 5, 82, 2001.
15. Reilly, D. and Harrison, T., Creative consulting: psychoneuroimmunology, the mind body, *Student Br. Med. J.*, 18, 312, 2002.
16. Nagashayana, N. et al., Association of L-DOPA with recovery following Ayurveda medication in Parkinson's disease, *J. Neurosci.*, 176, 124, 2000.
17. Srikanthamurthy, K.R., *Bhavprakash of Bhavmishra*, 1st ed., Krishnadas Academy, Varanasi, India, 1998.
18. Sachdev, K. et al., Recent advancement in *snehana, svedana* and *vamana* therapy with special reference to experimental study, in *The Holistic Principles of Ayurvedic Medicine*, 1st ed., Chaukhamba Sanskrit Pratishthan, Varanasi, India, 1998.
19. Rowan, J., Management of seizures in the elderly, *Pharmacotherapy*, 20, 178S, 2000.
20. Arroyo, S. and Kramer, G., Treating epilepsy in the elderly: safety consideration, *Drug Safety*, 24, 991, 2001.
21. Rantala, H., Tarkka, R., and Uhari, M., Preventive treatment for recurrent febrile seizures, *Ann. Med.*, 32, 177, 2000.
22. Chandrashekara, S., Anilkumar, T., and Jamuna, S., Complementary and alternative drug therapy in arthritis, *J. Assn. Physicians India*, 50, 225, 2002.
23. Mental and neurological disorders WHO fact sheet No. 265, Dec. 2001, *Indian J. Med. Sci.*, 56, 26, 2002.
24. Nayak, B., *Ayurmedline*, Ayurmedline, Bangalore, India, Jan–June 2001.
25. Malik, S., *Indian Drug Review*, Mediworld Publication Pvt. Ltd., New Delhi, India, May–June 2002.
26. Ramadasan, P., Chaudhary, S., Vaishampayne, S., and John, T.R., Stevens-Jhonson Syndrome due to Carbamazepine, *J. Assoc. Physicians India*, 48, 742, 2000.
27. Jallon, P. and Picard, F., Bodywight gain and anticonvulsants: a comparitive review, *Drug Safety*, 24, 969, 2001.
28. Bialer, M., Pharmacokinetic considerations in the design of better and safer new antiepileptic drugs, *J. Controlled Release*, 62, 187, 1999.
29. Schmitz, B., Psychiatric syndromes related to antiepileptic drugs, *Epilepsia*, 40, S65, 1999.
30. Shukla, S.D., Jain, S., Sharma, K., and Bhatnagar, M., Stress induced neuron degeneration and protective effects of *Semecarpus anacardium* Linn. and *Withania somnifera* Dunn. in hippocampus of albino rats: an ultrastructural study, *Indian J. Exp. Biol.*, 38, 1007, 2000.

31. Lele, R.D., Ayurveda (Ancient Indian system of medicine) and modern molecular medicine, *J. Assn. Physicians India*, 47, 625, 1999.
32. Aphale, A.A. et al., Subaute toxicity study of the combination of ginseng (Panax ginseng) and Ashwagandha (Withania somnifera) in rats: a safety assessment, *Indian J. Physiol. Pharmacol.*, 42, 299, 1998.
33. Mehta, A.K. et al., Pharmacological effects of *Withania somnifera* root extract on GABAA receptor complex, *Indian J. Med. Res.*, 94, 312, 1991.
34. Dwivedi, K.K. and Singh, R.H., Clinical trial of *medhya rasayana* drugs in apasmaara, in *The Holistic Principles of Ayurvedic Medicine*, 1st ed., Chaukhamba Sanskrit Pratishthan, Varanasi, India, 1998.
35. Shukia, B., Khanna, N.K., and Godhwani, J.L., Effect of *Brahmi rasayan* on the central nervous system, *J. Ethnopharmacol.*, 21, 65, 1987.
36. Koul, I.B. and Kapil, A., Evaluation of the liver protective potential of piperine, an active principle of black and long peppers, *Planta Medica*, 59, 413, 1993.
37. Pei, Y.Q., A review of pharmacology and clinical use of piperine and its derivatives, *Epilepsia*, 24, 177, 1983.
38. Hooge, R.D. et al., Anticonvulsant activity of piperine on seizures induced by excitatory amino acid receptor agonists, *Arzneim.-Forsch./Drug Res.*, 46, 557, 1996.
39. Johri, R.K. et al., Toxicity studies with potassium embelate, a new analgesic compound, *Indian J. Exp. Biol.*, 28, 213, 1990.
40. Vohora, S.B., Shah, S.A., and Dandiya, P.C., Central nervous system studies on an ethanol extract of *Acorus calamus* rhizomes, *J. Ethnopharmacol.*, 28, 53, 1990.
41. Prabhu, V., Karanth, K.S., and Rao, A., Effects of *Nardostachys jatamansi* on biogenic amines and inhibitory aminoacids in the rat brain, *Planta Medica*, 60, 114, 1994.
42. Sonavane, G.S., Palekar, R.C., Kasture, V.S., and Kasture, S.B., Anticonvulsant and behavioral actions of *Myristica fragrans* seeds, *Indian J. Pharmacol.*, 34, 332, 2002
43. Kasture, V.S., Deshmukh, V.K., and Chopde, C.T., Anxiolytic and anticonvulsive activity of *Sesbania grandiflora* leaves in experimental animals, *Phytother. Res.*, 16, 455, 2002.
44. Ganguly, D.K. and Malhotra, C.L., Some behavioral effects of an active fraction from *Herpestis monniera* Linn. (*Brahmi*), *Indian J. Med. Res.*, 55, 473, 1967.
45. Chopra, A. and Doiphode, V., Ayurvedic medicine, *Med. Clin. North Am.*, 86, 75, 2002.
46. Okamato, T. and Hino, O., Drug development with hints from traditional Indian Ayurveda medicine: hepatitis and rheumatoid arthritis as an example, *Int. J. Mol. Med.*, 6, 613, 2000.
47. Dandekar, U.P. et al., Analysis of a clinical important interaction between phenytoin and *shankhapushpi*, an ayurvedic preparation, *J. Ethnopharmacol.*, 35, 285, 1992.
48. Kshirsagar, N.A. et al., Phenytoin and Ayurvedic preparation-clinically important interaction in epileptic patients, *J. Assn. Physicians India*, 40, 354, 1992.
49. Garg, S.K. et al., Effect of Mentat on the pharmacokinetics of single and multiple doses of phenytoin in rabbits, *Neurol. India*, 47, 104, 1999.
50. Chen, L.C. et al., Drug utilization pattern of antiepileptic drugs and traditional Chinese medicines in a general hospital in Taiwan: a pharmaco-epidemiological study, *J. Clin. Pharm. Ther.*, 25, 125, 2000.
51. Koumaravelour, K. et al., Efffect of honey on Carbamazepine kinetics in rabbits, *Indian J. Exp. Biol.*, 40, 560, 2002.
52. Tripathi, Y.B., Molecular approach to Ayurveda, *Indian J. Exp. Biol.*, 38, 409, 2000.

25

Psychiatric Disorders

R.H. Singh and Lakshmi Chandra Mishra

CONTENTS

25.1 Introduction

The discipline of psychiatry according to Ayurveda has its roots in the four ancient books of knowledge called *Vedas of India*, where science and knowledge of an evil spirit (*bhutavidya*) is mentioned vividly. As a matter of fact, the word *bhutavidya* of *Vedas* refers to Ayurveda as a whole. There is no direct mention of *tridosa* doctrine (*vata, pitta,* and *kapha*) of Ayurveda in *Vedas*. As such, *bhutavidya* may be considered the mother of medicine as a whole in ancient India.[1]

0-8493-1366-X/04/$0.00+$1.50

Psychiatric disorders are very prevalent diseases. They accounted for 10 to 15% of the prescriptions written in 1996 in the U.S.[2] The diagnostic criteria for psychiatric disorders in the U.S. are described in the American Psychiatric Association's 2000-941 DSM IV TR publication, *Diagnostic and Statistical Manual of Mental Disorders*.[3] Since the mid-1950s, research and development efforts in drug therapies for psychiatric disorders have led to the discovery of many useful drugs.[2] These drugs, however, are known to have significant adverse side effects. Because Ayurvedic dietary herbal supplements are relatively safe, their use in managing various psychiatric disorders is explored here.

25.2 Basic Ayurvedic Concept of Psychiatry

The contemporary Ayurvedic psychiatry in terms of concepts consists of two components, namely:

1. Ayurvedic science of psychiatric disorders (*Ayurvediya manas roga vijnana*) or rational Ayurvedic psychiatry — This deals with clinical conditions where the disease and its treatment are based on fundamental principles of Ayurveda (i.e., theories of five elements [*pancamahabhuta*], *tridosa, triguna,* etc.). The diseases such as psychosis (*unmada*) and others are well characterized.
2. Demonology (science and knowledge of evil spirits) (*bhutavidya*) — This deals with psychiatric problems like psychosis (*bhutonmada, grahavesa*) in a nonconventional manner. Psychiatry emerged to the present scientific shape from demonology, where the disease and its treatment is not based on classical principles of Ayurveda and science (*vijnana*). Rather, it is based on paranormal factors like the doctrine of deeds (*karma*), planets (*graham*), evil spirits (*bhuta*), and others. The latter appears to be based more on astrology than on psychiatry. Sometimes this aspect of the psychiatric disorders, such as *bhutavidya,* is equated with demonology. It seems that different kinds of psychosis and effects of planets described in ancient texts are nothing but different forms of psychiatric syndromes or sets of behavioral alterations named symbolically after the name of different planets because of the similarity with their mythological descriptions. The element of demonology exists in Ayurveda but only symbolically.

In Ayurveda, the entire concept of life, health, and disease revolves around the classical theory (*loka-purusa samya*) that proclaims that the individual living being is a miniature replica of the universe; the universe (*loka*) and individuals (*purusa*) exist as a continuum of each other. The individual life entity is called *ayu,* which is four dimensia composed of physical, sensorial, mental, and spiritual attributes. The human being is provided not only with sensorial apparatus (*jnanendriyas*), but also with a highly dynamic psyche and mind (*manas*). According to Ayurveda, the mind is highly active but is unconscious (*acetana*). It derives its consciousness from the soul (*atma*) — an extension of the cosmic or divine consciousness.

The mind (*manas*) is further considered to have three dimensions in terms of the three properties or attributes (*gunas*): *sattva, rajas,* and *tamas*. The *rajas* represent activity and dynamism, whereas the *tamas* denotes inertia and darkness. *Sattva* is the state of pure mind with absolute balance when both the extreme qualities of mind, namely, *raja* and *tamas,* cease or merge into each other. It is believed that all mental illnesses are because of the *rajas* and *tamas*. These properties are also called mental (*manasa*) *dosas* in the same way as *vata, pitta,* and *kapha* are called body (*sarira*) *dosas* and all kinds of physical diseases are attributed to them.

In consideration of the *trigunas*,[4] Ayurveda postulates the idea that there can be three broad categories of mental personalities (*prakritis*): *sattvika prakrti, rajasa prakrti,* and *tamasa prakrt*.[5] These categories are further divided on the basis of finer considerations into 16 mental (*manasa*) personalities or mental traits. These 16 personality traits are characterized with unique features that may also predispose specific mental diseases simulating 16 personality factors (16 PF) of modern psychology.

The entire concept of the mind (*manas*) is psychological. Its neurophysiological attributes have not been described vividly in Ayurveda. However, the text *Bhela Samhita* states that the mind (*manas*) is located in the skull (*sirstalvantrgatam manah*). There are also references describing heart (*hrdaya*) as the seat of consciousness (*cetana*). Ayurvedic texts consider mental health a state of sensorial mental, intellectual, and spiritual well-being. Ill mental health is brought about essentially as a result of unwholesome interaction between the individual and his environment. This interaction operates through three fundamental factors: time rhythm (*kala*), intellect (*buddhi*), and sensorial inputs (*indriyartha*).

25.3 Etiology

Ayurveda believes in the theory of rebirth (*punarjanma*) and actions of past life (*karma*). Accordingly, clusters of mental illnesses primarily fall into two etiological areas: the hereditary and the environment.

Etiological factors in the diagnosis of psychiatric disorders are not clearly defined. Categorical relationships between disorders and the symptom constellation provide an important key in understanding how heterogeneous symptoms may descend upon a final common pathway. Consequently, a number of disorders exist as discrete mental disorders but rely on an aggregate of behavior that may be common among other families of mental disorders.

The role of environmental factors has not been adequately ruled out. In fact, socioeconomic, environmental, and dietary factors are currently considered causal, based on epidemiological studies for many diseases previously thought to be related to genetics (e.g., cancer).[6] The same may be true for psychiatric disorders.

25.4 Psychopathology

The psychopathology in Ayurveda is described by Charaka Samhita, Chapter 7 (*Nidana Sthana*), in a very systematic manner in terms of eight essential psychological factors considered to be centrally affected in all psychiatric disorders in varying degrees[7]:

1. Emotion, mood, affect (*mana*)
2. Thought and decision (*buddhi*)
3. Orientation (*sajna-jnana*)

4. Memory and learning (*Smrti*)
5. Desire (*bhakti*)
6. Habits (*sila*)
7. Psychomotor function (*cesta*)
8. Conduct and behavior (*acara*)

25.5 Clinical Description of Psychiatric Disorders

A wide range of psychiatric conditions and affective behaviors have been described in Ayurveda. Besides their aetiopathogenesis, the texts describe briefly but vividly the signs, symptoms, and behavioral alterations in different psychiatric diseases and their classifications. The psychiatric conditions described in original texts may be classified as follows:

1. Primary psychological conditions caused purely by *manasa dosas* (i.e., *rajas* and *tamas*). An example is the set of *manas dosas vikaras*[7]: lust (*kama*), anger (*krodha*), greed (*lobha*), delusion (*moha*), jealousy (*irsya*), pride (*mana*), eurphoria (*mada*), sorrow (*dukha*), grief (*soka*), anxiety (*cinta*), neurosis (*udvega*), fear (*bhaya*), and happiness (*harsa*).
2. Psychiatric conditions, neurological problems, and symptoms caused by the mixed pathology (*samprapti*) including both the body *dosas* (*vata, pitta, kapha*) and mental *dosas* (*raja, tama*). Examples include psychosis (*unmada*), convulsive diseases (*apasmara*), hysteria (*apatantraka*), obsession (*atattvabhinivesa*), vertigo (*bhrama*), drowsiness (*tandra*), neuresthenia (*klama*), comas (*mada-murccha-sanyas*), alcoholism (*madatyaya*), and hypochondriasis (*gadodvega*).
3. Personality (*prakrti*) disorders: There are 16 mental disorders (*manasa prakriti*) representing 16 types of behavior traits. When such personality behavior becomes overt and overrides the range of normalcy, the patient may have a psychiatric disorder.
4. Mental retardation (*buddhimandya*).
5. Neurological and behavioral problems of the elderly (*jara-janya manasa vikara*).
6. Psychosomatic diseases, where the cause of disease is mental and manifestation is somatic (*manodaihika vyadhis*,[*e.g.*, *sokatisara*]).

The psychiatric syndromes named symbolically after the name of planets (e.g., *bhutonmada* and *grahavesa*) warrant prayers (*daivavyapasraya cikitsa*). This is because herbal and purification treatments (*yuktivyapasraya cikitsa*) based on fundamental doctrines of Ayurveda are not possible.

In conventional medicine, mental diseases in general are characterized by altered behavior. The clinical diagnosis is done on the basis of the pattern of alteration of the behavior and certain associated signs and symptoms. Common psychiatric diseases described in the conventional medicine[8] and Ayurveda[7] are (1) psychosis (*unmada*), (2) depressive illness (*cittavasada*), (3) anxiety disorders (*cittodvega*), and (4) somatoform disorders, alcoholism, and drug abuse (*mada*). These diseases are briefly discussed here.

25.5.1 Psychosis

Psychosis is described in Ayurveda as a major psychiatric disease. There are several types identified in terms of the set of signs, symptoms, and the pattern of behavior alterations referable to the three *dosas* and their combinations.

A separate category of psychosis, described as *agantuja unmada* by Charaka and as *bhutonmada* by Susruta, forms an interesting dimension of Ayurvedic psychiatry. In this context about a dozen psychiatric syndromes are described and named after different planets or divinities (*grahas*). Thus, *bhutonmada* is a specialized aspect of Ayurvedic psychiatry using symbolic terms and need not be pushed into the realm of demonology.

In the conventional medicine, schizophrenia is a major psychotic (presence of hallucinations or delusions) illness. The major feature of schizophrenia is a decline in psychosocial functioning, with a tendency to move down in a person's social circle. Some patients may have acute full-blown symptoms, whereas others may have chronic and less severe symptoms. Characteristic symptoms are delusions, hallucinations, disorganized speech, grossly disorganized behavior, and hallucinations consisting of a voice or two voices that converse with each other and affect the behavior or thought of the patient. Prevalence of the disease is about 1% for lifetime risk. Schizophrenia affects both sexes equally. It affects all ages, although most cases are known to occur between the age of 15 and 35 years.[8]

25.5.2 Depressive Illness (*Cittavasada*)

Major clinical features of depressive disorders include persistent depressed mood, markedly diminished interest or pleasure, insomnia or too much sleep, psychomotor agitation, fatigue, loss of energy, diminished ability to think, and suicidal tendencies. An examination of the patient history does not reveal any organic factor or pathology or any family disaster to explain symptoms, nor does it reveal delusions, hallucinations in the past 2 weeks, or schizophrenia. In some cases, however, the family history may show biological or genetic propensity.

The mechanism responsible for depression is believed to be the decrease of catecholamine. This is based on the observations in 1950s that reserpine, a catecholamine and indolamine depleter, causes depression and drugs that replenish these amines are therapeutic; it was suggested that a reduction in the levels of these amines in the brain are related to depression. A specific cause responsible for the reduction in amine levels is not clear. It is possible that a thinking process in the cortex responding to an adverse physical or psychosocial environment may trigger the reduction in amine levels. Thus, the reduction in amine levels may be a manifestation of the disease and not the cause. Almost all antidepressant drugs are known to increase the availability of catecholamine and indolamine at the synapse in the central nervous system.[8]

25.5.3 Anxiety Disorders (*cittodvega*)

Major features of anxiety disorders include nervousness, sleeplessness, hypochondriasis, and somatic complaints. No age is immune to these disorders. Clinical symptoms may occur as an episode, such as paniclike anxiety, or may show chronic generalized anxiety. A panic anxiety episode may consist of following symptoms: shortness of breath, dizziness, unsteady feeling, fainting, accelerated heart rate, trembling, sweating, choking, nausea, depersonalization, paresthesia, hot flashes, chills, chest pain, fear of dying, and fear of going crazy. No clear etiology is known, but a cluster of cases in families indicates some genetic component similar to depression. However, physical and sociopsychological environmental factors must be considered. Neurophysiology and neurobiochemistry of anxiety disorders suggests the involvement of the noradrenergic system.[8]

25.5.4 Somatoform Disorders, Alcoholism, and Drug Abuse (*Mada*)

Somatoform disorders basically have one common characteristics: mimicry of medical diseases involving exaggeration of severity or disability accompanying actual medical illness. There is still no credible neurobiological basis for these disorders. Some examples of these diseases are listed below[8]:

1. Somatization disorder — This is a multisystem disorder characterized by complaints of pain, gastrointestinal, sexual problems, and pseudoneurologic problems. It begins early in life.
2. Hypochondriasis — Patients believe that they are going to contract some serious illness.
3. Conversion disorder — Patients mimic symptoms of neurological or medical illness and show dominant psychological factors as the cause.
4. Body dysmorphic disorder — Patients are concerned with an imagined defect in physical appearance.
5. Pain disorder — Patients complain of pain and indicate some dominant psychological factor as the cause.

Examples of somatiformlike disorders include the following:

1. Dissociative disorder — Patients show disrupted consciousness, memory, identity, or perception judged to be attributed to psychological factors.
2. Factitious disorder — Patients intentionally create physical and psychological signs of illness when no cause (financial gain, avoidance of responsibility, etc.) can be identified.
3. Malingering — Patients intentionally create false physical and psychological signs of illness and an identifiable cause (financial gain, avoidance of responsibility, and others).
4. Chronic fatigue syndrome — The syndrome has the basis in reports appeared in 1980s in the U.S. of pathologic fatiguability. Unconscious psychological factors are believed to be involved as important contributors.

25.6 Diagnosis of Psychiatric Disorders

The clinical examination in Ayurveda has two objectives: (1) to examine and assess the primary nature of the patient as an individual as opposed to a disease and his or her health (*rogi pariksha*) and (2) to examine and assess the nature and severity of the disease (*rog-parikhsa*). The examination of the patient is done by a 10-point interrogation (*dasavidha pariksa*):

1. Constitution (*prakriti*)
2. Morbidity (*vikrti*)
3. Quality of tissues (*sara*)
4. Body stucture (*samhanana*)
5. Anthropometry (*pramana*)
6. Adaptability (*satmya*)
7. Mental stamina (*sattva*)
8. Digestive power (*ahara sakti*)
9. Physical strength (*vyayama sakti*)
10. Age and aging (*vaya*)

The clinical examination includes an interview (*prasna pariksa*) with the patient, a reliable attendant, or relative. The physical examination of the patients (*pancendriya pariksa*) includes the following:

1. A general survey by eight-point examination (*astavidha pariksa*): pulse (*nadi*), urine (*mutra*), stool (*mala*), tongue (jihva), voice (*sabda*), skin (*sparsa*), eyes (netra), facies (*akrti*).
2. Systemic examination (*sadanga pariksa*) of the six parts of the body: head-neck, trunk, and the four limbs along with 13 channels (*srotamsi*) distributed over the entire body (*sadangas*). The examination of channels (*srotas*) with psychiatric patients must include the examination of mental channels (*manovaha srtoas*).

The clinical data available through the above methods are critically examined and evaluated in the light of the doctrine of Ayurvedic knowledge of clinical description, signs and symptoms, pathology, and diagnostic criteria (*pramana vijnana* and *nidana pancake, nidana, purvariipa, rupa, samprapti, upasaya-anupasaya*). The diagnosis is made not merely by name of a disease or syndrome, but in a descriptive way identifying the constitution, etiology, and abnormal personality (*prakrti, hetu, vikrti*); this includes *dosa* tissues (*dusya*) and seat of the vitiated *dosa* (*adhisthana*). The Ayurvedic physician pays special attention to the patient's environment, hereditary and genetic background, and original personality makeup in terms of *tridosa* and three personality properties (*triguna*).

25.7 Treatment

The Ayurvedic management of a psychiatric patient is carried out through three broad streams of therapy: (1) divine therapy (*Daivavyapasraya cikitsa*), (2) biological therapy (*Yuktivyapasraya cikitsa*), and (3) psychotherapy (*Sattvavajaya*). The divine therapy includes the use of religious activities (*mantra, japa*) and wearing of precious stones. Ayurvedic psychotherapy is practiced incorporating the principles of assurance therapy (*asviisana*), replacement of negative emotions with positive emotions, and psychological shock therapy. In addition, it includes encouraging the patient to find or develop a specific goal, purpose, or meaning in life; find a job that gives better job satisfaction; improve relationships with family members; contribute own share of responsibilities to the household;

maintain a healthy lifestyle with respect to daily routine (sleeping schedule and exercise); and join some sports activity, fitness club, and volunteer groups to help the community.

In biological therapy, the patient is subjected to biopurification by *pancakarma* in order to cleanse the channels of the body. This is followed by *salisamana* therapy or palliative treatment with the help of *ausadhi* (medicinal herbs and herbal formulas), *anna* (dietetics), and *vihara* (lifestyle). The drugs used in the treatment are mostly nootropic (*medhya*) herbs or herbomineral formulas or nootropic *rasayanas,* which are believed to act as brain tonics and adaptogens. The nootropic herbs are considered as specific molecular nutrients for the brain, affording a better mental health and leading to alleviation of behavioral alterations.[9] The *vajikarana* drugs such as *kapikacchu* and others are used in the treatment of depression. The entire Ayurvedic management is more health oriented than disease oriented. As such, there is a big scope of utilizing Ayurvedic approach and therapeutics as an adjunct to the disease-oriented therapy of modem psychiatry to afford a full treatment.

25.7.1 Ayurvedic Herbs and Herbal Formulas

Besides the nondrug approach to prevention and treatment of mental disorders, the Ayurvedic texts describe a large number of herbal and herbomineral formulas for treating mental diseases. Many of these formulas are still in popular use in the hands of a large number of Ayurvedic practitioners. The scientific validity of many of these herbs and herbal formulas drugs has been tested on scientific parameters, and several of these have been found effective.

Ayurveda describes a class of herbs termed as *medhya* herbs and *medhya rasayana.* All *medhya* and *medhya rasayana* drugs are claimed to be nutraceutical agents specific to neuronutrition. They are called *medhya* because they are beneficial for *medha* (i.e., intellect). All such herbs have been found to possess nootropic effect besides varying degrees of anxiolytic activity. In addition to other aspects of the rasayana effect, they bring about antistress effect and improve the memory and cognitive power. The popularly used *Medhya* herbs and commercially available herbal compound formulas are listed below:

Single Herbs	Herbal Formulas
1. *Sankhapuspi* (*Convolvulus pluricaulis*)	1. *Saraswatarista*
2. *Mandukaparni* (*Centella asiatica*)	2. *Aswagandharist*
3. *Brahami* (*Bacopa monnieri*)	3. *Smriti sagar rasa*
4. *Vaca* (*Acorus calamus*)	4. *Krisna chaturmukha rasa*
5. *Jatamansi* (*N. jatamansi*)	5. *Unmada gajankusa rasa*
6. *Ashwagandha* (*Withania somnifera*)	6. *Unmada gajakeshri rasa*
7. *Sarpagandha* (*Rauwolfia serpentina*)	
8. *Jyotismati* (*Celestrus panniculatus*)	
9. *Yasti madhu* (*Glycyrrhiza glabra*)	
10. *Guduchi* (*Tinospora cardifolia*)	

All these plants are tropical and grow in India and other tropical countries profusely. The recent clinical and laboratory studies conducted on these herbs have shown mild to moderate nootropic and antistress effects with high safety profile.[10–17]

In addition to the *medhya* herbs as mentioned above, it is pertinent to mention that the herbs of *vrisya* and *vajikarana* categories are also used in psychiatric care. *Vrisya* and *vajikarana* herbs are essentially aphrodisiacs and are commonly used for promotion of sexual stamina and virility. Some Ayurvedic physicians use this category of herbs for treating depression. The most popular herbal drug of this category is *kapikacchu* (*Mucuna pruriens*). The seeds of this plant, which are also edible as a vegetable, are used in the treatment of depression and also for treatment of Parkinsonism because of high levadopa (L-DOPA) content.

25.7.2 Nonherbal Therapies

The Ayurvedic classics describe *sattvavajaya* as one of the three major therapeutic streams of Ayurveda. *Sattvavajaya* is a special form of psychotherapy where the therapist attempts to divert the thought process of the patient from unwanted targets (*ahit bhawas*) to beneficial targets (*hita bhawas*). This is done through supportive therapy, assurance, and replacement of negative emotions by positive emotions.

In addition to this classic Ayurvedic psychotherapy, the role of yoga and meditation can not be over emphasized. Scientific evidence has already accumulated to suggest that several yogic practices have great psychorehabilitative and antistress effect.

Similarly, certain traditional practices of *keraliya panchakarma* (i.e., *sirodhara* and *sirobasti*) are used for treatment of chronic mental diseases and have good results. However, their mode of action has not yet been validated scientifically.

In conventional medicine, treating psychiatric disorders essentially consists of identifying and eliminating socioenvironmental factors and administration of antipsychotic drugs (neuroleptic drugs) similar to that in Ayurveda. The drugs used for the treatment of psychosis include phenothiazines, structurally similar thiozanthenes, and heterocyclic dibenzazepines; butyrophenones and diphenylbutylpiperdines; and indolones and other heterocyclic compounds. These drugs act via blocking the mesolimbic dopamine receptors. The adverse side effects of the drugs are as follows:

1. Acute spasm of the tongue, face, neck, or back may mimic seizures, not hysteria
2. Motor restlessness
3. Bradykinesia, rigidity, variable tremor, mask facies, and shuffling gait
4. Catatonia, stupor, fever, unstable blood pressure, and myoglobinemia can be fatal
5. Perioral tremor
6. Oral facial dyskinesia, widespread choreoathetosis, or dystonia
7. Agranulocytosis[8]

The pharmacologic agents available to treat depression disorders exert their antidepressant effect by inhibiting the reuptake of serotonin at presynaptic membrane selectively (fluoxetine) and the reuptake of both serotonin and norepinephrine or (imipramine), directly inhibiting monoaminao oxidase enzyme (phenelzine) or causing dopamine blockage (trazodone). These drugs provide symptomatic relief and remissions but do not cure the disease. The side effects of these drugs include dry mouth, constipation, postural hypotension, tachyarrhythmia, nervousness, insomnia, tremor, agitation, headache, weight loss, hypertensive crisis, and priapism.[2]

The drugs used for the treatment of anxiety disorders are primarily antihistamines and benzodiazepines. The adverse side effects of these drugs include dry mouth, mental confusion, addiction, ataxia, drowsiness, sedation, nervousness, headache, and bradycardia.[8]

No drug treatment should be given to patients suffering from somatoform disorders, alcoholism, or drug abuse (*mada*) unless there are secondary signs that require drug treatments. Attempts should be made to identify and eliminate sociopsychological factors and other environmental factors associated with the diseases. The psychiatrist and family members need to take care of the patient with assurances, spiritual guidance, and prayers.[8]

25.8 Prevention

Ayurveda places great emphasis on preventing diseases; psychiatric disorders are no exception. As a matter of fact, a healthy lifestyle, a healthy diet, balanced physical activities, living up to social and family responsibilities, enjoying work, regularly exercising, practicing a proper daily routine (*dincharya*), and keeping personal living spaces (such as bedrooms and cars) presentable and pleasing may prevent many psychiatric disorders, particularly if children are also raised with this lifestyle. According to Ayurveda, the human body is like a vehicle driven by the soul (spirit, *atma*). When the vehicle takes control of the travel, a disaster is bound to occur. One must not surrender his or her life to the body; the soul must drive the body.

25.9 Scientific Basis of Ayurvedic Therapies

Although the therapies mentioned above have been in traditional use for thousands of years, with the recent demand of evidence-based Ayurveda, modest efforts have been made to generate scientific evidence for the safety and efficacy of the traditional medications. Reports on such studies are accumulating in scientific journals. Some such studies are highlighted below.

25.9.1 Antistress Agents

A large number of Ayurvedic herbs have been described to possess the *medhya* effect. All such herbs are believed to have neuronutraceutical effect with varying degree of anxiolytic and antistress effect. The potentiation of barbiturate hypnosis by *sankhapuspi* (*C. pluricaulis*) in rats and the evidence of anxiolytic and adaptogenic effect of this drug in patients of anxiety and neurosis has been demonstrated.[18] In another study, similar effects for *mandukaparni* (*C. asiatica*) and *aswagandha* (*W. somnifera*) have been reported in animal models and in clinical settings, respectively.[19] The effect of *brahmi* (*B. monnieri*) in similar clinical and laboratory models was also investigated and was found to lower the level of anxiety and promote memory and adaptation.[11] Singh and associates screened a series of herbal therapies in albino rats for antistress effect by measuring swimming performance, changes in adrenal weight, and ascorbic acid and cortisol content of adrenal glands during stress; they also measured the incidence of stress ulcers in stomachs that were under the influence of herbs in stressed rats. The investigators found highly significant antistress effect in *ashwagandha* (*W. somnifera*) and *tulasi* (*O. sanctum*). These two drugs were found to be twice more effective than *P. ginseng* in terms of ED_{50}.[16,17]

25.9.2 Memory-Enhancing Agents

All *medhya rasayana* of Ayurveda are conceptually nootropic agents. Recent studies conducted on these herbs have shown evidence for this conceptual claim. Singh and Singh reported a memory-enhancing effect in *brahmi* (*B. monnieri*) followed by several studies conducted at the Central Drug Research Institute, Lucknow, India, by Dhawan and Associates in recent years characterizing active constituents of this plant responsible for the memory enhancing effect.[10,20]

25.9.3 Treatment of Residual Psychosis

With the advent of strong antipsychotic drugs in modern medicine, it is no longer difficult to control the acute episodes of psychotic disease. It is becoming more and more difficult, however, to take care of the long-term chronic residual phase of these diseases and their negative symptoms. Modern medicines are not suitable for such long-term use because of drug dependence and adverse side effects. In such cases, Ayurvedic medications are the only logical answer. Certain Ayurvedic herbs, particularly the polyherbomineral compounds like *smrti sagar rasa*[21,22] and *unmada gaja kesari rasa*, have shown encouraging results.[23]

25.9.4 Antidepressants and Mood Elevators

A number of Ayurvedic herbs, particularly the *vajikarana* formulas (Ayurvedic aphrodisiacs), have been evaluated for their possible role in the management of depressive illness. *Aswagandha* (*Withania somnifera*), *kapikacchu* (*Mucuna pruriens*), *jyotismati* (*Celeastrus paniculatus*), and *vaca* (*Acorus calamus*) have shown good results in pilot studies. In one study, *aswagandha* and *kapikacchu* used alone in patients of depressive illness exhibited an antidepressant effect when measured on the Hamilton Depression Rating Scale.[20] The potentiation of hypothermia effect of the agonist in *aswagandha*-treated animals suggests that *aswagandha* sensitizes serotonin (5-HTIA) autoreceptors. A similar effect was also found for *sankhapuspi* (*C. pluricaulis*).[20]

25.9.5 Geriatric Mental Health

Aging is generally associated with a range of psychological symptoms. The *rasayana* formulas of Ayurveda are the logical remedy. The antiaging effects of selected *rasayana* formulas like *aswagandha* (*W. somnifera*) and *tulasi* (*O. sanctum*) were evaluated by using a standardized biological age scale and brief psychiatric rating scale, memory span test, and mental fatigue rate.[24] It was observed that use of *aswagandha* and *tulasi* singly for a sample test period of 3 to 6 months exhibited notable beneficial effect in elderly individuals. Such an effect is attributed to the drugs' antistress and adaptogenic activities.

25.9.6 *Medhya Rasayana* and Mental Retardation

A varying degree of mental retardation is a major health hazard in children prevalent throughout the world and belong to divergent etiology. Besides self-recovery and compensation, there is no definite treatment for this condition in conventional Western medicine. But the Ayurvedic texts describe a range of restorative remedies (i.e., *rasayana*), especially for the promotion of mental health and cognitive functions. Such *rasayanas* are called *medhya rasayana*. It is claimed that such *rasayanas*, because of their nutritive impact on the brain, may help mentally retarded children. *Mandukaparni* (*C. asiatica*) is one of the four *medhya rasayanas* described by Charaka Samhita.[7] This drug is in traditional use and was studied preliminarily for its utility in mental retardation.[15] More recently, a clinical study on *mandukparni* in 30 mentally retarded children (6 to 18 years old), fulfilling the selection criteria for mental retardation and excluding any other major organic cause, was conducted.[14] These children received the *mandukparni* (whole plant granules) at a dose of 5 g twice/day for 6 months. The observations showed significant improvement in performance intelligence quotient, social quotient (measured by Vineland social maturity scale for behavior and social adoptability), immediate memory span, and reaction time. The authors concluded that such an effect of *mandukaparni* could be due to the *rasayana* effect of the drug both in terms of its microneuronutrient effect and its *srotas* (microvascular) effect by promoting the blood supply to the brain.

25.10 Summary and Conclusions

Mental health and ailments of psyche have been important considerations in the field of medicine from the very beginning. Ayurveda has a well-developed branch of psychiatry, and the principles and practices of mental health care which developed thousands of years ago are again drawing attention because of their unique holistic approaches. There is a need to integrate this novel wisdom into the mainstream of the health care delivery system of today.

References

1. Singh, R.H., *Ayurvediya Manas Vijnana*, Choukhamba Amara Bharati Prakashan, Varanasi, India, 1985.
2. Baldessarini, R.J., Drugs and the treatment of psychiatric disorders, in *Goodman and Gillman's The Pharmacological Basis of Therapeutics*, Hardman, J.G., Limbird, L.E., et al., Eds., McGraw-Hill, New York, 1996, chaps. 18 and 19.
3. American Psychiatric Association, *Diagnostic and Statistical Manual of Mental Disorders*, 4th ed., text revision, Washington, D.C., 2000.
4. Singh, R.H., Singh, M.B., and Udupa, K.N., A study of *tridosa* as neurohumours, *J. Res. Ayurveda Siddha*, 1(1), 1–20, 1979.
5. Udupa, K.N., Singh, R.H., Dubey, G.P., Rai, V., and Singh, M.B., Biochemical basis of psychosomatic constitution (prakriti), *Indian J. Med. Res.*, 63(7), 923, 1975.
6. Cotran, R.S., Kumar, V., and Collins, T., Neoplasia, in *Robins Pathological Basis of Disease*, Cotran, R.S., Kumar, V., and Collins, T., Eds., W.B. Saunders, New York, 1999, chap. 8.
7. *Charaka Smhita* (700 B.C.), translated by Sharma, P.V., Choukhamba Orientalia Varanasi, U.P., India.
8. Schiffer, R.B., Psychiatric disorders in medical practice, in *Cecil Text Book of Medicine*, Goldman, L. and Bennett, J.C., Eds., W.B. Saunders, Philadelphia, 2000, chap. 450.
9. Singh, R.H., Sinha, B.N., Sarkar, F.H., and Udupa, K.N., Comparative biochemical studies on the effect of *medhya rasayana* drugs on brain in rats, *J. Res. Indian Med.*, 14(3), 7–14, 1979.
10. Singh, H.K. and Dhawan, B.N., Neuropsychopharmacological study of B. monieri Linn. (brahmi), *Indian J. Pharmacol.*, 29, 5359–5365, 1997.
11. Singh, L. and Singh, R.H. (Sup), (1978): Studies on Psychotropic Effect of the Medhya Rasayan Drug, Brahmi (Bacopa Monieria), M.D. thesis (Kayachikitsa), Banaras Hindu University, Varanasi, India, 1978.
12. Singh, N., Study of anti-stress effect of plant drugs, *Ann. Natl. Acad. Indian Med.*, 1(1), 1987.
13. Singh, R.H., Singh, L., and Sen, S.P., Studies on medhya rasayan drug brahmi (Bacopa monnieri Linn.). II. Experimental studies, *J. Res. Indian Med.*, 14(3)1–6, 1979.

14. Agrawal, S.C. and Singh, R.H., Effect of *medhya rasayana* drug mandukaparni on cognitive functions and social adaptability of mentally retarded children, *J. Res. Ayurveda Siddha*, 18(3–4), 97–107, 1998.
15. Apparao, M.V.R., Srivastava, K., and Rao, K., The effect of mandukaparni (Centella asiation) on general mental ability of mentally retarded children, *J. Res. Indian Med.*, 8(4), 9–16, 1973.
16. Archana, R. and Namasivayam, A., Anti-stressor effect of Withania somnifera, *J. Ethnopharmacol.*, 64, 91–93, 1999.
17. Bhattacharya, S.K., Satyan, K.S., and Ghosal, S., Anxiolytic activity of glycowithanolides from Withania somnifera, *Indian J. Exp. Biol.*, 35, 236, 1997.
18. Mehta, A.K. and Singh, R.H. (Sup), Studies on the Psychotropic Effect of the *Medhya Rasayana* Drug: Shankhapuspi (Convolvulus Pluricaulis), M.D. thesis (Kayachikitsa), Banaras Hindu University, Varanasi, India, 1976
19. Mishra, B.K. and Singh, R.H. (Sup), Clinical and Experimental Evaluation of Medhya Rasayan Effect of Mandukaparni (Hydrocotyle Asiatica), M.D. thesis (Kayachikitsa), Banaras Hindu University, Varanasi, India, 1980.
20. Koirala, R.R. and Singh, R.H. (Sup), Clinical and Behavioural Study of Medhya Drugs on Brain Functions, M.D. thesis (Kayachikitsa), Banaras Hindu University, Varanasi, India, 1992.
21. Tripathi, J.S. and Singh, R.H. (Sup), A Clinical Study on Personality Factors in Cases of Residual Schizophrenia and Its Ayurvedic Management, M.D. thesis (Kayachikitsa), Banaras Hindu University, Varanasi, India, 1992.
22. Tripathi, K.M. and Singh, R.H. (Sup), A Study on Stress Profile and Personality Factors in Some Psychosomatic Disorders, Ph.D. thesis (Kayachikitsa), Banaras Hindu University, Varanasi, India, 1982.
23. Choudhuri, O. and Singh, R.H. (Sup), Development of an Ayurvedic Regimen for the Management of Residual Schizophrenia, M.D. thesis (Kayachikitsa), Banaras Hindu University, Varanasi, India, 2001.
24. Dwivedi, K.K. and Singh, R.H. (Sup), A Study on Psychiatric Symptoms of Geriatric Patients and Response to Ayurvedic Therapy, Ph.D. thesis (Kayachikitsa), Banaras Hindu University, Varanasi, India, 1997.

26

Parkinson's Disease (Kampa Vata)

Lakshmi Chandra Mishra and R.H. Singh

CONTENTS

26.1 Introduction

According to Ayurveda, most of the diseases of the *vata* system are essentially the conditions of degenerative diseases of the nervous system. As many as 80 kinds of *vata* diseases are described in Charak Samhita.[1] The syndrome of parkinsonism is commonly compared with *kampa vata* (*kampa* literally means tremors). The syndrome was comprehensively described by James Parkinson in 1817, but the review of much early literature would show that syndromes strikingly similar to parkinsonism were already known and were categorized among the *vata* diseases in Ayurveda.

Parkinson's disease (PD) is prevalent all over the world and has no definitive treatment in conventional medicine except for the palliative prescription of anticholinergics together with levodopa and dopadecarboxylase inhibitor. The Ayurvedic treatment strategy is to combat *vata dosa* and to sustain neuronutrition by *rasayana* remedies. This chapter discusses *vata* diseases (neurological diseases) as a class with emphasis on Ayurvedic therapies of PD and a possible scientific basis for the therapeutic effect.

26.2 Etiology

As discussed in Chapter 2, Ayurveda adopts a holistic approach to the understanding of whole body physiology by explaining the body functions in terms of three biofactors called

0-8493-1366-X/04/$0.00+$1.50

tridosa (*vata*, *pitta*, and *kapha*). In all applied considerations, the *vata* system of the *tridosa* doctrine represents neuroscience in Ayurveda. The *vata dosa* is responsible for the entire neurophysiological phenomena operating in the body.[1] There are five major components of *vata* systems: *prana, udana, vyana, samana,* and *apana*. These components are responsible for five different aspects of neural functions at five different levels in the body. When the *vata dosa* looses its equilibrium due to a wide range of aetiological factors, including tissue degeneration and damage (*dhatu ksaya*) and neuro-obstructive diathesis (*margavarana*), it leads to the development of 80 types of *vata* diseases or neurological diseases.

The etiopathogenesis of PD is not precisely known in conventional medicine, but it is understood to be caused by lesions in the basal ganglia and is especially associated with the damage to the interconnecting system between substantia nigra and corpus stratum. Specific etiology of PD is related to aging, and it develops in people over 50 years old. There is no specific genetic component involved in most cases, but mutation in the gene for alpha synuclein has been linked to PD in some cases.[2] Exposure to environmental chemicals may cause damage to basal ganglia and brain stem resulting in parkinsonism. For example, exposure to 1-methyl 4-phenyl-1, 2, 3, 6-tetrahydropyridine, a contaminant present in a psychoactive meperidine analog, can cause an acute onset of parkinsonism symptoms and the associated destruction of substantia nigra.

26.3 Pathology

In Ayurveda, no specific structural pathology of PD is described other than its identification as a *vata dosa* disease.

In conventional medicine, PD is described as a chronic progressive disease of extra pyramidal system of the brain where voluntary movement is disturbed with the appearance of involuntary movements and altered muscle tone. The pathology of PD essentially involves a loss of pigmented dopaminergic neurons in the substantia nigra pars compacta (SNPC) of the brain with the appearance of intracellular inclusions known as Lewy bodies.[3,4] SNPC provides dopaminergic innervation to the dopamine content (caudate and putamen). Early studies have shown 80% reduction in the dopamine content of the striatum. This reduction parallels a loss of neurons in the SNPC, indicating that dopamine loss may be the cause of PD symptoms and that replacement of dopamine could be helpful.[5,6] The major symptoms of PD are related to the deficiency of dopamine. Cholinergic nucleus basilis degeneration is believed to be related to dementia that affects many patients. Noradrenergic locus nucleus degeneration is believed to be associated with the facial expression of freezing and with depression.[7]

26.4 Classification of *Vata* Disorders

The *vata* diseases as described in Ayurvedic classics include a wide range of neurological morbidities, including inflammatory, degenerative, obstructive, and functional. The *vata* diseases may manifest as neural hyperfunctioning (*vata vriddhi*), neural hypofunctioning (*vata ksaya*), or masked functioning (*avarana*). It is not possible to innumerate and classify all 80 types of *vata* diseases here. However, Ayurvedic texts describe the etiology, symptomatology, and treatment of a variety of paralytic conditions, painful neuropathies, conditions with tremors, and involuntary movements and convulsions in detail. PD is one of those diseases. The descriptions of these conditions in Ayurveda are very similar to those described in conventional medicine. Some of these conditions are listed here as examples.

1. Paralysis and paresis — Facial paralysis (*ardita*), hemiplegias (*pakavadha*), paraplegias (*adharanga vata*), quadruplegi (*sarvauga vata*), and others
2. Painful neuropathies — Sciatica (*gridhrasi*), limb cramp (*khalli*), brachial neuritis (*avavahuka* and *viswachi*), trigeminal neuralgia (*siragrah*), lumbago (*kati-sula/pristha-sula*), cervical neuropathy (*manyastambh*), peripheral neuritis (*rasagata vata*), and others
3. Coordination disorders and convulsive diseases: parkinsonism, tremors, choreas (*kampa vata*), convulsive neuropathies (*aksepa*), epilepsies (*apasmara*), pseudo seizure disorders (*apatantraka*), and others
4. Visceral neuropathies — A large number of diseases and syndromes related to the neuropathy of different visceral organs of the digestive system, urogenital system, and sensory organs as described in Ayurveda

26.5 Clinical Features and Diagnosis of Parkinson's Disease

Clinical features of *kampa vata* in Ayurveda are similar to those described for parkinsonism and Huntington chorea in conventional medicine. These are the two most important neurodegenerative diseases of the basal ganglia and brain stem.[8] These diseases are frequently associated with movement disorders, rigidity, abnormal posturing, and involuntary movements marked by fine disorganized and random movements of the extremities (usually the hands and to a lesser extent proximal limb and muscles). The four main features of parkinsonism are (1) bradykinesia (abnormal slowness of voluntary movements, often associated with diminution of the range of movements), (2) muscular rigidity, (3) resting tremor, and (4) postural imbalance (leading to disturbance of gait and falling).[9] These features are also seen in other conditions, such as idiopathic PD, progressive supranuclear palsy, and corticobasal degeneration, with common damage to the nigro-striatal dopaminergic system.

Other symptoms of PD are related to mood, intellect, and the autonomic nervous system. These symptoms are hypophonic disarthria, monotonous speech pattern, difficulty in getting in and out of a chair or a bed, shuffling gait with short steps, decreased automatic movements, and arm swing. The resting tremors are slow, regular oscillations (3 to 6/sec) that usually cease during voluntary movements of the affected part, though occasionally the tremors may be of action type. Tremors are exacerbated by fatigue and cold; they can also affect the lips, lower jaw, and tongue. Tremors may be a dominant feature in some patients, whereas postural instability may be dominant in others.[7]

Other PD-like conditions can be differentiated from PD on the basis of a low to no degree of tremor and poor response to levodopa. The good response to levodopa in PD is because dopamine receptors are preserved in PD, but they are decreased in other PD-like conditions.

26.6 Prognosis

In Ayurveda, the prognosis of PD is not specifically given. Most *vata* diseases are not curable, but the patient may be able to live with the disease with certain degree of inconvenience and difficulties. As the disease progresses, patients develop rigidity and cannot take care of themselves. In extreme cases, death may occur from the patient's inability to breath, resulting in aspiration pneumonia or pulmonary embolism. Ayurvedic therapies available can make life much easier and increase life expectancy. Treatment with pharmacologic agents or direct electrical stimulation of target areas (thalamus, subthalamic nucleus, or globus pallidus) can provide relief in symptoms, good functional mobility for many years, and a substantial increase in life expectancy.[9]

26.7 Treatment

Ayurveda takes a unique approach to the management of the above-mentioned neuropathies with a special emphasis on eliminating their causes by *panchakarma*, physiotherapy, and medicinal treatment with the help of a wide range of herbal and herbomineral drugs. Ayurveda describes a large number of nootropic drugs (stimulating to mental activity, causing cerebral or intellectual activity) and nervous system tonics (i.e., rasayanas in the treatment of *vata* diseases). *Panchakarma* therapy is especially advocated in the treatment of neurological diseases. Using different kinds of oil massage (*snehana–abhyanga*) and medicated heat treatment (hot room) (*swedana*) is very efficacious. Besides special treatments like *sirovasti* and *sirodhara, vasti* therapy is indicated in such diseases and administered in the form of a specially planned therapeutic enema. With all this, contemporary Ayurvedic medicine claims good success in the practice of neuromedicine.

Being a neurodegenerative disease, parkinsonism is essentially treated by *rasayana* or a rejuvenative approach in Ayurveda.[10,11] The *rasayana* drugs of Ayurveda are essentially nutraceutical agents, and the *medhya rasayana* are specific neuronutrients or nervine tonics with nootropic effect. *Aswagandha* (*Withania somnifera*), *brahmi* (*Bocopa monnieri*), *mandukaparni* (*Centella asiatica*), and *bala* (*Cida cordifolia*) are the common classical drugs advocated for this purpose. This is because Ayurveda considers such movement disorders under *vata vyadhi*, and in common practice the term *kampa vata* is used to describe the syndrome. The strategy is to combat *vata dosa* and to sustain neuronutrition by *rasayana* remedies. *Kapikacchu* (*Mucuna pruriens*), an edible legume and popular Ayurvedic aphrodisiac, has also been used in the hands of Ayurvedic practitioners for treating *kampa vata*. With the recent discovery that *Mucuna pruriens* seeds are a highly rich source of levodopa, the use of *kapikacchu* in *kampa vata* has tremendously increased. *Kapikacchu* (*Atmagupta*) has been traditionally used for treating tremor disorders in Ayurveda.[12]

In conventional medicine, the treatment of PD is primarily based on increasing the levels of dopamine in SNPC. Carbidopa and levodopa, dopamine receptor agonists (pergolide and bromocriptine), and monoamino oxidase inhibitor (selegiline) are used to maintain the levels of dopamine. The other less-used drugs are muscarinic receptor antagonists and amentidine, an antiviral agent. The common side effects of levodopa are psychiatric problems, dyskinesis, and the wearing-off-effect (loss of effectiveness). The pharmacological treatments are only symptomatic; they do not change the progression of the disease. If used skillfully, these drugs may dramatically improve the quality of daily life and functional ability. Another treatment option is surgery. The main surgical approach commonly used is pallidotomy (incision or partial destruction of globus pallidus) and high-frequency deep-brain stimulation with an electrode implanted in one of these target areas: thalamus, subthalamic nucleus, or globus pallidus. These procedures are effective in providing relief from major symptoms and improving the quality of daily life but do not alter the course of the disease.[7,13]

26.8 Scientific Basis

The levodopa content of *M. pruriens* appears to be the basis for the therapeutic effect. MP endogenously accumulates L-dihydroxyphenylalanine in the range between 0.2 and 2.0% on a dry-weight basis in tissue culture.[14] In a clinical trial, HP-200 made from MP was found to be an effective treatment for patients with PD.[15]

A concoction of powdered *M. pruriens* seeds, *Hyoscyamus reticulatus* seeds, *W. somnifera* roots, and *C. cordifolia* roots in cow's milk was clinically tried in 18 diagnosed patients with PD.[16] Of these 18 patients, 13 cases underwent biopurificatory (*panchakarma*) procedures for 28 days and palliative therapy for 56 days, whereas the remaining 5 patients underwent palliative therapy alone for 84 days. The former group showed significant improvement in daily activities. Symptomatically, they showed a better response in tremor, bradykinesia, stiffness, and cramps as compared with the latter group. Salivation increased in both groups. Chemical analysis of the concoction revealed about 200 mg of levodopa per dose. The study shows the importance of cleansing therapy in Ayurveda medication before palliative therapy. It also confirms the usefulness of some Ayurvedic herbal preparations in PD.[17]

In an interesting study, PD was treated with the compound Parkino at 20 ml twice/day for 8 weeks.[18] The response was assessed symptomatically in terms of the subjective feelings of the patient, degree of involuntary movements, and facial expressions. All the patients exhibited highly significant improvement in symptoms during the first 2 to 4 weeks of treatment. However, during subsequent intervals, no further improvement was noted.

26.9 Summary and Conclusions

The review clearly indicates that PD patients can benefit from Ayurvedic therapies by using *M. pruriens* and *panchakarma*. Future research needs to focus on integrating Ayurvedic therapies with conventional therapies in treating PD.

References

1. Charak Samhita (700 B.C.), translated by Sharma, P.V., Choukhamba Orientalia, Varanasi, India.
2. Polymeropoulous, M.H. et al., Mutation in the alpha-synuclein gene identified in families with Parkinson's disease, *Science*, 276, 204, 1997.
3. Gibb, W.R., Neuropathology of Parkinson's disease and related syndromes, *Neurol. Clin.*, 10, 361, 1992.
4. Rempfer, R., Crook, R., Houlden, H., Duff, K., Hutton, M., Roberts, G.W., Raghavan, R., Perry, R., and Hardy, J., Parkinson's disease, but not Alzheimer's disease: Lewy body variant associated with mutant alleles at cytochrome P450 gene, *Lancet*, 344, 815, 1994
5. Cotzia, G.C., Papavasiliou, P.S., and Gellens, R., Modification of parkinsonism-chronic treatment with L-DOPA, *N.Engl. J. Med.*, 280, 337, 1969.
6. Hornykiewicz, O., Dopamine in the basal ganglia, *Br. Med. Bull.*, 29, 172, 1973
7. Jankovic, J., Parkinsonism, in *Cecil Textbook of Medicine*, Goldman, L. and Bennett, J.C., Eds., W.B. Saunders, New York, 2000, chap. 460.
8. Girolami, U.D., Anthony, D.C., and Frosch, M.P., The central nervous system, in *Robbin's Pathologic Basis of Disease*, Cotran, R.S., Kumar, V., and Collins, T., Eds., W.B. Saunders, New York, 1999, chap. 30.
9. Diamond, S.G., Markham, C.H., Hoehn, M.M., McDowell, F.H., and Muenter, M.D., Multicenter study of Parkinson mortality with early versus later dopa treatment, *Ann. Neurol.*, 22, 8, 1987.
10. Gourie-Devi, M. and Venkataram, B.S., Concept of disorders of muscles in Charaka Samhita an ancient Indian medical treatise-relevance in modern myology, *Neurology* (India), 31, 13–14, 1983.
11. Gourie-Devi, M., Ramn, M.G., and Venkataram, B.S., Treatment of Parkinson's disease in Ayurveda, *J. R. Soc. Med.*, 84, 491–492, 1991.
12. Manyam, B.V., Paralysis agitans and levodopa in "Ayurveda": ancient Indian medical treatise, *Movement Disorders*, 5, 47, 1990.
13. Standaert, D.G. and Young, A.B., Treatment of central nervous system disorders, in *Goodman & Gillman's The Pharacological Basis of Therapeutics*, Hardman, J.G., Limbird, L.E., Molinoff, P.B., Ruddon, R.W., and Gillman, A.G., Eds., McGraw-Hill, New York, 1996, chap. 22.
14. Pras, N., Woerdenbag, H.J., Batterman, S., Visser, J.F., and Van Uden, W., Mucuna pruriens: improvement of the biotechnological production of the anti-Parkinson drug L-dopa by plant cell selection, *Pharm. World Sci.*, 15(6), 263, 1993.
15. Anon., An alternative medicine treatment for Parkinson's disease: results of a multicenter clinical trial. HP-200 in Parkinson's disease study group, *J. Alt. Complement. Med.*, 1, 249, Fall 1995.
16. Schleibs, R., Liebmann, A., Bhattacharya, S.K., Kumar, A., Ghosal, S., and Bigle, V., Systemic administration of defined extracts from Withania somnifera and shilajit differentially affects cholinergic but not glutamatergic and GABAergic markers with rat brain, *Neurochem. Int.*, 30, 181–190, 1997.
17. Nagashayana, N., Sankarankutty, P., Nampoothiri, M.R., Mohan, P.K., and Mohanakumar, K.P.J., Association of L-DOPA with recovery following Ayurveda medication in Parkinson's disease, *Neurol., Sci.*, 176, 124, 2000.
18. Srividya, M. et al., Lead case study on Kampavata treated with the compound Parkino, presented to World Ayurveda Congress, Kochin, Kerala, India, 2002.

27

Male Reproductive Dysfunction

Mohammad Abdulkadar Akbarsha, Appian Subramoniam, and Viswanatha Menon Madhavachandran

CONTENTS

27.1 Introduction

The role of the male in the sexual process and reproduction is twofold: (1) to successfully perform sexual intercourse, deriving pleasure for himself and satisfying the female partner,

0-8493-1366-X/04/$0.00+$1.50

and (2) to contribute the sperm for successful fertilization of the ovum toward procreation. The problem of male infertility and impotency is increasing day by day. The global incidence of couple infertility is estimated at 10 to 15%.[1] The contribution of the male factor alone to couple infertility is believed to be about 20%.[2] Between 20 and 30 million American men suffer from some degree of sexual dysfunction, and a comparative figure generally applies worldwide.[3] Further, there are several lines of evidence to suggest that sperm counts are decreasing globally[4] and the incidence of erectile dysfunction is also on the increase.[5] The increase in male factor infertility in recent times is believed to be caused by altered lifestyle, stressful living conditions, diverse pollutants, certain prescription and several nonprescription drugs, dietary toxins, and certain nutritional deficiencies.[6–21] The causative factors produce many types of derangements that directly or indirectly cause various kinds sexual dysfunction.

The remedy for male sexual dysfunction in modern medicine is limited. The fact remains that, other than correction of obstruction, infections, varicocele, and certain endocrine abnormalities, in most cases there is practically no successful therapeutic measure for male infertility or erectile dysfunction except for surgical implants. The allopathic drugs used for erectile dysfunction are believed to produce side effects and affect other physiological processes and, ultimately, general health.[22] Ayurveda realized the problem of male sexual dysfunction thousands of years ago and developed a separate speciality, namely, reproductive medicine (*vaajeekarana*). It realized, among other things, the role of the nervous system, cardiovascular system, and psychological aspects of fertility and male sexual performance; it has also recommended an appropriate use of plant-based remedies, a proper lifestyle, and nutritious diet for improving overall health and treating male infertility and erectile dysfunction. Over 600 plants are described in the original Ayurvedic compendia like *Charak Samhita* and *Sushruta Samhita*. The potential of Ayurvedic and other traditional medicinal plants in the development of invaluable standardized phytomedicines and allopathic type of drugs is great, particularly in the context of male sexual dysfunction.

This chapter is an attempt to review the Ayurvedic concepts of male sexual dysfunction and the potential of Ayurvedic treatments for the same, with plant-based remedies as seen in the classical Ayurvedic treatises as well as in the modern practice. An attempt has also been made to review the pharmacological and biochemical studies on the plants and plant products that are in use in Ayurvedic therapy for problems in male reproduction. The need for more elaborate scientific investigations on the Ayurvedic therapy for male sexual dysfunction is emphasized.

27.2 Male Reproductive Dysfunction

The description of several ailments relating to male reproduction in Ayurveda has relevance to the modern science and clinical practices. *Charak Samhita* is perhaps the earliest medical treatise recognizing that the semen released during orgasm at the time of sexual intercourse is responsible for the development of the embryo and that defective semen is incapable of producing the fetus. Male reproductive disorders, as dealt with in classical Ayurvedic literatures, can be due to two major causes: (1) defective semen and (2) impotence (*viryalpata* or *klaibyam*).

27.2.1 Defective Semen

Ayurveda describes semen as oily, viscous, nonslimy, sweet, and nonburning with the smell of honey. It is white with a glaze similar to honey, dehydrated butter (ghee), or til (*Sesamum orientale*) oil. The total quantity of semen during ejaculation is 2 to 4 oz. Semen can become defective due to different causes. Excessive indulgence in sex or having sex at wrong times, masturbation, excessive exercise, eating an excess of bitter, astringent, salty, sour, or hot foods, old age, anxiety, grief, suspicion, fear, anger, exorcism, emaciation from disease, and suppression of natural urges and wounds can lead to the derangement of *tridosas* of tissues. This derangement can reach the semen-producing organs and carrying channels causing semen defects.

According to Ayurveda there are eight types of defective semen: *vatarethas, pittarethas, kapharethas, kunaparethas, grandhirethas, poothipooyarethas, ksheenarethas,* and *moothrapureesharethas*. The definitions, etiology, and prognosis of and treatments for each are furnished in Table 27.1.

27.2.2 Causes of Impotence

Main causes of impotence are basically (1) impaired and deficient semen (see Section 27.2.1) and (2) erectile dysfunction.

Erectile dysfunction (*dhwajabhangam*) results from ingesting excess, sour, salty, heavy, incompatible, and unsuitable foods, and drinking excess water. Other causes are irregular meals, excess use of milk and milk products, weakness from illness, defective seminal tract, excessive discharge, coitus with animals, and failing to clean the penis and injured genitals. Diet and lifestyle are emphasized as the causative factors for erectile dysfunction in addition to genetic causes.

There are five types of erectile dysfunction: *vatajam, pittajam, kaphajam, rakthajam,* and *sannipathajam*; detailed information about each is furnished in Table 27.2.

Old age often causes diminished semen and is related to deficiency of the seven body tissues or transformations (*dhathus*).

27.2.3 Eunuchs (*Napumsak*)

Sushruta Samhita characterizes five types of eunuchs: *asyeka, saugandhikam, kumbheeka, eershyakam,* and *shandakam* (Table 27.3). These eunuchs are to be inferred essentially as male perversion. Perhaps these eunuchs, except *shandakam*, shall have no relevance in the modern context. *Charak Samhita* describes eight types of eunuchs: *dviretha, pavanednriya, samskaravahi, narashanda, nareeshanda, vakri, eershyabhirathi,* and *vatheekashanda* (Table 27.4). Although most etiology part may not be acceptable in modern science, at least these types are parallel with modern clinical practices.

27.3 Treatment

Considering the gravity of male infertility, one part of octapartite Ayurvedic therapeutic speciality called semen therapy (*beeja poshana*) is devoted to the therapy for male infertility.

TABLE 27.1

Eight Types of Defective Semen as Identified in Ayurveda

Type	Definition	Etiology	Prognosis	Treatment
Vatarethas	Dark-colored frothy semen; painful ejaculation	*Vata*; vitiated by wrong lifestyle and food habits	Easily curable	Oliation, fomentation, purgation, catheterization, enema through penis, etc., along with medicines like *jeevaneeya ghrutham, chyavan prash*, and *shilajit*
Pittarethas	Yellow-colored very hot semen; burning sensation and pain during ejaculation	*Pitta*; vitiated by wrong lifestyle and food habits	Easily curable	Oliation, fomentation, catheterization, enema through penis, etc., along with medicines like *jeevaneya ghrutham, chyavan prash*, and *shilajit*
Kapharethas	Whitish, slimy, semen; obstructed and painful ejaculation	*Kapha*; vitiated by wrong lifestyle and food habits	Easily curable	Oliation, fomentation, purgation, catheterization, enema through penis, etc., along with medicines like *jeevaneya ghrutham, chyavan prash*, and *shilajit*
Kunaparethas	Cadaver-smelling semen; increased in volume	Vitiated by excessive coitus, injury, wound and by wrong lifestyle and food habits, leading to deterioration of quality of blood	Curable	*Woodfordia floribunda*, *Acacia catechu*, *Punica granatum* (fruit cover), and *Terminalia arjuna* (bark) prepared in butter
Grandirethas	Tissue-like semisolid semen; obstructed and painful ejaculation	*Kapha* and *vata* viatiated by wrong lifestyle and food habits	Curable	*Kaempferia galanga*, or *Rotula aquatica* (root), or ash of *Butea monosperma* prepared in ghee
Poothipooyarethas	Puslike and malodorous semen	*Pitta* and *kapha* vitiated by wrong lifestyle and food habits	Curable	*Parooshakadi ganam* or *nyagrodhadi ganam* prepared in ghee
Ksheenarethas	Decreased quantity and quality of semen; delayed ejaculation; blood stains in semen	*Vata* and *pitta* vitiated by excessive coitus, excessive exercise, wrong lifestyle and food habits	Curable	*Panchakarma rasayana* and *vajeekarana* treatment
Moothrapure-esharethas	Semen smells like urine and feces	All three *dosas*, vitiated by wrong lifestyle and food habits	Incurable	—

The basic principle of treatment in Ayurveda is to assist the body to heal itself. The Ayurvedic fundamental principles of repletion (*samtarpana* and *brmhana*) and depletion (*apatarpana* and *langhana*), consisting of radical (*sodhana*) and conservation (*samana*) treatments, apply to therapy for male sexual dysfunction, also. Radical therapy adopts techniques to drain the waste materials of different body compartments through the nearest channel in a system-friendly manner. Radical therapy, followed by repletion and reproductive medicine therapy, can probably improve the male reproductive function by cre-

TABLE 27.2

Classification of Erectile Dysfunction in Ayurveda

Types	Features
Vatajam	Effusion, pain, redness
Pittajam	Carbuncles and pus
Kaphajam	Increased penis size, lesions, discharge with reddish or dark color, ring-like processes near the root of penis
Rakthajam	Fever, burning sensation, vertigo, dizziness and vomiting; blackish red, red, or blue discharge
Sannipathajam (all the *dosas* acting together)	Pain and burning sensation in urinary bladder, testicles, and seminal vesicles; white and slimy discharge will be present; penis effused; eventually gets infected with pathogens; foul smell; rotted tip of the penis; entire penis and testicles can rot and wither off

TABLE 27.3

Eunuchs According to *Sushruta Samhita*

Type	Feature	Etiology
Asyeka	Erection occurs only when one drinks the semen of another person	Due to quantitative inadequacy of semen and *rethas*
Saugandikam	Erection occurs only when one smells the vagina or penis	Birth in a malodorous vagina
Kumbheeka	Erection occurs only when another person enters him through the anus	Not mentioned
Eershyakam	Erection occurs only when one sees another person making love	Not mentioned
Shandakam	Person has body structure and behavior of a woman	Due to father making love lying on his back

ating an optimal environment for spermatogenesis and improving intratesticular availability of nutrients.

The concept of radical therapy is highly relevant today in the light of studies emerging with evidence that the real culprits of infertility are the various tissue toxins (gonadotoxins).[15] These chemicals mimic hormones and impair their secretion, resulting in disruption of the normal physiological processes. Ayurveda recognizes the concept of weak toxins and it considers these toxins as one of the causes of subfertility.

As has been explained earlier, the etiology of the various diseases in Ayurvedic perspective is to be traced to the three basic states of the body (the *tridosas*), namely, *vata*, *pitta*, and *kapha*. Any aspect of male sexual dysfunction shall be reflection of any one or more of the *tridosas*. In fact, onset of a disease is due to an upset of the equilibrium of the three *dosas* and the seven tissues or the body transformation processes.

Charak Samhita recognizes the semen-producing and -transmitting parts of the body (*sukravahastrotas*). Depletion of hormones (*ojas*) and disruption in the semen-producing and -transmitting organs can lead to one or more of the manifestations of male sexual dysfunction. Hormones are considered to be the physical expression of consciousness in the body and play a role in immunity and procreation. The Ayurvedic remedy for male

TABLE 27.4

Eunuchs According to *Charak Samhita*

Type	Feature	Etiology
Dviretha	Person having physical characteristics of a man but behaves like a woman	Zygote produced with sperm and ovum having equal dominance
Pavanendriya	Person has erection but no ejaculation	Testicles of fetus destroyed by *vata*
Samskaravahi	Person has damaged seminal vesicles	Seminal vesicles damaged by *vata* due to vitiation of *dosas*), accident, or by birth
Narashanda	Male with weak sexual urges, poor semen volume, poor ejaculation, or has no interest in sexual intercourse	Father should have had these qualities
Nareeshanda	Female with weak sexual urges, poor menstrual flow, or no interest in sexual intercourse	Mother should have had these qualities
Vakri	No erection at all	Either the mother had little interest in sexual intercourse or sperm of father had weak sexual urges
Eershyabhirathi	Erection occurs only when one sees another person making love	Male and female getting angry during coitus
Vatheekashanda	Due to *in utero* destruction of testicles; azoospermic	Vitiated by *agni* or *vata*, testicles destroyed during early pregnancy

sexual dysfunction is aimed not only at the immediate etiological factors of the disease, but also toward improving the hormonal status of the body. For example, according to Charaka, in the case of seminal debility a patient must first be prepared for the therapy through cleansing the body by purgation and, if necessary, by vomiting. Then he must be given liquid diet and gradually transferred to the natural food so as to improve the body's overall health. The specific treatment for increasing the semen and the aphrodisiacs can be practiced either concurrently or in sequence. This is very clearly reflected in the various combinations of herbals and other traditional medicinal ingredients in the various Ayurvedic formulations for male sexual dysfunction.

27.3.1 Polyherbal Formulations

27.3.1.1 Classic Formulas

Among the several polyherbal formulas in the Ayurvedic system of medicine, such as *ghrutham, rasayana, kashyam, lehyam, etc.*, each formula has one or more ingredients that can take care of male sexual debility. Information about a few of the most important classical Ayurvedic polyherbal formulations is furnished in Table 27.5, and more detailed information is found in classic texts.

Ashtangahrudayam, in the volume *Utharasthanam*, lists several combinations of herbals and other ingredients for management of male reproductive dysfunction (Table 27.6). In the modern practice, the formulations have been changed or altered by the individual Ayurvredic practitioners, based on their experiences.

27.3.1.2 Nonclassic Formulas

Although the classical Ayurvedic approach in therapy is still practiced, there has been a rewarding blend of the Ayurvedic approach and the modern allopathic approach through adopting phytochemistry and pharmacology. Further, though the birthplace of

TABLE 27.5

Classical Polyherbal Ayurvedic Formulations Used in Treating Male Sexual Debility

No.	Name	Textbook Reference
1	*Chyavan prash*	*Ashtangahrudayam*
2	*Kalyanaka ghrutham*	*Ashtangahrudayam*
3	*Phalasarpsis*	*Ashtangahrudayam*
4	*Sathavaryadi ghrutham*	*Sahasrayogam*
5	*Sukumaram ghrutham*	*Ashtangahrudayam*
6	*Kalyanakam kashayam*	*Sahasrayogam*
7	*Sukumaram kashayam*	*Ashtangahrudayam*
8	*Vidaryadi kashayam*	*Ashtangahrudayam*
9	*Sukumaram lehyam*	*Ashtangahrudayam*
10	*Vidaryadi lehyam*	*Ashtangahrudayam*
11	*Narasimha rasayanam*	*Ashtangahrudayam*
12	*Sathavari gulam*	*Sahasrayogam*
13	*Ashwagandhadi lehyam*	*Bhaishajyaratnavali*
14	*Amruthaprasa rasayanam*	*Ashtangahrudayam*
15	*Ashwagandharishtam*	*Bhaishajyaratnavali*
16	*Dhasamoolarishtam*	*Bhaishajyaratnavali*
17	*Jeevaneya ganam*	*Ashtangahrudayam*
18	*Nyagrodhadi ganam*	*Ashtangahrudayam*
19	*Parooshskadi ganam*	*Ashtangahrudayam*
20	*Bala thailam*	*Sahasrayogam*

Note: Only some of the Ayurvedic manufacturers, who produce generic Ayurvedic preparations, have all these products. Examples include (1) Vaidyarethnam P.S. Varier's Arya vaidhya sala, Kottakal, Malappuram District, Kerala, India; (2) Vaidyarethnam Oushadasala, Thaikkattuseri, Ollur, Thirusur District, Kerala, India; (3) Nagarjuna Herbal Concentrates Ltd., Kalayanthani, Thodupuzha, Kerala, India.

Ayurveda is India, it has come to be adopted worldwide in which traditional medicine processes of the different regions of the world have been blended. Currently, many patent formulas are the blend of Ayurvedic herbs along with some herbs in other countries. In this process of blending, micronutrients and hormones are also managed. A few such combinations are currently marketed, and their trade names are in Table 27.7. As evident in the following section, very few of these medicinal plants have been subjected to pharmacological testing.

27.4 Scientific Basis

27.4.1 Ayurvedic Herbs

One of the major pitfalls in Ayurvedic therapy in general, and for male sexual dysfunction in particular, is that there is very little research with regard to pharmacological testing and clinical trials. Further, as could be seen from the various chapters in this book, the same herb (e.g., *Withania somnifera*, *Asparagus racemosus*, *Tribulus terrestris*, etc.) is used therapeutically for several ailments. Within this limitation an attempt has been made to review the scientific investigations made on a few of the herbals consistently used as remedials in male sexual dysfunction in the various combinations.

TABLE 27.6

Ayurvedic Formulations for the Treatment of Male Reproductive Dysfunction (Ashtanga Hrudayam, Utharasthanam)

Combination	Ingredients
Combination 1: To increase the power of erection and number of coitus	*Taccharum munja* (root), *Saccharum officinarum* (stem), *Desmostachya bipinnata* (whole plant), *Desmostachys* spp., *Adenia hondala* (tuber), *Vetiveria zizanoides* (root), *Solanum surattense, Malaxis acuminata* (wet stem), *Malaxis muscifera* (wet stem), *Sida rhombifolia* (root and leaves), *Polygonatum cirrhifolium, Polygonatum vertcillatum* (root stock), *Fritillaria roylei* (stem), *Lilium polyphyllum* (bulb), *Atylosia goensis* (seed), *Phaseolus trilobus* (seed), *Asparagus racemosus* (tuber), *Withania somnifera* (tuber), Vellooppam, *Mucuna pruriens* (seed), *Boerhaavia diffusa* (whole plant), *Coccinia grandis* (root), *Ipomoea paniculata* (tuber), *Holostemma ada-kodien* (tuber), *Cassia absus* (seed), *Alpinia somnifera* (rhizome), *Tribulus terrestris* (fruit), *Glycyrrhiza glabra* (root), *Desmodium gangeticum* (root), *Phaseolus roxburghii* (seed), *Emblica officinalis* (fruit), cow's milk, *Ficus racemosa* (fruit), *Piper longum* (dried spike), *Scindapsus officinalis* (dried spike), *Vitis vinifera* (fruit), *Phoenix dactylifera, Madhuca longifolia* (flower), sugar, *Curcuma angustifolia* (rhizome), *Piper nigrum, Cinnamomum zeylanicum* (bark), *Cinnamomum tamala* (leaves), *Elettaria cardamomum* (seed), *Mesua ferrea* (flower) honey
Combination 2: For vitality	*Ipomoea paniculata* (tuber), *Piper longum* (dried spike), *Oryza* sp. (seed), *Buchanania lanzan, Hygrophila auriculata* (seed), *Mucuna pruriens* (seed), honey, sugar, ghee
Combination 3: For vitality	*Mucuna pruriens* (seed), *Triticum aestivum* (seed), cow's milk, ghee, honey
Combination 4: For vitality	Cow's milk, ghee, honey, *Phaseolus mungo* (seed)
Combination 5: For vitality	*Mucuna pruriens* (seed), cow's milk, *Sesamum indicum* (seed), sugar
Combination 6: For vitality	*Ipomoea paniculata* (tuber), ghee, honey
Combination 7: For senile impotence	*Emblica officinalis* (fruit), ghee, sugar, cow's milk, *Piper longum*
Combination 8: To quicken ejaculation	*Glycyrrhiza glabra* (root), ghee, cow's milk, honey
Combination 9: For impotence	*Pistacia integerrima* (galls), cow's milk, ghee, sugar
Combination 10: To increase sperm count	*Holostemma ada-kodien* (tuber), cow's milk, ghee, honey
Combination 11: To prolong coitus	*Curculigo orchioides* (tuber), *Asparagus racemosus* (tuber), sugar, cow's milk
Combination 12. Senile impotence	Watery portion of curd, sugar, *Oryza* sp.
Combination 13: Senile impotence	*Tribulus terrestris* (fruit), *Hygrophila auriculata* (seed), *Phaseolus roxburghii* (seed), *Mucuna pruriens (seed), Asparagus racemosus* (tuber), cow's milk

Note: Information in parentheses refers to the part used.

27.4.1.1 Asparagus racemosus

Asparagus racemosus is considered as an aphrodisiac to both males and females.[23] In traditional medicine, the plant is used as a refringent, demulcent, diuretic, aphrodisiac, anticeptic, alterative, antidiarrheal, antidysentery, and galactagogue agent. It is also used for nervous and rheumatic complaints. The roots are rejuvenating and carminative; they are also used as an appetizer, stomachic, and tonic.

27.4.1.2 Cynomorium coccineum

The aqueous extract of this plant increased the weight of the testes, diameter of the seminiferous tubules, and the number of tubular cell layers in immature rats. It also elicited notable spermatogenesis in the immature rats. However, serum testosterone and follicle

TABLE 27.7

Aphrodisiac Formulations Available in the Market

Product	Ingredients	Contact
Adam's Secrets	Yohimbe, *Avena sativa*, androstenedione, saw palmetto, guarana, taurine, Siberian ginseng, *Tribulus terrestris*	E-mail: info@adamssecrets.com
ArginMax for Men	L-Arginine; ginseng; ginkgo; vitamins A, C, E, B-complex; selenium, zinc, niacin	Web: www.arginmax.com
Ascend for Men	Oats, nettle, saw palmetto, damiana, zinc	Web: www.herbalremedies.com
BetterMan	Radix ginseng (ginseng root), *Rhizoma dioscoreae* (yam rhizomes), *Radix paeoniae* alba (white peony root), *Herba epimedii* (aerial parts of epimedium), *Cornu cervi* pantotrichum (deer antler), *Radix astragali* (astragalus root), *Poria cocos* (poria fungus), *Radix morindae* officinalis (morinda root), *Fructus corni* (Cornus fruit), cortex eucommiac (wood cotton bark), *Radix angelicae* sinensis (dong quai root), *Fructus lycii* (wolfberry fruit), *Radix rehmanniae* (rehmannia root), rhizoma chuanxiong (Szechuan Lovage root), *Fructus schisandrae* (Schisandra fruit), *Acanthopanax senticosus* (Siberian ginseng), *Cynomorium songaricum* rupr (fleshy stem of cynomorium), cortex cinnamomi (cinnamon bark)	Web: www.worldclassnutrition/ phonoremor.html
Count Plus	*Mucuna pruriens, Withania somnifera, Holostemma adakodien, Sida rhombifolia, Curculigo orchioides, Asparagus racemosus, Hygrophila auriculata, Glycyrhiza glabra,* cow's milk, ghee	E-mail: nhcltdpa@md5.vsnl.net.in
Endow Plus	Yohimbe, damiana, guarana, wild oats, sarsparilla, ginkgo biloba, saw palmetto	Web: www.tiger-one.com
HerbalArouse–M	Zinc, selenium, manganese, *Lepidium meyenii* (extract), L-Arginine, L-Methionine, ginkgo biloba (extract), *Eleutherococcus senticosus* (extract), *Withania somnifera* (extract), *Scocolens forskohilii* (extract), *Tribulus terrestris* (extract), *Lirosma ovata* (extract), *Avena sativa* (extract), gelatin, *Tilophora indica* (extract), bioperine (piperine), bovine orchic substance, magnesium, dihydroepiandrosterone	Web: www.healingedge.net
Horny Goat Weed	*Epimedium grandiflorum* (horny goat weed), *Lepidium meyenii* (maca pure), *Mucuna pruriens, Polypodium vulgare*	Web: www.pinnaclebody.com
Horny Goat Weed Capsules	*Epimedium grandifolium* (extract), *Schisandra chinensis* (extract), Psoralia coryflora (extract)	E-mail: cielo@cieloherbals.com
Horny Goat Weed Plus	*Epimedium sagittatum* (horny goat weed), *Tribulus terrestris* (puncture vine), *Ptychopetalum uncinatum* (muira puama), *Avena sativa* (wild oats), *Turnera diffusa* (damiana), Korean ginseng, acanthopanax senticosus (Siberian ginseng), gingko biloba, nettle, vitamin B6, zinc	Web: www.discountnaturalherbd.com

TABLE 27.7 (continued)

Aphrodisiac Formulations Available in the Market

Product	Ingredients	Contact
Libido-X	Tea tree oil, yohimbe, damiana, saw palmetto, passion flower, Chinese hibiscus	Web: www.male-sexual-enhancement.com
Nirvana	*Tribulus terrestris, Mucuna pruriens, Withania somnifera, Matthiola incana, Cherianthus cheiri, Salvia haematodes, Centaura behen*	Web: www.herbal-nirvana.com
Teenex Capsules	*Withania somnifera (ashwagandh), Mucuna pruriens* (cow hage), *trivang, Nux vomuca, Hygrophila spinosa, shilajit, Myristica fragrans, Ancyclus pyrephrum*, mikardhwaj, *Crocus sativus* (saffron)	E-mail: odpl@sancharnet.in
Vibro Plus	*Ptychopetalum uncinatum* (muira pauma root), catuaba, Jamaican ginger, echinacea, *Turnea diffusa* (damiana), panax ginseng (ginseng), *Avena sativa* (wild oat), cayenne, schizandra, yohimbe bark	E-mail: vhssales@viable-herbal.com
Vigor™	Borage oil, organic flaxseed oil, puncture vine, *Withania somnifera* (extract), gingko biloba (extract), zinc sulphate, vitamin E, gingerol, pyridoxine HCl, folic acid	Fax: (713) 683-8796/920-1917 E-mail: Jac53@prodigy.net
Vita Sex	*Epimedium sagittatum* (horny goats weed), *Tribulus terrestris* (puncture vine), *Ptychopetalum uncinatum* (muira puama), *Eleutherococcus senticosus* (Siberian ginseng), *Withania somnifera* (ashwagandha), *Turnera diffusa* (damiana), *Lepidium meyenii* (maca), Smilax officinalis (sarsaparilla), ginkgo biloba	E-mail: health@feelgoodnatural.com

Source: From various Web sources. Constituents are listed as found in their respective Web sites. The authors do not hold responsibility to the accuracy; the list is not exhaustive but only indicative.

stimulating hormone (FSH) levels were lowered in the treated animals. It was suggessted that the plant extract may have direct spermatogenic effect on the seminiferous tubules of the immature rats, presumably by exerting a testosterone-like effect. This plant extract is better than *Withania somnifera* in this respect.[24]

In 25-day-old rats, extracts of *Cynomorium coccineum* elicited significant changes in gonodotrophin levels coupled with a significant increase in the ovarian weight and profound folliculogenesis. In 7-day-old animals, these changes were not observed.[25,26]

No citable clinical studies for this plant showing curative effects for male sexual dysfunction were found.

27.4.1.3 Mucuna pruriens

Mucuna pruriens seed powder, when administrated at the dose of 75 mg/kg/day, increased the sexual activity of the male albino rats considerably. The different components of copulatory behavior, including mount frequency, mount latency, intromission frequency, and intromission latency, were found to be influenced by the test drug. The plant contains, among other things, levadopa (L-DOPA), which is reported to arouse sexual desire in patients suffering from Parkinson's disease.[27]

Earlier, the total alkaloids from the seeds of *M. pruriens*, composed of five alkaloidal bases, were found to increase the population of spermatozoa and weight of the testes, seminal vesicles, and prostate in the albino rat. Isolation of various chemical constituents has been reported. Beta sitosterol has been isolated from unsaponisable part of the petroleum ether extract of the seeds.[28,29] No citable clinical studies for this plant showing curative effects for male sexual dysfunction were found.

27.4.1.4 *Piper longum*

In Ayurveda and folk medicine, *Piper longum* fruit is an important ingredient of herbal mixtures used as aphrodisiacs and sexual tonics. This is also supported by animal experiments. Acute (2-h) and chornic (90-day) oral toxicity studies of the ethanolic extract of *Piper longum* were carried out in mice. *Piper longum* extract (0.1 g/kg for 90 days) caused a significant increase in the weight of the lungs and spleen in the treated animals. Interestingly, the extract induced a significant increase in the weight of the reproductive organs, sperm motility, and sperm count but failed to elicit any spermatotoxic effect.[30] However, it exerted antifertility effect in female rats.[31] No citable clinical studies for this plant showing curative effects for male sexual dysfunction were found.

27.4.1.5 *Tribulus terrestris*

Tribulus terrestris is used as a diuretic, cardiotonic, aphrodisiac, emollient, appetiser, expectorant, laxative, etc. It is also used to cure cough, asthma, anemia, and inflammation, and in treatment of male urinary problems and impotence.[32] *Tribulus terrestris* extract has been found to increase testosterone and spermatogenesis in male animals.[33]

Tribulus terrestris extract (2.5 to 10 mg/kg) treatment for 8 weeks daily resulted in an increase in the relaxation of penile tissue isolated from treated animals compared with that in the control. The relaxant response to electrical field simulation, acetyl choline, and nitroglycerin in noradrenaline-treated precoxified corpus cavernosal tissue from the treated group was found to be higher compared with that in the control. It was concluded that the enhanced relaxant effect observed was probably due to an increase in the release of nitric oxide from the endothelium and nitrinergic nerve endings, which may account for its claim as an aphrodisiac.[34]

The alkaloids isolated from *T. terrestris*, harmane and nor-harmane (54 mg/kg), caused limb paresis which, in some sheep, was body-side based. It was proposed that these alkaloids accumulate in tryptamine-associated neurons of the central nervous system (CNS) during months of tribulus feeding and gradually interact irreversibly with a specific neuronal gene dexoribonucleic acid sequence.[35]

A recent study has shown that protodioscin, a phytochemical in *T. terrestris*, improves sexual desire and enhances erection via the conversion of protodioscin to dehydroepiandrosterone.[36–38] No citable clinical study for this plant showing curative effects for male sexual dysfunction was found.

27.4.1.6 *Tricopus zeylanicus*

Recently, it has been shown that the ethanol extract of *Tricopus zeylanicus* has aphrodisiac activity in male mice as evidenced by an increase in the number of mounts and mating performance. Repeated daily administration was more effective than a single dose. The pups fathered by the treated mice were found to be normal with respect to fetal growth, litter size, and sex ratio.[39] No citable clinical studies for this plant showing curative effects for male sexual dysfunction were found.

27.4.1.7 *Vanda tessellata*

Screening of orchids for aphrodisiac activity in male mice resulted in the identification of remarkable aphrodisiac activity in *Vanda tessellata*. The flower and, to some extent, the root (but not the leaf) were found to stimulate the mounting behavior of male mice. This activity was found in the alcoholic extract of the flower. The flower extract (50 or 200 mg/kg) increased mating performance in mice. The pups fathered by the extract-treated mice were found to be normal with an increasing trend in the male/female ratio of the pups. Preliminary toxicity studies have shown no conspicuous toxicity in mice.[40,41] No citable clinical studies for this plant showing curative effects for male sexual dysfunction were found.

27.4.1.8 *Withania somnifera*

Recent studies have shown that the aqueous extract of *Withania somnifera* (*ashwagandha*) increased the testicular weight, the diameter of seminiferous tubules, and the number of seminiferous tubular cell layers in the immature rats. Further, the extract of the plant elicited notable spermatogenesis in the rat. However, serum testosterone and FSH levels were lower, whereas the luteinizing hormome (LH) level was higher in the treated animals. It was concluded that the extract has a direct spermatogenic influence on the seminiferous tubules of immature rats, presumably by exerting a testosterone-like effect.[24] An investigation was conducted to test the curative property of *W. somnifera* root powder in the context of derangements in spermatogenesis caused by treatment of the fungicide carbendazim (methyl 2–benzimidazole carbomate) in Wistar rats. It was found that when the root powder was suspended in milk and fed through oral route to the affected rats, spermatogenesis was restored to the full status (Akbarsha and Kadalmani, unpublished observation). No citable clinical studies for this plant showing curative effect for male sexual dysfunction were found.

27.4.1.9 *Shilajit, the Black Asphaltum*

Shilajit, a popular incredient in several Ayurvedic preparations, is considered an aphrodisiac. It has been suggested that it be taken with *Withania somnifera* in order to combat sexual weakness.[23]

27.4.1.10 *Zingiber officinale*

Studies on experimental animals indicate that *Z. officinalis* (ginger) significantly increases sperm counts and motility.[42]

27.4.2 Non-Ayurvedic Herbs

The following herbs are not cited in Ayurveda but are used in other countries, such as the U.S., to treat male sexual dysfunction.

27.4.2.1 *Ginseng*

Ginseng is one of the plants subjected to a fairly extensive scientific investigation for application in male sexual dysfunction. The studies have concerned three ginseng plants, *Panax ginseng* (Asian ginseng), *P. quinquefolium* (American ginseng), and *Ganoderma japonicum* (Korean red ginseng). Ginsenosides, which are glycosidic compounds, in the ginseng plant, are the active compounds under consideration. These compounds are, by and large, antioxidants and enhance nitric oxide (NO) synthesis in the endothelium of many organs, including the corpus cavernosum, which is the erectile tissue of the penis. Ginsenosides also enhance acetylcholine-induced and transmural nerve stimulation-activated relaxation associated with increased tissue cyclic guanosinemonophosphate. Both these properties appear to qualify ginsenosides as male aphrodisiacs.[43] However, it is important to test the efficacy of ginseng in humans by means of appropriately designed double-blind, placebo-controlled clinical studies in a large scale and under the various causative conditions of infertility and erectile dysfunction.[44]

27.4.2.1.1 Animal Studies

Under the influence of ginseng, male mice began ejaculation earlier and repeated the action more often in a 45-min observation period and deposited more copulation plugs in 10 days.[45] Male rats that were administered American ginseng were stimulated in copulatory behavior,[46] unaccompanied by any change in the circulating levels of testosterone and LH. The prolactin level was reduced, suggesting that ginsenosides affect the pituitary gland directly.[47] In a different approach, it was shown that daily treatment of mice with an extract of Asian ginseng (2.5 to 100 mg/kg intraperitoneally [i.p.]) or ginsenoside Rg1 (2.5 to 10 mg/kg i.p.) produced a dose-related increase in the number of mice displaying copulatory behavior; ginsenosides Rb1, Rb2, and Ro did not have any effect.[48] *In vivo* and *in vitro* studies on the corpus cavernosal endothelium of rabbit showed that ginsenosides enhanced the release of NO.[49,50] Ginsenosides also enhance acetylcholine-induced and transmural nerve stimulation-elicited relaxation in the rabbit corpus cavernosum.[49] These results suggest that the effects of ginseng extract on corpus caverenosum tissue are mediated by the release of NO from the endothelial cells and perivisceral nerves.[47]

There is at least one animal study that does not recommend the use of ginseng in male sexual dysfunction.[51] In this study, feeding male rats with a diet supplemented with the ginseng extract G115 produced little change in the sexual performance.

27.4.2.1.2 Clinical Studies

There are two reports of clinical studies testing the efficacy of Korean red ginseng in treating erectile dysfunction. The first study[52] consisted of a total of 90 patients in 3 groups of 30 each (ginseng-treated, placebo-controlled, and trazodone [a proerectile drug treated]). It was reported that in the ginseng-treated patients, changes in early detumescence and erectile parameters, such as penile rigidity and girth, libido, and patient satisfaction, were significantly higher than in the other groups, and the overall therapeutic efficiencies on erectile dysfunction were 60% for ginseng group and 30% for placebo- and trazodone-treated groups. The second investigation[53] was a double-blind, placebo-controlled, crossover study in which a total of 45 patients with clinically diagnosed erectile dysfunction were enrolled. The treatment dosage was 900 mg of Korean ginseng or placebo, 3 times/day for first 8 weeks; this was followed by a 2-week wash-out period where the patients received crossover treatment. It was shown that ginseng treatment increased penetration, maintenance, and Rigiscan test outcome.

27.4.2.2 Yohimbe

The bark of *yohimbe* (*Pausinistalia yohimbe*), an African tree, is the source of yohimbine hydrochloride; in short, yohimbine is an indolequinolonic alkaloid. It has been used historically for several years as a treatment for male and female sexual dysfunction.[54]

Yohimbine is an established alpha 2-adrenoceptor antagonist.[55] Its action at the CNS and the central endocrine mechanisms is believed to increase sexual arousal.[56,57]

27.4.2.2.1 Animal Studies

In an early study of the male rat, it was shown that yohimbine increased mounting performance, the percentage of male rats ejaculating in their first heterosexual encounter, and induction of copulatory behavior in sexually inactive male rats.[56] It was later shown that yohimbine treatment caused a decrease in the ejaculatory latency, postejaculatory interval, and intercopulatory interval.[58] In a more recent study, male golden hamsters were administered i.p. with yohimbine at a single dose of 2 mg/kg body weight 30 min prior to a number of sexual behavior tests. It was found in the treated animals, when compared with the saline-injected controls, that aspects of male sexual behavior, including ejaculatory frequency, were increased.[59]

27.4.2.2.2 Clinical Studies

There are a few clinical reports encouraging the use of yohimbine in erectile dysfunction.[60–69] A few authors have opined that these studies are poorly designed trials, that yohimbine does not appear to have any modest therapeutic benefit over placebo,[54,70] and that the drug has not yet been subjected to scientifically rigorous clinical trials.[71] In the most recent clinical studys of 18 men between the ages 40 to 80 years, who were not active smokers,[72] were given doses of 5.4 mg of yohimbine three times/day for 4 weeks; the doses were then increased to 10.8 mg three times/day for another 4 weeks. Results showed that 50% of patients had a positive effect, an improvement over the already reported success histories.[60,61,64,65] An earlier clinical study[69] also supports the view that yohimbine could be therapeutic in the case of nonorganismic impotence. Another study[73] in Brazil examined 22 patients with organismic impotence, all serving as placebo control for 1 month, who were later treated with 100 mg of yohimbine once a day for 1 month. Results did not encourage the use of yohimbine in male sexual dysfunction, supporting the view of Danjou et al.[74]

27.4.2.3 *Lepedium meyenii* (Maca)

Lepedium meyenii is a domesticated crop of the Andean Mountains of Central Peru, cultivated at an altitude of 3000 m and above. Its subterranean part (hypocotyle) is edible and highly valued for its nutritive value. For several hundred years it has been used by the Andean Indians as food and folk medicine and used to increase the fertility and sexual performance of men and women. There have been a few attempts of scientific investigation on the application of this plant as a male aphrodisiac and as a curative of sexual dysfunction.

27.4.2.3.1 Animal Studies

Purified lipidic fraction of the alcoholic extract of dried maca roots was produced into two formulae, namely, M-01 and M-02, differing in the concentration of macaene and macamide. Along with a few additional and new compounds, both formulae were administered to male mice for 22 days, and the mice were allowed to mate with virgin female mice. The sexual performance of the treated male mice almost doubled. In the same report, a test on the latent period of erection (LPE) in the rats with erectile dysfunction revealed that the purified maca products at 180 and 1800 mg/kg body weight were improving the erectile function in the testis-removed rats, as demonstrated by the decrease in LPE. The study revealed, for the first time, an aphrodisiac activity of *L. meyenii*.[75] In a parallel study,[76,77] *L. meyenii* pulverized root (standardized to 0.6% macamides and macaenes), prepared in saline, was administered to male rats through a gastric tube at a daily dose of 15 and 75 mg/kg (acute and chronic doses, respectively) for 15 days. It was shown that the treatment significantly improved the sexual performance parameters of the treated rats.

A third study[78] was concerned with the spermatogenesis in adult male rats. Male rats receiving aqueous extract of maca root (66.7 mg/ml) twice/day for 14 consecutive days showed increased weight of the testes and epididymis and in the length and frequency of stages IX–XIV seminiferous tubules and a decrease in the stages I–VI. Results indicate that *L. meyenii* root invigorates spermatogenesis acting on its initial stages.

27.4.2.3.2 *Clinical Studies*

In the only clinical study,[79] a 4-month oral treatment was conducted on 9 men 24 to 44 years old with *L. meyenii* tablets (1500 or 3000 mg of maca). Results showed increased seminal volume, sperm count per ejaculation, motile sperm count, and sperm motility; the response was not related with any alteration in the serum hormones. The study has limitation in respect of sample size and lack of placebo control.

27.5 Future Perspectives

From the foregoing review it is evident that Ayurveda/phytotherapy has the potential to become into effective therapy for male sexual dysfunction. Additional research is required in order to make it acceptable to health-care providers as an alternative to conventional medicine. It is likely that because sex, infertility, and impotence are highly personal and embarrassing issues, several commercial establishments sought to profit from these problems with cheap advertisements to lure the suffering men. The question of heavy metal concentration in some of these preparations and the likely consequence on the general health are also of concern.[80,81]

The application of the various therapeutic modalities in the abrogation of male sexual dysfunction needs to be related to the various etiological categories of male sexual dysfunction. Most of the scientific studies, among those conducted so far, have been concerned with impotence and aphrodisiacs. There is an urgent need to conduct scientific studies on the phytochemical therapy for male infertility such as the aspects connected with sperm and the mechanism of action at the cellular and molecular levels.

Acknowledgments

The authors place on record the authoritative contribution of Dr. T.V. Narayanan and Shri Sasi Varier, Ashtanga Ayurveda Sala, Tiruchirappalli, India, in the preparation of the Ayurvedic portion of the manuscript. The help rendered by S. Anandhi, R. Girija, Sr., Jancy M. George, and B. Kadalmani, doctoral students of M.A. Akbarsha, in the compilation and verification of the data, are heartily acknowledged. The financial assistance from the Department of Science and Technology, Government of India, to M.A. Akbarsha, to study the male reproductive effects of phytotherapeutics (Grant No. SP/SC/C-31/98) is also acknowledged. A. Subramoniam thanks Dr. G.M. Nair, Director, TGBRI, and V.M.

Madhavachandran thanks Shri Devadas Namboodiripad, Managing Director, Nagarjuna Herbal Concentrates Ltd., respectively, for the permission to participate in the review and their support. The technical support of S. Sudhakar is heartily acknowledged.

References

1. Krausz, C. and Forti, G., Clinical aspects of male infertility, in *The Genetic Basis of Male Infertility*, McElreavey, K., Ed., Springer-Verlag, New York, 2000, p. 1.
2. World Health Organization, Towards more objectivity in diagnosis and management of male infertility, *Int. J. Androl.*, 7, 1, 1987.
3. Hellstrom, W.J.G., Preface, in *Male Infertility and Sexual Dysfunction*, Hellstrom, W.J.G., Ed., Springer-Verlag, New York, 1997, p. ix.
4. Carlsen, E. et al., Evidence for decreasing quality of semen during past 50 years, *Br. Med. J.*, 305, 609, 1992.
5. Seftel, A.D., Challenges in oral therapy for erectile dysfunction, *J. Androl.*, 23, 729, 2002.
6. Hess, R.A., Effects of environmental toxicants on the efferent ducts, epididymis and fertility, *J. Reprod. Fertil.*, 53, 247, 1998.
7. McClure, R.D., Office evaluation of the infertile men, in *Male Infertility and Sexual Dysfunction*, Hellstrom, W.J.G., Ed., Springer-Verlag, New York, 1997, p. 22.
8. Stanley, A. and Akbarsha, M.A., Ultrastructural changes in the Leydig cell on treatment with vincristine, *Cytobios*, 79, 51, 1994.
9. Akbarsha, M. A. and Averal, H. I., Epididymis as a target organ for the toxic effect of vincristine: light microscopic changes in the epididymal epithelial cell types, *Biomed. Lett.*, 54, 133, 1996.
10. Cooke, P.S., Peterson, R.E., and Hess, R.A., Endocrine disruptors, in *Handbook of Toxicologic Pathology*, 2nd ed., Vol. 1, Academic Press, London, 2002, p. 501.
11. Akbarsha, M.A. and Sivasamy, P., Male reproductive toxicity of phosphamidon: histopathological changes in epididymis, *Indian J. Exp. Biol.*, 36, 34, 1998.
12. Agnes, V.F. and Akbarsha, M.A., Pale vacuolated epithelial cells in epididymis of aflatoxin-treated mice, *Reproduction*, 122, 629, 2001.
13. Akbarsha, M.A. et al., Spermatotoxic effect of carbendazim, *Indian J. Exp. Biol.*, 39, 921, 2001.
14. Degen, G.H. and Bolt, H.M., Endocrine disruptors: update on xenoestrogens, *Int. Arch. Occup. Environ. Health*, 73, 433, 2000.
15. Gray, L.E., Xenoendocrine disruptors: laboratory studies on male reproductive effects, *Toxicol. Lett.*, 102, 331, 1998.
16. Morley, J.E., Impotence, *Am. J. Med.*, 80, 897, 1986.
17. Miller, M.A. and Morgan, R.J., Eicosanoids, erections and erectile dysfunction, *Prostaglandins Leucotrienes and Essential Fatty Acids*, 51, 1, 1994.
18. Thomas, J. A., Diet: micronutrients and the prostate gland, *Nutr. Rev.*, 57, 95, 1999.
19. Khedun, S.M., Naicker, T., and Maharaj, B., Zn, hydrochlorothiazide, and sexual dysfunction, *Cent. Afr. J. Med.*, 41, 312, 1995.
20. Ahlborg, B., Ekelund, L.G., and Nilsson, C.G., Effect of potassium-magnesium aspartate on the capacity for prolonged exercise in man, *Acta Physiol. Scand.*, 74, 238, 1968.
21. Seftel, A.D. and Althof, S.E., Premature ejaculation, in *Male Infertility and Sexual Dysfunction*, Hellstrom, W.J.G., Ed., Springer-Verlag, New York, 1997, 356.
22. Vitezic, D. and Pelcic, J.M., Erectile dysfunction: oral pharmacotherapy options, *Int. J. Clin. Pharmacol. Ther.*, 40, 393, 2002.
23. Nadkarni, K.M., *Indian Materia Medica*, Vols. 1 & 2, Popular Prakasham Pvt. Ltd., Bombay, India, 1976.
24. Abdel-Magied, E.M., Abdel-Rahman, H.A., and Harraz, F.M., The effect of aqueous extracts of Cynomorium coccineum and Withania somnifera on testicular development in immature Wistar rats, *J. Ethnopharmacol.*, 75, 1, 2001.

25. Al-Qarawi, A.A. et al., The effect of extracts of Cynomorium coccineum and Withania somnifera on gonadotrophins and ovarian follicles of immature Wistar rats, *Phytother. Res.*, 14, 288, 2000.
26. Abdel-Rehman, H.A. et al., The effect of the aquous extract of Cynomorium coccineum on the epididymal sperm pattern of the rat, *Phytother. Res.*, 13, 248, 1999.
27. Anantha Kumar, K.V. et al., Aphrodisiac activity of the seeds of Mucuna pruriens, *Indian Drugs*, 31, 321, 1994.
28. Nair, P.V. and Pillai, K.S.M., Bulletin Central Research Institute, University of Tranvancore (Trivandrum), 3 A(1), 83, 1954.
29. Pillai, K.S.M. and Anantharaman, R., Bulletin Central Research Institute, University of Tranvancore (Trivandrum), 4 A(1), 41, 1955.
30. Shah, A.H. et al., Toxicity studies in mice of common spices, Cinnamomum zeylanicum bark and Piper longum fruits, *Plant Foods Human Nutr.*, S2, 231, 1998.
31. Kholkute, S.D., Kekare, M.B., and Munshi, S.R., Antifertility effects of the fruits of Piper longum in female rats, *Indian J. Exp. Biol.*, 17, 289, 1979.
32. Warrier, P.K., Nambiar, V.P.K., and Ramankutty, C., Eds., *Indian Medicinal Plants: A Compendium of 500 Species*, Vols. 1–5, Orient Longman Ltd., Madras, India, 1994–1996.
33. Georgiev, P., Dimitrov, M., and Vitanov, S., Effect of Tribestan (from Tribulus terrestris) on plasma testosterone and spermatogenesis in male lambs and rams, *Veterinarna Sbirka*, 86, 20, 1988.
34. Adaikan, P.G. et al., Proerectile pharmacological effects of Tribulus terrestris extract on the rabbit corpus cavernosum, *Ann. Acad. Med.* (Singapore), 29, 22, 2000.
35. Bourke, C.A., Stevents, G.R., and Carrigan, M.J., Locomotor effects in sheep of alkaloids identified in Australian Tribulus terrestris, *Aus. Vet. J.*, 69, 163, 1992.
36. Adimoelja, A., Phytochemicals and the breakthrough of traditional herbs in the management of sexual dysfunctions, *Int. J. Androl.*, 23, 82, 2000.
37. Adimoelja, A. and Adaikan, P.J., Protodioscin from herbal plant Tribulus terrestris L. improves male sexual function possibly via DHEA, *Int. J. Impotence Res.*, 91, S64, 1997.
38. Gauthaman, K., Adaikan, P.G., and Prasad, R.N.V., Aphrodisiac properties of Tribulus terrestris extract (protodioscin) in normal and castrated rats, *Life Sci.*, 71, 1385, 2002.
39. Subramoniam, A. et al., Aphrodisiac property of Trichopus zeylanicus extract in male mice, *J. Ethnopharmacol.*, 57, 21, 1997.
40. Suresh Kumar, P.K., Subramoniam, A., and Pushpangadan, P., Aphrodisiac activity of Vanda tessellata (Roxf) root extract in male mice, *Indian J. Pharmacol.*, 32, 300, 2000.
41. Suresh Kumar, P.K., Ethnobotanical Investigation and Search for Aphrodisiac and Anticancer Activities from Wild orchids of Western Ghat region of Kerala, Ph.D. thesis, University of Kerala, India, 2001.
42. Qureshi, S., Shah, A.H., Tariq, M., and Ageel, A.M., Studies on herbal aphrodisiacs used in Arab system of medicines, *Am. J. Clin. Med.*, 17(1-2), 57, 1989.
43. Sandroni, P., Aphrodisiacs, past and present: a historical review, *Clin. Auton. Res.*, 11, 303, 2001.
44. Gillis, C.N., Panax ginseng pharmacology: a nitric oxide link?, *Biochem. Pharmacol.*, 54, 1, 1997.
45. Kim, C. et al., Influence of ginseng on mating behavior of male rats, *Am. J. Clin. Med.*, 4, 163, 1976.
46. Murphy, L.L. et al., Effect of American ginseng (Panax quinquefolium) on male copulatory behavior in the rat, *Physiol. Behav.*, 64, 445, 1998.
47. Murphy, L.L. and Lee, T.J.-F., Ginseng, sex behavior and nitric oxide, *Ann. N.Y. Acad. Sci.*, 962, 372, 2002.
48. Yoshimura, H., Kimura, N., and Sugiura, K., Preventive effcts of various ginseng saponins on the development of copulatory disorders induced by prolonged individual housing in male mice, *Meth. Find. Exp. Clin. Pharmacol.*, 20, 59, 1998.
49. Chen, X. and Lee, T.J., Ginsenosides-induced nitric oxide-mediated relaxation of the rabbit corpus cavernosum, *Br. J. Pharmacol.*, 115, 15, 1995.
50. Choi, Y.D., Xin, X.C., and Choi, H.K., Effect of Korean red ginseng on the rabbit corpus cavernosal smooth muscle, *Int. J. Impotency Res.*, 10, 37, 1998.

51. Hess, F.G. et al., Reproduction study in rats or ginseng extract G115, *Food. Chem. Toxicol.*, 20, 189, 1982.
52. Choi, H.K., Seong, D.H., and Rha, K.H., Clinical efficacy of Korean red ginseng for erectile dysfunction, *Int. J. Impotency Res.*, 7, 181, 1995.
53. Hong, B. et al., A double-blind crossover study evaluating the efficacy of Korean red ginseng in patients with erectile dysfunction: a preliminary report, *J. Urol.*, 168, 2070, 2002.
54. Riley, A.J. et al., Yohimbine in the treatment of erectile disorder, *Br. J. Clin. Pract.*, 48, 133, 1994.
55. Clark, J.T. et al., Enhancement of sexual motivation in male rats by yohimbine, *Science*, 225, 847, 1984.
56. Doherty, P.C., Oral, transdermal, and transurethral therapies for erectile dysfunction, in *Male Infertility and Sexual Dysfunction*, Hellstrom, W.J.G., Ed., Springer-Verlag, New York, 1997, p. 452.
57. Giuliano, F. and Rampin, O., Alpha receptors in the central nervous system and its effects on erection, *J. Androl.*, 20, 683, 1999.
58. Clark, J., Smith, E.R., and Davidson, J., Evidence for the modulation of sexual behavior by alfa adrenoceptors in male rats, *Neuroendocrinology*, 41, 36, 1985.
59. Arteaga, M. et al., Effects of yohimbine and apomorphine on the male sexual behavior pattern of the golden hamster (Mesocricetus auratus), *Eur. Neuropsychopharmacol.*, 12, 39, 2002.
60. Morales, A. et al., Nonhormonal pharmacological treatment of organic impotence, *J. Urol.*, 128, 45, 1982.
61. Morales, A. et al., Is yohimbine effective in treatment of organic impotence? Results of a controlled trial, *J. Urol.*, 137, 1168, 1987.
62. Reid, K. et al., Double-blind trial of yohimbine in treatment of psychogenic impotence, *Lancet*, 2, 421, 1987.
63. Riley, A.J. et al., Double blind trial of yohimbine hydrochloride in the treatment of erection inadequacy, *Sex Marital Ther.*, 4, 17, 1989.
64. Susset, J.G. et al., Effect of yohimbine hydrochloride on erectile impotence: a double-blind trial, *J. Urol.*, 141, 1360, 1989.
65. Sonda, L.P., Mazo, R., and Chancellor, M.B., The role of yohimbine for the treatment of erectile impotence, *J. Sexual Marital Ther.*, 16, 15, 1990.
66. Hollander, E. and McCarley, A., Yohimbine treatment of sexual side effects induced by serotonin reuptake blockers, *J. Clin. Psychiatr.*, 53, 207, 1992.
67. Jacobsen, F.M., Fluoxetine-induced sexual dysfunction and an open trial of yohimbine, *J. Clin. Psychiatr.*, 53, 119, 1992.
68. Carey, M.P. and Johnson, B.T., Effectiveness of yohimbine in the treatment of erectile disorder: four meta-analytic integrations, *Arch. Sexual Behav.*, 25, 341, 1996.
69. Mann, K. et al., Effects of yohimbine on sexual experiences and nocturnal penile tumescence and rigidity in erectile dysfunction, *Arch. Sexual Behav.*, 25, 1, 1996.
70. Rowland, D.L., Kallan, K., and Slob, A.K., Yohimbine, erectile capacity and sexual response in men, *Arch. Sexual Behav.*, 26, 49, 1997.
71. Morales, A., Yohimbine in erectile dysfunction: the facts, *Int. J. Impotency Res.*, 12(Suppl. 1), S70, 2000.
72. Guay, A.T. et al., Yohimbine treatment of organic erectile dysfunction in a dose escalation trial, *Int. J. Impotency Res.*, 14, 25, 2002.
73. Teloken, C. et al., Therapeutic effects of high dose yohimbine hydrochloride on organic erectile dysfunction, *J. Urol.*, 159, 122, 1998.
74. Danjou, P. et al., Assessment of erectogenic properties of apomorphine and yohimbine in man, *Br. J. Clin. Pharmacol.*, 26, 733, 1988.
75. Zheng, B.L. et al., Effect of a lipidic extract from Lepidium meyenii on sexual behavior in mice and rats, *Urology*, 55, 598, 2000.
76. Cicero, A.F.G., Bandieri, E., and Arletti, R., Lepidium meyenii Walp. improves sexual behavior in male rats independently from its action on spontaneous locomotor activity, *J. Ethnopharmacol.*, 75, 225, 2001.
77. Cicero, A.F. et al., Hexanic Maca extract improves rat sexual performance more effectively than methanolic and chloroform Maca extracts, *Andrologia*, 34, 177, 2002.

78. Gonzales, G.F. et al., Effect of Lepidium meyenii roots on spermatogenesis of male rats, *Asian J. Androl.*, 3, 231, 2001.
79. Gonzales, G.F. et al., Lepidium meyenii (Maca) improved semen parameters in adult men, *Asian J. Androl.*, 3, 301, 2001.
80. Ernst, E., Heavy metals in traditional Indian remedies, *Eur. J. Clin. Pharmacol.*, 57, 891, 2002.
81. Ernst, E., Toxic heavy metals and undeclared drugs in Asian herbal medicines, *Trends Pharmacol. Sci.*, 23, 136, 2002.

28

Raktaja Krimis (Dermatophytes)

Mahendra K. Rai, Nandkishore J. Chikhale, Manjusha J. Choukhande, and Milind N. Dudhane

CONTENTS

28.1 Introduction

Raktaja krimis have been described as very minute (invisible with naked eyes) on the basis of the description available in Ayurvedic texts. Their corelation can be made with the dermatophytic fungi, causing superficial infections in man and animals. In Ayurveda, *krimis* of a particular group are responsible for hair loss from the head, face, and other parts of the body; the distortion of nails (*kesha, shamarshu, nakha, loma dhwansa*), hair-raising sensation of a person after a horrific situation (*roma harsha*); itching and pain in the wounds (*vranna, kandu, toda*); a creeping sensation (*sansarpa*); and the eating away of the skin, vessels, ligaments, muscles, and cartilage (*twak, shirasnayu, mansa, tarunasthi bhakshanana*).

0-8493-1366-X/04/$0.00+$1.50

The word *krimi* originated from Dhatu *kramu pad vikccep* (*kramyati sarpati*), meaning that which moves with legs. But this derivation of *krimi* does not include all the *krimis* because there are several *krimis* described in *vedas* and Ayurvedic texts that are without legs. Therefore, they cannot be included in the group of *krimi* according to above definition. However, *yaskacharya* has defined *krimi* as *kravyamedati*, which means the organisms that eat and grow on raw flesh.

28.2 Historical Background

Krimi has been classified as external (*bahya*) and internal (*abhyantra*) in most of the Ayurvedic texts, except *Sushrutra Samhita* and *Bhela Samhita*. As compared with other texts, a detailed classification of *krimi* is found in *Charak Samhita*. The classification of *sahaja krimi* is given in *Charak Samhita*. Bhela, who was a prudent student of maharishi Attreya, did not give any account of external *krimi*. It seems that external krimis are probably a personal contribution of *Agnivesha*, which was universally accepted by later scholars. The classification of *krimi* by *Kashyap Samhita* is found only in the treatment chapter.

In *Charak Samhita*, *raktaja krimis* have been explained up to a certain extent. On the contrary, Sushrutra did not pay any attention to the health problems. Sharma et al.[3] proposed close similarity of *raktaja krimis* with microbes and parasites. Some *raktaja krimis* can be compared with dermatophytes (etymologically the plants of skin) of the fungal kingdom.

This chapter will focus on the scientific basis of *raktaja krimis* as described in Ayurveda.

28.3 Etiology of *Raktaj Krimis*

According to Sushruta, the *kapha* and *pitta* of the body are aggravated by several factors. Examples include eating before the digesting the previous meal; excessively using any indigestible, uncongenial, incompatible, or filthy articles of fare sedentary habits; eating cold, heavy, or fatty meals; sleeping during the day; and excessively using *masha* (meat). In modern system of diagnosis, the minute *krimis* are supposed to be the following species: *Epidermophyton* (1 species), *Microsporum* (14 species), and *Trichophyton* (20 species).

28.4 Clinical Description

28.4.1 Symptoms of *Dadrukustha*

The *dadrukustha* (ringworm caused by dermatophytes) have coloration of linseed flowers or copper. They are also serpigerous and full of eruptions.

The general features of this disease are elevated, spherical, itching, and slowly growing patches. Other types of *kustha* may be considered as tuberculoid leprosy, piodermas, psoriasis, melanodermas, and erysepales. These types are incurable or difficult to treat according to Ayurveda.

28.5 Classification of *Krami Roga*

Acharya Charak and Sushrut mentioned a special chapter on diseases caused by *krimis*, and classified them into seven types of *purisaj*, six types of *kaphaj*, and seven types of *raktaja*. *Raktaja krimis* circulates in the blood and eventually produce disease symptoms in skin. In Ayurveda, Sushrutra has focused more elaborately on *krimi*. According to him, raktaja *krimi* cannot be seen with the naked eye. He has mentioned seven types of *kustha* (skin disease):

1. *Arunkustha* (due to *vata*)
2. *Udumbarkustha*
3. *Krishyajivhakustha*
4. *Kapalkustha*
5. *Kakanakakustha* (due to *pitta*)
6. *Pandarika*
7. *Padrukustha* (due to *kapha*)

Out of these seven types, *dadrukustha* is curable with Ayurvedic treatment. Nomenclature given by Sharma et al.[3] is given below.

Ayurvedic Nomenclature	Mycological Nomenclature	Term
Keshad	*Trichophyton* sp.	Dermatophyte
Lomada	*Microsporum* sp.	Dermatophyte
Nakhada	*Epidermophyton* sp. *Trichophyton* sp.	Dermatophyte

Mycological Types and Species

Raktaja Krimi (Dermatophyte)	Selected Species
Epidermophyton	*E. stockdale, E. floccosum*
Microsporum	*M. audouinii, M. canis, M. gypseum, M. fulvum, M. nanum*
Trichophyton	*T. tonsurans, T. mentagrophytes, T. rubrum, T. schoenleimii, T. soudanes*

28.5.1 Dermatophytes

Dermatophytes (*derma* = skin, *phyton* = plant) are a highly specialized group of keratinophilic fungi that utilizes keratin of the skin. They are also known as ring-worm fungi and tinea infections. More than 40 dermatophyte species are known to exist.[1,2,4] The three types of dermatophytes (ringworm) — geophilic, zoophilic, and anthropophilic — are shown below:

Geophilic	Zoophilic	Anthropophilic
Soil as a substrate	Parasitizes on animals and may also cause infections in man	Parasitizes on man
Microsporum gypseum, Trichophyton ajelloi, T. terrestre	*Microsporum canis, Trichophyton verrucosum, T. mentagrophytes*	*Microsporum audouinii, E. floccosum, T. rubrum, T. tonsurans, T. violaceum*

Dermatophytes have also been isolated from air, public swimming pools, and barbershops.

28.5.1.1 Clinical Types

The infection caused by dermatophytes is clinically known as tinea infections. These can be categorized as follows:

28.5.1.1.1 *Tinea pedis*

This type of infection is also known as athlete's foot or ringworm of the foot. The causal organism involved in *Tinea pedis* are *Trichophyton rubrum* and *T. mentagrophytes.*

28.5.1.1.2 *Tinea unguinum*

The ringworm of the nails is referred to as *Tinea unguinum* or onychomycosis. Such infections generally occur in nails that are deformed due to the pressure of tight shoes. The species usually responsible for onychomycosis are *T. rubrum* and *T. mentagrophytes.*

28.5.1.1.3 *Tinea corporis*

The ringworm of the glabrous skin is called *Tinea corporis* or *Tinea circinata.* It is characterized by a circular lesion exhibiting varying degrees of inflammation. The infection is usually caused by *T. rubrum, M. canis,* and *T. mentagrophytes.*

28.5.1.1.4 *Tinea imbricata*

Tinea imbricata (*dadru*) is a common infection in tropical areas. It is characterized by lesions that are originally circinate but which become irregular and coalescent and do not heal at the center. The causal organism is usually *T. concentricum.*

28.5.1.1.5 *Tinea barbae*

It is also called ringworm of the beard, barber's itch, or sycosis. *Tinea barbae* is a foliculitis of the beard and rarely infects the face and neck. *T. verrucosum* of *Tinea barbae* is transmitted from cattle, whereas *T. mentagrophytes* is transmitted from horse or dog.

28.5.1.1.6 *Tinea favosa*

It is commonly known as favus and is a severe type of chronic ringworm. The causal organisms of favus are *T. schoenieinii, T. violaceum,* and *M. gypseum.*

28.5.1.1.7 *Tinea cruris*

This infection is also known as Dhobi's itch, ringworm of the groin, jock itch, or eczema marginatum. *Tinea cruris* is an acute or chronic infection usually severely pruritic dermatophytosis of the groin. The lesions are generally caused by *Epidermophyton floccosum* and various species of *Trichophyton* with special reference to *T. rubrum.*

28.5.1.1.8 Tinea capitis

This infection is usually known as ringworm of the scalp. *Tinea capitis* includes dry, diffuse, and scaly lesions of the scalp. Generally, it is caused by *T. tonsurans, T. violaceum, T. schoeninileinii, T. mentagrophytes, T. audouinii,* and *M. canis.*

28.5.1.1.9 Mycological Types

There are three main genera or mycological types: *Epidermophyton, Microsporum,* and *Trichophyton.* These genera have been classified purely on the basis of mycology.

28.5.1.1.9.1 Epidermophyton — The genus *Epidermophyton* includes only one valid species, *E. floccosum,* which is a good example of anthropophilic dermatophyte. Another species named *E. stockdale* is yet to be recognized. It was reported from only one soil sample. It produces club-shaped macroaleuriospores that are 59.5–2 × 12.9–3.0 μm with two to nine cells. *E. floccosum* rarely parasitizes lower animals. It lives in human and is transmitted from man to man by direct and indirect contact. *E. floccosum* is a cosmopolitan fungus in distribution and invades only human nails and skin. It is not capable of invading human hair. The teleomorphic state of *E. floccosum* is unknown.

The genus *Epidermophyton* is characterized by large, fusiform that obovate and smooth, multiseptate asexual spores known as macroaleuriospores. They are produced in bunches of two or three. They measure 20–40 × 6–3 μm with two to four cells. The microaleuriospores are not formed.

28.5.1.1.9.2 Microsporum — There are 15 species of *Microsporum,* which can be categorized on the basis of natural habitat into three broad groups. Eight of them live saprophytically in soil (geophilic). *M. boulardi* is reported only from the African republic of Guinea. There is only one report of *M. boulardi.* The majority of the species of dermatophtes produce two types of conidia in culture. The smaller, pyriform to obovate conidia are known as microaleuriospores; the larger conidia are called macroaleuriospores which are multiseptate, echinulate, variable in size and shape (fusiform to obovate), and thin or thick walled. They are born singly or in hyphae. The length of conidia are 5 to 100 μm and width 3 to 8 μm, with two to five cells. The type species of *Microsporum* is *M. audouinii.* The important species include *M. audouinii, M. canis, M. gypseum, M. fulvum,* and *M. nanum.*

28.5.1.1.9.3 Trichophyton — Macroaleuriospores are smooth and either thin or thick-walled and range from clavate to fusiform in shape. They are born singly or in clusters. Microaleuriospores are spherical either pyriform or clavate and are borne singly or in chains (in grapelike bunches). The genus *Trichophyton* has 25 valid species. The type species is *T. tonsurans.*

Some important species are *T. equinum* (teleomorph unknown), *T. mentagrophytes* (teleomorph *Arthoderma benhamiae, A. vanbreuseghemii*), *T. rubrum* (teleomorph unknown), *T. schoenleimii* (teleomorph unknown), *T. soudanes* (teleomorph unknown), *T. verrucosum* (teleomorph unknown), and *T. violaceum* (teleomorph-unknown). The common names of fungal diseases are listed in Table 28.1.

TABLE 28.1

Common Names of Fungal Diseases and Corresponding Meanings

General Term	Meaning
Tinea infections	Dermatophytes
Tinea pedis	Ringworm of foot
Tinea unguinum/onychomycosis	Ringworm of the nails
Tinea corporis	Ringworm of glabrous skin
Tinea imbricata	Originally circinate but which become irregular and coalescent
Tinea barbae	Ringworm of the beard
Tinea favosa	
Tinea cruris	Severe type of chronic ringworm
Tinea capitis	Ringworm of the groin
	Ringworm of the scalp

28.6 Diagnostic Methods

The method of diagnosis in the ancient period was according to sign and symptoms of the disease, because pathological investigations were not possible. Generally round, bluish, or reddish spots are formed on the skin. Sometimes boils or eruptions may also be produced. The spots generally spread and sometimes coalesce with other spots to form irregular bigger spots.

In conventional medicine, *krami rogas* are diagnosed by the following laboratory test methods: potassium hydroxide (KOH) squash tests, culture techniques, agar blocks technique.

28.7 Treatment

28.7.1 Ayurvedic Therapies

There are various medicines used in Ayurveda for the cure of *raktaja krimis*. Some of them are described below.

28.7.1.1 Plant-Based Natural Oils

1. *Mahamarichadi taila* — This oil is also prepared from natural products. It is used in all kinds of skin infections, such as boils, ringworm, etc. It consists of *kali marich* (*Piper longum*), *hartal*, *Sweta nishoth*, *lal chandan* (*Santalum* sp.), *nagarmotha* (*Cyperus scarious*), *manasnil*, *jatamansi* (*Nardostachys jatamansi*), *daruhaldi* (*Berberis* sp.), *haldi*, *indrayanmula* (*Citrullus colocynthis*), *kanermula* (*Nerium* sp.), *kuth* (*Saussurea lappa*), *arka* (*Calotropis gigantea*), *dugdha*, and *vatsanabha*.
2. *Laghu-vis-garva taila* — This oil is used in cutaneous infections. It is extracted from *Argemone mexicana* Linn. (Papaveraceae), *Nardostachys jatamansi* DC (Valerianaceae),

Terminalia chebula Retz. (Combretaceae), *Ricinus communis* Linn. (Euphorbiaceae), *Plumbago zeylanica* Linn. (Plumbaginaceae), *Curcuma longa* Linn. (Scitaminae), and *Saussurea lappa* Clarke (Asteraceae).

3. *Karanjadi Taila* — The oil is extracted from *Pongamia pinnata* (Linn.) Merr. (Fabaceae). It is useful in various kinds of skin infections, including ringworm (dermatophytes). It consists of seeds of *karanj* (*Pongamia pinnata*), *kuth, chitrakmul* (*Plumbago zeylanica*), *chameli puspa* (*Jasminum* sp.), and *Kaner* (*Nerium oleander* L.).
4. Ring-ring — This oil is used for ringworm infections caused by fungi. It is also useful for other cutaneous infections.
5. *Dadrughni-Vati* — This tablet is prepared from *chakramarda* (*Cassia tora* Linn.). It is used for all kinds of skin infections, ringworm, and white spots.
6. V-Gel: This gel is useful in vaginitis, vaginal candidiasis and other fungal infections of the vagina. Each gram of V-Gel contains: extracts of *triphala* (4.0 mg), *satapatri* (*Rosa damascena* Syn. *R. centifolia;* 3.6 mg), ela (*Elettaria cardamomum;* 3.6 mg), *punarnava* (*Boerhaavia diffusa;* 3.6 mg), *shaileyam* (*Parmelia perlata;* 2.0 mg), *nirgundi* (*Vitex negundo;* 1.6 mg), and *Haridra* (*Curcuma longa;* 1.6 mg). The drug is manufactured by Himalayan Herbal Products Co.
7. *Sankhpushpi taila* — This oil includes extract and oil from the plant *Evolvulus alsinoides.* It is used for ringworm, particularly for infections of scalp (*Tinea capitis*) in children. It is also used to cure scabies and other cutaneous infections.
8. *Tuvarakadi taila* — The oil is extracted from *Hydnocarpus laurifolia*, a plant of tropical origin. It is also known as *chalmongra taila.* The oil is used to cure all kinds of cutaneous fungal infections. The oil is sold in the market. Upadhyay[11] reported that *Trichophyton mentagrophytes* was very much sensitive to essential oil of *H. laurifolia.*
9. *Chopchinyadi churna* (powder) — This powder is used for all kinds of skin infections.

28.7.1.2 Role of Different Elements

Certain elements like sulfur, mercury, and copper are used in the treatment of mycotic infections. The metals and nonmetals are used in combination with a powdered mixture of *amla* (*Emblica officinalis*), *baheda* (*Terminalia belerica*), and *harada* (*Terminalia chebula*) referred to as *triphala churna* (powder of three fruits). The formulas that contain different compositions of these herbs and minerals are *arogyavardhini, gandhak-rasayana,* and *sukhshura triphala.*

28.7.2 Conventional Medicine Approach

Oral administration of griseofulvin is the best treatment for dermatophytosis in general and for *Tinea pedis* in particular. Earlier, the treatment depended only upon topical application of medicines. Sometimes, results are not favorable with griseofulvin and topical therapy is required. At present, a combination of oral administration of griseofulvin and topical antifungal agents are the main therapies.[6]

In onychomycosis, topical therapy is not successful because the causal pathogen does not respond well to griseofulvin. The patient does not feel relief even if the nail is removed surgically because the growing nail will continuously get infected. Griseofulvin used regularly for consecutive months gives promising results because it acts slowly. Topical application is important in such cases. The current most effective and acceptable preparations are imidazole ointments, such as clotrimazole, miconazole, or ketoconazole, which are frequently used. Oral administration of ketoconazole is recommended in some countries but not in Japan; the rate of hepatic disorders is too high there.

Terbinafine is used as an antimycotic agent, which does not cause hepatic disorders. If terbinafine is orally administered once a day, high concentrations in blood can be achieved.[7] The transfer of this drug from blood to skin is sufficient enough to be effective.[8] For deep-seated mycosis, fluconazole is administered. Another drug used is amphotericin B, a polyene-based antimycotic. It is used for the cure of fungal infections like aspergillosis, blastomycoses, candidasis cryptococcosis, histoplasmosis, and paracoccidiodomycosis. Fluorcytosine is used especially in Candidasis or in combination therapy. It inhibits DNA and RNA synthesis. Terbinafine and naftifine are both allylamines used against dermatomycoses and mucosal infections. They inhibit ergosterol biosynthesis by blocking squalene epoxidase.

Azoles include ketoconazole, miconazole, itraconazole, and fluconazole. These are known as imidazoles. They are used for the cure of blastomycosis, coccidiodomycosis, histoplasmosis, and paracoccidiodomycosis and inhibit ergosterol biosynthesis by blocking 14-demethylation of lanosterol. Such infections should also be treated with systemic antibacterial antibiotics because secondary bacterial infection may occur. During the recent years, many antifungal agents were introduced only for topical application owing to their toxicity. Today, a mostly broad spectrum of antifungal agents are preferred.

Increasingly, allergic reactions of the skin are observed today. One reason is the high rate of sensitization power of these antimycotics. There are some adverse reactions such as gastrointestinal and hepatic disorders and photo sensitivity reactions particularly by griseofulvin and ketoconazole.[6] Allergic contact dermatitis due to these new antimycotic agents of imidazole family is rare. Another problem is the use of application.

28.8 Scientific Basis

Dadrughni-vati is a well-known antifungal agent in Ayurveda. The drug is extracted from pawar (*Cassia tora*), a plant of the Fabaceae family. In Sanskrita it is known as *chakramard*, meaning killer of ringworm. An antifungal phytochemical chrysophanic acid-5-anthrone was isolated by Acharya and Chatterjee.[35] *Trichophyton mentagrophytes*, a fungus responsible for causing ringworm infections, can be inhibited by oil of *Hydnocarpus laurifolia* at 1:4 dilution, which is equal to 0.125 μg/ml dilution of miconazole nitrate, followed by seed oil of *Derris indica* (*Pongamia pinnata*) at 1:2 dilution (0.25 μg/ml miconazole nitrate). *Epidermophyton floccosum*, another causal fungus of ringworm, was reported to be the most sensitive to oil of *H. laurifolia*.[11]

Argemone mexicana, Ricinus communis, and *Plumbago zeylanica* are included in *Laghu-visgarva taila* (oil). All the three plants are highly antifungal. Roots of *Plumbago zeylanica* are utilized by people of India and China against skin diseases.[36,37] The plant extract was found to be active against causal organisms of ringworm fungi.[11] The *karanjadi taila* is extracted from *karanj* (*Pongamia pinnata*). The oil was reported as high antifungal agent.[29] *Bakuchi taila* is extracted from *Psoralea corylifolia.* The plant is reported to contain antimycotic potential. It showed remarkable activity against *Trichophyton mentagrophytes* and *Epidermophyton floccosum*.[11] V-Gel has been very effective in ringworm infections, particularly in severe vaginitis.[38-40]

Ayurvedic plants are currently being studied for their antidermatophyte activity to find better treatment for skin infections. Plants are extracted either by boiling in water or by soxhlet extraction procedures. The extracts are evaluated for their minimum inhibitory concentration (MIC). Colony-forming units of a test fungus are determined in a sabouraud dextrose agar medium, which is prepared and sterilized at 15 lb for 15 min. The MIC of the plant extract is then determined in this system. The commonly used methods are a dry-weight method, in which the actual weight of the harvested fungus is weighed at the end of the incubation period, and the disc diffusion method, in which the effect of the extract placed in the center of the plates is measured on the growth of the fungus by the area of the growth.

There have been numerous studies on the plants used for antidematophyte activity. The antifungal activity of nonvolatile constituents of higher plants has been reviewed earlier by many workers.[9–14] Many plants produce essential oils as secondary metabolites. Their exact role in the life processes of the plant is unknown. A review of literature reveals that a large number of essential oils were reported to possess fungitoxic activity.[15–34] Most members of the Asteraceae family are known to contain essential oils that usually have antifungal and cytotoxic sesquiterpene lactones.

28.8.1 Why Ayurvedic Drugs for *Raktaja Krimis*?

Ayurvedic therapy for *raktaja krimis* is mostly based on essential oils and plant extracts. These oils are very effective and are aromatic. The patient feels comfortable with this kind of therapy. The essential oil therapy has become more important after the invasion of secondary infections in dreaded diseases like AIDS and cancer. The risk of opportunistic pathogens is increasing day by day in such patients because of the immunocompromising capacity of the hosts. Generally, the secondary infections are caused by yeasts like *Candida albicans* and other filamentous fungi including Alternaria, Curvularia, Phoma, and Fusarium. The oil provides a soothing experience after application on skin and also avoids infections caused by opportunistic pathogens. Moreover, the drugs are relatively cheaper, easily available, and do not have side effects; in most antifungal drugs (allopathy), such as imidazoles, there can be side effects. These ointments are chemical based and not natural like the essential oils used in Ayurvedic therapy.

28.9 Conclusions

The drugs of Ayurveda have a tremendous effect on human beings, as these drugs are natural and easily available. In the case of *raktaja krimis*, most drugs are prescribed for topical application because dermatophytes generally infect the dermis of the human beings. There has been a great need to revitalize this system. Most plants used in Ayurveda are becoming rare and some of them are threatened. Oils present in herbs need to be evaluated in order to know their validity for topical application. The sensitivity of *raktaja krimis* to many oils extracted from herbs have already been evaluated in different parts of the world.

References

1. Rebell, G. and Taplin, D., *Dermatophytes: Their Recognition and Identification,* University of Miami Press, Coral Gables, FL, 1970.
2. Currah, R.S., Taxonomy of the onygenales: arthrodermataceae, gymnoascaceae, myxotrichaceae and onygenaceae, *Mycotaxon,* 24, 1, 1985.
3. Sharma, R., Chaturvedi, C., and Tiwari, P.V., Intestinal parasites: an ayurvedic approach, *J. Res. Educ. Ind. Med.,* 6(1–2), 27, 1987.
4. Harmsen, D., Schwinn, A., Brocker, E.B., and Frosch, M., Molecular differentiation of dermatophytic fungi, *Mycoses,* 42, 67, 1999.
5. Gentles, J.C., Experimental ringworm in guinea pigs; oral treatment with griseofulvin, *Nature,* 182, 476, 1958.
6. Tanuma, H., Pathogenesis and treatment of hyperkeratotic tinea pedis in Japan, *Mycoses,* 42, 21, 1999.
7. Hay, R.J., Antifungal drugs-an introduction, *J. Dermatol. Treat.,* 1(Suppl. 2), 1, 1990.
8. Lever, L.R., Dykes, P.J., and Finaly, A.Y., How orally administered terbinafine reaches the stratum corneum, *J. Dermatol. Treat,* 1(Suppl. 2), 23, 1990.
9. Dekker, J., Antibiotics, in *Fungicides: An Advance Treatise,* Vol. 2, Torgeson, D.C., Ed., Academic Press, New York, 1969, p. 580.
10. Thapliyal, P.N. and Nene, Y.L., Inhibition of plant pathogens by higher plant substances, *J. Sci. Indian Res.,* 26, 289, 1969.
11. Upadhyay, S.K., Studies on Ethnomedicinal Plants of Chhindwara District with Special Reference to Search for Antimycotic Activity against Superficial Mycosis, Ph.D. thesis, Dr. H.S. Gour University, Sagar, M.P., 1993.
12. Fawcett, C.H. and Spencer, D.M., Plant chemotherapy with natural products, *Ann. Rev. Phytopathol.,* 8, 403, 1970.
13. Dixit, S.N. and Tripathi, S.C., Antifungal antibiotics from higher plants, in *Recent Advances in the Biology of Micro-organisms,* Bilgrami, K.S. and Vyas, K.M., Eds., Bisen Singh Mahendra Pal Singh, Dehra Dun, India, 1970, pp. 519.
14. Mahadevan, A., *Biochemical Aspects of Plant Disease Resistance.* Part I. *Performed Inhibitory Substances — Prohibitins,* Today and Tomorrow's Printers and Publishers, New Delhi, India, 1982.
15. Barnes, G.L., *In vitro* toxicity of various fixed and essential oils of Pecan scab fungus *Fusicladium effusum, Plant. Dis. Rep.,* 47, 114, 1963.
16. Korta, J. and Starzyk, J., Investigation on antibiotic properties of essential oils of certain species of umbelliferae, *Acta Botinica Cravoviensia,* 6, 149, 1963.
17. Maruzzella, J.C., The effect of perfume oils on the growth of phytopathogenic fungi, *Plant Dis. Rep.,* 47, 756, 1963.
18. Hiller, K., Antimicrobial substances in flowering plants — a review, *Pharmazie,* 19, 167, 1964.
19. Birch, A.J., Some natural antifungal agents, *Chem. Ind.,* p. 1173, 1966.
20. Korbely, I. and Florian, E., Effects of essential oils on *Candida albicans, Gyogyszereszet,* 15, 462, 1971.
21. Garg, S.C., Antifungal activity of some essential oils, *Indian J. Pharm.,* 36, 46, 1974.
22. Zutschi, S.K. and Mehta, S.C., Screening of some essential oils for antifungal properties, *Indian Drugs Pharm.,* 12, 13, 1977.
23. Goutam, M.P., Jain, P.C., and Singh, K.V., Activity of some essential oils against dermatophytes, *Indian Drugs,* 17, 269, 1980.
24. Jain, P.C., Jain, C.K., and Jain, K., A note on the activity of odoriferous compound against dermatophytes, *Indian Drugs,* 17(12), 397, 1980.
25. Deshmukh, S.K., Jain, P.C., and Agrawal, S.C., A note on mycotoxicity of some essential oils, *Fitoterapia,* 67, 295, 1986.
26. Singh, K.V. and Deshmukh, S.K., Volatile constituents from members of Liliaceae and spore germination of *Microsporum gypseum* complexes, *Fitoterapia,* 55(5), 297, 1984.

27. Kishore, N. and Dwivedi, R.S., Fungitoxicity of the essential oil of *Tagetes erecta* L. against *Pythium aphanidermatum* Fitz., the damping-off pathogen, *Flavour Fragrance J., V,* 6(4), 291, 1991.
28. Jain, P.C. and Agarwal, S.C., Activity of plant extract against some keratinophilic species of *Nannizzia, Indian Drugs,* 13(12), 25, 1976.
29. Perrucci, S., Mancianti, F., Cioni, P.L., Flamini, G., Morelli, I., and Macchioni, G., *In vitro* antibacterial activity of essential oils against some isolates of *Microsporum canis* and *Microsporum gypseum, Planta Med.,* 60, 184, 1994.
30. Mwosu, M.O. and Okafor, J.L., Preliminary studies of the antifungal activities of some medicinal plants againts Basidiobolus and some other pathogenic fungi, *Mycoses,* 38 (5–6), 191, 1995.
31. Goren, N., Voerdenbag, H.J., and Johansson, B.C., Cytotoxic and antibacterial activities of sesquiterpene lactones isolated from *Tanacetum praeteritum* sub sp. *praeteritum, Planta Med.,* 62, 419, 1996.
32. Gopallakrishnan, G., Banumathi, B., and Suresh, G., Evaluation of the antifungal activity of natural xanthones from *Garcinia mangostana* and their synthetic derivatives, *J. Nat. Prod.,* 60(5), 519, 1997.
33. Calpouzos, L., Oils, in *Fungicides,* Vol. 2, Torgeson, D.C., Ed., Academic Press, London, 1969, p. 367.
34. Rai, M.K., Qureshi, S., and Pandey, A.K., *In vitro* susceptibility of opportunistic *Fusarium* spp. to essential oils, *Mycoses,* 42(1,2), 97, 1999.
35. Acharya, T.K. and Chatterjee, I.B., Isolation of chrysophonic acid-5-anthrone: a fungicidal compound from *Cassia tora* Linn., *Sci. Cult.,* 40(7), 316, 1974.
36. Shen-ji, P., Preliminary study of ethnobotany in Xixhuang Banna Peoples Republic of China, *J. Ethnopharmacol.,* 13, 223–230, 1985.
37. Sebastian, M.K. and Bhandari, M.M., Medico-ethnobotany of Mount Abu, Rajasthan, India, *J. Ethnopharmacol.,* 13, 121–137, 1985.
38. Kulkarni, R., Kashalikar, N., et al. Clinical evaluation of PD-959vaginal gel: an open trial, *The Antiseptic,* 97, 400–401, 2000.
39. Umadevi, K. and Swarup, A., Efficacy of V-Gel (PD-959Gel) in abnormal vaginal discharge, *Asian J. Obstet. Gynecol. Pract.,* 3, 68, 1999.
40. Singh, R., Vaginitis. I. Evaluation of V-Gel in vaginitis and cervicitis, *The Antiseptic,* 98, 6, 2001.

29

Eye Diseases

Aashish S. Phadke

CONTENTS

0-8493-1366-X/04/$0.00+$1.50

29.1 Introduction

One of the subspecialties of Ayurveda is *shalakyatantra,* which includes diseases of the eye, ear, nose, and throat.[1] In this chapter, management of common eye disorders are discussed along with available scientific information that seems to support various Ayurvedic therapies.

29.2 Anatomy of the Eye in Ayurveda

In intrauterine development of the eye, *pitta dosa,* especially *Alochaka pitta,* is a major contributor along with *kapha* for the development of blood vessels and related structures of circulatory system (*Raktavaha srotasa*).[1,2] Of five basic elements, the fire element (*teja mahabhoot*) is predominant in the formation of the eye. The differentiation of the eye starts during the fourth month of pregnancy.[3] The description of eye development in Ayurveda is very much similar to that known in conventional medicine at this time.[4] The eye is made up of five orbits (*mandal*), six junctions (*sandhi*), and six coats (*patal*).[5] The orbits in sequence are as follows: (1) orbit of eyelashes, (2) eyelids, (3) sclera and sclerotic circular margin, (4) corneal area, (5) underneath portion of iris, and (6) pupillary zone or circular area of pupil. The junctions include (1) junction of eye lashes with lids; (2) fornices (singular-fornix), where bulbar conjunctiva gets attached to palpebral conjunctiva; (3) sclerocorneal junction or limbus; (4) pupillary margin; (5) inner canthus; and (6) outer canthus.

Six coats (*patal*) are differentiated as two external and four internal. The external two coats are the upper eyelid and lower eyelid. (Although one may not be able to replace all ayurvedic terms with modern medical term, effort has been made to give more appropriate parallel terms.) The first internal coat is sclera (*tejojalashrit patal*). It is the outermost coat and consists an aqueous humor (*tejojal*). Other important areas in this layer are the whites of eyes (*shwetapatal*) and the cornea (*karnika*). The second internal coat is the choroid (*mamsashrit patal*), a fleshy coat that has been indicated at times as *krishnapatal*. Important structures in this coat are the choroid (*kalaka*), cilliary body (*upataraka*), pupil (*tara*), and iris (*taraka*). Medas patal is the third internal coat. Some scholars consider this as the lens (*drishtimani*) and vitreous humor (*sandrajala*). The fourth internal coat is the retina (*asthipatal* or *drishtipatal*). This coat is said to be placed midway between *krishnapatal* and *medas patal*. Some scholars consider this coat as the pupil (*drihti*), whereas others consider it as the entire retina.[6]

29.3 Etiology of Eye Disorders

Etiological factors of eye disorders discussed in Ayurveda[7,8] are the following:

1. Constant exposure to cold water
2. Exposure to cold immediately after exposure to heat
3. Constant watching of distant objects
4. Alteration in sleep pattern
5. Tensions
6. Excessive exercise
7. Crying
8. Anger
9. Trauma
10. Consuming sour preparations in excess
11. Controlling essential urges
12. Increased amount of sudation
13. Exposure to gases or fumes, e.g., pollutant on roadways or from industries
14. Purification measures (*panchakarma* [e.g., induced emesis in excess])
15. Observing microscopic objects for long periods

In traumatic eye disorders, the traumatic lesion causes vitiation of *dosas* in the eye.

29.4 Pathogenesis of Eye Disorders

Vitiated *dosas* move upward to the eyes, invade various channels, and lead to malfunctioning of various substructures of the eye. The vitiated *dosas*, especially the *pita dosa*, propagate through the channels or vessels (*srotasa*) toward the head region. They enter various parts of the eye such as the lids, junction, sclera, iris, choroids, cilliary body, pupil, and retina and cause a variety of eye diseases.[9,10]

29.5 Clinical Features of Eye Disorders

The general symptoms of eye disorders[11] are the following:

1. Eyes with muddy discharge
2. Hazy cornea or sclera
3. Congestion of eye
4. Sticking of lids due to eye discharge (due to *kapha*)

5. Heaviness of the lids or eyes (due to *kapha*)
6. Burning sensation or hot feeling of eyes (due to *pitta*)
7. Pricking pain in eyes (due to *vata*)
8. Hyperemia of eyes (in *rakta* predominance)
9. Foreign body sensation
10. Pain in lids
11. Visual disturbances
12. Difficulty in eye movement
13. Difficulty in closing or opening of eye
14. Impaired visual perception

29.6 Classification of Eye Disorders

Ayurvedic texts describe 76 to 96 ocular diseases and have several systems of classification, namely, based on vitiated *dosas* (67), therapeutic management (76), or anatomical structure based (76).[12–15] The structure-based classification closely resembles the classification mentioned in conventional medicine. The diseases are also characterized based on prognosis: curable, difficult to cure, and incurable. An attempt is made to translate Ayurvedic names of eye disorders, but Ayurvedic scholars of eye diseases may disagree on some of the translations.

29.7 Symptoms, Etiology, Pathology, and Management of Eye Disorders

The management of some of the eye disorders in Ayurvedic texts is very similar to contemporary modern ophthalmology. Only six diseases are selected as examples of Ayurvedic management in this chapter: (1) conjunctivitis (*abhishyanda*), (2) glaucoma (*adhimantha*), (3) trichiasis (*pakshmakopa*), (4) chalazion (*utsangini* and *lagan*), (5) cataract (*kaphaja linganash*), and (6) miscellaneous diseases (*Drishtigata vyadhi*). Formulations used in the management of eye diseases are given in Table 29.1.

29.7.1 Conjunctivitis (*Abhishyanda*)

According to Ayurvedic texts, conjunctivitis (*abhishyanda* or *syandam*) refers to a condition in which there mainly exists a congestion in general of all channels situated above the level of clavicle (collar bone) and specifically that of the eye.[15,16] According to modern ophthalmology, inflammation of conjunctiva characterized by redness of the eye and conjunctival discharge is known as conjunctivitis.[17] According to Ayurvedic texts, it is considered to be one of the major causes for eye disorders. If not treated, in time it can lead to other severe ocular disorders similar to those known in conventional medicine.[18,19]

TABLE 29.1

Formulations Used in the Management of Eye Diseases

Formula Name	Text Reference	Manufacturer[a]
Triphala ghrita	*Siddha yoga sangraha* *Sahasrayogam*	BAB, AVS
Mahatriphala ghrita	*Siddha yoga sangraha* *Sahasrayogam*	AVP
Shatavaryadi ghrita	*Bharat bhaishajya ratnakara*	AVP, AVS
Saptamruta yoga	*Siddha yoga sangraha*	BAB
Punarnavashtak kwatha	*Sharangdhara samhita*	BAB, ZP, SP
Rasanjana	*Sharangdhara samhita*	Classic formula manufacturers
Paradanaga rasanjana	*Netra roga vidnyana*	Classic formula manufacturers
Punarnavanjana	*Netra roga vidnyana*	Classic formula manufacturers
Netrashani rasa	*Netra roga vidnyana*	Classic formula manufacturers
Marichyadi yoga	*Yoga ratnakara*	Classic formula manufacturers
Nibapatranetrabindu	*Dravyaguna vidnyana*	Classic formula manufacturers
I-tone eyedrops	Patented and proprietary drug	DP
Ophthacre eyedrops	Patented and proprietary drug	HDC

[a]AVP = Arya Vaidya Pharmacy, Coimbtore, India; AVS = Arya Vaidya Sala, Kottakal, Kerala, India; BAB = Baidyanatha Ayurveda Bhavana, Nagpur, India; DP = Dey's Pharmaceuticals, Calcutta, India; HDC = Himalaya Drug Company, Banglore, India; SP = Sandu Pharmaceuticals, Mumbai, India; ZP = Zandu Pharmaceuticals, Mumbai, India.

29.7.1.1 Symptoms

The common symptoms of conjunctivitis are muddiness of eyes, inflammation of eyes, epiphora or discharge, itching of eyes, heaviness of the eyes, pain in the eyes, burring of the eyes, and congestion of eyes.[20,21] Ayurvedic scholars defined this disease as an infectious disease (*aupasargika roga*)[22] and classified it into four types of conjunctivitis: *vataja abhishyanda, pittaja abhishyanda, kaphaja abhishyanda,* and *raktaja abhishyanda*. Descriptions of each are listed below.[23]

1. Subacute catarrhal conjunctivitis and catarrhal conjunctivitis (*vataja*) — Symptoms include pricking pain in the eye, stiffness of the appendages of eye (e.g., lids), horripilation, foreign body sensation, roughness, headache, dryness in eye, cool lacrimation, and slight oedema of eye. These symptoms are relieved with oleation and heat treatment.[24]
2. Acute catarrhal conjunctivitis (*pittaja*) — Symptoms include burning sensation of the eye, suppuration or pus formation, feeling of smokiness, blackish lids, chemosis, edematous lids, aggregation of exudates within the eye, and a feeling of extreme heat. These conditions are relieved with cool therapies.[25]
3. Catarrhal conjunctivitis or purulent conjunctivitis or mucopurulent conjunctivitis (*kaphaja*) — Symptoms include heaviness in and around eyes, swelling of the eyes, itching of eyes, sticking of the lids due to purulent or mucopurulent discharge, feeling drowsy, and loss of taste. These conditions are relieved with hot therapies.[26]
4. Acute mucopurulent conjunctivitis (*raktaja*) — Symptoms include red lacrimation along with a pus or blood-stained discharge, red eye, or the entire eye appears to be red with red capillaries. Symptomatology is similar to the *pittaja* type.[27]

29.7.1.2 Treatment

Patients should be protected from external factors like fumes, dust, bright sunlight, etc. Treatment of conjunctivitis is done in two phases; one is specific for a chronic condition (*amavastha*) and the other is specific for acute condition phase (*teevravastha*).[28,29] In the chronic phase, the therapy is directed toward toxic waste materials in the body, which can continue up to 4 to 5 days with the same preliminary practices before advising *panchakarma* procedures such as fasting (*langhan*), sudation therapy (*swedan*), applying a layer of thin medicament paste on the lid of the affected eye (*pralepa*), and eating bitter foods to cause elimination of toxic materials into the gut. During this treatment, patients are asked to avoid heavy meals, bathing, intake of decoction, and eye ointment and liners.

After treating the chronic phase (*samavastha*), the patient is given treatment in the phase after the toxic materials are eliminated (*niramavastha*). The treatment includes two aspects: (1) local therapy and (2) general therapy. Certain local therapeutic modalities used in *niramavastha* are *tarpana, putapaka, parisheka,* eyedrops (*ashchyotana*), eye powder (*anjanna*), medicated smoking (*dhoomra*), and nasal drops (*shirobasti, nasya*). Drugs used for treatment of conjunctivitis according to vitiated *dosa,* particularly in the form of eyedrops, are described here. In general therapy, one has to undergo *panchakarma* therapy to eliminate the vitiated *dosa* from the gut and body and its further aggregation and bring them to equilibrium. The specific procedures of general therapy are given only if necessary. The following decoctions are cleaned and filtered through a very fine filter and used as eyedrops.

29.7.1.2.1 Vataja Type

1. *Brihat panchamool* or *brihati* (*Solonum indicum*), *erand* (*Ricinus communis*), and *shigru* (*Moringa olifera*) in decoction form
2. *Nimbapatra* (*Azadirrhacta indica*) and *lodhra* (*Symplcos racemosus*)
3. *Saindhav* (salt), *pippali* (*Piper longum*), *wala* (*Andropogan vetiveria*), and *yashtimadhu* (*Glycerrhyza glabra*) processed with medicated milk (*siddha dugdha*)

29.7.1.2.2 Pittaja Type

1. *Kamal* (*Nymphea* spp.), *neelakamal* (*Nymphea* spp.), *amalki* (*Phyllanthus embelicus*), *kantakari* (*Solanum xanthocarpum*), *brihati* (*Solanum indicum*), *dashmool, shatavari* (*Asparagus racemosus*), *talispatra* (*Abies webbiana*), and *manjishtha* (*Rubia cordifolia*) in decoction form
2. *Chandan* (*Santalinum album*), *manjishtha* (*Rubia cordifilia*), *yashtimadhu* (*Glycerrhyza glabra*), lodhra (*Symplocos racemosus*), *surarnagarik,* and honey; used in painful conditions of the eye

29.7.1.2.3 Kaphaja Type

1. Decoction of roots and bark of *bilva* (*Aegel marmelos*), *kantakari* (*Solanum xanthocarpum*), and *aragvadha* (*Cassia fistula*)
2. Decoction of *shunthi* (*Zinziber officinalis*), *triphala* (mixture of fruits of three myrobalans, neem (*Azadiracta indica*), *vasa* (*Adhatoda vasika*), and *lodhra* (*Symplocos racemosus*)

29.7.1.2.4 Raktaja Type

A decoction for treating this type includes eyedrops made up of *stree stanya* (breast milk), mixture of *musta* (*Cyperus rotandus*) and *jyeshthamadhu* (*Glycirrhiza glabza*) in rain water, and *lodhra* (*Symplocos racemosus*) in dehydrated butter from cow's milk (ghee). This is all mixed with water along with triphala and sugar.

A great difference does not exist with regard to the current Ayurvedic therapy and that of traditional practice (textual therapy). However certain formulations cannot be prepared today because of the unavailability of certain ingredients or because of difficulties in proper identification of certain ingredients. Many Ayurvedic physicians use Ayurvedic commercial eyedrops in the treatment of conjunctivitis such as Ophthacare Eyedrops (Himalaya Drug Company, Banglore, India) or Itone Eyedrops (Dey's Pharmaceutical, Calcutta, India). These products are made under sterile conditions instead of having the companies make their own.

In contemporary ophthalmology, there are various approaches to treating different types of conjunctivitis. Basically, usage of antimicrobial preparations and antiallergics have a major role in the treatment of conjunctivitis.

Ayurveda is especially useful when patients have nonspecific conjunctivitis or have resistance to existing antibiotic preparations. With these types of patients, the use of Ayurvedic therapy either alone or as an adjuvant therapy is useful.

29.7.2 Glaucoma (*Adhimantha*)

According to Ayurvedic texts, glaucoma (*adhimantha*) is an ocular disorder characterized by pain in the eye with a particularly churning or throbbing type of pain. The pain is very severe as if the eye is being scooped out, crushed, or churned.[30,31] According to modern ophthalmology, glaucoma is a symptomatic condition where there is pain in the eye because of increase in the intraocular pressure of the eyeball. Glaucoma is a condition of the eye in which the ocular tension is raised above the normal. The tension becomes high because of the faulty drainage of the aqueous humor. The tension of the eye is variable in health and is usually between 16 to 23 mmHg measured by the Schiotz tonometer.[32]

29.7.2.1 Etiology

According to Ayurveda, if a case of conjunctivitis (*abhishyanda*) is not treated in time, it may lead to glaucoma (*adhimantha*).[33]

29.7.2.2 Classification of Glaucoma

According to Ayurveda, glaucoma can be classified into four types (*dosa*-based classification): *vataja, pittaja, kaphaja,* and *raktaja adhimantha*.[34] As per modern contemporary ophthalmology, there are various approaches of classification of glaucoma. Examples include primary and secondary glaucoma, acquired and congenital glaucoma, acute and chronic glaucoma, and open-angle and angle-closure glaucoma.[35]

29.7.2.3 Symptoms

29.7.2.3.1 Vataja Type

With *vataja* type of glaucoma,[36] there is a severe feeling of pain at the eyebrows, temple region, and in the half portion of the head (of the side of an affected eye). There is congestion, muddiness of cornea, tinnitus, and vertigo.

29.7.2.3.2 *Pittaja Type*

Symptoms of the *pittaja* type of glaucoma[37] include severe pain in the eyes as if they were being burnt by fire or a caustic chemical (*kshara*). The eyes have red capillary network throughout and are liver-colored. They are watery with edematous lids, and there is a burning sensation at the head region. The patient is often unconscious.

29.7.2.3.3 *Kaphaja Type*

With the *kaphaja* type of glaucoma,[38] the eyes are heavy, with secretion, edema, echimosis, excessive lacrimation, cold and sticky discharge, hypersensitivity, and headache. The patient sees things as smoky, dirty, and imperfect (suggestive of halos). Other symptoms include a sunken cornea and bulged sclera (suggestive of shallow angle of anterior chamber).

29.7.2.3.4 *Raktaja Adhimantha Type*

Symptoms of the *raktaja adhimantha* type of glaucoma[39] include severe pain in the eyes with tenderness, blood-stained discharge, redness, and ciliary congestion. The patient visualizes colors and flames.

29.7.2.4 Prognosis

If not treated in time, there is a possibility of blindness. According to ancient Ayurvedic texts, one may lose sight within 7 days in the *kaphaj* type, 6 days in *vataj*, 5 days in *raktaj adhimantha*, and 3 days or sudden loss (*tatkal*) in the *pittaj* type.[40] It is also the understanding in modern ophthalmology that if the glaucoma is not treated properly or remains untreated, irreversible loss of visual field may occur, which can lead to blindness.

29.7.2.5 Treatment

Ayurveda has two lines of treatment for glaucoma: general and specific.[41–43]

29.7.2.5.1 *General Line of Treatment*

The patient is advised to rest the affected eye and is given sudation, proper diet, and induced medicated purgation at the period of exacerbation of the disease. The patient should avoid intake of liquors and excess sleep. Detoxification methods (*panchakarma*) such as the oleation, sudation, and induced medicated purgation or enema are advised to eliminate vitiated *dosas* that are responsible for the problem. Another unique technique advised traditionally is bloodletting, where leeches are applied around the temporal region. This technique is not currently popular. The patient is advised to take meat soups with ghee, oils, fats, and bone marrows and processed milk medicated with drugs such as *meshashringi* (*Gymnea sylvestris*) and *ajamoda* (*Carum roxburghianum*). The patient is given *triphala* ghee orally after food. During the acute pain phase, the patient is given *kapitha* medicated milk or *brihat panchamool siddha* ghee or milk.

29.7.2.5.2 *Specific Line of Treatment*

Many physicians prescribe specific formulations such as *punarnavashtaka kwatha, chandraprabha vati, laghu malini vasanta rasa, mahatriphala ghrita, saptamruta loha,* and many other Ayurvedic medicines orally for treatment, and certain medicaments are applied locally as ophthalmic preparation (*anjanas*). The following ophthalmic preparations are applied gently on palpebral conjunctiva: *parad nag rasanjana* and *punarnava anjana*.

29.7.2.5.3 *Cauterization (Agnikarma)*

Cauterization is done only when there is no relief from other recommended medication. Cauterization is a form of heat therapy. Heat is applied by a special hot metal rod placed in-between the eyebrows or at the lateral ends of the eyebrows. This procedure is currently not practiced.

Ghee is applied to these spots, and the wound is then treated with a paste made of 125 mg of common salt and ten leaves of neem (*Azadirrhacta indica*). If a patient comes with a higher degree of intraocular pressure (IOP), the first line of therapy recommended to Ayurvedic eye departments is surgical procedures (antiglaucoma surgeries [AGS]). For fresh cases with mild to moderate increase in the IOP, Ayurvedic physicians provide Ayurvedic therapy.

In conventional ophthalmology, the treatment of glaucoma includes the use of diuretics, meotic agents (e.g., pilocarpine), and the latest antiglaucoma drugs (e.g., Timolol maleate) as a conservative therapy. Treatment can also include various surgical procedures (AGS) such as iridectomy, cyclodiathermy, and trabeculectomy.[44]

29.7.3 Trichiasis and Entropion (*Pakshmakopa* and *Antarvyavartana*)

29.7.3.1 Pathogenesis

Vata, *pitta*, and *kapha* in their aggravated stages cause dryness and pointed eyelashes. The involvement of *vata* causes the eyelashes to turn inside, touching the sclera and cornea and giving rise to friction and irritation of these surfaces.[45] Trichiasis involves inversion of a varying numbers of eyelashes, so that they rub against the cornea (eyelid margins are in the normal position). The misdirected eyelashes cause mechanical irritation and injury to the cornea, with pain, lacrimation, photophobia, and ulceration.[46]

29.7.3.2 Treatment

Ayurveda recommends removal of the defective eyelashes.[47] Again, there is a similarity in the Ayurvedic treatment with the modern therapeutic approach of removing the eye lashes with the epilation forcep.[48] The contraction of the lid may also cause the above problem. In modern ophthalmology, this can be compared with trichiasis and entropion, respectively. Surgical procedures for trichiasis (*pakshmakopa*) and entropion (*pakshmasankocha* or *antarvyavartana*) discussed by various Aayurvedic scholars are similar to those of the modern surgical procedure of tarsorrhaphy.[49] In practice, Ayurvedic physicians apply certain pastes on eyelashes or use epilation forceps to epilate the hair follicle of eye lashes. In case of entropion or ectropion, modern surgery usually is recommended.

29.7.4 Chalazion (*Utsangini* and *Lagan*) (Internal Hordeolum, Tarsal Cyst, and Meibomian Cyst)

This consists of a swelling of the meibomian gland following an obstruction of its duct accompanied by chronic inflammation in the surrounding tarsus. More than one chalazion may occur at the same time.[50]

29.7.4.1 Pathogenesis

According to Ayurveda, this condition is due to vitiation of all the three *dosas* (*tridohadushti*) and vitiation of the blood (*raktadushti*).[51]

29.7.4.2 Symptoms

The signs and symptoms are itching and pain. In addition, when the eye is opened there is discharge similar to egg yolk.[52]

29.7.4.3 Treatment

The recommended treatment in both conventional medicine and Ayurveda is surgery. The Ayurvedic practitioner uses the paste of herbal ingredients such as *hirakasis, trikatu, rasanjana,* and *saindhava* mixed with honey to heal the wound.[53]

29.7.5 Cataract (*Kaphaja Linganasha*)

Cataract is a well-identified and characterized eye disorder in Ayurveda. *Linganash* is a term derived from two words: *linga* (funtion) and *nash* (destruction). When there is destruction of the function of the eye, the lens becomes opaque and is known as *linganasha*.[54] Opacification (formation of opacities) in the crystalline lens is known as cataract.[55] Ayurveda recognizes three stages of cataract: initial blurred vision stage or refractive error (*timir*), immature cataract (kacha), and cataract (*kaphaja linganasha*). These stages are not recognized contemporary medicine. Ayurvedic physicians refer these patients to conventional-medicine doctors for the latest procedures, such as intraocular lens implantations, which are far superior and effective to deal with this condition.

29.7.5.1 Treatment

Although the following methods are not practiced today, the descriptions below are given to show how surgery was practiced thousands of years ago.[57–60]

Ayurveda mentions preoperative procedures (*poorvakarma*), main operative procedures (*pradhana karma*), and post-operative procedures (*pashchat karma*). The procedure describes piercing the globe at a particular position, specifically at the intersection of two thirds of the limbal side and one third of the outer canthal side. This is where a thin rodlike instrument (*shalaka*) is used to prick in such a way that it does not disturb other important appendages of the eye or blood vessels of the eye; it reaches straight to the opaque lens (*drushtimani*) and produces a typical sound when watery secretions of *linganasha dosa* (liquified lenticular matter) come out. This is somewhat similar to the latest approach of surgery, the phacoemulsification procedure. The procedure needs to be done in such a way that the patient is able to see objects like fingers (*anguli*) and threads (*tantu*) clearly. The eye is covered with a dressing of medicated ghee and is properly bandaged.

Ayurveda also describes the complications resulting from a surgery performed by an inexperienced surgeon (e.g., breaking of the lens in several pieces or lens falling back into vitreous chamber) and how to remedy them.

Ayurvedic ophthalmic surgeons currently follow all modern methods of treatment, including conventional modern drugs for anesthesia. Surgeons also undertake procedures like intraocular lens (IOL) implants as well for cataract.

29.7.6 Miscellaneous Eye Disorders (*Drishtigat Vyadhi*)

Ayurveda mentions 12 disorders of *drishtigat vyadhi*.[56] Six types are *linganasha* and the other six disorders include *nakulandhya* (eye looks like those of a cat under a flashlight). The pupil gives a bright light suggestive of retinoblastoma of the eye or glioma of the retina. According to Ayurveda and conventional medicine, it is an incurable disease. Enucleation of the eyeball should be undertaken as soon as possible. In descriptions of *patalgat dushti*, equivalents of vitreous degenerations, cobwebs, mosquitoes, refractive errors, diplopias, and even clues towards retinal detachments are found. A certain description given by *Vagbhatacharya* for timir specifically points to hypermetropia and myopia. In *tritiya patalgat dushti*, references are indicative of conditions similar to retinal detachments.

29.8 Scientific Basis

An attempt is made here to review the existing scientific literature on Ayurvedic ophthalmology. The references are taken from different sources such as research journals, postgraduate theses, and Internet databases. Some references do not have details, but they are cited only to show that there has been an interest.

29.8.1 Clinical Studies

29.8.1.1 Conjunctivitis

1. Neem eyedrops on viral conjunctivitis (*netrabhishyanda* by *nimbapatra netrabindu*) —The drops were prepared in the department of the *shalakyatantra*. There were 30 patients of viral conjunctivitis who were treated for 3 weeks with sterilized eyedrops prepared from the extract of leaves of *Azadirrhacta indica*. The improvement was statistically significant.[61]
2. Ophthacare eyedrops (a herbal formulation manufactured by Himalaya Drug Company) — An open multicentric clinical trial was conducted in patients suffering from various ophthalmic disorders, namely conjunctivitis, conjunctival xerosis (dry eye), acute dacryocystitis, and degenerative conditions (e.g., pterygium and pinguecula), and in postoperative patients of cataract with Ophthacare. The formula contains chemical ingredieents (details not available) from *Carum copticum, Terminalia belerica, Emblica officinalis, Curcuma longa, Ocimum sanctum, Cinnamonum camphora, Rosa damascena*, and *meldespumapum*. These herbs reportedly possess anti-infective and anti-inflammatory properties.[62]
3. Second study on Ophthacare eyedrops — This was a comparative, double-blind, multicentric-randomized, placebo-controlled clinical trial that included 157 patients suffering from different eye ailments: cataract dry eye syndrome, ocular asthenia, refractive errors, and allergic conjunctivitis with a herbal eyedrop preparation and placebo. In both dry eye syndrome and ocular asthenia, the herbal eyedrop preparation was promising. In a few cataract patients, the vision seemed to improve. No analysis of the data was given. In early myopia, it seems to correct the refractive errors whereas in high myopic conditions it controlled the progressive deteriorations. Subjective improvements were also noted with hypermetropia, presbyopia, and astigmatism. Its healing capacity in allergic conjunctivitis was

certainly better than placebo. It had no short-term or long-term side effects and is considered to be a useful drug in all conditions studied.[63]

29.8.2 Refractive Errors

Although there are no direct references available on refractive errors in ancient Ayurvedic texts, some of the texts are indicative of refractive disorders. Available studies in this area are described below.

1. *Saptamrut loha* and *yashad bhasma* on refractive errors — Although details of the study are not available, the results were reported to be encouraging.[64]
2. *Saptamrut loha*, *Yashtimadhu ghruta*, *Shatavari ghruta*, *Punarnavadi yoga*, and *Pathyadi kwatha* — The author of this chapter has treated many patients with refractive disorders such as high myopia and high hypermetropia by using these formulas with encouraging results at The Center of Ayurveda and Panchakarma Therapy, Eye Care Clinic.

Some studies done at postgraduate institutes of Ayurveda in India by postgraduate students and others on different eye disorders such as trachoma, pterygium, blephritis, corneal ulcer, and retinal disorders are presented here.

29.8.2.1 Trachoma (Pothaki)

As per Ayurvedic texts,[65] trachoma consists of multiple projections that are reddish on the inner side of the lid (on palpebral conjunctiva).These symptoms are combined with profuse eye discharge, pain, itching, and heaviness in eyes.

According to modern medicine, trachoma (granular conjunctivitis or granular eyelids) is a specific contagious disease of the conjunctiva and cornea. It is chronic and characterized by a subepithelial infiltration of the conjunctiva by a cellular granulation tissue, which is responsible for the presence of the typical follicles or granulations.

29.8.2.2 Therapeutic Efficacy of Shobhanjana Eyedrops in Trachoma (Pothaki)

In one unpublished study,[66] there were 30 patients with trachoma, where 22 patients in the prefollicular stage of trachoma and 8 patients in the follicular stage of trachoma. All patients were treated with the eyedrops for 8 weeks. There were 25 patients (85%) who showed complete relief, 3 patients (10%) who have moderate relief, and 2 patients (5%) who showed no relief.

29.8.2.3 Pterygium (Arma)

As per Ayurvedic texts,[67] this is a disease of sclera (*shwetamandala*). It is a triangular growth from either the inner or outer canthus heading toward the limbus. Ayurveda classifies it into five types.

According to modern ophthalmology, pterygium is a threefold of conjunctiva. It occupies the interpalpebral fissure extending from the inner or outer part of the bulbar conjunctiva on the cornea, and the base spreads out and merges with the subconjunctival tissue.

In Ayurvedic texts, there is mention of both surgical and medical treatment of pterygium. Thirty patients of Pterigyum were treated with *Marichyadi yoga* (containing marich [*Piper nigrum*] and triturated with the juice of kesharaj [*Eclipta alba*]) for 4 weeks at one of the institutes by a postgraduate student. Results were encouraging in 75% of the cases.[68]

29.8.2.4 Corneal Ulcer (Savarna Shukra)[69]

As per Ayurvedic texts, there is an ulceration of the cornea (*krishnapatal*) because of vitiated increased *pitta*; it is circular in shape, with a little depression on the area of ulcer bed, and it is surrounded by neovascularization. There is pain, redness, and overlacrimation of the ulcer-affected eye. According to modern ophthalmology, the break of the continuous lining of the epithelial line of the cornea is known as a corneal ulcer. There are various causes attributed to the formation of the corneal ulcers.

Yashtimadhu ghruta (medicated ghee composed of *amalki* [*Phyllanthus embelicus*], *haritaki* [*Terminalia chebula*], *bhibhitaki* [*Terminalia belerica*], *musta* [*Cyperus rotandus*], and *haridra* [*Curcuma longa*]) was investigated in 30 patients with corneal ulcers by a postgraduate student at one of the institutes. Significant healing activity was noted within 6 to 7 days ($p < 0.05$).[70]

29.8.2.5 Blepharitis (Klinnavratma)

As per Ayurvedic texts,[71] Blepharitis (*klinnavartma*) is explained as two types: simple blepharitis (*Pralinna vartma*) and ulcerative blepharitis (*aklinna vartma*). In simple blepharitis there is swelling of the lids, sticky blood-stained discharge from eyes, and pain and itching of the eyelids. This is a *kaphaja* disorder. In ulcerative blepharitis, there are ulcerations at the level of edges of the eyelids, which may lead to entropion if not treated correctly. According to modern ophthalmology, blepharitis is a chronic inflammatory condition of the margin of the eyelids. It occurs in two forms: nonulcerative (squamous blepharitis) and ulcerative.

In one clinical study[72] done at the institute by postgraduate students, *rasanjanadi rasakriya* (ointment containing *daruharidra* [*Berberis aristata*] processed in goat's milk) was used to treat 30 patients with blephritis by external application. The ointment (*anjan*) showed healing activity, reduced edema, discharge, itching, and pricking pain within the first week. The results were significant ($p < 0.05$).

29.8.2.6 Retinal Disorders

29.8.2.6.1 Diabetic Retinopathy

Fifteen patients of diabetic retinopathy (a complication of diabetes mellitus) were given *Vasant kusumakar Rasa*; the other 15 patients were given a placebo for a 12-week period. There was a good improvement in, seven cases, no change observed in seven cases, and deterioration in the condition observed in one case. One case of those seven cases improved. This case initially had retinopathy and showed no evidence of the diabetic retinopathy, but a complete cure was seen at the end of the study. Three cases showed marked improvement, whereas two cases showed marginal improvement. There was no significant change noticed in the biochemical parameters at the end of the therapy.[73]

29.8.2.6.2 Retinitis Pigmentosa

In an open prospective study[74] on 15 cases of retinitis pigmentosa having less than 3 ft of vision, 2 cases were screened with electroretinography and visual-evoked potential studies in both pre- and posttherapy. The drugs used in the study were *shatavaryadi ghrita, netryatarpaka yoga*, and *mahatraiphal ghrita*, along with certain herbal combinations of *punarnava, yashtimadhu, amalki*, and other herbs. Treatment was given in either form, orally or locally. *Ghrita* were used locally. All these preparations were prepared at the Center of Ayurveda and Panchakarma Therapy, Eye Care Clinic. Nine patients completed the study, of which four showed a marked improvement in the visual acuity, four showed moderate improvement, and one patient showed no change.

29.8.3 Studies on Special Therapeutic Procedures

One of the Ayurvedic *panchakarma* therapies used in Ayurvedic ophthalmology is *tarpana* (eye is kept in medicated ghee for a given predetermined period while keeping the patient in a supine position). A preliminary study[75] was conducted by the author of this chapter on 25 healthy volunteers to assess this therapy's safety profile. Certain parameters such as IOP, temperature, pulse, respiration, blood pressure, and other common ocular symptoms and signs were observed for possible adverse effects. No serious adverse effect were noticed and no significant results were obtained.

29.8.4 Biological Studies

The anticonjunctival activity of the *punarnava* (*Borehaavia diffusa*) and neem (*Azadirachta indica*) was assessed by preparing water extracts and testing them on the experimental model of bacterial conjunctivitis in rats. The experimental study revealed that both extracts as well as marketed gentamicin eyedrops showed statistically significant anticonjunctival activity. Herbal extracts showed comparable effect with the established drug, Gentamycin.[76]

29.8.5 Antimicrobial Activities of Herbs Used in the Treatment of Eye Disorders

A study of *in vitro* antibacterial activity of extracts from the plants *T. chebula, E. alba,* and *O. sanctum* was carried out by disk diffusion technique. All showed activity against human pathogenic Gram-positive and Gram-negative bacteria. The activity against salmonella organisms was shown only by *T. chebula*; the action against shigella organisms was shown by *T. chebula* and *E. alha,* but not by *O. sanctum*. The widest spectrum of antibacterial activity was shown by *T. chebula*. It was also most potent. The antibacterial spectrum of *E. alba* was between that of *T. chebula* and *O. sanctum*. The narrowest spectrum of antibacterial activity was observed in *O. sanctum*.[77]

Eugenia aromatica (lavanga) (clove) has been studied for its antibacterial activity. Clove oil inhibited tuberculosis at 1:80 dilution. Ethanol extracts of clove inhibited the growth of *C. botulinum*. The extracts were also found to be effective against several Gram-positive and Gram-negative microorganisms tested on agar media at 5000 ppm.[78]

The chloroform extract of *Azadirachta indica* (neem) oil has been found to be fungicidal for common skin pathogens *Trichphyton* spp. The essential oil has shown antibacterial activity against *Staph. aureus, E. coli., S. pyogenes,* etc. *A. flavus* and other fungi are also susceptible to neem oil. Neem has known to have antiviral properties.

The volatile oil from the fruit of *Piper nigrum* (*Maricha*) showed antifungal activity.[79] A crystalline fraction obtained from bark of *Symplocos racemosa* Roxb. (*Lodhra*) is found to inhibit the growth of staphylococci.[80] Cold water extract of the fruit of *Terminalia belerica* Roxb. (*bibhitaka*) was found to posses antibacterial activity.[81] *Curcuma longa* (*haridra*) exhibits antimicrobial activity; sodium curcuminate in a dilution of 1:1 million inhibited micrococcus pyogenes.[82]

29.8.6 Anti-Inflammatory Activity of Herbs Used in the Treatment of Eye Disorders

The anti-inflammatory activity of various extracts of roots of *Boerhaavia diffusa* Linn. were studied in carragenin-induced edema and formaldehyde-induced arthritis in albino rats. Acetone extract showed most the potent anti-inflammatory effect.[83]

Commiphora mukul (*Guggul*) has been extensively studied for its anti-inflammatory effects. The steroidal component of Fraction A of the petroleum ether extract has marked antiarthritic effect comparable with that of hydrocortisone and more potent than phenyl-butazone.[84]

Water extract of *Curcuma lona* Linn. (*haridra*) showed significant anti-inflammatory activity in acute carrageenin-induced edema. Active principle curcumin showed anti-inflammatory activity similar with cortisone and phenylbutazone in carrageenin-induced edema in rats with an equivalent dose.[85]

Acknowledgments

I would like to thank Dr. Amita Manu, Dr. Ashish Mungantiwar, and Dr. Lakshmi Mishra for their valuable help in developing this chapter. I also acknowledge all institutes, authors of papers, and editors of various journals cited in this chapter.

References

1. Sushrutacharya, *Sushruta Samhita, Ayurvedatatvasandipika*, Hindi commentary by Kaviraj, A.S., Chaukhamba Sanskrit Series Office, Varanasi, India, 1959, *Uttartantram*, chap. 1/5, p. 2.
2. Vartak, S.G., *Doshadhatumalavidnyanam* (Sanskrit), 1st ed., Atreya Prakashana, 1968, p. 45.
3. Padmawar, R., *Netrarogavidnyana*, 3rd ed., Shri Baidyanath Ayurved Bhavan Ltd., Nagpur, India, 1989, p. 5
4. Munje, B.S., *Netrachikitsa* (Sanskrit), 2nd ed., Shri Baidyanath Ayurved Bhavan Ltd., Nagpur, India, 1976, p. 12.
5. Sushrutacharya, *Sushruta Samhita, Ayurvedatatvasandipika*, Hindi commentary by Kaviraj, A.S., Chaukhamba Sanskrit Series Office, Varanasi, India, 1959, *Uttartantram*, chap. 1/14, p. 7.
6. Padmawar, R., *Netrarogavidnyana*, Shri Baidyanath Ayurved Bhavan Ltd., 3rd ed., Nagpur, India, 1989, p. 17.
7. Sushrutacharya, *Sushruta Samhita, Ayurvedatatvasandipika*, Hindi commentary by Kaviraj, A.S., Chaukhamba Sanskrit Series Office, Varanasi, India, 1959, *Uttartantram*, chap. 1/26–27, p. 11.
8. Dwivedi, R., *Shalakyatantra (Nimitantra)*, 9th ed., Chaukhamba Sanskrit Series Office, Varanasi, India, 1991, p. 436.
9. Dwivedi, R., *Shalakyatantra (Nimitantra)*, 9th ed., Chaukhamba Sanskrit Series Office, Varanasi, India, 1991, p. 444.
10. Sushrutacharya, *Sushruta Samhita, Ayurvedatatvasandipika*, Hindi commentary by Kaviraj, A.S., Chaukhamba Sanskrit Series Office, Varanasi, India, 1959, *Uttartantram*, chap. 1/20, p. 10.
11. Sushrutacharya, *Sushruta Samhita, Ayurvedatatvasandipika*, Hindi commentary by Kaviraj, A.S., Chaukhamba Sanskrit Series Office, Varanasi, India, 1959, *Uttartantram*, chap. 1/20–23, p. 11.

12. Sushrutacharya, *Sushruta Samhita, Ayurvedatatvasandipika,* Hindi commentary by Kaviraj, A.S., Chaukhamba Sanskrit Series Office, Varanasi, India, 1959, *Uttartantram,* chap. 1/28–45, pp. 12, 13.
13. Padmawar, R., *Netrarogavidnyana,* 3rd ed., Shri Baidyanath Ayurved Bhavan Ltd., Nagpur, India, 1989, p. 44.
14. Dwivedi, R., *Shalakyatantra (Nimitantra),* 9th ed., Chaukhamba Sanskrit Series Office, Varanasi, India, 1991, p. 429.
15. Vagbhatacharya, *Ashtanga Sangraha,* commentary by Kunte, A.M., Chaukhamba Orientalia, *Uttartantram,* chap. 16, p. 456.
16. Padmawar, R., *Netrarogavidnyana,* 3rd ed., Shri Baidyanath Ayurved Bhavan Ltd., Nagpur, India, 1989, p. 45.
17. Lyle, T., Cross, A., and Cook, C., *May & Worth's Manual of Diseases of the Eye,* 1st Indian ed., CBS Publishers & Distributors, Delhi, India, 1985, p. 142.
18. Sushrutacharya, *Sushruta Samhita, Ayurvedatatvasandipika,* Hindi commentary by Kaviraj, A.S., Chaukhamba Sanskrit Series Office, Varanasi, India, 1959, *Uttartantram,* chap. 6/5, p. 26.
19. Lyle, T., Cross, A., and Cook, C., *May & Worth's Manual of Diseases of the Eye,* 1st Indian ed., CBS Publishers & Distributors, Delhi, India, 1985, p. 156.
20. Padmawar, R., *Netrarogavidnyana,* 3rd ed., Shri Baidyanath Ayurved Bhavan Ltd., Nagpur, India, 1989, p. 47.
21. Dwivedi, R., *Shalakyatantra (Nimitantra),* 9th ed., Chaukhamba Sanskrit Series Office, Varanasi, India, 1991, p. 590.
22. Dwivedi, R., *Shalakyatantra (Nimitantra),* 9th ed., Chaukhamba Sanskrit Series Office, Varanasi, India, 1991, p. 591.
23. Padmawar, R., *Netrarogavidnyana,* 3rd ed., Shri Baidyanath Ayurved Bhavan Ltd., Nagpur, India, 1989, p. 46.
24. Sushrutacharya, *Sushruta Samhita, Ayurvedatatvasandipika,* Hindi commentary by Kaviraj, A.S., Chaukhamba Sanskrit Series Office, Varanasi, India, 1959, *Uttartantram,* chap. 6/6, p. 26.
25. Sushrutacharya, *Sushruta Samhita, Ayurvedatatvasandipika,* Hindi commentary by Kaviraj, A.S., Chaukhamba Sanskrit Series Office, Varanasi, India, 1959, *Uttartantram,* chap. 6/7, p. 26.
26. Sushrutacharya, *Sushruta Samhita, Ayurvedatatvasandipika,* Hindi commentary by Kaviraj, A.S., Chaukhamba Sanskrit Series Office, Varanasi, India, 1959, *Uttartantram,* chap. 6/8, p. 26.
27. Sushrutacharya, *Sushruta Samhita, Ayurvedatatvasandipika,* Hindi commentary by Kaviraj, A.S., Chaukhamba Sanskrit Series Office, Varanasi, India, 1959, *Uttartantram,* chap. 6/9, p. 26.
28. Padmawar, R., *Netrarogavidnyana,* 3rd ed., Shri Baidyanath Ayurved Bhavan Ltd., Nagpur, India, 1989, p. 48.
29. Dwivedi, R., *Shalakyatantra (Nimitantra),* 9th ed., Chaukhamba Sanskrit Series Office, Varanasi, India, 1991, p. 594.
30. Sushrutacharya, *Sushruta Samhita, Ayurvedatatvasandipika,* Hindi commentary by Kaviraj, A.S., Chaukhamba Sanskrit Series Office, Varanasi, India, 1959, *Uttartantram,* chap. 6/10–11, p. 27.
31. Sushrutacharya, *Sushruta Samhita, Ayurvedatatvasandipika,* Hindi commentary by Kaviraj, A.S., Chaukhamba Sanskrit Series Office, Varanasi, India, 1959, *Uttartantram,* chap. 6/12–13, p. 27.
32. Lyle, T., Cross, A., and Cook, C., *May & Worth's Manual of Diseases of the Eye,* 1st Indian ed., CBS Publishers & Distributors, Delhi, India, 1985, p. 364.
33. Sushrutacharya, *Sushruta Samhita, Ayurvedatatvasandipika,* Hindi commentary by Kaviraj, A.S., Chaukhamba Sanskrit Series Office, Varanasi, India, 1959, *Uttartantram,* chap. 6/10–11, p. 27.
34. Padmawar, R., *Netrarogavidnyana,* 3rd ed., Shri Baidyanath Ayurved Bhavan Ltd., Nagpur, India, 1989, p. 56.
35. Lyle, T., Cross, A., and Cook, C., *May & Worth's Manual of Diseases of the Eye,* 1st Indian ed., CBS Publishers & Distributors, Delhi, India, 1985, p. 369.
36. Sushrutacharya, *Sushruta Samhita, Ayurvedatatvasandipika,* Hindi commentary by Kaviraj, A.S., Chaukhamba Sanskrit Series Office, Varanasi, India, 1959, *Uttartantram,* chap. 6/12–13, p. 27.
37. Sushrutacharya, *Sushruta Samhita, Ayurvedatatvasandipika,* Hindi commentary by Kaviraj, A.S., Chaukhamba Sanskrit Series Office, Varanasi, India, 1959, *Uttartantram,* chap. 6/14–15, p. 28.
38. Sushrutacharya, *Sushruta Samhita, Ayurvedatatvasandipika,* Hindi commentary by Kaviraj, A.S., Chaukhamba Sanskrit Series Office, Varanasi, India, 1959, *Uttartantram,* chap. 6/16–17, p. 28.

39. Sushrutacharya, *Sushruta Samhita, Ayurvedatatvasandipika*, Hindi commentary by Kaviraj, A.S., Chaukhamba Sanskrit Series Office, Varanasi, India, 1959, *Uttartantram*, chap. 6/18–19, p. 28.
40. Sushrutacharya, *Sushruta Samhita, Ayurvedatatvasandipika*, Hindi commentary by Kaviraj, A.S., Chaukhamba Sanskrit Series Office, Varanasi, India, 1959, *Uttartantram*, chap. 6/20, p. 28.
41. Padmawar, R., *Netrarogavidnyana*, 3rd ed., Shri Baidyanath Ayurved Bhavan Ltd., Nagpur, India, 1989, p. 63.
42. Dwivedi, R., *Shalakyatantra (Nimitantra)*, 9th ed., Chaukhamba Sanskrit Series Office, Varanasi, India, 1991, p. 88.
43. Padmawar, R., *Netrarogavidnyana*, 3rd ed., Shri Baidyanath Ayurved Bhavan Ltd., Nagpur, India, 1989, p. 66.
44. Lyle, T., Cross, A., and Cook, C., *May & Worth's Manual of Diseases of the Eye*, 1st Indian ed., CBS Publishers & Distributors, Delhi, India, 1985, p. 387.
45. Padmawar, R., *Netrarogavidnyana*, 3rd ed., Shri Baidyanath Ayurved Bhavan Ltd., Nagpur, India, 1989, p. 64.
46. Lyle, T., Cross, A., and Cook, C., *May & Worth's Manual of Diseases of the Eye*, 1st Indian ed., CBS Publishers & Distributors, Delhi, India, 1985, p. 65.
47. Padmawar, R., *Netrarogavidnyana*, 3rd ed., Shri Baidyanath Ayurved Bhavan Ltd., Nagpur, India, 1989, p. 65.
48. Lyle, T., Cross, A., and Cook, C., *May & Worth's Manual of Diseases of the Eye*, 1st Indian ed., CBS Publishers & Distributors, Delhi, India, 1985, p. 80.
49. Dwivedi, R., *Shalakyatantra (Nimitantra)*, 9th ed., Chaukhamba Sanskrit Series Office, Varanasi, India, 1991, p. 525.
50. Lyle, T., Cross, A., and Cook, C., *May & Worth's Manual of Diseases of the Eye*, 1st Indian ed., CBS Publishers & Distributors, Delhi, India, 1985, p. 67.
51. Padmawar, R., *Netrarogavidnyana*, 3rd ed., Shri Baidyanath Ayurved Bhavan Ltd., Nagpur, India, 1989, p. 68.
52. Padmawar, R., *Netrarogavidnyana*, 3rd ed., Shri Baidyanath Ayurved Bhavan Ltd., Nagpur, India, 1989, p. 69.
53. Padmawar, R., *Netrarogavidnyana*, 3rd ed., Shri Baidyanath Ayurved Bhavan Ltd., Nagpur, India, 1989, p. 70.
54. Padmawar, R., *Netrarogavidnyana*, 3rd ed., Shri Baidyanath Ayurved Bhavan Ltd., Nagpur, India, 1989, p. 10.
55. Lyle, T., Cross, A., and Cook, C., *May & Worth's Manual of Diseases of the Eye*, 1st Indian ed., CBS Publishers & Distributors, Delhi, India, 1985, p. 253.
56. Padmawar, R., *Netrarogavidnyana*, 3rd ed., Shri Baidyanath Ayurved Bhavan Ltd., Nagpur, India, 1989, p. 100.
57. Padmawar, R., *Netrarogavidnyana*, 3rd ed., Shri Baidyanath Ayurved Bhavan Ltd., Nagpur, India, 1989, p. 111.
58. Sushrutacharya, *Sushruta Samhita, Ayurvedatatvasandipika*, Hindi commentary by Kaviraj, A.S., Chaukhamba Sanskrit Series Office, Varanasi, India, 1959, *Uttartantram*, chap. 17/55–99, p. 63.
59. Dwivedi, R., *Shalakyatantra (Nimitantra)*, 9th ed., Chaukhamba Sanskrit Series Office, Varanasi, India, 1991, p. 568.
60. Lyle, T., Cross, A., and Cook, C., *May & Worth's Manual of Diseases of the Eye*, 1st Indian ed., CBS Publishers & Distributors, Delhi, India, 1985, p. 306.
61. Salunke, A., Clinical study of *Netrabhishyanda* by *Nimbapatra Netrabindu Ashchyotana*. (Study on 30 patients of viral conjunctivitis using sterilized eye drops prepared from the extract of leaves of *Azadirrhacta indica*), M.D. thesis (Ayurveda), University of Mumbai, India, 1996.
62. Biswas, N.R. et al., Evaluation of Ophthacare eye drops: a herbal formulation in the management of various ophthalmic disorders, *Phytotherapy Res.*, 7, 618, 2001.
63. Biswas, N.R. et al., Comparative double blind multicentric randomised placebo controlled clinical trial of a herbal preparation of eye drops in some ocular ailments, *J. Indian Med. Assn.*, 943, 101–102, 1996.
64. Srinivasulu, C., Comparative evaluation of the effect of the *saptamrut loha* & *yashad bhasma* on refractive errors, M.D. thesis (Ayurveda), Banaras Hindu University, Varanasi, India, 1980.

65. Dwivedi, R., *Shalakyatantra (Nimitantra)*, 9th ed., Chaukhamba Sanskrit Series Office, Varanasi, India, 1991, p. 525.
66. Lahankar, M., Therapeutic Efficacy of *Shobhanjana* Eye Drops in Trachoma (Pothaki), M.D. thesis (Ayurveda), University of Mumbai, India, 1996.
67. Padmawar, R., *Netrarogavidnyana*, 3rd ed., Shri Baidyanath Ayurved Bhavan Ltd., Nagpur, India, 1989, p. 100.
68. Surve, S., A Clinical Evaluation of *Marichyadi yoga* on Pterygium (*Marichyadi yogaka Armapar adhyayana*), M.D. thesis (Ayurveda), University of Mumbai, India, 1997.
69. Dwivedi, R., *Shalakyatantra (Nimitantra)*, 9th ed., Chaukhamba Sanskrit Series Office, Varanasi, India, 1991, p. 568.
70. Dudhat, S., A Clinical Evaluation of Yashthimadhu Ghrita on Corneal Ulcers (*Savrana shukla vyadhimen Yashtimadhu Ghrutka Prayogika adhyayana*), M.D. thesis (Ayurveda), University of Mumbai, India, 1997.
71. Padmawar, R., *Netrarogavidnyana*, 3rd ed., Shri Baidyanath Ayurved Bhavan Ltd., Nagpur, India, 1989, p. 74.
72. Padvi, V., A clinical study of *Rasanjanadi rasakriya* on ulcerative blephritis (*Rasanjanadi Rasakriya ya Anjanacha Klinnavartma ya vyadhivara honara parinama eka adhyayana*), M.D. thesis (Ayurveda), University of Mumbai, India, 1999.
73. Tamboli, S., A Clinical Evaluation of *Vasant Kusumakara Rasa* in *Prameha Upadrava* with Special Reference to Diabetic Neuropathy and Diabetic Retinopathy, M.D. thesis (Ayurveda), University of Mumbai, India, 2001.
74. Phadke, A., A Clinical Evaluation of Cases of Retinitis Pigmentosa (R.P.) with the Management of Ayurvedic Composite Therapy, paper presented at national conference of NIMA, Mumbai, India, 2001.
75. Phadke, A., A Critical Study on Safety of a Unique Therapeutic Modality of Ayurvedic *Panchakarma* therapy, *Tarpana*, paper presented on pre conference workshop on research methodology of ayurvedic medicine, Update Ayurveda, Seth G.S. Medical College & K.E.M. Hospital, Mumbai, India, 1999.
76. Khadilkar, M., Phytochemical and Pharmacological Investigation of Water Extracts of *Boerhaavia diffusa* (*Punarnava*) & *Azadirachta indica* (*neem*) in Experimentally Induced Conjunctivitis, M.Pharm. thesis, S.N.D.T. Womens University, Mumbai, India, 1998.
77. Phadke, S.A. and Kulkarni, S.D., Screening of in vitro antibacterial activity of *Terminaliachebula, Eclapta alba* and *Ocimum sanctum*, *Indian J. Med. Sci.*, 43(5), 113, 1989.
78. Board of editors, *Selected Medicinal Plants of India* (A Monograph of Identity, Safety and Clinical Usage), compiled by Bharatiya Vidya Bhavan's S.P.A.R.C. Mumbai for Chemexcil, Basic Chemicals, Pharmaceuticals and Cosmetics Export Promotion Council, Bombay, India, set up by Ministry of Commerce, Government of India, 1992, p. 149.
79. Board of editors, *Selected Medicinal Plants of India* (A Monograph of Identity, Safety and Clinical Usage), compiled by Bharatiya Vidya Bhavan's S.P.A.R.C. Mumbai for Chemexcil, Basic Chemicals, Pharmaceuticals and Cosmetics Export Promotion Council, Bombay, India, set up by Ministry of Commerce, Government of India, 1992, p. 201.
80. Board of editors, *Selected Medicinal Plants of India* (A Monograph of Identity, Safety and Clinical Usage), compiled by Bharatiya Vidya Bhavan's S.P.A.R.C. Mumbai for Chemexcil, Basic Chemicals, Pharmaceuticals and Cosmetics Export Promotion Council, Bombay, India, set up by Ministry of Commerce, Government of India, 1992, p. 303.
81. Board of editors, *Selected Medicinal Plants of India* (A Monograph of Identity, Safety and Clinical Usage), compiled by Bharatiya Vidya Bhavan's S.P.A.R.C. Mumbai for Chemexcil, Basic Chemicals, Pharmaceuticals and Cosmetics Export Promotion Council, Bombay, India, set up by Ministry of Commerce, Government of India, 1992, p. 317.
82. Board of editors, *Selected Medicinal Plants of India* (A Monograph of Identity, Safety and Clinical Usage), compiled by Bharatiya Vidya Bhavan's S.P.A.R.C. Mumbai for Chemexcil, Basic Chemicals, Pharmaceuticals and Cosmetics Export Promotion Council, Bombay, India, set up by Ministry of Commerce, Government of India, 1992, p. 123.

83. Board of editors, *Selected Medicinal Plants of India* (A Monograph of Identity, Safety and Clinical Usage), compiled by Bharatiya Vidya Bhavan's S.P.A.R.C. Mumbai for Chemexcil, Basic Chemicals, Pharmaceuticals and Cosmetics Export Promotion Council, Bombay, India, set up by Ministry of Commerce, Government of India, 1992, p. 57.
84. Board of editors, *Selected Medicinal Plants of India* (A Monograph of Identity, Safety and Clinical Usage), compiled by Bharatiya Vidya Bhavan's S.P.A.R.C. Mumbai for Chemexcil, Basic Chemicals, Pharmaceuticals and Cosmetics Export Promotion Council, Bombay, India, set up by Ministry of Commerce, Government of India, 1992, p. 105.
85. Board of editors, *Selected Medicinal Plants of India* (A Monograph of Identity, Safety and Clinical Usage), compiled by Bharatiya Vidya Bhavan's S.P.A.R.C. Mumbai for Chemexcil, Basic Chemicals, Pharmaceuticals and Cosmetics Export Promotion Council, Bombay, India, set up by Ministry of Commerce, Government of India, 1992, p. 121.

30

Ischemic Heart Disease

Karunakaran Gauthaman and Lakshmi Chandra Mishra

CONTENTS

0-8493-1366-X/04/$0.00+$1.50

30.1 Introduction

Ischemic heart disease (IHD) is a leading cause of morbidity and mortality in the Western world. Cardiovascular disease (CVD), particularly IHD, has become a worldwide health problem affecting all economic groups of society and is responsible for 25% of all deaths in the world. The mortality due to CVD ranges from 16 to 50% in the developing and developed countries. Because 78% of all deaths in the world occur in the developing countries, the absolute number of deaths is very high in these areas. Due to such high incidence, IHD is now considered a modern epidemic.[1]

Considering the huge burden of IHD management, there has been a continuous attempt to develop drugs that will delay the development and halt the progress of the disease. In this regard, there is great potential for identifying outstanding Ayurvedic components or its active principles, especially in consideration of the fact that such substances may provide maximum benefit with cost effectiveness, minimum side effects, and enhancement of patient compliance.

The focus of this chapter will be to explore the scientific basis for the Ayurvedic treatment of IHD with herbs, herbal formulae, and dietary interventions by using modern technologies with a view to establishing a scientific rationale for therapeutic acceptance. The modes of administration and the associated lifestyle changes required for the treatment to be effective will be described.

30.2 Definition

In Ayurveda, IHD, or *hridroga*, is clinically characterized by chest pain produced by increased workload on the heart. The pain is felt mostly over the sternum. The pain spreads toward the left side of the chest and radiates to the left arm, neck, and upper part of the abdomen. There are several types depending upon the characteristic features of the pain. If the pain is acute and has a shifting nature, it is known as *vatika* heart disease. If it is associated with a burning sensation, it is called *pitaja* heart disease. If the pain is mild and is associated with heaviness, nausea, and cough, it is called *kaphaja* heart disease.

In modern medicine, IHD is characterized by the atherosclerotic narrowing of the lumen of coronary arteries and reduction in the blood flow to the heart muscle. The symptoms described are the same as described in Ayurveda. There may be a burning sensation in the chest radiating to the arms, back, abdomen, and jaw; there may also be a pressure — a feeling of tightness within the chest or a feeling of heaviness. These symptoms arise under physical or emotional exertion; later on they appear in the resting state.

30.3 Clinical Description

One of the classical Ayurvedic texts, *Rugviniscaya,* lists a variety of symptoms of heart diseases often experienced by patients:

1. Stiffness of the cardiac region (*hrdayayama*)
2. Stabbing pain in the heart region (*hrdaya dirana*)
3. Heaviness of heart (*hrdaya gautaca*)
4. Weakness of heart (*hridayaksobha* or *hrdaya klams* or *hridaya upahata*)
5. Cutting pain in the heart (*hrdayapatna*)
6. Fluttering of the heart (*hrdayanirmathana*)
7. Pericardial discomfort (*hridaya pidana*)
8. Pain in the heart (*hridayaruja*)
9. Feeling of emptiness of heart (*hridaya sunyata*)
10. Cutting pain in the heart region (*hridaya sphotana*)
11. Pericardial suppression (*hridayastambha*)
12. Heaviness of heart (*hridayastyana* or *hrtstyana*)
13. Pricking pain in the pericardium (*hridayatoda*)
14. Cardiac pain (*hridayavyadha, hrdsula*)
15. Burning sensation in the region of the heart (*hrddaha*)
16. Discomfort in the pericardium (*hrdgraha*)
17. Tachycardia and pericardial muscular twitching (*hrtkampa*)
18. Pericardial pain (*hrdruk*)
19. Pricking pain in the pericardial region (*hrdisula*)
20. Tachycardia (*hrdvega*)
21. Pain and discomfort in the region of the heart (*hrtpida*)

There are five clinical descriptions of ischemic heart disease according to Ayurveda based on vitiated *dosas* and other causes: (1) *vataja,* (2) *pitaja,* (3) *kaphaja,* (4) *Tridosaja,* and (5) *kramija* (caused by worms or parasite infections).

30.3.1 Vataja Heart Disease

The features of *vataja* heart diseases are a stretching, pinching, grinding, cracking, and tearing types of pain in the heart. The other symptoms seen are abnormal complexion, fainting, fever, cough, hiccups, dyspnea, distaste in mouth, thirst, mental confusion, vomiting, excitement of *kapha* and consequent distress, anorexia, palpitation, wasting, tearing, obstructed movement, severe pricking, piercing, bursting, constricting, or splitting pain, dryness, immobility, emptiness, increased heart rate, unfounded helplessness, grief or fear, tremors, body contractions, dislike for noise, obstructed breathing, dark rings around the eyes, hypersensitivity, and attacks of fear, anxiety, worry, and fainting.

30.3.2 *Pittaja* Heart Disease

Pittaja heart disease is characterized by morbid thirst, heating sensation, burning sensation, cardiac fatigue, a feeling of being inside a smoke-filled place, fainting, sweating, and dryness of the mouth. Other symptoms are feeling of being in a dark place, distress, mental confusion, terror, heat, pyrexia, dizziness, acidity, exhaustion, vomiting (sourness), yellowish skin, eyes, and stool, fever, and flushed or bloodshot eyes.

30.3.3 *Kaphaja* Heart Disease

Kaphaja heart disease is characterized by heaviness, excessive salivation, anorexia, stiffness, suppression of the power of digestion, and sweet taste in the mouth. The movements of the heart become obstructed by *kapha*, which gives the feeling of dullness, fever, cough, and drowsiness. The other features are stiffness feeling of the heart, expectorating mucus, excess of sleep, lassitude, fever, cardiac edema, and heaviness of the limbs.

30.3.4 *Tridosaja* Heart Disease

This type of heart disease is characterized by the manifestation of symptoms of all the three varieties of heart diseases related to three *dosas* described above. The main symptoms are constricting pain and discomfort as a result of the vitiation of all three *dosas* simultaneously, spitting of sticky mucus, stabbing pain, colic pain, sensation as if entering into darkness, anorexia, grayish coloration of eyes, and dryness.

30.3.5 *Kramija* Heart Disease

If a patient suffering from this type of heart disease consumes oils, milk, and jaggery, then nodules (*granthis*) appear on and around the area of the heart, and fluids (*rasa*) located there become sticky. Because of this stickiness, germs appear. The patients shows dark discoloration around the eyes, dry irritated skin, and excess mucus expectoration; the patient is prone to fainting.

In modern medicine, the clinical descriptions of IHD are angina, myocardial infarction, chronic postischemic cardiac failure, and sudden ischemic cardiac death.

30.3.6 Angina

The pain that occurs during periods of myocardial ischemia consists of retrosternal constricting discomfort that may radiate to the arms, throat, or jaw; it is associated with shortness of breath. Three types of angina syndromes are clinically recognized: stable angina, unstable angina, and variant angina.[2]

30.3.6.1 Stable Angina

Stable angina may be provoked by any stimulus that increases myocardial oxygen demand through increments in blood pressure or heart rate. Typically, it is provoked by exertion (e.g., exercise, hurrying, or sexual activity) or emotions (e.g., stress, anger, fright, or frustration) and is relieved within 2 to 10 min by resting. Symptoms are usually worse in the morning shortly after getting up, probably because the blood pressure is at its peak level at this time of the day; symptoms tend to worsen in cold weather and also after a heavy meal, which increases heart rate. Patients seek medical help for troublesome or fighting chest discomfort, usually described as heaviness, pressure, squeezing, smothering, or choking; it is rarely described as frank pain. This symptom is usually crescendo or decrescendo and lasts 1 to 5 min. Angina can radiate to the left shoulder and to both arms, especially to the ulnar surfaces of the forearm and hand. It can also radiate to the back, neck, jaw, teeth, and epigastrium.[2]

30.3.6.2 Unstable Angina

This is accompanied by objective electrocardiographic evidence of transient myocardial ischemia (chest pain associated with [ST] segment changes in electrocardiogram [ECG] or T-wave inversions). It is mostly associated with critical stenoses in one or more major epicardial coronary arteries. The following three groups of patients may be said to have unstable angina: (1) patients with new onset (<2 months) angina that is severe or frequent (≥3 episode/day), (2) patients with accelerating angina (i.e., those with chronic stable angina who developed angina that is distinctly more frequent, severe, prolonged, or precipitated by less exertion), and (3) those with angina at rest. Unstable angina may be primary (i.e., occurs in the absence of an extra cardiac condition that has intensified myocardial ischemia, such as anemia, fever, infection, tachyarrhythmias, emotional stress, or hypoxemia). Unstable angina may also develop shortly after myocardial infarction.[2]

30.3.6.3 Variant Angina

This unusual angina symptom is characterized by an unprovoked episode of chest pain which may be associated with ST segment depression in the ECG. IHD is present in 70% of cases, but the remainder of the coronary arteries appears normal. An exaggerated increase in coronary arterial tone (spasm) has been demonstrated in these patients during attacks of angina. These patients are at risk of cardiac arrhythmias, and prolonged attacks of spasm may result in myocardial infarction. The spasm is usually of focal distribution, and even in the absence of coronary artery disease, it can restrict flow sufficiently to produce profound myocardial ischemia.

30.3.7 Myocardial Infarction

In myocardial infarction, the pain is deep and visceral. Patients describe it as a heavy, squeezing, and crushing feeling in the chest around the area of the heart. It is similar in character to the discomfort of angina pectoris, but is usually more severe and lasts longer. Typically, the pain involves the central portion of the chest and radiates to the left arm. Less common sites of radiation are the abdomen, back, lower jaw, and neck. The location of the pain beneath the xiphoid and the patients' denial of heart attack are two main causes responsible for the mistaken diagnosis of indigestion. The pain of myocardial infarction may radiate as high as the occipital area but not below the umbilicus. Weakness, sweating, nausea, vomiting, giddiness, and anxiety often accompany the pain. The discomfort usually commences when the patient is at rest. When the pain begins during a period of exertion, in contrast to angina pectoris, it usually does not subside with cessation of activity. Other less common symptoms, with or without pain, include sudden loss of consciousness, a confused state, a sensation of profound weakness, the appearance of an arrhythmia, evidence of peripheral embolism, or an unexplained drop in arterial pressure. [3]

30.3.8 Sudden Ischemic Cardiac Death

Sudden ischemic cardiac death occurs due to abrupt rupture of an atheromatous plaque and coronary thrombosis along with left ventricular failure.[4]

30.4 History and Epidemiology

Heart diseases are well described in Ayuravedic texts. *Charaka Samhita*, compiled during 10th century A.D., describes the reasons for cardiac problems and the means for their prevention as follows:

> Cardiac diseases of *kapha* type are born by the intake of fatty meals and over eating, and also by excessive indulgence in sleep, sedentary habits.
>
> The person desiring to be protected from the adverse effects upon his heart, coronary blood vessels, and the contents thereof should particularly avoid all that causes mental affliction.
>
> **Charaka Sutra, 30/13**

Modern medicine has provided excellent tertiary care and means for the treatment in the form of very effective drugs, angioplasty procedures, radio therapeutics, and sophisticated advanced surgical techniques that can beneficially treat CVD. Despite declines in mortality in the past 2 decades, occlusive atherosclerotic coronary artery disease remains a major cause of morbidity and mortality all over the world. The overall mortality from coronary artery disease has declined by almost 50% since reaching its peak in the mid 1960s. Nonetheless, there is still an excess of 500,000 deaths annually in the U.S. attributable to coronary artery disease. The incidence of myocardial infarction, the most dramatic manifestation of coronary artery disease, remains alarmingly high. Up to 1,500,000 persons sustain a myocardial infarction each year in India; unfortunately, many of them die suddenly, and only 50% survive long enough to receive hospital care.[1]

30.4.1 Public Health Scenario

Three of trends of IHD are observed[1]:

1. In the U.S., where the epidemic started as early as 1920, the death rate due to IHD is declining without change in morbidity since 1968. Similar trends can be seen in Australia, New Zealand, and Canada.

2. In countries where the epidemic started late, either no change is noticed or there is an increase in the incidence and mortality. Most of the European countries fall into this category.
3. The developing countries have started experiencing the epidemic only recently; no clear trend can be described due to the short period. India is in the third category of trend of IHD. Some of the major surveys conducted indicate that the prevalence of IHD ranges from 22.8 to 65.4/1000 in males and 17.3 to 47.8/1000 in females worldwide. With a progressive adaptation of a Westernized lifestyle and increasing life expectancy, India is experiencing both a health and an epidemiological transition with the progressive decline in mortality rate and disability; this is attributable to infectious disease and nutritional deficiencies and is accompanied by the emergences of lifestyle related to other chronic disease epidemics.[5]

It has been projected by the World Bank Health Sectoral Priority Review that in India, CVD alone will account for 33.5% of deaths at all ages by 2015. There is, therefore, sufficient cause of concern that CVD will be the major public health threat by the end of the millennium (Ministry of Health and Family Welfare, Government of India).

30.5 Etiology

In Ayurveda, *kapha* (atherosclerosis) is the major underlying mechanism of heart diseases. The major causes mentioned are unhealthy lifestyle, lack of physical exercise, excessive indulgence in sleep, and sedentary habits.

In conventional medicine, the etiopathogenesis of IHD includes hyperlipidemia, increased waist-hip ratio, hypertension, insulin resistance, stress, smoking, alcoholism, and environmental pollution. Risk factors are causally related to the development of IHD but do not imply that they are causal to all IHD; they merely indicate that they are the determinants of the disease in a sufficiently large number of individuals in the population studied.

30.5.1 Risk Factors for Ischemic Heart Disease

The differences in the incidence and prevalence of coronary artery disease among countries have stimulated the search for factors that might predict the development of the disease. These are now referred to as risk factors. They include not only the physiochemical characteristics of the individuals, but also certain aspects of lifestyle such as diet, smoking, and behavior patterns. It is hoped that the discovery of such risk factors might help in the effort to prevent coronary heart disease. According to the World Health Organization (WHO) (1985), the major modifiable risk factors associated with IHD are serum cholesterol, cigarette smoking, high blood pressure, obesity, lack of physical activity, and diabetes.

It is recognized that the association of these variables with the disease did not establish any etiological relationship. Unfortunately, a high proportion of patients who develop CVD do not have any treatable risk factors. Furthermore, a large proportion of patients with risk factors do not develop the disease. Most of the reversible risk factors are predictive of coronary artery disease only in relatively young people; this suggests that in older people the disease process is principally related to aging rather than one of the avoidable risk factors.

30.6 Pathogenesis and Pathology

In Ayurvedic texts, the causes of IHD are the intake of excessively hot, heavy, sour, astringent, and bitter food; physical exhaustion; injury; habitually taking food before the previous meal is digested; worry; and suppression of natural urges. When vitiated *dosas* located in the heart afflict blood (*rasa dhatu*) to cause pain in cardiac region, the condition is called heart disease. It is caused by the obstruction to the coronary arteries (*dhamanis*) of the heart muscles. Because the heart muscles consume a huge amount of energy, they need ceaseless nourishment, meaning they demand a good supply of blood. Any impairment of these blood vessels interferes with adequate blood flow to the heart muscles. If its blood flow is significantly diminished, then the heart signals its difficulties by registering pain or discomfort in the chest. The *vata* located in the heart being obstructed by *kapha* and *pitta* interacts with blood nutrients (*rasa*), causing pain, fainting, and (cardiac) obstruction.

In conventional medicine, IHD implies structural and functional abnormalities of the heart as a consequence of an inadequate supply of blood to its tissue. The heart suffers from ischemia when the blood supply to the heart is decreased, either due to increased demand or decreased supply or more commonly due to a combination of both these factors. Ischemia is caused by the insufficiency of oxygen and reduced availability of nutrient substrates and inadequate removal of metabolites.[4] Once IHD develops, the cells of the cardiac muscles suffer from a lack of O_2 and nutrition, which may be critically low. The condition is manifested as angina pain. This critical reduction of blood supply is corrected either spontaneously, by resting, or by drugs. In conditions like unstable angina and acute myocardial infarction, more aggressive intervention procedures like thrombolytic drugs and surgical procedures are required to restore coronary blood flow.[6]

IHD is composed of four clinical syndromes caused by myocardial ischemia: angina pectoris, acute myocardial infarction, chronic postischemic cardiac failure, and sudden ischemic cardiac death.[4] The four major pathogenic components of IHD are based primarily on the consideration that the chronic atherosclerotic background determines manifestation and outcomes of IHD. In addition, the components are also based on multiple acute stimuli that cause transient or persistent myocardial ischemia and the heart's response to ischemia. The pathogenic components of IHD, with their individual etiologic and pathogenic components, collectively cause the four major ischemic syndromes and determine their outcomes. The most common cause of IHD is atherosclerotic, the narrowing of the coronary arteries.

30.6.1 Atherosclerosis

This is a pathological condition that underlines several important disorders, including coronary artery disease, cerebrovascular disease, and disease of aorta and peripheral arterial circulation. It involves lesions of the intimal layer of the wall of epicardial coronary arteries regardless of its nature or pathogenetic and etiologic mechanism. Serum lipids play a significant role in the genesis and progression of atherosclerosis; low-density lipoprotein (LDL) cholesterol is an especially strong atherogen. Recently, it has been documented that oxidation of LDL molecules is needed for its atherogenic action.[7,8]

The variable severity of coronary atherosclerosis may result from various types of intimal injury, a variable combination of smooth muscle cell proliferation and lipid ground substance deposition, fibrinogen and fibrin deposition, and from thrombus organization. Stimuli may suddenly reduce regional coronary blood flow, transiently or persistently causing coronary constriction, thrombosis, or both. Weaker stimuli may be sufficient to cause ischemia in the presence of a severe atherosclerotic background. Flow limiting stenosis can reduce the coronary flow reserves and cause ischemia when the increase in myocardial demand is excessive. The responses of the heart to ischemic insult in terms of the development of collateral blood flow are angina, ischemia, necrosis, heart failure, and fatal arrhythmias. Of these components of IHD, undoubtedly the most important is the development of ischemic stimuli. The chronic atherosclerotic background and the response of the heart predispose or modulate the effects of ischemic stimuli.

30.6.2 Natural Course of Myocardial Ischemia

Inadequate oxygenation causes disturbances in the cardiac function. When ischemic events are transient, they may cause angina pectoris. If prolonged, they can lead to irreversible injury to the affected part (myocardial infarction). Reestablishment of blood flow or reperfusion, either spontaneous or drug- or surgery-induced, constitutes the only rational therapeutic option for IHD. But it is an established fact that reperfusion of the ischemic myocardium carries with it some detrimental effects that contribute significantly to the delayed or loss of functional recovery of the heart.[9] The whole phenomenon has given birth to a well-known entity called ischemic reperfusion injury.[10,11]

Ischemic reperfusion injury is responsible for delayed or loss of recovery of cardiac function depending on the duration and extent of preceding ischemia. If the ischemic period is brief and is not associated with any irreversible myocardial injury, reperfusion can cause myocardial stunning or postischemic myocardial dysfunction of a relatively short duration (weeks to months). On the other hand, reperfusion of irreversibly injured myocardial cells causes permanent loss of cardiac function. It is now well established that ischemic-reperfusion injury plays a major role in the natural course of almost all forms of IHD, such as exercise-induced angina, variant angina, unstable angina, acute myocardial infarction with early reperfusion, coronary angioplasty, coronary graft surgery, and cardiac transplant.[6]

30.7 Diagnosis and Prognosis

Ayurvedic diagnosis of heart diseases is made by observing the clinical features, description, history, location, and characteristics of the pain as described in Section 30.3. In modern medicine, IHD is diagnosed by physical and laboratory examinations, ECG, stress testing (treadmill testing), and coronary arteriography.

30.7.1 Physical Examination

The patient's appearance may reveal signs of risk factors associated with atherosclerosis or diabetic lesions along with signs of anemia, thyroid disease, and cigarette smoking. Palpitation can reveal thickened or absent peripheral arterial pulse, which are signs of cardiac enlargement and abnormal enlargement of cardiac impulse. Examination of the eyes may reveal increased light reflexes and arteriovenous nicking as evidence of hypertension, whereas auscultation can uncover arterial bruits; a third or fourth heart sound; and, if acute ischemia or previous myocardial infarction has impaired papillary muscle function, a late epical systolic murmur. These disorders may cause angina even in the absence of coronary artery disease.

30.7.2 Laboratory Examination

Urine is examined for evidence of diabetes mellitus and renal disease. Blood is examined for measurements of lipids (cholesterol, total HDL, and LDL), glucose, creatinine kinase, and lactate. A chest x-ray is performed to find gross structural changes secondary to IHD (i.e., cardiac enlargement, ventricular aneurysm, or signs of heart failure). Chest fluoroscopy is done to identify the calcification of the coronary arteries.

30.7.3 Electrocardiogram

A 12-lead ECG recorded at rest is normal in about half of the patients with typical angina pectoris, but there may be signs of an old myocardial infarction. Serial tracings are particularly useful to look for past or evolving myocardial infarction. They show repolarization abnormalities (i.e., T-wave and ST segment changes) and intraventricular conduction disturbances at rest, which are suggestive of ischemic heart disease; they are nonspecific, because they can also occur in pericardial, myocardial, and valvular heart disease. Typical ST segment and T-wave changes that accompany episodes of angina pectoris and disappear thereafter are more specific.

30.7.4 Stress Testing

The most widely used test in the diagnosis of IHD involves recording the 12-lead ECG before, during, and after exercise on a treadmill or using a bicycle ergometer. The test consists of a standardized incremental increase in external workload while the patient's ECG, symptoms, and arm blood pressure are continuously monitored. Performance is usually symptom limited and the test is discontinued upon evidence of chest discomfort, severe shortness of breath, dizziness, and fatigue.

30.7.5 Coronary Arteriography

This invasive diagnostic method outlines the coronary anatomy and can be used to detect important evidence of coronary artherosclerosis to assess the severity of obstructive lesions in the major arteries. Coronary arteriography is indicated for the following:

1. Patients with chronic stable or unstable angina pectoris who are severely symptomatic despite medical therapy and being considered for revascularization (i.e.,

percutaneous transluminal coronary angioplasty or coronary artery bypass graft surgery)

2. Patients with troublesome symptoms that present diagnostic difficulties in whom there is need to confirm or rule out the diagnosis of coronary artery disease
3. Patients suspected of having left main stem or three-vessel coronary artery disease based on signs of severe ischemia on noninvasive testing, regardless of the presence or severity of symptoms

30.7.6 Echocardiography

A two-dimensional echocardiography records the image of the left ventricle (LV), which can identify regional wall motion abnormalities due to myocardial infarction or persistent ischemia. This test can also be used as an aid in the diagnosis of IHD.

30.8 Therapy

In Ayurvedic texts, the treatment for all heart diseases is offered to promote biofire (*agni*) and to purify the channels by *panchakarma* in addition to using natural palliative herbs that have hypolipdemic and antistress activity. For heart diseases with a specific vitiated *dosa,* herbs known to mitigate that *dosa* are given in the form of a decoction or medicated ghee. These herbs are listed in Appendix 2.

A few examples of decoctions, medicated ghee, paste, and powders for each type of heart disease as given in *Ashtanghradaya Samhita* text are cited here just to show the historic use of the formulas. Some of these formulas are still used.

30.8.1 *Vataja* Heart Disease

1. Water decoction of *punarnava* (*Boerhovia diffusa*), *devadaru*, *pancamula*, *rasna* (*Pluchea lanceolata*), barley grains, *bilva* (*Aegle marmelos*), *kulattha* (*Dolichos biflorus*), and *kola*
2. Medicated ghee prepared with the paste of *haritaki* (*Terminalia chebula*), *sunthi*, (*Zinziber officinale*), *puskaramula* (*Iris germanica*), *vayahstha*, *guduci* (*Tinospora cardifolia*), *kayastha*, *amalaki* (*Tinospora cardifolia)*, salt, and asafetida
3. Powder of *dadima* (*Punica grantum*), black salt, *sunthi*, asafetida, and *amlavetasa*
4. Paste of *puskarahva*, *sathi* (*Hedychium spicatum*), *sunthi*, root of *bijapura* and *haritaki* mixed with *ksara* (*yavaksara*), and ghee
5. Decoction of *yavani, salt, ksara, vaca* (*Acorus calamus*), *ajaji* (*Cuminum cyminum*), *ausadha, putidaru, bijahva, palasa, sathi*, and *pauskara*
6. Powder of *pancakola* (*pippali, pippalimula, cavya, citraka, nagra*), *sathi* (*Hedychium spicatum*), *pathya, guda* (jaggery, molasses), *bijahva*, and *pauskara* made into a paste with *varuni* (a kind of liquor) fried in *yamaka* (mixture of oil and ghee) and added with salt
7. Decoction of *sunthi* or *varuni*, thin liquor of *dadhi* (curds), or fermented water boiled with corn and made into a drink

8. *Bala taila* or *sukumara* or *satapaka yasti taila* or *mahasneha*
9. Decoction or paste of *rasna, jinaka, jivanti* (*Leptedenia reticulate*), *bala* (*Sida cordifolia*), *vyaghri, punarnava, bharangi* (*Cleodendron serratum*), *sthira* (*Desmodium gangeticum*), *vaca*, and *vyosa*, one fourth part of *dadhi*, and sour liquids
10. Warm oil mixed with *sauviraka*, curd water, buttermilk, and salt
11. Paste of *puskaramula, sunthi*, and *sati* mixed with alkali, water, dehydrated butter, and salt
12. The paste of *haritaki, sathi, puskaramula, pancakola*, and *matulunga* fried in *yamaka* and with jaggery, clear wine, and salt
13. *Pippalyadi curna* is given along with the decoction of *triphala, dhanyamla* (a sour drink), decoction of *kulattha*, curd, *madya* (alcoholic drink), *asava* (a type of fermented drink). The constituents are powders of *pippali, ela, vaca*, asafetida, *yavaksara, saindhava, sauvarcala, sunthi*, and *ajmoda* (*Carium roxburghiana*).

30.8.2 *Pittaja* Heart Disease

1. The treatment is directed to mitigate *pitta*. Purgation is given with the juice of *draksa* (*Vitis vinifera*), *Iksu* (*Saccharum officinarum*), *sita* (*Santalum album*), ksaudra, and *parusaka*. Along with this emetic therapy is given with *sriparni, madhuka* (*Glycyrrhiza glabra*), honey, sugar, and jaggery and is mixed with water.
2. Medicated ghee is prepared with the decoction or paste of *sreyasi*, sugar, *draksa, jivaka, rsabhaka, utpala, balam kharjura, kakoli* and *meda yugma* with milk, and ghee.
3. Medicated ghee is prepared with the decoction or paste of *prapaundarika, madhuka, bisagranthi, kaseruka, sunthi, saivala*, and milk.
4. Milk is boiled with the decoction of the bark of *T. arjuna* along with the sugar and decoction of *Pancamula*, or *Madhuka*.
5. Powder of the bark of *Terminalia arjuna* along with ghee, milk, or jaggery.

30.8.3 *Kaphaja* Heart Disease

The patient suffering from *kaphaja hridroga* is given emetic therapy with the help of the decoction of *vaca* and *nimba* and *pippalyadi curna*. A decoction of *T. arjuna*, as well as other treatment given for *kaphaja* heart disease, is given as a palliative treatment.

30.8.4 *Tridosaja* Heart Disease

The patient is given a fasting therapy followed by a diet that is suitable for all three *dosas*. After ascertaining less aggravated, more aggravated, and moderately aggravated *dosas*, the patient is given the following therapies that will balance all *dosas*:

1. Wheat flour and *T. arjuna* bark powder boiled with oil, ghee, and jaggery and a diet of milk as well as rice
2. A mixture of equal parts of fine powder of asafetida, *ugragandha* (*Acorus calamus*), vida, *visva, krsna, kustha* (*Soussera lappa*), citraka (*Plumbago zeylanica*), and *yav ksara* mixed with sufficient quantity of *sauvarcala* and *puskaramula* along with barley
3. Decoction of *dasamula* mixed with salt and *ksara* (alkali preparation)

4. A mixture of equal parts of fine powder of *patha, vaca, yava, haritiki, amlaki* (*Phyllanthus emblica*), *vetasa, duralabha* (*Fagonia arabica*), *citraka, tryusana, triphala, sathi, puskaramula, tintidi, dadima* (*Punica grantum*), and root of *motulunga*

30.8.5 Parasitic (*Kramija*) Heart Disease

The patients are given rice cooked with meat and ghee along with curd and *patala*. After 3 days, purgation therapy is given. *Dhanyamla* mixed with herbs, salt, *ajaji*, sugar, and *vidanga* is also prescribed.

1. *Vallabha ghrta* — Ghee should be cooked with 50 matured fruits of *haritaki* and two *palas* of *sauvarcala* (a kind of salt).
2. *Baladya ghrta* — Ghee is cooked with the decoction of *bala, nagabala,* and *T. arjuna* and one fourth in quantity of the paste of yastimadhu (*Glycyrrhiza glabra*). (It is good in *rakta-pitta* condition.)
3. *Arjuna Ghrta* — Ghee is cooked with the paste and juice (or decoction) of *T. arjuna.*

Most of the Ayurvedic formulations contain the bark of *T. arjuna*. It is one of the most popular Ayurvedic herbs being used by the Ayurvedic practitioners for the prevention and management of various CVDs. The stem bark of this plant is used for medicinal purposes. This herb has been scientifically evaluated and has sufficient data to support its use in IHD. The other herbs found useful in IHD are *Aloe vera, Coleus forskohlli, Inula recemosa, Andrographis panicilata, Centella asiatica, Piper longum, Picrorhiza kurrora,* and *Commiphora mukul.* These herbs have also been scientifically evaluated and found to be useful in the management of IHD. Patent herbal formulas such as Abna, Hartone, and Lipistat that contain several herbs are also commercially available.

30.9 Scientific Basis

Pharmacological and clinical investigations are reviewed to explore the scientific basis for the use of Ayurvedic therapies. Clinical and biological studies on several botanicals, including *Crataegus oxycantha, T. arjuna, Inula racemosa,* and *Astragalus membranaceus*, have been reviewed and found to have therapeutic benefit for the treatment of CVD.[12] The studies are primarily focused on cardioprotective effects against chemical or biological injuries of the heart. The effects studied include anticoagulant, angiogenic, antiatherosclerotic, anti-infarction, blood vessel endothelium protection, and anticholesterol. All these effects are, directly or indirectly, cardioprotective. They can be useful in the management of IHD.

30.9.1 *Terminalia arjuna*

30.9.1.1 Animal Studies

T. arjuna has been a major treatment for IHD in Ayurveda. Because anticoagulants have been found useful in IHD, *T. arjuna* was investigated for a possible anticoagulant activity. An emulsion of *T. arjuna* bark powder (10 g/kg) was given to rabbits orally for 7 days at the dosage of 10 g/kg body weight. The treatment caused a significant increase in prothrombin time (20 sec vs. 10.01 sec) and decrease in platelet count (44 vs. 473/thousand). In a similar study[13–15] with the alcoholic extract, there was no change in prothrombin time.

A water-soluble portion of the total alcoholic extract of *T. arjuna* was found to cause an increase in the force of contraction of a frog heart.[16] In later studies,[17,18] both negative and positive ionotropic effects were observed in isolated perfused frog and rabbit hearts and isolated frog and rat atria. It was suggested that the extract consists of a mixture of subsatances capable of exerting both positive and negative ionotropic effects.[19] The aqueous extract of *T. arjuna* was also found to produce dose-dependent sustained hypotension and bradycardia in dogs.[20] Intracerebroventricular and intravertebral injection of the extract in chloralose anesthetized dogs caused hypotension and bradycardia in doses as small as 1/10th and 1/20th, respectively, of the intravenous dose. Prior bilateral vagotomy blocked the bradycardia, associated hypotension, and the ability of the intravertebral dose of *T. arjuna* to produce these effects in a lower dose. These observations led the authors to propose that the active constituent in the extract acts centrally.[20] The hypotensive effect of the alcoholic extract in dogs is abolished by pretreatment with atropine.[17]

Subsequently, a study[19] on the isolated rat thoracic aorta showed that the aqueous extract caused contraction of the aorta followed by relaxation. The initial contraction was blocked by propranolol, whereas the vaso relaxant effect was unaffected. Similarly, in another study,[21] both the aqueous extract as well as the fraction of the extract containing tannin-related compounds (F_2), produced hypotensive effects. The hypotensive effect of F_2 was not affected by pretreatment of rats with propranolol but was attenuated by pretreatment with atropine. The authors suggested that the hypotensive effect of F2 may be mediated by cholinergic mechanisms. In another study,[22] it was observed that aortic prostaglandin E_2–like (PGE_2) activity was enhanced in ischemic rabbit aorta pretreated with *T. arjuna.* This finding is significant because PGE_2 causes coronary vasodilatation, and this may explain the beneficial effect of *T. arjuna* in patients with cornary artery disease (CAD). In a subsequent study,[23] myocardial ischemia in rabbits was produced by isoproternol infusion and confirmed by ECG and later by histopathological examination. In this study, the onset of ischemia and its severity were both reduced by *T. arjuna. Abana*, an herbal formula containing *T. arjuna,* significantly increased creatinine phosphokinase (CPK), glutamate oxaloacetate transaminase (GOT), glutamate pyruvate transaminase (GPT), and gamma-glutamyltranspeptidase (γ-GT) in serum following myocardial necrosis.[24] The study also showed that 90% of the protection against reduction in glycogen levels in ischemic rats was provided by *T. arjuna*. The beneficial effect of abana was further evident from the reduction in mitochondrial enzymes, such as γ-GT and sorbitol dehydrogenase (SDH), by 44 and 48%, respectively.

T. arjuna has also been reported to possess significant hypolipidemic effect in rabbits fed *T. arjuna* bark for 3 months.[23] In another study,[25,26] it was shown that rabbits fed *T. arjuna* along with a high-cholesterol diet showed a lesser increase in total cholesterol and triglycerides and no change in high-density lipoprotein (HDL) cholesterol as compared with control rabbits. In addition, treating hypercholesterolemic rabbits with *T. arjuna* led to a marked reduction in total cholesterol and triglycerides as well as elevation in HDL-cholesterol as compared with hypercholesterolemic control rabbits. The chronic oral administration of *T. arjuna* was found to augment the endogenous antioxidant compounds of rat heart and also prevented oxidative stress associated with myocardial ischemic reperfusion injury.[27] In a recent study,[28] pre- and posttreatment of rats with arjunolic acid, a new triterpene and a potent active principle from the bark of *T. arjuna*, provided significant cardiac protection in isoproterenol induced myocardial necrosis in the rats.

30.9.1.2 Clinical Studies

The usefulness of *T. arjuna* in IHD has been confirmed in many clinical studies.[29–31] In one study,[32] *T. arjuna* was found to be a mild diuretic without any cardiotonic action, but in another study it was reported to be beneficial.[33] A decoction prepared from the bark of *T. arjuna* was administered to patients of chronic heart failure (CHF), essential hypertension, and cirrhosis of the liver. The decoction showed clinical improvement in 42, 62, and 40% of patients, respectively.[33] Improvement in CHF substantiated earlier claims of its cardiotonic property. On the basis of the description in *Chakradutta Samhita* (an Ayurvedic text) that *T. arjuna* bark powder with milk, water, or ghee causes relief in heart pain,[34,35] a clinical trial in 12 patients with angina pectoris and hemiplegia following cerebral thrombosis was conducted.[17] A total dose of 20 g of crude bark powder of *T. arjuna* was administered to the patients in divided doses for 1 month. At the end of this period, approximately 80% of the patients showed increase in prothrombin time (24.3 ± 2.65 sec vs. 13.4 ± 1.22 sec; $p < 0.001$) along with some degree of functional improvement. *T. arjuna* was also reported to provide marked improvement in a case of Stokes-Adam's attack following chest pain after 3 months of therapy.[17]

T. arjuna was further tested in 30 patients with stable angina pectoris.[35] These patients were administered 25 mg/kg body weight dose of *T. arjuna* bark powder divided into three doses per day. The mean anginal frequency by the end of 3 months had declined (1.57 ± 1.28 vs. 3.47 ± 1.04/day). By the end of 1 month, 10% of patients did not require sublingual nitrate. There was concurrent reduction in systolic blood pressure ($p < 0.001$) without much change in the diastolic blood pressure. Electrocardiographic improvement in terms of reduction in the depth of Q- and T-waves and changes in ST segment configuration, decrease in heart rate, and correction of rhythm disturbance (particularly ventricular premature contraction) was also noted. Biochemical parameters, such as plasma catecholamines, plasma cortisol, blood sugar, and serum cholesterol had declined. A significant reduction in body weight was also evident.[35]

In a double-blind study[36] in 30 patients of decompensated rheumatic valvular heart disease, treatment with 200 mg of *T. arjuna* improved LV fraction significantly (54.41 ± 11.62 vs. 41.47 ± 8.62%; $p < 0.001$). The exercise duration, as obtained on bike ergometry, improved from 98.5 ± 44.2 sec to 178.7 ± 6.1 sec. Heart size also decreased significantly. In a subsequent study,[37] 500 mg of *T. arjuna* extract was administered twice daily in 25 patients with CAD. After 3 months of therapy, reduction in grade of positivity of a treadmill test response was observed in 6 patients. Also, improvement in exercise tolerance was evident with concurrent reduction in frequency of anginal attacks and use of sublingual nitrates.

In another similar study,[38] 500 mg *T. arjuna* was administered twice daily to 20 patients; 15 had stable angina pectoris (Group A) and 5 had unstable angina pectoris (Group B). In both these groups, patients experienced a reduction in anginal frequency and increase in LV ejection fraction (39.7 ± 9.93 vs. 36.2 ± 10.08%). Group A cases also exhibited a decline in mean systolic blood pressure and body mass index. Treadmill testing on 10 patients of stable angina pectoris showed reversion from moderate to mild changes after 3 months of therapy. The target heart rate during exercise could be achieved without significant chest pain.

In a double-blind, crossover design, placebo-controlled study,[39] 500 mg of aqueous and alcoholic extract of the bark of *T. arjuna* was administered every 8 h to 12 patients of refractory chronic CHF (New York Heart Association [NYHA] class IV). It was given in addition to maximal tolerable doses of conventional therapy (i.e., digitalis, diuretics, and vasodilators). In this study, *T. arjuna* therapy as compared with placebo was associated with the following improvements:

1. Symptoms and signs of heart failure
2. Improvement in NYHA classes (class III vs. class IV)
3. Decrease in echo-LV end diastolic (125.28 ± 27.91 vs. 134.56 ± 29.71 ml/m^2; $p < 0.005$) and end systolic volume (81.06 ± 24.6 vs. 94.1 ± 24.62 ml/m^2; $p < 0.005$) indices
4. Increase in left ventricular stroke volume index (44.21 ± 11.92 vs. 40.45 ± 11.56 ml/m^2; $p < 0.005$)
5. Increase in left ventricular ejection fractions (35.33 ± 7.85 vs. 30.24 ± 7.13%; $p < 0.005$)

These patients were followed up with *T. arjuna* therapy for another 20 to 28 months (mean 24 months) during phase II of the study. There was further improvement in symptoms, signs, effort tolerance, and NYHA class.[39]

The adjuvant *T. arjuna* therapy has been found to reduce LV mass (140.62 ± 55.65 vs. 159.18 ± 51.11 g/m^2) and frequency of angina pectoris (1.08 ± 1.08 vs. 3.5 ± 1.98) per day. Besides these findings, it also improved LV ejection fraction (52.67 ± 12.32 vs. 42.25 ± 9.96%).[40] Similar observations have been reported in a recent open study[41] conducted on 20 patients of hypertension. Oral administration of Abana, a compound formulation containing *T. arjuna* (30 mg/tablet), resulted in significant reduction of the systolic blood pressure, ECG LV internal diameter, posterior wall thickness, and interventricular septum thickness.[41] The reduction in LV mass was seen from 18 weeks onward and lasted through 42 weeks. Compared with these observations, the decrease in LV mass was found at 12 weeks and maintained up to 36 weeks in those patients who were kept on propranolol.

In an open comparative trial[42] of safety and efficacy of Hartone (herbal product containing TA) in stable angina pectoris patients, 10 patients were given Hartone 2 capsules twice daily for 6 weeks and 1 capsule twice daily for the next 6 weeks. Hematological and biochemical investigations to assess safety were carried out on days 0, 42, and 84. A serum lipid profile was done before and after therapy. Efficacy was based on the reduction in the number of angina episodes and improvement in stress test. These results were compared with 10 patients of stable angina pectoris on isosorbide mononitrate (ISMN) (20 mg twice/day). In this study, Hartone afforded symptomatic relief in 80% of patients and ISMN in 70%. The number of angina attacks was reduced from 79 to 24/week by Hartone and from 26 to 7/week by ISMN. Although patients of both groups showed improvement in several stress test parameters compared with baseline, the difference was not statistically significant. Hartone improved blood pressure response to stress test in two patients and ejection fraction in one. Hartone was better tolerated than ISMN and showed no evidence of hepatic or renal impairment. Its effects on lipid profile were not consistent. The authors of the study suggested that Hartone is a safe and effective antianginal agent comparable with ISMN and is better tolerated.[42]

In a double-blind, placebo-controlled crossover study[43] comparing *T. arjuna* with ISMN in chronic stable angina patients, 58 male patients with chronic stable angina (NYHA class II-III) with evidence of provocable ischemia on the treadmill exercise test received *T. arjuna* (500 mg), isosorbide mononitrate (40 mg/day), or a matching placebo for 1 week each, separated by a wash-out period of at least 3 days. The patients underwent clinical, biochemical, and treadmill exercise evaluation at the end of each therapy; the scores were compared during the three therapy periods. *T. arjuna* therapy was associated with a significant decrease in the frequency of angina and need for isosorbide dinitrate (5.69 ± 6.91 mg/week in the treated group vs. 18.22 ± 9.29 mg/week in the placebo therapy; $p < 0.005$). The treadmill exercise test parameters improved significantly during therapy with *T. arjuna* compared with those with placebo. The total duration of exercise increased (6.14 ± 2.51 vs. 4.76 ± 2.38 min; $p < 0.005$), maximal ST depression during the longest equivalent stages of submaximal exercise decreased (1.41 ± 0.55 vs. 2.21 ± 0.56 mm; $p < 0.005$), time to recovery decreased (6.49 ± 2.37 vs. 9.27 ± 3.39 min; $p < 0.005$), and higher double products were achieved (25.75 ± 4.81 vs. 23.11 ± 4.83 × 10^3; $p < 0.005$) during the *T. arjuna* therapy. Similar improvements in clinical and treadmill exercise test parameters were observed with ISMN compared with placebo therapy. No significant differences were observed in clinical or treadmill exercise test parameters when *T. arjuna* and ISMN therapies were compared. No significant untoward effects were reported during *T. arjuna* therapy. *T. arjuna* bark extract (500 mg) given every 8 h to patients with stable angina with provocable ischemia on treadmill exercise. The treatment led to an improvement in clinical and treadmill exercise parameters as compared with placebo therapy. These benefits were similar to those observed with ISMN (40 mg/day) therapy and the extract was well tolerated.[43]

The antioxidant and hypocholesterolaemic effects of *T. arjuna* bark powder was compared with a known antioxidant, vitamin E, in a randomized controlled trial.[44] One hundred five patients with coronary heart disease were recruited and separated into 3 groups of 35 each using a Latin-square design.[44] The groups were matched for age, lifestyle and dietary variables, clinical diagnosis, and drug treatment status. None of the patients took lipid-lowering drugs. Supplemental vitamins were stopped for 1 month before the study began, and American Heart Association Step II dietary advice was given to all. At baseline, total cholesterol, triglycerides, HDL and LDL cholesterol, and lipid peroxide estimated as thiobarbituric acid reactive substances were determined. Group I received placebo capsules, Group II received vitamin E capsules (400 units/day), and Group III received fine powder of *T. arjuna* tree bark (500 mg/day) in capsules. Lipids and lipid peroxide levels were determined at 30 days follow-up. The response rate in various groups varied from 86 to 91%. No significant changes in total HDL, LDL cholesterol, and triglycerides levels were seen in Groups I and II (paired t-test $p < 0.05$). In Group III (*T. arjuna*-treated group) there was a significant decrease in total cholesterol (9.7 ± 12.7%) and LDL cholesterol (15.8 ± 25.6%) (paired t-test $p < 0.01$). Lipid peroxide levels decreased significantly in both treatment groups ($p < 0.01$). This decrease was more in the vitamin E group (36.4 ± 17.7%) as compared with the *T. arjuna*-treated group (29.3 ± 18.9%). In this study, *T. arjuna* exhibited a significant antioxidant effect that was comparable with vitamin E. In addition, it also had a significant hypocholesterolemic effect.[44]

In toxicological studies[13] conducted in rats and rabbits, no histopathological changes in the heart, liver, and kidney of these animals were evident even after they had been administered 10 g/kg body weight of *T. arjuna* orally for 40 days. The LD_{50} of *T. arjuna* extract was 2.5 g/kg by intraperitoneally in albino mice.[20] It appears that mice are more sensitive to *T. arjuna* than are rats and rabbits.

In various clinical studies,[38] *T. arjuna* has been used in the dose of 1 to 2 g/day, and this dose was found to be the optimum in patients with CAD. At this dose, it is well tolerated.[37] However, some patients complained of mild gastritis, headache, and constipation.[39] No metabolic, renal, and hepatic toxicity has been reported even when patients were administered *T. arjuna* for more than 24 months.[39]

30.9.2 *Aloe vera*

In an *in vitro* study,[45] angiogenic activity of *Aloe vera* gel was investigated by using the most active fraction (F_3) from dichloromethane extract of *Aloe vera* gel. The F_3 increased the proliferation of calf pulmonary artery endothelial (CPAE) cells. In addition, it induced CPAE cells to invade type 1 collagen gel and form a capillary-like tube in an *in vitro* angiogenesis assay; it also increased the invasion of CPAE cells into matrigel through an *in vitro* invasion assay. F_3 also increased the effect on the messenger ribonucleic acid expression of proteolytic enzymes, which are the key participants in regulation of extracellular matrix degradation.

In a clinical study,[46] 5000 patients with atheromatous heart disease presented as angina pectoris were studied over a period of 5 years with diet containing *Aloe vera* and husk of isabgol. The dietary treatment increased HDL and produced a marked reduction in total serum cholesterol, serum triglycerides, fasting and postprandial blood sugar levels in diabetic patients, and total lipids. The clinical profile showed a reduction in the frequency of anginal attacks; gradually, the doses of the drugs, such as verapamil, nifedipine, beta-blockers, and nitrates, were reduced. Diabetic patients benefited the most. Although the exact mechanism of the action of the above two herbs is not known, it appears that they probably act through their high fiber contents. Both these herbs should be further studied. No undesirable side effects were noted.

30.9.3 *Coleus forskohlii*

C. forskohlii (CF) has been used in Ayurvedic medicine for heart diseases, spasmodic pain, painful micturition, and convulsions. Forskolin, an alkaloid isolated from CF, inhibits adenosine di-phosphate (ADP)-induced and collagen-induced platelet aggregation in human and rat platelet-rich plasma.[47] These studies demonstrated an important role of plasma adenosine, a natural antiplatelet and vasodilatory agent produced by vascular endothelium, in the antiplatelet activity of forskolin. Findings also proved that the effect can be greatly potentiated by the clinically used drugs dipyridamole and dilazep. The anticoagulant effect of *C. forskohlii* may be helpful in IHD.

Coleonol, a diterpene isolated from *C. forskohlii*, has been shown to lower the blood pressure of anesthetized cats and rats and of spontaneously hypertensive rats due to relaxation of the vascular smooth muscle.[48] In small doses it showed a positive inotropic effect on isolated rabbit hearts as well as on cat hearts *in vivo*. Coleonol also exhibits nonspecific spasmolytic activity on the smooth muscle of the gastrointestinal tract in various species but not on the bronchial musculature of guinea pig. Large doses of coleonol have a depressant action on the central nervous system. The positive ionotropic effect of *C. forskohlii* provides the rationale for its use in IHD. In another study,[49] forskolin activated a membrane bound adenylatecyclase and a cytoplasmic cAMP-dependent protein kinase to a much higher degree than does isoprenaline. The authors postulated that the adenylatecyclase activation may be correlated with the positive inotropic effect via an enhanced calcium uptake by the heart muscle cell.

30.9.4 *Inula recemosa*

The effects of *I. recemosa* on biochemical parameters in rats with myocardial infarction induced by isoprenaline injection was investigated.[50] The effects on circulating GOT, LDH, CPK, cAMP, cortisol, pyruvate, lactate glucose, and cardiac cAMP adenyl cyclase levels were gradually increased, and serum and cardiac cAMP-PDE levels were gradually decreased from 1 to 120 h after the first injection of isoprenaline. The rats pretreated with ciplar (beta-blocker) or *pushkarmula* (indigenous drug) showed fewer changes as compared with untreated infarcted rats. Posttreatment with *I. recemosa* also produced similar results. *I. recemosa* was found to be more effective given before infarction induction rather than given after infarction induction.

30.9.5 *Andrographis paniculata* (*Kirata*)

A. paniculata (AP) (*Kirata*) was investigated in seven infarction-induced dogs to study the protective effect.[51] One hour after the development of myocardial infarction by formation of thrombus, aqueous extract of AP was injected intravenously. Six infarction-induced dogs served as the control group. As compared with the control group, the treated group showed increased levels of prostacyclin (PG12), inhibition of thromboxane A2 (TXA2), elevated cAMP in platelets, lowered creatine kinase isoenzyme MB (CK-MB) peak, shortened euglobulin lysis time (ELT), decreased release of platelet beta-(1-4)galactosyl transferase (beta-GT) and inhibited platelet maximum aggregation rate, reduced size of the ischemic area recorded by epicardial ECG, and a lowered amplitude of ST segment elevation; a Q-wave appeared in only one dog. Pathologically, the myocardial structure surrounding the initial ischemic area became relatively normal, whereas the degree of myocardial degeneration and necrosis in the central part of the ischemic area was mild. These data suggest that AP may limit the expansion of ischemic focus, exert marked protective effect on reversibly ischemic myocardium, and demonstrate a weak fibrinolytic action. These observations support the use of AP in Ayurvedic therapies of IHD.

The effect of AP and fish oil was further studied on atherosclerotic stenosis and restenosis after coronary angioplasty in dogs.[52] Preliminary results showed that AP can significantly relieve atherosclerotic iliac artery stenosis induced by both deendothelialization and high cholesterol diet. The authors concluded that AP may play an important role in preventing restenosis after coronary angioplasty, and fish oil may be useful in reducing the extent of restenosis after coronary angioplasty. AP has also been shown to alleviate the ischemia-reperfusion injury in experimental dogs.[53] As compared with a control ischemia group, the AP-treated group showed reversal of the changes in the following parameters: superoxide dismutase (SOD), malondialdehyde (MDA), Ca2+ in myocardial cells, and ultrastructural changes of myocardial tissues. The observations were confirmed in additional studies.[54]

A component (API0134) of AP was studied in an experimental atherosclerotic rabbit model to determine the effects on on nitric oxide, endothelin, cyclic guanosine monophosphate, lipid peroxide, and superoxide dismutase. The study showed that API0134 possesses the effects of antioxidation, preserving endothelial function, and maintaining the balance of NO/ET. *A. paniculata* crude extracts were further fractionated and studied for various cardiovascular activities, mainly the hypotensive and the antithrombotic effects.[55,56]

30.9.6 Lipistat

Lipistat is made up of equal proportions of extracts of *T. arjuna*, *I. racemosa* Hook, and latex of *C. mukul*. The formula was given to rats at different doses (225, 350, 450 mg/kg) orally daily for 6 days/week for 60 days.[58] Thereafter, the rats were subjected to isoproterenol-(ISO) induced (85 mg/kg, s.c. for 2 days) myocardial necrosis. Gross and microscopic examinations (histopathology) were done along with estimations of myocardial tissue high energy phosphates stores and lactate content. The study showed protective effect of the formula. The authors suggested that the formula may be potentially useful in the prevention of IHD.

30.9.7 *Centella asiatica*

The effects of the total triterpenic fraction of *C. asiatica* on serum levels of the uronic acids and lysosomal enzymes involved in mucopolysaccharide metabolism (beta-glycuronidase, beta-*N*-acetylglucosaminidase, arylsulfatase) in patients with varicose veins were studied.[58] The results of this trial provide an indirect confirmation of regulatory effects of the extract of *C. asiatica* on metabolism in the connective tissue of the vascular wall and thus may prove useful in treatment of IHD. Total triterpenic fraction of *C. asiatica* has been found effective in improving venous wall alterations in chronic venous hypertension and in protecting the venous endothelium.[59]

30.9.8 *Piper longum*

An amide, dehydropipernonaline, isolated from *P. longum* has been shown to have coronary vasorelaxant activity.[60]

30.9.9 *Picrorhiza kurrora*

The ethanol extract of *P. kurrora* rhizomes and roots was found to exhibit a cardioprotective effect on ISO-induced myocardial infarction in rats as measured by lipid metabolism in serum and heart tissue.[61]

30.9.10 *Commiphora mukul*

Hypercholesterolemia is a known risk factor for IHD. In a clinical trial[62] with 61 hypercholesterolemia patients, 31 patients were given guggulipid, representing 50 mg of guggul sterones, and 30 patients were given placebo capsules twice daily for 24 weeks. The compliance of patients was greater than 96%. In the treated group, total cholesterol level decreased by 11.7%, the LDL by 12.5%, triglycerides by 12.0%, and the total cholesterol/HDL cholesterol ratio by 11.1% as compared with baseline levels; the levels were unchanged in the placebo group. The lipid peroxides, indicating oxidative stress, declined 33.3% in the guggulipid group without any decrease in the placebo group. The combined effect of diet and guggulipid at 36 weeks was as great as the reported lipid-lowering effect of modern drugs. After a wash-out period of another 12 weeks, changes in blood lipoproteins were reversed in the guggulipid group without any changes in the placebo group. Side effects of guggulipid were headache, mild nausea, eructation, and hiccups in a few patients. In another similar study,[63] guggulipid also showed similar results.

30.10 Summary and Discussion

In recent years, considerable attention has been paid to the utilization of traditional systems of medicine including Ayurveda in the management of IHD. WHO has recommended utilization of alternative forms of medicine for total health care. *T. arjuna* is one of several popular Ayurvedic herbs already being utilized by the Ayurvedic practitioners for the prevention and management of IHD. Other herbs with great potential to improve quality of life of individuals with IHD and that are commonly used are *Aloe vera, Cole forskohlii, Inula recemosa, Andrographis paniculata, Centella asiatica, Piper longum, Picrorhiza kurrora,* and *Commiphora mukul.* The experimental data available supports their use in IHD.

According to Ayurveda, IHD is the outcome of faulty diet and stressful lifestyle which leads to an *ama* state (i.e., hyperlipidemia) leading further to *dhamani praticaya* (thickening of arteries) and *dhamani kathinya* (hardening of arteries), resulting into angio-obstruction and aggravation of *vata dosa* showing chest pain and angina. The principle treatment is to promote *agni* (biofire) and to purify the channels by *panchakarma* in addition to the use of natural palliative drugs that have cardiotonic, hypotensive, hypolipidemic, and anticoagulant properties. The recent studies show that *T. arjuna* has shown varying degrees of cardioprotective effect as evaluated in terms of being cardio tonic, hypotensive, hypolipidemic, and anticoagulant. Toxicity studies show that *T. arjuna* is a safe and effective herb in the treatment of IHD without any harmful side effects.

In modern medicine, the treatment of IHD involves expensive and chronic drug therapy or equally expensive interventional procedures, such as thrombolytic therapy and surgical recanalization. Reperfusion injuries and undesired side effects of drugs are the major drawbacks of the conventional therapies. There is a vast and untapped source of medicinal plants with cardioprotective effects used in Ayurvedic therapies. The recent research on *T. arjuna* and other Ayurvedic herbs suggests a better cost-effective and socially acceptable therapeutic option for IHD.

The drugs mentioned in this chapter have been used in the treatment of heart disease for thousands of years. The current research data show that they can be utilized effectively in deadly heart diseases, including IHD. The relief provided by *T. arjuna* in angina and its effect on ST segment changes and T-wave depression in IHD are quite impressive. The Ayurvedic herbs discussed in this chapter have the potential of improving quality of life, while avoiding the side effects of conventional treatment. LV function improvement by *T. arjuna* in IHD cannot be overlooked, especially in view of the fact that IHD has an annual mortality rate of 40% under conventional treatment. The widespread use of *T. arjuna* and the other herbs can improve the quality of life in individuals with IHD and potentially save millions of lives.

References

1. Pedoe, H.T., Ischemic heart disease, in *Epidemiology of Diseases,* Miller, D.L. and Farmer, R.T.D., Eds., Blackwell, Oxford, 1982.
2. Therous, P., Angina pectoris, in *Cecil's Textbook of Medicine,* Goldman, L. and Bennett, J.C., Eds., W.B. Saunders, New York, chap. 59.
3. Sobel, E.S., Acute myocardial infarction, in *Cecil's Textbook of Medicine,* Goldman, L. and Bennett, J.C., Eds., W.B. Saunders, New York, chap. 60.
4. Schoen, J.F., The heart, in *Robbins Pathologic Basis of Disease,* Cotran, R.S., Kumar, V., and Collins, T., Eds., W.B. Saunders, New York, 1999, chap. 13.
5. Dewan, B.D., Malhotra, K.C., and Gupta, S.P., Epidemiological study of coronary heart disease in rural community in Haryana, *Indian Heart J.,* 26, 68, 1974.
6. Bolli, R., Basic and clinical aspects of myocardial stunning, *Prog Cardiovasc Dis.,* 40, 477, 1998.
7. Carpenter, K.L.H., Taylor, S.E., Vander Veen, C., William Sen, B.K., Ballamtine, J.A., and Mitchinson, M.J., Lipids and oxidized lipids in human atherosclerotic lesion at different stages of development, *Biochem. Biophy. Acta,* 1256, 141, 1995.

8. Mitchinson, M.J., Is lipid oxidation essential for atherogenesis?, *J. Clin. Pathol.*, 50, 268, 1997.
9. Bolli, R., Mechanism of myocardial stunning and its clinical relevance, *Circulation*, 82, 723, 1990.
10. Braunwald, E. and Kloner, R., Myocardial reperfusion: a double edge sword, *J. Clin. Invest.*, 76, 1713, 1985.
11. Hearse, D. and Bolli, R., Reperfusion induced injury: manifestation, mechanism and clinical relevance, *Cardiovasc. Res.*, 26, 101, 1992.
12. Miller, A.L., Botanical influences on cardiovascular disease, *Alter. Med. Rev.*, 3, 422, 1998.
13. Chaturvedi, P.N., A Study on the Effect of an Indigenous Drug *Arjuna* (*Terminalia arjuna* W & A) on arterial thrombosis and ischemic heart disease, thesis (Doctor of Ayurvedic Medicine), Banaras Hindu University, Varanasi, U.P., India, 1967.
14. Gupta, L.P., Sen, S.P., and Udupa, K.N., Pharmacognostical and pharmacological studies on *Terminalia arjuna*, *J. Res. Indian Med. Yoga Homeopathy*, 11, 16, 1976.
15. Wahal, P.K., A preliminary report on the inhibitory effect of Abana on platelet aggregation and adhesiveness in cases of coronary heart disease and hypertension, *Probe*, 30, 312, 1991.
16. Gupta, L.P., Studies on Cardiac Muscle Regeneration under the Influence of Certain Indigenous Drugs, Ph.D. thesis, Banaras Hindu University, Varanasi, U.P., India, 1974.
17. Srivastava, R.D., Dwivedi, S., Sreenivasan, K.K., and Chandrashekhar, C.N., Cardiovascular effects of *Terminalia* species of plants, *Indian Drugs*, 29, 144, 1992.
18. Radhakrishnan, R., Wadsworth, R.M., and Gray, A.I., *Terminalia arjuna*: an Ayurvedic cardiotonic, increases contractile force of rat isolated atria, *Phytotherapy Res.*, 7, 443, 1993.
19. Karamsetty, M., Ferrie, T.J., Kane, K.A., and Gray, A.I., Effects of an aqueous extract of *Terminalia arjuna* on isolated rat and thoracic aorta, *Phytotherapy Res.*, 9, 575, 1995.
20. Singh, N., Kapur, K.K., Singh, S.P., Shankar, K., Sinha, J.N., and Kohli, R.P., Mechanism of cardiovascular action of *Terminalia arjuna*, *Planta Medica*, 45, 102, 1982.
21. Takahashi, S., Tanaka, H., Hano, Y., Ito, K., Nomura, T., and Shigenobu, K., Hypotensive effecting rats of hydrophilic extract from *Terminalia arjuna* containing tannin-related compounds, *Phytotherapy Res.*, 11, 424, 1997.
22. Dwivedi, S., Chansouria, J.P.N., Somani, P.N., and Udupa, K.N., Influence of certain indigenous drugs on the PGE-like activity in the ischemic rabbit aorta, *Indian Drugs*, 24, 378, 1987.
23. Dwivedi, S., Somani, P.N., Chansouria, J.P.N., and Udupa, K.N., Cardioprotective effects of certain indigenous drugs in myocardial ischemia in rabbits, *Indian J. Exp. Biol.*, 26, 969, 1988.
24. Tandon, S., Rastogi, R., and Kapoor, N.K., Protection by abana: a herbomineral preparation, against myocardial necrosis in rats induced by isoproterenol, *Phytotherapy Res.*, 10, 263, 1995.
25. Tiwari, A.K., Gode, J.D., and Dubey, G.P., Effect of *Terminalia arjuna* on lipid profiles of rabbit fed hypercholesterolemic diet, *Int. J. Crude Drug Res.*, 28, 43, 1990.
26. Alpana, R., Laurai, P., Gupta, R., Kumar, P., and Sharma, V.N., Hypocholesterolaemic effects of *Terminalia arjuna* tree bark, *J. Ethnopharmacol.*, 55, 165, 1997.
27. Gauthaman, K., Maulik, M., Kumari, R., Manchanda, S.C., Dinda, A.K., and Maulik, S.K., Effect of chronic treatment with bark of *Terminalia arjuna*: a study on the isolated ischemic reperfused rat heart, *J. Ethnopharmacol.*, 75, 197, 2001.
28. Sumitra, M., Manikandan, P., Kumar, D.A., Arutselvan, N., Balakrishna, K., Manohar, B.M., and Puvanakrishnan, R., Experimental myocardial necrosis in rats: role of arjunolic acid on platelet aggregation, coagulation and antioxidant status, *Mol. Cell Biochem.*, 224, 135, 2001.
29. Ghosal, L.M., *Terminalia arjuna*, Ph.D. thesis, Calcutta University, Calcutta, India, 1909.
30. Kirtikar, K.R., Basu, B.D., and Combretaceae, N.O., *Terminalia arjuna*, in *Indian Medicinal Plants*, 2nd ed., Vol. 2, Kirtikar, K.R. and Basu, B.D., Eds., Allahabad Press, Allahabad, U.P. India, 1935, pp. 1023–1028.
31. Chopra, R.N. and Ghosh, S., *Terminalia arjuna*: its chemistry, pharmacology and therapeutic action, *Indian Med. Gazette*, 64, 70, 1929.
32. Caius, J.S., Mhaskar, K.S., and Issacs, M., A comparative study of the dried barks of the commoner Indian species of genus, *Terminalia*, *Indian Med. Res. Memoirs*, 16, 51, 1930.
33. Colabawalla, H.M., An evaluation of the cardiotonic and other properties of *Terminalia arjuna*, *Indian Heart*, 3, 205, 1951.
34. Bajpayee, J., Ed., *Chakradutta*, 1st ed., Venkateshwar Press, Bombay, India, 1959.

35. Dwivedi, S. and Udupa, N., *Terminalia arjuna*: pharmacogonosy, phytochemistry, pharmacology and clinical use: a review, *Fitoterapia*, 60, 413, 1989.
36. Antani, J.A., Gandhi, S., and Antani, N.J., *Terminalia arjuna* in congestive heart failure (abstr.), *J. Assoc. Physicians India*, 39, 801, 1991.
37. Jain, V., Poonia, A., Agarwal, R.P., Panwar, R.B., Kochar, D.K., and Mishra, S.N., Effect of *Terminalia arjuna* in patients of angina pectoris (a clinical trial), *Indian Med. Gazette* (New Series), 36, 56, 1992.
38. Dwivedi, S. and Agarwal, M.P., Antianginal and cardioprotective effects of *Terminalia arjuna*, an indigenous drug in coronary artery disease, *J. Assoc. Physicians India*, 42, 287, 1994.
39. Bharani, A., Ganguly, A., and Bhargava, K.D., Salutary effect of *Terminalia arjuna* in patients with severe refractory heart failure, *Indian J. Cardiol.*, 49, 191, 1995.
40. Dwivedi, S. and Jauhari, R., Beneficial effects of *Terminalia arjuna* in coronary artery disease, *Indian Heart J.*, 49, 507, 1997.
41. Yegnanarayan, R., Sangle, S.A., Sirsikar, S.S, and Mitra, D.K., Regression of cardiac hypertrophy in hypertensive patients: comparison of Abana with propranolol, *Phytotherapy Res.*, 11, 257, 1997.
42. Kumar, P.U., Adhikari, P., Pereira, P., and Bhat, P., Safety and efficacy of Hartone in stable angina pectoris — an open comparative trial, *J. Assoc. Physicians India*, 47(7), 685, 1999.
43. Bharani, A., Ganguli, A., Mathur, L.K., Jamra, Y., and Raman, P.G., Efficacy of *Terminalia arjuna* in chronic stable angina: a double-blind, placebo-controlled, crossover study comparing *Terminalia arjuna* with isosorbide mononitrate, *Indian Heart J.*, 54, 170, 2002.
44. Gupta, R., Singhal, S., Goyle, A., and Sharma, V.N., Antioxidant and hypocholesterolaemic effects of *Terminalia Arjuna* tree-bark powder: a randomized placebo-controlled trial, *J. Assn. Physicians India*, 49, 231, 2001.
45. Lee, M.J., Lee, O.H., Yoon, S.H., Lee, S.K., Chung, M.H., Park, Y.I., Sung, C.K., Choi, J.S., and Kim, K.W., In vitro angiogenic activity of Aloe vera gel on calf pulmonary artery endothelial (CPAE) cells, *Arch. Pharm. Res.*, 21, 260, 1998.
46. Agarwal, O.P., Prevention of atheromatous heart disease, *Angiology*, 36, 485, 1985.
47. Agarwal, K.C., Zielinski, B.A., and Maitra, R.S., Significance of plasma adenosine in the antiplatelet activity of forskolin:potentiation by dipyridamole and dilazep, *Thromb. Haemost.*, 61, 106, 1989.
48. Dubey, M.P., Srimal, R.C., Nityanand, S., and Dhawan, B.N., Pharmacological studies on coleonol, a hypotensive diterpene from Coleus forskohlii, *J. Ethnopharmacol.*, 3, 1, 1981.
49. Metzger, H. and Lindner, E., The positive inotropic-acting forskolin, a potent adenylate cyclase activator, *Arzneimittelforschung*, 31(8), 1248, 1981.
50. Patel, V., Banu, N., Ojha, J.K., Malhotra, O.P., and Udupa, K.N., Effect of indigenous drug (Pushkarmula) on experimentally induced myocardial infarction in rats, *Act. Nerv. Super (Praha)*, 6(Pt 2), 387, 1982.
51. Zhao, H.Y. and Fang, W.Y., Protective effects of *Andrographis paniculata* nees on post-infarction myocardium in experimental dogs, *J. Tongji Med. Univ.*, 10, 212, 1990.
52. Wang, D.W. and Zhao, H.Y., Experimental studies on prevention of atherosclerotic arterial stenosis and restenosis after angioplasty with *Andrographis paniculata* Nees and fish oil, *J. Tongji Med. Univ.*, 13, 193, 1993.
53. Guo, Z.L., Zhao, H.Y., and Zheng, XH., The effect of *Andrographis paniculata* Nees (APN) in alleviating the myocardial ischemic reperfusion injury, *J. Tongji Med. Univ.*, 14, 49, 1994.
54. Guo, Z.L., Zhao, H.Y., and Zheng, X.H., An experimental study of the mechanism of *Andrographis paniculata* Nees (APN) in alleviating the Ca(2+)-overloading in the process of myocardial ischemic reperfusion, *J. Tongji Med. Univ.*, 15, 205, 1995.
55. Zhang, C.Y. and Tan, B.K., Mechanisms of cardiovascular activity of *Andrographis paniculata* in the anaesthetized rat, *J. Ethnopharmacol.*, 56, 97, 1997.
56. Zhang, C., Kuroyangi, M., and Tan, B.K., Cardiovascular activity of 14-deoxy-11,12-didehydroandrographolide in the anaesthetized rat and isolated right atria, *Pharmacol. Res.*, 38, 413, 1998.

57. Seth, S.D., Maulik, M., Katiyar, C.K., and Maulik, S.K., Role of Lipistat in protection against isoproterenol induced myocardial necrosis in rats: a biochemical and histopathological study, *Indian J. Physiol. Pharmacol.*, 42, 101, 1998.
58. Arpaia, M.R., Ferrone, R., Amitrano, M., Nappo, C., Leonardo, G., and del Guercio, R., Effects of *Centella asiatica* extract on mucopolysaccharide metabolism in subjects with varicose veins, *Int. J. Clin. Pharmacol. Res.*, 10, 229, 1990.
59. Incandela, L., Cesarone, M.R., Cacchio, M., De Sanctis, M.T., Santavenere, C., D'Auro, M.G., Bucci, M., and Belcaro, G., Total triterpenic fraction of Centella asiatica in chronic venous insufficiency and in high-perfusion microangiopathy, *Angiology*, 52(Suppl. 2), S9, 2001.
60. Shoji, N., Umeyama, A., Saito, N., Takemoto, T., Kajiwara, A., and Ohizumi, Dehydropipernonaline, an amide possessing coronary vasodilating activity,isolated from *Piper longum* L., *J. Pharm. Sci.*, 75, 1188, 1986.
61. Senthil Kumar, S.H., Anandan, R., Devaki, T., and Santhosh Kumar, M., Cardioprotective effects of *Picrorrhiza kurroa* against isoproterenol-induced myocardial stress in rats, *Fitoterapia,* 72, 402, 2001.
62. Singh, R.B., Niaz, M.A., and Ghosh, S., Hypolipidemic and antioxidant effects of *Commiphora mukul* as an adjunct to dietary therapy in patients with hypercholesterolemia, *Cardiovasc. Drugs Ther.*, 8, 659, 1994.
63. Arora, R.B., Das, D., Kapoor, S.C., and Sharma, R.C., Effect of some fractions of *Commiphora mukul* on various serum lipid levels in hypercholesterolemic chicks and their effectiveness in myocardial infarction in rats, *Indian J. Exp. Biol.*, 11, 166, 1973.

31

Urolithiasis (Mutrashmari)

Venigalla Sridevi, I. Rajya Lakshmi, and I. Sanjeeva Rao

CONTENTS

0-8493-1366-X/04/$0.00+$1.50

31.1 Introduction

Formation of stones in the urinary tract is a global phenomenon and is described in ancient Ayurvedic scriptures as *mutraashamari*. It is said to be one of the eight most troublesome diseases (*mahaorgas*).[1] Ayurvedic texts have classified the stones according to *dosic* profiles, namely, *vata-*, *pitta-*, or *kapha*-related and others. Here we have to interpret that the very mention of *dosic* involvement is indicative of the biochemical influences in the formation of stones.

The formation of a stone (calculus) can be at any level in the urinary system. These stones are most frequently formed in the kidney, but they pass farther down the urinary tract toward the bladder. They are intensely painful as they pass along the ureters and out through the urethra.

There are useful management and herbal treatments for urolithiasis that have been currently investigated extensively. The main aim of this chapter is to summarize the management of urolithiasis with herbs, herbal formulations, and dietary and lifestyle inventions; to understand the Ayurvedic concept of urolithiasis; and to explore the scientific basis of Ayurvedic therapies.

31.2 Epidemiology

The overall probability of forming stones varies in different parts of the world. The risk of developing urolithiasis in normal adults appears to be lower in Asia (1 to 5%) than in Europe (5 to 9%) and in North America (12% in Canada, 13% in the U.S.). The highest risk was reported in Saudi Arabia (20.1%).[2] The compositions of stones and their location in the urinary tract, bladder, or kidneys may also significantly differ in different countries. Moreover, in the same region, the clinical and metabolic patterns of stone disease can change over time. In India, bladder stones accounted for 30% of all urinary stones in 1965, but their prevalence had dropped to 5% in 1985. Concurrently, the chemical composition of stones in the upper urinary tract changed; the prevalence of calcium oxalate stones rose from 26 to 82%, and the prevalance of struvite stones fell from 20 to 5%.[3] In Japan, bladder stones decreased from 50 to 5% from 1950 to 1985.[4] In Portugal, over a 20-year period, the prevalence of calcium stones rose from 64 to 82%, struvite stones decreased from 14 to 3%, and uric acid stones decreased from 19 to 12%.[5]

31.3 Definition

Urolithiasis is defined as a stone or stonelike hard substance formed in the urinary tract. The definition is consistent with current knowledge of urolithiasis — the accretion of hard, solid, nonmetallic minerals in the urinary tract consisting of a nucleus of organic material around which urinary salts are deposited in concentric layers.

31.4 Clinical Description

A renal calculus is similar to that of the kadamba flower. It is three-layered, resembles a stone, and is either hard or smooth in texture.[6] The prodromal signs and symptoms described in Ayurvedic texts consist of severe pain around or near the urinary bladder region, suprapubic region, internal urethral orifice, testicles, and in the penis. Common symptoms include distension of urinary bladder, fever, anorexia, dense and turbid urine, dysuria, fatigue, and odor of urine resembling the smell of a sheep.[15,16]

The major clinical features described are pain in the umbilical and suprapubic regions and in the penis; obstructed urinary flow; split voiding of urine; hematuria; honey colored or yellowish red urine, turbid urine; sandlike particles passing along with urine; pain aggravated by jumping, swimming, riding a horse or camel, climbing in upward direction; and polyurea.[17–19]

All these clinical features are very much similar to those currently known. In conventional medicine, clinical features of stones vary according to their size, shape, and location of the stone and the nature of underlying condition. The most common complaint is intermittent dull pain in the loin or back increased by movement. Proteins, red cells, or leucocytes may appear in the urine.

31.4.1 Clinical Features According to the Location of the Calculi

31.4.1.1 Renal Calculus

Pain is characterized by a fixed dull ache in the angle between the lower border of the last rib and lateral border of sacro spinalis. Pain is also felt anteriorly in the corresponding hypochondriac region. Pain worsens with movement like running, jumping, and climbing up stairs and eases with rest. Sudden gripping pain is felt in the loin and tends to radiate toward the groin. Patients may experience fitful sleep because of pain. Pain may be associated with hematuria and may be complained of either during or after an attack.

31.4.1.2 Ureteric Calculus

Ureteric colic starts as soon as the stone enters into the pelviureteric junction and recurs at shorter or longer intervals as long as the stone remains in the ureter. Ureteric colic ceases when the stone is ejected into the bladder or impacted in the ureter. When the stone is present in the upper one third of the ureter, pain starts in the loin or near the renal angle and gradually radiates to the groin. Pain is gripping and starts suddenly. The patient experiences fitful sleep because of pain, which is often associated with hematuria and may be complained of either during or after an attack. When the stone is at a lower level, pain commences rather anteriorly just above the iliac crest and is referred along the two branches of the genitofemoral nerve to the testis in males, labia majora females, and anteromedial aspect of the thigh in both sexes. When the stones enter into the intramural part of the ureter in males, pain is referred to the tip of the penis, and the patient complains of strangury.

When the stone is impacted, colic ceases; a dull ache arises according to the site of impaction. Such pain varies in intensity, and it increases with exercise and is relieved by rest.

31.4.1.3 Vesical Calculus

With increased frequency of micturition, pain is often referred to the tip of penis or the labia majora and becomes aggravated by running and jolting. Children may scream and pull the prepuce for pain after micturition and experience hematuria at end of the micturition.

31.5 Etiology

In Ayurveda the causes of urinary calculi are mainly nonadoption of the purificatory measures such as emesis, purgation, and medicated enemas in order to eliminate the vitiated *dosas* (toxic materials) and practice of unhealthy diets and lifestyles. These factors are responsible for the formation of calculi.[7–10] They are primarily classified into two categories: unhealthy diet or excessive physical activity.

In conventional medicine, there are three primary factors considered responsible for stone formation. They are the supersaturation of stone-forming compounds in urine, the presence of chemical or physical stimuli in urine that promote stone formation, and the inadequate amount of compounds in urine that inhibit stone formation (e.g., magnesium, citrate).

Categories of specific risk factors for stone formation are listed below.[11]

1. Diet associated with stone formation — Vitamin A deficiency; a high-oxalate diet rich in purine levels; a diet high in protein from animal sources, glucose, or sucrose; etc.
2. Medication associated with stone formation — Calcium supplements, vitamin D supplements, ascorbic acid in megadoses (4 g/day), sulfonamides, triamterene, indinavir, etc.
3. Diseases associated with stone formation — Hyperparathyroidism, renal tubular acidosis (complete or partial), jejunoileal bypass, Crohn's disease, intestinal resection, malabsorptive conditions, sarcoidosis, hyperthyroidism, etc.
4. Anatomical abnormalities associated with stone formation — Tubular ectasia (MSK), pelviureteral junction obstruction, calix diverticulum or calyceal cyst, ureteral stricture, vesicoureteral reflux, horseshoe kidney, etc.

The additional risk factors include habitually low urine volume, high urine excretion of calcium, uric acid and oxalate, low urine pH (uric acid and cystine are less soluble in acid urine), and high urine pH (struvite and calcium phosphate are less soluble in alkaline urine). Some of the biochemical processes not only become relevant here, but also lay the basis for the drug therapy.

The stone is the outcome of accretion of inorganic material around an organic nidus not soluble in its own solution. Urine that is an end-point excreta, in a liquid form, represents the biochemical status of a person's metabolism. For example, in normal urine, nephrocalcin is an acidic glycoprotein, rich in ϒ-carboxy glutamic acid, which inhibits calcium oxalate crystal growth. The nephrocalcin present in the organic matrix of calcium oxalate kidney stones resembles the nephrocalcin present in the urine of the patient from whom the stone was removed, but it differs from the nephrocalcin in normal urine. The stone's former nephrocalcin lacks 'ϒ'-carboxy glutamic acid, which reduces to air-water interfacial films that are less stable than those formed by nephrocalcin from normal urine. It is safe to presume that the alteration of the biochemical quality of urine can help in the prevention of stone formation. The biochemical quality of urine can change with the quality and quantity of fluid inputs, the type of diets, and the constitutional factors. This in turn can play a great role in the formation or nonformation of stones in the urine. Ayurveda suggests a number of herbs and herbal preparations for stone breakdown. It is possible that the therapeutic agents are capable of altering the chemical composition of the urine and its pH.

31.6 Pathology

In Ayurveda, the concept of renal calculi pathogenesis is indicated as when the *kapha dosa* is vitiated because of the etiological factors, *kapha* reaches to the urinary system and, with the help of *vata* and *pitta dosas,* dries up and forms the calculus.[12] There is another similar opinion regarding the pathogenesis of urolithiasis.[13]

Urinary concretions may vary greatly in size. There may be particles like sand anywhere in the urinary tract or large stones in the bladder. Staghorn calculi fill the whole pelvis and branch into the calyces and are usually associated with pyelonephritis. Deposits may also be present throughout the renal parenchyma, giving rise to nephrocalcinosis.[14]

31.7 Classification of Renal Calculi

Ayurvedic texts have described four types of urinary calculi: *sleshmaashmari, pittaashmari, vataashmari,* and *sukraashmari.*[20]

1. *Sleshmaashmari* — In *sleshmaashmari,* stones are white, unctuous, and as big as a hen's egg. They produce symptoms such as dysuria, cutting, incising, pricking pain, heaviness, and a cold sensation over area the bladder region.
2. *Pittaashmari* — In *pittaashmari,* stones are reddish, yellowish, and blackish and resemble the color of honey. They produce a sucking type of pain, burning sensation, a warm feeling over the bladder region, and *ushnavata.*
3. *Vataashmari* — In *vataashmari,* stones are dusty in color, hard, irregular, rough and nodular or spiny like the kadamba flower. Patients experience severe pain (and may scream); pull out the prepuce; and have difficulty when passing flatus, urine, and stools.
4. *Sukraashmari* — *Sukraashmari* occurs in adults only. It is due to suppression of ejaculation for months or years and frequent coitus or coitus interruption. The semen to be ejaculated will be obstructed, condensed, and brought in-between the scrotum and penis (prostatic part of the urethra) by *vata.* This causes dysuria, scrotal swelling, and lower abdominal pain. The special characteristic of *sukraashmari* is that handling can dissolve it.

In conventional medicine, urinary calculi are classified according to their chemical components. Examples include uric acid and urates, calcium oxalates calcium and ammonio-magnesium phosphate (Struvite), cystine, combinations of the preceding items, and drugs or their metabolites (e.g., phenytoin, triamterene). Descriptions of these components are highlighted below.

1. The uric acid stone is moderately hard and brown. It is usually multiple, typically faceted, occurs in acid urine, and shows concentric rings on the cut surface. The uric acid usually combines with urates and sometimes with oxalates to form opaque stones.
2. The oxalate stone is the most common form of calculus and consists of calcium oxalate. It is extremely hard and the surface is rough and sometimes spiny (mulberry calculus). It causes marked irritation due to rough surface and becomes dark in color due to bloodstains. The outer layers often contain urates, which are usually a single crystal, and give an exceptionally good shadow on radiography.
3. The phosphatic stone consists of calcium phosphate and triple phosphates (ammonio-magnesium phosphate). It is white, smooth, chalky, and is easily broken up; occurs in alkaline urine; and is easily distinguishable from other types. It often fills the renal calyces taking on their shape such as stag horn calculus. In alkaline urine it grows rapidly because it is smooth; a phosphatic calculus gives rise to few symptoms until it attains a large size. Deposits of phosphates are often formed on the surface of uric acid and oxalate stone due to changes in chemical characteristics of the urine as a result of infection.
4. The uric acid and oxalates stones occur away from gross infection in the renal pelvis and sometimes in the bladder as primary stones. The phosphatic stones that form as a result of infection usually in the bladder, but sometimes in the renal pelvis, are known as secondary stones.
5. Cystine calculi are hexagonal, white, translucent, and occur in acid urine. They are soft like bees wax, pink or yellow when first removed, and change color to a greenish hue on exposure to air and light. They are radio-opaque due to the sulfur atom.
6. Xanthene calculi are extremely rare. They are smooth, round, brick red, and show lamella structure.

It should be noted that with the Ayurvedic description of urinary stones, *sleshmaashmari* can be correlated with the phosphatic stone and *pittaashmari* can be correlated with urate stones, *vataashmari* can be correlated with oxalate stones, and *sukraashmari* can be correlated with spermolith or seminal concretions of conventional medicine.

31.8 Diagnosis

After taking a detailed history, diagnosis is made on the basis of laboratory investigations and diagnostic imaging for mere confirmation.

31.8.1 Laboratory Investigations

The routine laboratory investigation includes examination of the urinary sediment and a dipstick test for red cells, white cells, nitrate, pH of the urine, and measurement of serum creatinine. In patients with fever, an analysis of C-reactive protein, a white blood cell count, and a urine culture are carried out. In cases of vomiting, serum sodium and serum potassium should be measured. To exclude metabolic risk factors, it is important to measure the serum calcium and serum urate.

31.8.2 Diagnostic Imaging

Routine examination involves a plain film of kidneys, ureters, and bladder plus an ultrasound examination or an excretory pyelography (urography). The latter examination must not be carried out in patients with an allergy to contrast media, serum creatinine (>200 μmol/l), or treatment with metformine and myelomatosis. Other special examinations that can be useful in diagnosis are spiral (helical) unenhanced computered tomography (CT), retrograde and antegrade pyelography, and scintigraphy. Because of the risk of impaired renal function due to lactic acidosis, the antidiabetic drug metformine should be stopped 2 to 3 days before administration of iodine containing contrast medium. Spiral (helical) CT is a new noninvasive technique that might be considered in case iodine containing contrast medium cannot be administered.[21]

Health conditions frequently associated with stone formation are as follows[22]:

1. Obstruction and infection of urinary tract
2. Climate or occupation giving rise to high concentration of constituent materials in the urine and reduced urine volume
3. Hypercalciuria
4. Hyperoxaluria
5. Inherited disorders (e.g., cystinuria, xanthinuria, gout)

31.9 Prognosis

From an Ayurvedic perspective, except for *sukraashmari* or seminal concretions, the other three types are manageable by surgery. If the renal calculus is associated with swelling in the scrotum and umbilical region, retention of urine with severe pain, and passing of urine with fine particles, the condition is said to be incurable.[23] In conventional medicine, prognosis of renal calculi is generally good. Occasionally, death or significant morbidity occurs, but most of the patients recover.

31.10 Treatment

The management of urolithiasis in Ayurveda basically includes herbal formulas, alkaline liquid, and surgical procedures. Newly formed calculi can be cured by herbal formulas, but chronic calculi has to be treated surgically. Oiling, induced sweating, medicated emesis, purgation and enemas should be given in the prodromal state of the disease only in order to cure it completely.[24]

31.10.1 Type of Management

31.10.1.1 Shamana Therapy

Palliative treatment includes administration of herbal drugs and herbal formulas orally. The palliative drugs used to treat renal calculi are analgesic, diuretic, and linthnotriptic agent and are able to balance *vata*. Preparations of *varuna, gokshura, pashana bheda, shilajitu, ela, veerataru, brihati, kantakari, yava kshara, kushmanda, trapusa, hazrul yahud bhasma,* etc. are commonly used in renal calculi.

A list of commonly used formulations is in Table 31.1.

31.10.1.2 Shodhana Therapy

Cleansing treatment includes *prepanchkarma* procedures such as external and internal oleation and induced sweating, and *panchakarma* procedures, such as medicated emesis, purgation, and enemas. Most of the Ayurvedic classics recommend medicated enemas for the treatment of urolithiasis. *Saindhavadi taila niruha vasti*[25] and *vrushadi asthapana vasti*[26] are generally used in renal calculi. The idea here is that transmucosal fluxes are encouraged away from the kidney for removal of unwanted metabolites, thereby reducing the ionic load on the kidney filtration system. This may be considered as a type of dialysis procedure.

31.10.1.3 Alkali Therapy

Most of the alkaline materials (*kshara*) act as diuretics, lithotriptic, alkalizer, and antispasmodic agents. These pharmacological activities are shown to be effective in the management of different symptoms of urolithiasis. Examples include *palasa kshara, yava kshara,* and *mulaka kshara.*

31.10.2 Medical Management[27]

31.10.2.1 Vataashmari Treatment

A decoction is made for the following drugs: *pashana bheda, vasuka, ashmantaka, satavari, gokshura, brihati, kantakari, bhramhi, artagala, usira, kubjaka, vrukshadani, bhalluka,* and *varuna,* and fruits of *saka, yava, kulutha, kola,* and *kataka*. To this *ushakadi* group of drugs, *kalka* (paste) is added and thus *ghrita* is prepared. This preparation immediately destroys *vatashmari*.

Kshara (alkali), gruels, soups, decoctions, milk preparations, and food prepared from this *vata*-allaying group of substances should be administered.

31.10.2.2 Pittaashmari Treatment

A decoction is made for the following drugs: *kusa, kasa, sara, morata, pasana bheda, satavari, pashana bheda, vidari, varahi, shalimula, trikantaka, bhalluka, patala, patha, kuruntika, punarnava,* and *shirisha*. *Ghritha* has to be prepared by using the above drugs' decoctions to which *silajit, madhuka,* seeds of *indivara* and *trapusa,* and seeds of *eravaruka* are added.

TABLE 31.1

Some of Important Formulations Mentioned in Ayurvedic Texts

No.	Medicine	Doses, Vehicle, and Duration	Reference[a]	Manufacturer
1	*Gokshuradi guggulu*	3 g/day with *pashana bheda kwatha*	AF Sec. 5:3	Amrita, Arkashala, Baidyanath, Indian Medical Practitioner's Co-operative Pharmacy & Stores, Kerala Ayurvedic Pharmacy Ltd., Sandu, Zandu
2	*Ashmari hara kashaya churna*	48 g/day	AF Sec. 4:3	—
3	*Varuna kwatha churna*	48 g/day	AF Sec. 4:22	—
4	*Trikantaka ghritha*	12 g/day with warm water or warm milk	AF Sec. 6:15	Kottakal
5	*Vatsyamayantaka ghritha*	12 g/day with warm milk	AF Sec. 6:40	Arya Vaidya Pharma, Kottakal
6	*Mulaka kshara*	1 g/day with water	AF Sec. 10:10	Dindayal, Prabhat
7	*Yava kshara*	$^1/_2$–1 g/day with water		Dindayal, Prabhat
8	*Palasha kshara*	$^1/_2$–1 g/day with water	AF Sec. 10:9	—
9	*Chandra prabha vati*	250–500 mg two times/day with water, milk, or ginger powder	AF Sec. 12:10	Arya Vaidya Pharma, Dabur, Dindayal, Dhootpapeshwar, Nagarjuna, etc.
10	*Sweta Parpati*	725 mg–1.25 g two times/day with coconut water or cold water	AF Sec. 12:2	—
11	*Hazrul yahud bhsama*	500 mg–1 g two times/day with *ashmari hara kashaya*	AF Sec. 14:4	—
12	*Trivikrama ras*	250 mg two times/day with *beejapuraka nimba moola twak* and water	AF Sec. 16:24	Bhuvaneshwari
13	*Sukramatraka vati*	500 mg with juice of pomagranate, goat's milk, or water	AF Sec. 12:29	—
14	*Vishnu Tailam*	Internal and external application	AF Sec. 8:15	—
15	*Brihat Saindhavadya Tailam*	External application	AF Sec. 8:40	—

[a]All references are from *The Ayurvedic Formulary of India* (AF), a Government of India Publication.

Alkalis, gruels, soups, decoctions, milk, and foods prepared from these *pitta*-allaying groups of substances should be administered.

31.10.2.3 Sleshmashmari Treatment

Drugs of this decoction include *varunadi gana, guggulu, ela, harenuka, kushta,* and drugs of *bhdraadi gana, maricha, chitraka,* and *devadaru.* The decoction, added with paste of the *ushakadi* group of drugs, has to be taken along with dehydrated butter. This preparation provides relief from *sleshmaashmari.*

Alkalies, gruels, soups, decoctions, milk preparations, and food prepared from these *kapha*-balancing groups of substances should be administered. Karpasa flowers, *ankola, nirmali, saka,* and *indivara* fruits powder have to be taken internally with water and jaggery; this mixture quickly reduces blood sugar levels. *Gokshura, talamuli, ajamoda,* roots of *kadamba,* and *adraka* are taken with wine or hot water to remove calculi. *Gokshura* seeds powder with honey should be taken with milk for 1 week to disintegrate the calculi.

31.10.2.4 Sukraashmari Treatment

If seminal concretions or fine particles spontaneously come in the urethra, they should be removed by the *badisha* instrument (a hook). After the wound is healed, the patient is advised not to undertake any physical activity, such as horse riding.

31.10.2.5 Alkali Treatment[28]

In Ayurvedic texts, it is advocated that a formulation with medicated *ghrita* and *kshara* is made from the drugs mentioned above.

Kshara (alkali) prepared from pastes of *tila, apamarga, kadali, palasa,* and *yava* administered as a drink quickly relieves the symptoms. *Kshara* prepared from *patala* and *karavera* can also be effective.

Patients suffering from pain should be given milk processed with the above drugs or *triphala* groups or with *punarnava* as a drink. The drugs of the *veerataru* group can be administered by all modes.

31.10.2.6 Surgical Treatment

The surgical procedure (*shastra karma*) depicted in the classical texts may be presented as follows.[29]

First, the patient should be cleansed of the vitiated *dosas*. Then the patient, who is strong enough and is not nervous, should be laid flat with the upper part of his body resting on the lap of another person sitting on a knee-high plank facing east; the patient's waist should be raised by cushions and his knees and ankles flexed and tied together by straps (lithotomy position). After massaging the left side of the well-oiled umbilical region, pressure should be applied first below the navel until the stone comes down. Introduce the lubricated index and middle fingers into the rectum below the perineal raphe. Thereafter, with manipulation and force bring the stone down between the rectum and the penis. Keeping the bladder tense and distended so as to obliterate the folds, the stone is pressed hard by fingers so that it becomes prominent like a tumor.[39]

An incision of about the size of the stone is then made just a few millimeters away from the perineal raphe on the left side. Some surgeons prefer the incision on the right side for the sake of technical convenience. Precautions should be taken so that the stone does not get broken or crushed. Even a small particle left behind can increase in size. The stone is then removed with an *agravaktra* instrument (small-tipped forceps, like mosquito forceps).

In females, as the uterus is situated very near the urinary bladder posteriorly, the incision should be directed upward. An incision in the bladder made at one place for the removal of a stone heals well. After removal of the stone, the patient is put in a tub of hot water and sedated to avoid any blood filling the urinary bladder. If the bladder does fill with blood, it is irrigated through a catheter with the decoction of the latex trees.

The decoction of the latex trees administered as an irrigating fluid through a catheter also removes the stones and the blood from the bladder.

31.10.3 Postoperative Management

To purify the urinary tract after an operation, the patient is given sufficient jaggery-based preparations. The patient is taken out of the tub, and honey and ghee are applied to the wound. The patient is given warm gruel processed with urine-purifying substances twice daily for 3 nights. After 3 nights, milk with treacle and small quantities of well-cooked rice is given to eat for 10 nights. After 10 nights, the patient is given sudation therapy either by oils or by liquids. The wound is washed with the decoction of latex trees.

The paste of *lodhra*, *madhuka*, *manjista*, and *prapaundrika* is applied to the wound. An oil or *ghrita* prepared from same substances along with *haridra* should also be anointed over the wound.

In case blood coagulates, it should be managed by bladder washes. If urine does not come out from its natural passage even after 7 nights, the wounds should be treated by heat treatment (cautery) according to the described method. When urine starts flowing along its natural passage, the patient should be treated by bladder washes, enemas of medicated decoctions, and medicated oils and given preparations made of jaggery to eat.

31.10.4 Management of Urolithiasis in Modern Medicine

The immediate treatment of loin pain or renal colic is bedrest and application of warmth to the site of pain. Pain relief can be achieved by administering the following agents: Diclophenac sodium, Indomethacin, Hydromorphone (Hydrochloride+atropin sulfate [Dilaudid-Atropin®]), Methamizol, Penta-zocin, and Tramadol. Treatment is started with an NSAID and changed to an alternative drug if the pain persists. Hydromorphone and other opiates without simultaneous administration of atropine should be avoided. Diclophenac sodium affects glomerular filtration rate in patients with reduced renal function but not in patients with normal renal function.[30] When pain relief cannot be achieved by medical means, drainage by stenting or percutaneous nephrostomy or by stone removal is performed.

The medical therapy depends on the type of stone produced. The therapeutic agents that are generally used in renal calculi are alkalinizing agents (sodium citrate and citric acid, sodium citrate, and potassium citrate mixture), diuretics (hydrochlorothiazide), chelating agents (cellulose sodium phosphate), and Xanthine oxidase inhibitors (Allopurinol).

31.11 Prevention

Ayurvedic texts provide detailed information regarding the dietary habits and lifestyles that are to be adopted in renal calculi. It is advised to take whole rice, wheat, barley, horse gram, green gram, matured pumpkin, *varuna,* ginger, *gokshura* and amaranthus, flesh of birds residing on dry soil or barren land, and measures such as medicated enemas, emesis, purgation, fasting or light diet, and sudation. The intake of sour, dry, and heavy foods, food substances that cause indigestion, and unwholesome food items should be avoided.[31,32]

In conventional medicine, the dietary habits are not much emphasized, but in some conditions some general advice is given. In idiopathic calcium nephrocalcinosis, patients are advised to maintain adequate fluid intake to produce at least 2 l/day of urine, maintain adequate calcium intake (at least recommended daily allowances) from food sources, cut down intake of animal protein, cut sodium intake 4 g/day (170 meq), cut sucrose intake, increase dietary K intake, avoid grapefruit juice, and avoid unnecessary vitamin C. Coffee, tea, and alcoholic beverages should neither be avoided nor encouraged.[33]

31.12 Scientific Basis for the Use of Ayurvedic Drugs in Urolithiasis

31.12.1 Clinical Studies

1. In one study[34] with 30 cases of nephrouretero lithiasis, 17 cases were given 1 g of *swetaparpati* with 50 ml of *kuluttha kwatha* three times/day for 1 month. Marked improvement was noticed in different symptoms and pathological findings after the course of the therapy. Radiological investigations revealed expulsions of ureteric calculi were much more than those of renal calculi.
2. In another study,[35] 50 patients with urolithiasis (24 patients with renal calculus and 26 patients with ureteric calculus) were given *palasa kshara* in the dose of 1 g three times/day for 30 days. On the basis of radiological findings, the drug is said to be more effective in the expulsion of ureteric calculi as compared with renal calculi.
3. In one clinical study[36] consisting 30 urolithiasis patients (14 patients with renal calculi and 16 patients with ureteric calculi), 1 g of *sveta parpati* with 50 ml of *pasanabheda* and *gokshuru kwatha* was given three times/day for 3 weeks. The study indicated significant effect in majority of the cases. The x-ray findings indicated the clearance of the stone. Some of the stones had also passed through urine during the course of treatment.
4. A study[37] was conducted with 71 patients suffering from urolithiasis (*ashmari*) who were diagnosed by kidney, ureter, and bladder intravenous pyelography (KUB, IVP). They were treated with juice of the core of the pseudostem of *Musa paradisiaca* Linn. and *Musa sapientum* Linn. A significant segment of them passed out calculi of varying size after consuming the drugs for 2 weeks. The recurrence of stone formation was also prevented by the treatment. The author concludes that the plant material is quite effective in curing urolithiasis, especially of the calcium oxalate variety.
5. Of a total 110 cases, 30 cases were included in group A-1 and treated with *sveta parpati, pasanabheda,* and *gokshuru*; 30 cases were included in group A-2 and treated with *sveta parpati* and *kulutha kwatha*; and 50 cases were included in group B and treated with *palasa-ksara*. On the basis of the radiological evidence and clinical pathological criteria, it was concluded that the drug combinations in groups A-1 and A-2 had very good lithotriptic, diuretic, alkaliser, coagulant, and *vata shamaka* properties. The drug combination in group A-2 showed better lithotriptic action than that in group A-1. The drugs in group B have diuretic, linthnotriptic, and alkalizer properties and also have an antispasmodic effect. The radiological findings indicate that almost all the three therapies proved more effective in the expulsion of ureteric calculi as compared with the nephrotic calculi.[38]

6. One hundred cases of nephroureterolithiasis were treated with Cystone tablets (Himalaya Drug Company) in four different combinations (plenty of fluids by mouth, forced diuresis, antispasmodics, and antispasmodic-forced diuresis) for 1 year. The therapy with Cystone tablets and fluids given orally gave 76% positive results. The therapy with Cystone tablets combined with forced diuresis revealed 80% positive results, whereas antispasmodics combined with fluids given orally showed 20% positive results. Therapies with antispasmodics in combination with forced diuresis showed 28% positive results. The study indicates that forced diuresis alone is not as effective as the therapy with Cystone tablets alone in the treatment of nephroureterolithiasis. The mechanism action of Cystone could be attributed to any of its pharmacologic agents: diuretic, spasmolytic action, effect on crystalloid and colloid balance, and disintegrating action on the binding mucin. As Cystone contains no toxic ingredients, no side effects were observed even with prolonged therapy for 6 months.[39]

31.12.2 Pharmacological Studies

31.12.2.1 Varuna (Cratevea nurvala)

1. The cytoprotective action of lupeol isolated from *Crataeva nurvala* stem bark against free radical toxicity has been investigated in experimental urolithiasis. The increase in lipid per oxidation and super oxide dismutase activity, associated with decreased catalase activity and glutathione level, are the salient features observed in tissues of stone-forming rats. Lupeol administration induced a remarkable decrease in kidney oxalate level and also was effective in counteracting the free-radical toxicity by bringing about a significant decrease in peroxidative levels and an increase in antioxidant status. The antioxidant property of lupeol and its cytoprotective action against free-radical toxicity has also been studied.[40]
2. The antiurolithiatic activity in the crude extract of *C. nurvala* has already been examined. Further fractionation of this extract led to the isolation of the active constituent lupeol (Lup 20(29)-en-3beta-ol). Antiurolithiatic activity of lupeol was assessed in rats by observing the weight of the stone, biochemical analysis of serum and urine, and histopathology of bladder and kidney. Lupeol not only prevented the formation of vesicle calculi, but also reduced the size of the preformed stones.[41]
3. Male albino rats (100 ~10 g) were fed daily with a 3% glycolic acid solution (1 g/kg) orally for 4 weeks. It caused the deposition of lithogenic constituents, calcium and oxalate in kidneys, in significant amounts and induced hyperoxaluria, hypercalciuria, and hypercrystalluria. Oral administration of ethanolic extract of *C. nurvala* (stem bark) at the dose levels of 25, 50, and 100 mg/kg for 4 weeks showed 12 to 54% protection against the deposition of stone-forming constituents in the kidney and against hyperoxaluria, hypercalciuria, and hypercrystalluria. Similarly, lupeol, the active constituent of *C. nurvala,* was also found to be active. At an oral dose of 10, 25, and 50 mg/kg for 4 weeks, it showed 24 to 63% activity. The increased urinary excretion of the crystalline constituents, found in the stone-forming rats, was nearly normalized by lupeol treatment in a dose-dependent manner.[42]

31.12.2.2 Gokshura (Tribulus terrestris)

An ethanolic extract of the fruits of *T. terrestris* showed significant dose-dependent protection against urolithiasis induced by glass-bead implantation in albino rats. On subsequent fractionation of the ethanol extract, maximum activity was localized in the 10% aqueous methanol fraction. It provided significant protection against the deposition of calculogenic material around the glass bead. It also protected leucocytosis and elevation in serum urea levels. Further fractionation lead to decreased activity. This could be either due to the loss of active compounds during fractionation or the antiurolithiatic activity of *T. terrestris* being a combined effect of several constituents present in the methanolic fraction.[43]

31.12.2.3 Pashanabheda (Bergenea ligulata)

Acetone extract of the root bark of *B. ligulata* has been subjected to preliminary pharmacological investigations. Observations indicate that the extract contains components possessing sedative action, potentates analgesia induced by a subanalgesic dose of morphine, and anti-inflammatory activity comparable with that of aspirin. The extract was devoid of possessing antilithiatic activity but exhibited a mild diuretic effect when tested on rats and dogs.[44]

31.13 Discussion and Conclusions

The epidemiology shows that there is a wide variation in the occurrence of urolithiasis in various countries. There are also many variations in the chemical composition of stones. Basically, it is a physicochemical phenomena involving the nature of urine and the accretion of minerals. It is interesting to note that the stone former's nephrocalcin lacks ϒ-carboxy glutamic acid. This chapter provides a number of herbal treatments that provide scope for research into their ability to alter the chemical composition of the urine, making the stone vulnerable for dissolution. This is a very fruitful area for future research for metabolic management of the patients, particularly after surgical removal of the stone.

31.14 Future Research Areas

Biochemical and biophysical characters of the body's metabolism involving hydrokinetics and dispersal of organic waste matter in urolithiasis is a potentially fruitful area. This may give leads for phytotherapy intervention suited to rectify the aberration.

References

1. Susruta, *Susrutha Samhita*, Part 1, 8th ed., commentary by Shastri, K.A., Chowkhamba Sanskrit Sansthan, Chowkhamba, Varanasi, India, Samvat, 1993, Sutra sthanam 126, chap. 33.
2. Robertson, W.G. and Hughes, H., Epidemiology of urinary stone disease in Saudi Arabia, in *Urolithiasis*, Ryall, R., Bais, R., Marshall, V.R., Rofe, A.M., Smith, L.H., and Walker, V.R., Eds., Plenum Press, New York, 1994, pp. 453–455.
3. Thind, S.K., Sidhu, H., et al., Chronological variation in chemical composition of urinary calculi between 1965-68 and 1982-86 on North-Western India, in *Urolithiasis*, Walker, V.R., Sutton, R.A.L., Cameron, E.C.B., Pak, C.Y.C., and Robertson, W.G., Eds., Plenum Press, New York, 1989, pp. 673–675.

4. Yoshida, O., Okada, Y., et al., Descriptive epidemiology of urolithiasis in Japan, in *Urolithiasis,* Walker, V.R., Sutton, R.A.L., Cameron, E.C.B., Pak, C.Y.C., and Robertson, W.G., Eds., Plenum Press, New York, 1989, pp. 651–654.
5. Reis Santos, J.M., Composition of urinary calculi in the south of Portugal, in *Urolithiasis,* Ryall, R., Bais, R., Marshall, V.R., Rofe, A.M., Smith, L.H., and Walker, V.R., Eds., Plenum Press, New York, 1994, pp. 465–467.
6. Agnivesa, *Charaka Samhita,* 3rd ed., revised by Charaka and Dridhabala, with the Ayurvedia-Deepika commentary of Chakrapanidatta, Trikamji, V.J. and Pandurang, S., Eds., Nirnaya Sagar Press, Bombay, India, 1941, Chikitsa sthana 599, chap. 26.
7. Susruta, *Susrutha Samhita,* Part 1, 8th ed., commentary by Shastri, K.A., Chowkhamba Sanskrit Sansthan, Chowkhamba, Varanasi, India, Samvat, 1993, Nidana sthanam 240, chap. 3.
8. Agnivesa, *Charaka Samhita,* 3rd ed., revised by Charaka and Dridhabala, with the Ayurvedia-Deepika commentary of Chakrapanidatta, Trikamji, V.J. and Pandurang, S., Eds., Nirnaya Sagar Press, Bombay, 1941, Chikitsa sthana 599, chap. 26.
9. Vagbhatta, *Astanga Hridayam,* 6th ed., collated by AnnaMoreswar Kunte and Krisna Ramachandra Satri, edited by Hari Shastri Paradkar, Panduranga Jawaji, Nirnaya Sagar Presee, Bombay, 1939, Nidana sthana 498, chap. 9.
10. Vrudha Jivaka, *Kashyapa Samhita,* revised by Vatsya, The Chowkhamba Sanskrit Series Office, Banara, 1953, Chikitsa sthana, p. 120.
11. Tiselius, H.G., Ackermann, P., et al., Guidelines on urolithiasis, *Eur. Urol.,* 40, 363, 2001.
12. Susruta, *Susrutha Samhita,* Part 1, 8th ed., commentary by Shastri, K. Ambikadatta, Chowkhamba Sanskrit Sansthan, Chowkhamba, Varanasi, India, Samvat, 1993, Nidana sthanam 243, chap. 3.
13. Agnivesa, *Charaka Samhita,* 3rd ed., revised by Charaka and Dridhabala, with the Ayurvedia-Deepika commentary of Chakrapanidatta, Trikamji, V.J. and Pandurang, S., Eds., Nirnaya Sagar Press, Bombay, 1941, Chikitsa sthana 599, chap. 26.
14. Davidson, S., *Principles and Practices of Medicine,* 16th ed., Christopher, R.W. and Bouchier, I.A.D., Eds., Churchil Livingstone, Edinburgh, 1991, chap. 12.
15. Susruta, *Susrutha Samhita,* Part 1, 8th ed., commentary by Shastri, K. Ambikadatta, Chowkhamba Sanskrit Sansthan, Chowkhamba, Varanasi, India, Samvat, 1993, Nidana sthanam 240, chap. 3.
16. Madhavkar, *Madhava Nidana,* Charyulu, G., Ed., Ayurveda Ashram, Chennapuri, India, 1958, p. 230 (Telugu).
17. Susruta, *Susrutha Samhita,* Part 1, 8th ed., commentary by Shastri, K.A., Chowkhamba Sanskrit Sansthan, Chowkhamba, Varanasi, India, Samvat, 1993, Nidana sthanam 241, chap. 3.
18. Agnivesa, *Charaka Samhita,* 3rd ed., Revised by Charaka and Dridhabala, with the Ayurvedia-Deepika commentary of Chakrapanidatta, Trikamji, V.J. and Pandurang, S., Eds., Nirnaya Sagar Press, Bombay, India, 1941, Chikitsa sthana 599, chap. 26.
19. Vagbhatta, *Astanga Hridayam,* 6th ed., collated by Kunte, A.M. and Satri, K.S.; Paradkar, H.S. and Panduranga, J., Eds., Nirnaya Sagar Press, Bombay, India, 1939, Nidana sthana 498, chap.9.
20. Susruta, *Susrutha Samhita,* Part 1, 8th ed., commentary by Shastri, K.A., Chowkhamba Sanskrit Sansthan, Chowkhamba, Varanasi, India, Samvat, 1993, Nidana sthanam 241, chap. 3.
21. Mindelzun, R.E. and Jeffrey, R.B., An enhanced helical CT for evaluating acute abdominal pain — a little more cost, a lot more information, *Radiology,* 205, 43, 1997.
22. Davidson, S., *Principles and Practices of Medicine,* 16th ed., Christopher, R.W. and Bouchier, I.A.D., Eds., Churchil Livingstone, Edinburgh, 1991, chap. 12.
23. Susruta, *Susrutha Samhita,* Part 1, 8th ed., commentary by Shastri, K.A., Chowkhamba Sanskrit Sansthan, Chowkhamba, Varanasi, Samvat 1993, Sutra sthanam 227, chap. 33.
24. Susruta, *Susrutha Samhita,* Part 1, 8th ed., Commentary by Shastri, K., Ambikadatta, Chowkhamba Sanskrit Sansthan, Chowkhamba, Varanasi, Samvat 1993, Chikitsa sthanam 41 chap. 7.
25. Agnivesa, *Charaka Samhita,* 3rd ed., Revised by Charaka and Dridhabala, with the Ayurvedia-Deepika commentary of Chakrapanidatta, Trikamji, V.J. and Pandurang, S., Eds., Nirnaya Sagar Press, Bombay, India, 1941, Siddi sthana 698, chap. 4.

26. Susruta, *Susrutha Samhita*, Part 1, 8th ed., commentary by Shastri, K.A., Chowkhamba Sanskrit Sansthan, Chowkhamba, Varanasi, India, Samvat, 1993, Chikitsa sthanam 45 and 46, chap. 38.
27. Susruta, *Susrutha Samhita*, Part 1, 8th ed., commentary by Shastri, K.A., Chowkhamba Sanskrit Sansthan, Chowkhamba, Varanasi, India, Samvat, 1993, Chikitsa sthana 41, chap. 7.
28. Susruta, *Susrutha Samhita*, Part 1, 8th ed., commentary by Shastri, K.A., Chowkhamba Sanskrit Sansthan, Chowkhamba, Varanasi, India, Samvat, 1993, Chikitsa sthana 42, chap. 7.
29. Susruta, *Susrutha Samhita*, Part 1, 8th ed., commentary by Shastri, K.A., Chowkhamba Sanskrit Sansthan, Chowkhamba, Varanasi, India, Samvat, 1993, Chikitsa sthana 42–44, chap. 7.
30. Cohen, E., Hofner, R., et al., Comparison of ketorolac and di-clofenac in the treatment of renal colic, *Eur. J. Clin. Pharmacol.*, 54, 455, 1998.
31. Govinda Das, *Bhaishjya Ratnavali* with Vidyotanai commentary, commentary by Shastri, K.A., Chowkhamba Sanskrit Sansthan, Chowkhamba, Varanasi, India, 1983, chap. 36, p. 506.
32. Yogaratnakar, *Yogaratnakah,* Shastri, S.S., Ed., Chowkhamba Sanskrit Santhana, Varnasi, India, 1939, p. 506.
33. Curhan, G.C. and Stampfer, M.J., Beverages, diet and prevention of kidney stones, Author's reply, *Am. J. Kidney Dis.*, 33, 398, 1999.
34. Kumar, A. et al., To evaluate the effect of Ayurvedic drugs (an herbo mineral combination of Sveta parpati with Kulatha kwatha in the management of Mutrasmari), *J. Res. Ayurveda Siddha*, 16, 1–2, 1995.
35. Kumar, A. et al., To evaluate the effect of *Palasa Kshara* in the management of *Mutrasmari, J. Res. Ayurveda Siddha*, 16, 1–2, 1995.
36. Sannd, B.N. et al., To evaluate the effect of Ayurvedic drugs Sveta parpati with Pasanabheda and Gokshuru in the management of Mutrasmari (urolithiasis), *J. Res. Ayurveda Siddha*, 14, 3–4, 1993.
37. Gopakumara Pillai, R. et al., The core of the pseudostem of musa (kadali) in the treatment of urinary stones, *Ancient Sci. Life*, 15, 1, 1995.
38. Kumar, N., To evaluate the therapeutic efficacy of different drug schedules in the management of nephro-uretro calculi, *Semin. Res. Ayurveda Siddha*, CCRAS, New Delhi, India, 24, 20, 1995 (Eng.).
39. Misgar, M.S., Controlled trial in 100 cases with nephro-uretero-lithiasis by Cystone: an indigenous drug and other advocated methods, *Curr. Med. Pract.*, 26(11), 327, 1982.
40. Baskar, R., Malini, M.L., et al., Effect of lupeol isolated from Crataeva nurvala stem bark against free radical induced toxicity in experimental Urolithiasi, *Fitoterapia*, 67, 121, 1996.
41. Anand, R., Patnaik, G.K., et al., Antiurolithiatic activity of lupeol, the active constituent isolated from Crateva nurvala, *Phytotherapy Res.*, 8, 417, 1994.
42. Anand, R., Patnaik, G.K., et al., Effect of *Crateva nurvala* on calcium oxa-late Nephrolithiasis and hyperoxaluria, paper presented in XXV Annual Conference of Indian Pharmacological Society, Muzaffarpur, Dec. 6–8, 1992, *Indian J. Pharmacol.*, 25, 12, 1993.
43. Anand, R. and Patnaik, G.K., Activity of certain fractions of *Tribulus terrestris* fruits against experimentally induced urolithiasis in rats, *Indian J. Exp. Biol.*, 32, 548, 1994.
44. Gupta, S.C. and Sharma, V.N., Some pharmacological observations on root bark of *Bergenia ligulata (Pakhan-bheda)*, paper presented at the sixth Annual conference of the Indian Pharmacological Society, Hissar Dec. 30, 1973 to Jan. 1, 1974, *Indian. J. Pharmacol.*, 6, 17, 1974.

32

Gynecological Diseases

Manjusha Vinjamury, Natesh Nagashayana, Sivarama P. Vinjamury, and Betsy B. Singh

CONTENTS

0-8493-1366-X/04/$0.00+$1.50

32.1 Introduction

Women's health is a topic of concern in the medical field, as women are an important factor in the reproduction of healthy progeny. The environmental factors, fast-changing lifestyles, and various addictions (drug abuse) as well as excess use of drugs (like steroids) have endangered their health.[1] More than 4.5 million women (ages 18 to 50) report at least one chronic gynecological condition each year.[2] It is estimated that 30 to 40% of women have premenstrual syndrome (PMS) with symptoms severe enough to impair their daily activities.[3] Infertility affected 6.1 million people in 1997 (about 10% of the reproductive age population), up from 4.6 million in 1988.[4]

Currently available therapies, which advocate greater use of antibiotics, steroids, or surgery, may not be an ultimate answer for a woman's ill health.[5,6] So, alternative systems of medicine such as Ayurveda could be an option. *Streeroga* and *prasutitantra* (obstetrics and gynecology) is one of the eight branches of Ayurveda.[7] Women's disorders are described as diseases of female genitalia (*Yonivyapad*).[8] Some people perceive *yoni* as vagina, but that is just the literal meaning. The real meaning comprises the whole female reproductive system. *Yoniyapad* consists of diseases of *yoni* and *stanaroga* (diseases of breast). The major ailments described in conventional medicine such as amenorrhea, dysmenorrhea, and menorrhagia come under this category and are discussed here along with breast diseases. Uterine and breast cancers (*raktagulma, mamsarbuda, stanarbuda*) are dealt with under a different category and are not the subject of this chapter. Etiopathogenensis, diagnosis, prognosis, and treatment of all women's diseases including pregnancy, prenatal, postnatal health, and childcare are described in detail in this section.[8] This chapter deals with the treatment and management of major gynecological disorders based on clinical, laboratory, or pharmacological research.

32.2 Classification

There are 20 types of gynecological disorders (*yonirogas*).[8]

1. Menorrhagia (*asruja*)
2. Amenorrhea (*arajaska*)
3. Vaginitis (*acharana*)
4. Excessive sexual indulgence (*aticharana*)
5. Loss of libido (*prakcharana*)
6. Leukorrhea (*upapluta*)
7. Sexually transmitted diseases (*paripluta*)
8. Dysmenorrhea (*udavartini*)
9. Uterine polyp (*karnini*)
10. Bad obstetric history (*putraghni*)
11. Vaginal atrophy (*antarmukhi*)
12. Atrophy of uterus-congenital anomaly (*soochimukhi*)
13. Vaginal dryness (*shushka*)
14. Small uterus (*vamini*)
15. Sterility (*shandhi*)
16. Prolapse of vaginal walls or uterus (*mahayoni*)
17. *Vataja*
18. *Pittaja*
19. *Kaphaja*
20. *Sannipataja*

These disorders are also considered predisposing factors of infertility. Traditionally, it is believed that women suffering from these disorders cannot receive or hold semen (*shukra*) and hence cannot conceive. Apart from these complaints, there are some separate entities such as abnormal vaginal bleeding (*pradara*) and infertility (*vandhyatva*) that are described in detail. Uterine fibroid, myoma, breast cancer, and endometriosis are categorized under different headings like *gulma, arbuda,* etc. in the Ayurvedic classics and are not listed under gynecological diseases.[8] Neoplasms are not discussed in this chapter. Even women's diseases are a vast topic, which comprises various ailments of reproductive organs and associated organs such as the endocrine system. It is not possible to describe all of them because of the constraint of space and scope of this textbook. The major diseases that affect a majority of the female population are discussed in this chapter.

32.3 Etiopathogenesis

According to Ayurveda, women who violate proper diet and lifestyle are more prone to ill health.[9] Heavy, slimy, and excessive intake of sweet, acid, salty, sour, and incompatible foods, lack of exercise, excessive sleep, laziness, daytime naps, and overeating are some of the general causative factors of gynecological disorders.[10] Women's diseases can also occur due to external causes that are beyond one's purview. One has to remember that specific *dosa*-aggravating or -depleting factors (mentioned elsewhere in the textbook) could also be contributory factors to gynecological diseases in addition to those mentioned above. Essentially, all these factors cause an imbalance in the body tissues and organs and make them prone to infections or internal pathology.[11] For any pathogenesis there are two essential factors: structural and functional. The disease could originate from structural changes and then bring about functional changes or vice versa. In this context, an increase or deficiency (imbalance) of the three basic entities, *vata*, *pitta*, and *kapha*, lead to the vitiation of the related structure or tissue of the genitourinary system.[11]

As *dosas* become aggravated they develop pathogenesis in three different manners. When *vata* is aggravated, it dries up the organ or tissues absorbing necessary unctuousness and water in the tissue and makes the surface rough due to its innate rough (*rooksha*) property. In an excited state, the *vata* becomes hypermotile (*chala*) and travels in all directions. For example, this excited state of *vata* can expel the excretory products in excess, like in menorrhagia, or move them upward and stop the normal expulsion that causes pain in the local area (e.g., dysmenorrhea). *Apana vayu* is the type of *vata* that is involved basically in menstrual disorders.

Pitta, in an aggravated state, also absorbs water and creates excess heat, burning sensation, and inflammation in the organ. It also interferes with clotting because of its hot and liquefying properties and may cause excess flow as in menorrhagia. *Kapha*, when out of balance, obstructs the channels because of its slimy and heavy property. It disturbs proper metabolism and stops or delays functions like ovulation and menstruation as in amenorrhea. It can also produce heaviness, coldness, and sluggishness in the body as well as in the local area. Some fungal infections in the vaginal area or vulval region may be attributed to imbalance in *kapha* where itching (*kandu*) is the major symptom.[11]

An imbalance of a single *dosa* or combination of *dosas* residing in the genitourinary system may cause a gynecological disorder in women.

32.4 Clinical Features

There is no clear-cut description of clinical symptoms for all gynecological disorders in Ayurveda. The symptoms are usually based on the affected *dosas*.[8] The characteristic properties of each *dosa* reflected during an ailment are utilized by the physician for easy diagnosis and treatment of the gynecological disorder.

32.5 Diagnosis and Prognosis

Diagnosis of gynecological disorders is also based on the same principles of Ayurveda as are any other disease.[12] The history of the disease, its aggravating and relieving factors, its predominant symptoms, and the patient's personal and family history, pulse, tongue, diet, and lifestyle are all taken into consideration to diagnose the type, subtype, and stage of the specific gynecological ailment. Currently, Ayurvedic physicians in India are also using the modern diagnostic procedures such as blood chemistries, hormonal assays, x-ray, ultrasound, computered tomography scan, and magnetic resonance imaging for proper diagnosis and staging of the disease.

32.6 Treatment

The Ayurvedic approach of treatment is always holistic and works at both psycho and somatic levels. As most of the women's diseases are psychosomatic, Ayurvedic therapy has been often found to be effective in treating gynecological disorders. The first goal of treatment is to relieve the symptoms and give comfort, which is followed by alleviation or control of disease. The treatment comprises internal and external therapies.[7,8] Internally, clearing the channels, correcting *dosa* imbalance, and improving internal environment of the system is emphasized. Internal cleansing, if required, is usually done through *panchakarma* therapy. External modalities such as oleation (*snehana*), fomentation (*swedana*), medicated enema (*basti*), and uterovesical douche (*uttara basti*) are also very effective in women's diseases and are usually combined with internal cleansing procedures.[13] However, they form the main treatment methods in some conditions. They help relieve the obstructions, pacify aggravated *dosas*, and give symptomatic relief reducing pain and tension. Compound formulas used for the treatment of gynecological diseases are listed in Table 32.1.

Usually this purification therapy is followed by the pacification by oral supplementation of Ayurvedic herbs or herbal formulas.[14] Ayurveda also emphasizes preventive measures using behavioral and dietary regimens to all gynecology patients, because both diet and lifestyle play important roles in the etiopathogenesis of the disease. It helps maintain the health and control the frequency and severity of the ailment. Ayurvedic treatment is comprehensive because it encompasses cleansing (detoxifying), pacification, mental health, diet, and behavioral therapy while treating gynecological disorders.

Specific details of seven gynecological disorders are described in detail below.

32.6.1 Amenorrhea

32.6.1.1 Etiopathogenesis

According to Ayurveda, aggravated *vata* and *pitta* affect blood by drying-up menstrual blood (*raja*), which ceases the regular flow of menses (*nashtartava* or *ksheenartava*).[8] General symptoms that are associated with this condition are emaciation and pallor. It suggests the deficiency of blood or a severely anemic condition and weakness.

Conventional medicine indicates that amenorrhea is due to a wide range of causes that include anatomic or structural and physiological or functional defects. It can be congenital or develop at a certain age because of a particular change. There can be a defect from the ovarian or uterine level to hypothalamus and pituitary level.[15]

32.6.1.1.1 Structural

Anatomically there are four major congenital anomalies: absence of uterus or some part of the vagina, failure of the vagina to develop, imperforate hymen, or intrauterine synechiae. All these consequently result in primary amenorrhea.

TABLE 32.1

Compound Formulas for Gynecological Disorders

Formula	Dosage
	Gynecological Diseases in General
Ashokarishtom	15–20 ml two times/day after meals with equal water
Pushyanuga choornam	3–5 g two times/day with rice water
Kumaryasavam/kumari kalpa	15–20 ml two times/day after meals with equal water
Phalakalyanaka ghrita	5–10 two times/day with milk or warm water
	Amenorrhea
Rajahpravartini vati	2 tablets two to three times/day with warm water or *kumaryasavam*
Nashtapushpantaka ras	Same as above
Jeerakadyarishtom	15–20 ml two times/day after meals with equal water
Chandraprabha vati	2 tablets two or three times/day with warm water or *kumaryasavam*
Kumaryasavam	15–20 ml two times/day with equal water after meals
	Dysmenorrhea
Rajahpravartini vati	2 tablets two or three times/day with warm water or *kumaryasavam*
Jeerakadyarishtom	15–20 ml two times/day after meals with equal water
Ashokarishtom	Same as above
Dhanwantharam thailam	For external application like massage
Kumaryasavam	15–20 ml two times/day with equal water
	Menorrhagia
Pradarantaka rasa/loha	2 tablets two or three times/day with warm water or *chandanasavam*
Chandanasavam	15–20 ml two times/day after meals with equal water
Chandrakala ras	2 tablets two or three times/day with warm water or *chandanasavam*
Bolabaddha ras	Same as above
Lodhrasavam	15–20 ml two times/day after meals with equal water
	Leukorrhea
Pushyanuga choorna	3–5 g two times/days with rice water
Chandraprabha vati	2 tablets two or three times/day with warm water or *chandanasavam* or *ashokarishtam*
Chandrakala ras	1–2 pills two times/day with warm water
Chandanasavam	15–20 ml two times/day after meals with equal water
Praval bhasma	120–240 mg two times/day with warm milk
	PMS
Ashokarishtom	15–20 ml two times/day after meals with equal water
Kumaryasavam	Same as above
Manasamitra vatakam	1 tablet one or two times/day
Ashwagandhadi choornam	3–5 g two times/day with rice water
	Infertility
Phala ghrita	5 ml two times/day with milk or warm water
Satavari kalpa	5–10 g two times/day with warm milk
Kumaryasavam	15–20 ml two times/day after meals with equal water
Ashokarishtom	Same as above
Jeevaniya rasayana	5–10 ml two times/day with milk or warm water
	Menopausal Syndrome
Ashokarishtom	15–20 ml two times/day after meals with equal water
Shatavari kalpa	5–10 g two times/day with warm milk
Panchagavya ghrita	5–10 ml two times/day with milk or warm water
Kalyanaka ghrita	Same as above
Chandanasavam	15–20 ml two times/day after meals with equal water
Chyavanaprasha	5–10 g with warm milk one time/day in the morning

32.6.1.1.2 Functional

Physiologically, after menarche, women have a menstrual flow every month because of ovulation secondary to certain hormonal changes. The leutinizing hormone (LH) -releasing hormone is the main hormone produced in hypothalamus that further releases the LH and the follicular stimulating hormone (FSH). These hormones are responsible for the process of ovulation and endometrial changes. There are also gonadotropins and estradiol that stimulate ovarian functions. A defect of any of these glands at any level of hormone production and at any age from puberty to menopause can cause amenorrhea.[1,15]

32.6.1.2 Clinical Features

Absence of menstrual cycle during the reproductive years is the clinical symptom according to both Ayurveda and conventional medicine.

32.6.1.3 Diagnosis and Prognosis

Diagnosis of amenorrhea is very complicated and requires a series of investigations and physical examinations. To reach a perfect diagnosis, a step-by-step evaluation is necessary from vaginal or uterine level to the hypothalamus. To detect the anatomical anomalies, a pelvic ultrasound or examination under anesthesia may be required in adolescent girls. The hormonal levels can be investigated to help determine the exact cause. Prognosis of amenorrhea is good. It is not a life-threatening disease and can be treated successfully in many cases.[15]

32.6.1.4 Treatment

According to Ayurvedic treatment, the major objective is to alleviate *vata* in amenorrhea. The therapy is composed of three stages: (1) cleansing therapy, (2) palliative therapy, and (3) advising a dietary regimen.

32.6.1.4.1 Cleansing Therapy (Shodhana)

Vasti (medicated enema), one of the detoxification procedures (*panchakarma*), is the *vata* alleviation treatment. *Vata*-pacifying herbs such as castor, sesame oil, meat soups, and milk can be used for the enema treatment.[8]

32.6.1.4.2 Palliative Therapy (Shamana)

This therapy works on two principles: one is to control *vata* and *pitta* and the other is to improve tissue status. In amenorrhea, blood is deficient, so supplements like iron (*loha*) and *Suvarna makshika* give good results in weak or anemic women. Where there is a hormonal imbalance, herbs like *Aloe vera, ashwagandha,* and black kohosh are more useful. *Ultakambal* (*Abroma augusta*), *vamsha* (*Bambusa arundinacea*), and *shana* (*Crotolaria junecea*) are the herbs described for inducing menstruation (*artavajanana*). Black pepper (*Piper nigrum*), long pepper (*Piper longum*), garlic (*Allium sativum*), ginger (*Zingiber officinale*), sesame (*Sesamum indicum*), and papaya (*Carica papaya*) are some of the stimulating herbs proved effective to induce menstruation. *Rajapravartini vati, Nashtapushpantaka rasa,* and *Chandraprabha vati* are some of the effective formulas to treat amenorrhea.[14]

Conventional treatment includes the induction of ovulation as the main goal of therapy. It is done with the help of the drugs such as bromocriptine, clomiphene citrate, and steroids. Some patients who are hypoestrogenic can be treated with progesterone and estrogen in combination.[15]

32.6.1.4.3 Dietary and Behavioral Regimen

Cold and heavy food, oily deep-fried food, and frozen food tend to increase the *vata dosa* in the body in general and might accumulate in the uteri of women suffering with amenorrhea; such foods also block the free flow of menstrual blood.[10] Foods such as potatoes and peas produce gas and constipation and need to be avoided. A sedentary lifestyle aggravates the disease. Light exercises such as *yogasanas* or walking are recommended.

32.6.2 Dysmenorrhea

Dysmenorrhea is a painful period or menstrual cramps. It is the most common complaint among all gynecological disorders. Because most women have some discomfort during the period, it is considered natural. It is named dysmenorrhea only when the pain is too severe and disturbs a woman's routine, and it is relieved only with medication.[15]

32.6.2.1 Etiopathogenesis

Ayurvedic literature attributes dysmenorrhea to the above-mentioned general causes as well as suppression of natural urges (sneezing, coughing, micturition, defecation, etc). These factors provoke *Apana vata* and disturb its natural route of a downward direction and start moving it in reverse or an upward direction. The change in direction of the *vata dosa* alters the menstrual blood flow. This results in painful and scanty menstruation. When the flow is proper without any obstruction, pain is relieved.[10]

In conventional medicine, the prostaglandin theory is currently more accepted as the causal explanation for dysmenorrhea, although endometriosis or adhesions can also cause dysmenorrhea. It is believed that women with dysmenorrhea have much higher concentrations of prostaglandin.[15]

32.6.2.2 Clinical Features

The symptoms are cramping and spasmodic pain in the lower abdomen which may spread over to the gluteal region, thighs, and lower back. Generalized pelvic tenderness is usually present. Nausea, diarrhea, or constipation and headaches are the other common symptoms. Vomiting or fainting may occur in some cases.[3,15]

32.6.2.3 Diagnosis and Prognosis

Because the pain and discomfort is subjective, diagnosis relies upon the proper history. It is also important to differentiate the primary diagnosis from the secondary one. For example, an underlying cause like endometriosis may create confusion or be missed. Prognosis of dysmenorrhea is good. It can be treated successfully with Ayurvedic single herbs or formulations in addition to making diet and lifestyle changes.[15]

32.6.2.4 Treatment

Ayurvedic treatment emphasizes sweating, cleansing douches, and medicated enemas. Oil therapy, including massage, is used to relieve any obstructions in the passage, relieve any spasms, facilitate free movement of *vata* in the proper direction, and enhance a proper menstrual flow. Gentle massage with sesame oil, *dhanwanthara thailam*, *narayan thailam*, or *kottamchukkadi thailam* is advised over the lower abdomen, pelvic region, and thighs. Sweating methods and fomentation remove the toxins and also relieve muscular spasms and tenderness. A medicated enema with a mixture of oil, milk, herbal paste, and decoction or tea also pacifies *vata* and reduces any flatulence, removes obstruction of fecal matter, and relieves the tension in the pelvic cavity. These three therapies together help relieve pain and discomfort in the pelvic region.[7,8]

32.6.2.4.1 Palliative Therapy

Pootikaranja (*Caesalpinia bonducella*) is a very effective herb for improving menstrual flow and relieving abdominal pain. It also checks nausea and vomiting along with clove or black pepper. *Bol,* or myrrh (*Commiphora myrrh*), is another effective drug used in this disease.[14]

The first aim of the conventional treatment is to relieve pain and discomfort. Analgesics such as codeine or parenteral medication in severe pain will serve the purpose. If the causative factor is prostaglandin as is currently hypothesized, antiprostaglandins (e.g., ibuprofen) are generally very effective. Cyclic administration of oral contraceptives in the lowest dosage is useful in many cases, especially if the patient cannot tolerate antiprostaglandins. In some cases of severe pain, medication does not help. When the underlying cause is endometriosis or adhesions, surgical treatment is recommended.[15]

32.6.2.4.2 Dietary and Behavioral Regimen

Hot, slightly oily, and light food containing digestive herbs such as ginger, pepper, clove, and cinnamon is advised. Light exercises, such as like walking or *yogasanas*, are beneficial.

32.6.3 Menorrhagia

Excessively heavy bleeding or prolonged periods are considered as menorrhagia. It is categorized under abnormal uterine bleeding.[15]

32.6.3.1 Etiopathogenesis

According to Ayurveda, the aggravated *pitta* vitiates blood (*rakta*) and causes overflow through *yoni*. This is named *asruja yoni*.[8]

In modern medicine, submucous myomas, complications of pregnancy, adenomyosis, endometrial hyperplasias, or malignant tumors are some of the causes. It is very difficult to determine the exact cause, and there may be more than one diagnosis present. Metrorrhagia (bleeding any time in-between the period), polymenorrhea (too frequent menstruation), and menometrorrhagia (frequent and intermediate bleeding) are other types of abnormal excess bleeding. Dysfunctional uterine bleeding is one more type that is without any pathologic cause; it is due to only hormonal imbalance. In this disorder, the endometrium outgrows its blood supply because of estrogen stimulation, breaks down, and sheds in an irregular manner.[15]

32.6.3.2 Clinical Features

The symptoms differ according to type. There are four types of *pradara*; three types are caused by a single *dosa* (*vata*, *pitta*, and *kapha*) and the fourth one is known as *sannipataja*.

1. *Vataja pradara* — Menstrual discharge is painful, frothy, thin, rough, dark, and graying or light red. The associated symptoms are intense pain in pelvic region, thighs, back, and sides of the chest.[7,8]
2. *Pittaja pradara* — This type of *pradara* is characterized by a dark red a with yellowish or bluish tinge; hot, continuous flow that is associated with a burning sensation; and redness in the local area. Excess thirst, vertigo, and fever are the general symptoms.

3. *Kaphaja pradara* — In this condition, menstrual discharge will be slimy, pale, thick, heavy, and unctuous with dull pain. General features are nausea, vomiting, anorexia, cough, and dyspnea.
4. *Sannipatika pradara* — *Sannipatika* refers to all three *dosas*, hence there will be a variety of severe symptoms. Examples include slimy, dark-red blood; hot, yellowish discharge; or discharge containing body fat or marrow. Flow will be continuous, resulting in extreme weakness and anemia. Thirst, a burning sensation, and fever are some of the general symptoms. They indicate that deep tissues in the body are involved. Therefore, one can infer the prognosis is worst.[3,10]

According to conventional medicine, the main symptom is heavy bleeding with clots and gushing. Many times it is prolonged more than 7 days. Usually it leads to anemia due to excessive blood loss. Severe weakness, pallor, cramps, and palpitations are usually associated with excess bleeding.[15]

32.6.3.3 Diagnosis and Prognosis

The number of sanitary napkins soaking per hour with passage of clots or prolonged periods more than 7 days is the salient feature used to make such a diagnosis. Diagnosis requires proper history, physical examinations to detect abdominal masses and so on, endometrial biopsy to rule out malignancy, ultrasonography, and hysterescopy to confirm the diagnosis and obtain a clear picture.[15,16]

32.6.3.4 Treatment

The external therapy includes the following:

1. A continuous thin flow of medicated oil (*dhara*), milk, or buttermilk on forehead or lower abdomen
2. Fomentation (*seka*)
3. Simple oil application (*abhyanga*)
4. A local application of drugs with cotton ball as a plug (*pichu*)

These external treatments are done to alleviate pain, stop the excess blood flow, and relax the patient. Internally *Saraca indica, Terminalia arjuna, Indian sarsaparila, Santalum album,* and *A. vera* are commonly used herbs. *Lodhrasavam, chandanasavam, kumaryasavam, ashokarishtom, chandrakala vati, bolabaddha ras,* and *pradarantak ras* are some of the most commonly used formulas.[14]

Takradhara (a continuous flow of buttermilk processed with *Cyperus rotundus* and *Emblica officinalis* is called a *Takradhara*)[17] was found effective in menorrhagia in a 10-day pilot study conducted in Maharashtra, India. Uterovaginal administration (*uttarabasti*) of a formulation named *kashmarya-kutaja ghrita* was found very effective in menorrhagia in a study conducted at Government Ayurveda College, Trivandrum, India. The duration of the study is not available.[18]

Pushyanuga churnam was found highly significant in menorrhagia at Government Ayurveda College, Trivandrum, India. In an animal study, the same formulation showed positive effects on endometrium, such as atrophy of hyperplastic endometrium. The investigators' details are not available. In a study conducted at Government Ayurveda College, Trivandrum,[19] *ashokarishtam* and *musalikhadiradi kwatha,* two multiherbal formulas, have been shown to be highly effective in normalizing the menstrual cycle as well as reducing associated symptoms such as palpitation, weakness, and myalgia. *Kutajashtaka lehyam*, a classical formula, was also found to be very effective in menorrhagia and dysfunctional uterine bleeding in a study with little details.[20]

A multiherbal formula containing *Saraca indica, A. vera, Cyperus rotundus,* etc. produced significant results in oligomenorrhea. Approximately 25% of women conceived during the study. This suggests that the formula may be significantly effective in helping infertility disorders.[21]

According to conventional medicine, conservative therapy is advised; when bleeding is not acute and life threatening, a hormonal therapy (e.g., oral contraceptives) can control the disease. If the cause is myoma or adenoma, the new growths are excised to save the uterus in childbearing age. Otherwise, a hysterectomy is the preferred treatment.[15]

32.6.3.4.1 Dietary and Behavioral Regimen

Women should avoid foods that are fried, greasy, spicy, and sour. Indian spices such as coriander, turmeric, mint, and anise seeds are recommended. Hot spices, garlic, ginger, and chilies and hot beverages such tea, coffee, and alcohol should be avoided. Green vegetables including zucchini, squash, cucumber, pumpkin, Indian gooseberry, and dates and soups of legumes and vegetables are recommended, as these have a cooling effect. Women should add fresh fruits (except citrus) and dairy products such as milk, fresh cottage cheese, and ghee (butter oil) to the diet. Pulses and grains are also very beneficial. Coconut water, barley water, and buttermilk are also good. Excessive stress and strain need to be avoided. Maintaining proper hygiene of the genital organs is of primary importance. A proper bowel movement everyday is also considered important. Relaxation of the mind is very important for menorrhagia as in any other disease.[3,8,12]

32.6.4 Leukorrhea

32.6.4.1 Etiopathogenesis

Leukorrhea is also called as *sweta pradara* in Ayurveda. This disease is caused by the imbalance of *vata* and *kapha dosa*. The production and transportation of fluids by the urogenital organs becomes disturbed and leads to leukorrhea.[8,10]

In conventional medicine, an abnormal vaginal discharge that is watery, cloudy, or white; thick or thin in consistency; and malodorous or odorless is a condition known as leukorrhea. When it is thin, clear, mucuslike, odorless, and not subsequently increased in quantity, it is considered normal. It is generally secreted before menstruation, due to sexual excitement, or due to emotional stress. Fungal, bacterial, and viral infections change the environment in the vagina and make it alkaline. An alkaline environment results in production of vaginal discharge. Foreign bodies also cause vaginal infections and discharge. There are several other causes that also cause this type of discharge (e.g., worms or ulcers).[15]

32.6.4.2 Clinical Features

According to Ayurveda, the main symptoms are a pale or white discharge from the vagina that is usually painful and thick or thin in consistency.

Western medicine attributes specific symptoms to specific causative agents. The discharge may be malodorous or show a change in color with fever if it is due to bacterial infections. In viral infections, discharge may be profuse and the cervix tender. In fungal infections, vulvar pruritis followed by burning urination and itching are the principal symptoms. Along with the profuse vaginal discharge, there may be symptoms like weakness, lower backache, leg pain, etc.[15]

32.6.4.3 Diagnosis and Prognosis

Diagnosis is dependent upon a proper history and pelvic examination. In addition, a pap smear is done to identify any pathogens and also to rule out any displasia. Prognosis is often very good except in the case of a malignancy of the cervix.[15]

32.6.4.4 Treatment

Ayurvedic treatment emphasizes the use of vaginal douches (*uttarbasti* or *yonidhavana*). These douches are intended to treat the uterus, fallopian tubes, and the external vagina. They act as local antibiotics, clear the blockages in the channel pathway, and pacify *dosas*.[8] The herbs used for douches are *Santalum album* (*chandana*), *Azadiracta indica* (*neem*), *Tinospora cordifolia* (*guduchi*), *Saraca indica* (*ashoka*), *Terminalia arjuna* (*Arjuna*), etc. Internally, ginger, cinnamon, fenugreek, gooseberry (*Emblica officinalis*), *Terminalia chebula*, and *Hemidesmus indicus* are the popular herbs. *Pushyanuga choorna, Chandraprabha vati, Chandrakala ras, Chandanasavam, loha*, and *praval bhasma* are some of the effective formulas.[14]

Conventional medicine treatment includes cleaning the genitalia; maintaining dryness, avoiding tight clothing, and occasionally douching. Infections can be treated with antibiotic drugs. In some cases, surgical intervention is necessary to eradicate infections.[15]

32.6.4.4.1 Dietary Regimen

Food should be simple, easily digestible, and taken at regular intervals. Excessive amounts of puddings, garlic, onion, pickles, potatoes, sour foods, and excessive fried and greasy foods are not recommended. Rice water (water collected after washing the raw rice) is a very useful remedy in this disease.[14]

32.6.5 Infertility

In Ayurveda, if the breasts, ovaries, and uterus are not well developed and the patient cannot ovulate, then it is considered primary infertility (*shandi yoni*).[8,10] Women with this condition cannot conceive due to a genetic defect. The monthly cycle may or may not be regular in such women. Decreased fertility (*vandhyatva*), which is also primary infertility, can be treated. Secondary infertility is known as *kakavandhya* according to Ayurveda.[7,8]

32.6.5.1 Etiopathogenesis

There are four major causes for primary infertility: systemic (*dosadhatu mediated*), congenital (*beejadosa*), vaginal and organic defects (*yonivyapat*), and idiopathic (*daiva*).[3,10]

Conventionally, infertility is attributed equally to both factors, male and female. In the female factor, congenital and acquired structural abnormalities, ovulatory defects, and a hormonal imbalance should be investigated. The psychological factor is a very important precipitating factor and needs to be considered.[15]

32.6.5.2 Clinical Features

No specific symptoms are seen in infertile patients that can differentiate them from other women who have not had problems conceiving. Infertility is defined as a failure to conceive after a year of regular intercourse without using any contraceptives. The infertility can be primary or secondary. Primary infertility refers to those who have never conceived. Secondary infertility applies to those who have conceived in the past. Although both partners are equally important in the act, there is more evidence of infertility due to abnormalities in the female reproductive system. The abnormality may be structural (e.g., developmental anomalies) or functional (e.g., hormonal imbalance). There are many diseases of various systems as underlying causative factors. Infertility is different than sterility. Sterility implies an intrinsic inability to conceive.[15] It resembles the concept of *shandhi yoni* in Ayurveda.

32.6.5.3 Diagnosis and Prognosis

History, pelvic examination, ultrasonography (USG), hysterosalpingogram, diagnostic laparoscopy, and blood examination are some of the investigations necessary to reach a proper diagnosis. Prognosis is dependent upon the cause. It is usually difficult to treat with total success in every patient.[15]

32.6.5.4 Treatment

Ayurvedic treatment differs according to etiopathogenesis. When infertility is due to congenital or idiopathic causes, it cannot be treated. It is clearly mentioned in the classical texts that when a woman has any local defect, she cannot conceive. Those disorders should be treated first and her menstrual cycle should be regular. Cleansing therapies are carried out using herbs and formulas that have a penetrating capacity (e.g., *Triphala/Trikatu kwatha, kshara taila*).[8] These therapies are advised to unblock the channels and make the tracts patent. Some uterine tonics and ovulation inducing herbs or formulas should be administered as a palliative therapy. The *jeevaniya gana, rasayana,* and *vajikarana* group of formulations not only enhance strength and vigor, but improve the internal environment of the reproductive system. Formulas such as *ashokarishta, phala ghrita,* and *shatavari kalpa* give excellent results. *Amalaki, guduchi, bala,* and *ashwagandha* are some of the uterine and ovarian tonics which promote fertility.[1,14]

Conventional treatment is offered at various levels. If infertility is due to anovulation, then using clomiphene citrate alone or in combination with some steroids or human gonadotrophins will be the best choice. In case of endometriosis or adhesions, surgical intervention is necessary. If cervical mucus is inadequate, it should be improved or introduced.[15]

Diet and lifestyle are not very specific. Eating healthy foods and doing some simple exercises (e.g., yoga) are believed to be beneficial according to the Ayurvedic treatment.

32.6.6 Premenstrual Syndrome (PMS)

32.6.6.1 Etiopathogenesis

In Ayurveda there is no specific information about this disease. The concept and symptoms can be perceived on the basis of *tridosa* theory. The symptoms like heaviness of breasts, change in appetite, nausea, vomiting, depression, and nervousness can be correlated to *kapha* imbalance. Aggravated *pitta* contributes to irritability, anxiety, anger, vomiting, headache, food cravings, and sleep disorders. Bloating of the stomach, pelvic pain, headache, difficulty in concentrating, sleep disorders, mood swings, and anxiety are the features of provoked *vata*.[11]

In the conventional medicine, though the exact cause of PMS is not yet known, the most popular theory is cyclic change in hormones or estrogen levels. Another cause is chemical changes in brain, especially seretonin levels. Some habits or addictions like eating salty food and consuming alcohol and cold beverages containing caffeine aggravate the problem.[1,15]

32.6.6.2 Clinical Features

PMS is a psychoneuroendocrinological disorder. It is characterized by physiological and psychological changes in the body before or during each menstrual period and is severe enough to disturb a woman's routine life. Approximately 75% of women suffer from PMS. Among them, 40% have a disturbed routine due to severity. The range of the symptoms is very high. Common physical symptoms include tenderness and heaviness of breasts, change in appetite and food cravings, nausea, vomiting, headache, pelvic pain, and bloating of the stomach. Common psychological symptoms include mood swings, depression, irritability, anger, sleep disorders, nervousness, anxiety, and difficulty concentrating.[2,15]

32.6.6.3 Diagnosis and Prognosis

PMS is diagnosed by using a proper history. No major investigations are required to diagnose PMS. From an Ayurvedic point of view, the symptoms are differentiated based on the *dosa* involved to choose the right remedy. Prognosis of PMS is good and is quite successful.

32.6.6.4 Treatment

Externally, oleation with sesame oil and fomentation with herbal decoctions give excellent results. In severe cases, medicated oil enema (*anuvasana basti*) is very beneficial (e.g., sesame oil and *dashamoola kwatha*).[8] Internally, *ashokarishtam* and *A. vera* in combination with some other drugs are used in Ayurvedic practice. For *vata* and *pitta* symptoms, *shatavari* (asparagus), *ashwagandha* (*Withania somnifera*), *amalaki* (Indian gooseberry), and *yashtimadhu* (licorice) work very well. To reduce *kapha* symptoms such as heaviness of breasts and fluid retention, herbs such as *triphala*, *trikatu* (pepper, ginger, and long pepper), and *vacha* (*Acorus calamus*) are very useful. *Jeerakadyarishtom, manasamitra vatakam, saraswatarishtam, shatavari kalpa,* and *kumaryasavam* are some of the effective herbal formulas.[10,14]

In conventional medicine, a definite treatment has not yet emerged as a definition, and the etiology of the disease is unclear. Symptomatic treatment can be given using sedatives, diuretics, laxatives, and analgesics. Progesterone or its derivatives are recommended to improve the condition.[15]

Women suffering from this disorder should specifically avoid *vata* aggravating a week before the menstruation. Examples include dried fish and dry meat, deep fried and very spicy foods, very cold foods, sprouts, beans, and potatoes.

32.6.7 Menopausal Syndrome

32.6.7.1 Etiopathogenesis

In Ayurveda, menopause is called *rajonivrutti*. It means that the menstrual flow stops forever. As this is a natural phenomenon, it is not considered a disorder in Ayurveda. However, a common understanding is that the three *dosas* are imbalanced during menopause. Symptoms of menopause can be correlated to change in *dosa* dynamics. Among the three *dosas, vata* is of prime importance. It is said that there is not a single disorder of the reproductive system without aggravated *vata*. Women generally reach menopause after the age of 45, which is when *vata* is dominant in the body. Pelvic region is a seat of *vata*. It usually becomes vitiated when monthly flow ceases. All pains, roughness of skin, etc. during menopausal age can be attributed to aggravated *vata*. Finally, *vata* can also provoke *kapha* and *pitta*. Symptoms such as heaviness of body, fluid retention, and hot flashes are some of the symptoms attributed to an imbalance in *kapha* and *pitta* during menopause.[3,10,11]

Modern medicine defines menopausal age as between 47 and 52. Menopause is exactly a last or final menstruation. Postmenopause refers to the phase that comes after menopause. Menopause occurs when oocytes responsive to gonadotropins disappear from the ovary, or the oocytes remaining do not respond to gonadotropins. When this phenomenon occurs at certain age due to hormonal imbalance (i.e., change in levels of concentration of FSH, estradiol, LH, etc.), it is called physiological menopause. If menopause is due to cessation of ovarian function because of surgery (e.g., hysterectomy, oophorectomy), then it is called as artificial menopause.[22,23]

32.6.7.2 Clinical Features

Symptoms start to show up from the pre- or perimenopausal period. The first and foremost symptom is the alteration of the menstrual cycle. Abrupt cessation is rare. The usual pattern is a gradual decrease in quantity, duration, and frequency of the menstrual flow. In some patients it is heavy or more frequent before menopause. Another common symptom is hot flashes. This is a feeling of excessive heat or burning sensation on the face, neck, chest, and back, sometimes followed by sweating. Many times it is preceded by pressure in the head or a headache. Other symptoms like regression of breasts, inadequate lubrication in vagina, urinary urgency or incontinence, loss of libido, sleep disturbances, or fatigue may be present. Psychological symptoms are also equally important, as they may disturb a woman's life. Mood swings, irritability, depression, anxiety, and dysphoria are common psychological changes during menopause. Additionally, there are some major metabolic changes that manifest in the body during in the postmenopausal period (e.g., osteoporosis and increased risk of heart attacks).[22,23]

32.6.7.3 Diagnosis and Prognosis

Menopausal syndrome is essentially diagnosed from the patient's age and history. Routine blood work will help differentiate the fluid retention in menopause from anemia and other disorders. Menopause can be treated successfully using Ayurvedic herbs and dietary advice.

32.6.7.4 Treatment

The major goal of the treatment is to reduce symptoms and discomfort as well as to enhance well-being and prevent cardiovascular changes or osteoporosis. No drastic cleansing procedures are advised to menopausal women. *Shirodhara* (continuous flow of medicated oil, decoctions, or buttermilk on the head) and gentle a body massage are advised, as these treatments relieve muscle spasms, pains, burning, and restlessness. Internally, *chandanasava, ushirasavam,* and *draksharishtom* are some of the drugs that reduce hot flashes, burning, and urinary incontinence. *Shatavari, vidari,* and *kumari* are the herbs that reduce fatigue and vaginal dryness and give a *rasayana* effect. For psycological symptoms, like irritability, anxiety, or depression, there are very effective drugs like *brahmi, vacha, jyotishmati,* and *shankhapushpi* or formulas such as *panchagavya ghrita, kalyanaka ghrita,* stresscom cap, and *manasmitra vatakam.* On the whole, *Saraca indica* (*ashoka*) is the herb of choice that takes care of most of the problems.[3,8,14]

The American Association of Clinical Endocrinologists recommends hormone replacement therapy (HRT) as a preventive medicine for menopausal syndrome. HRT relieves menopausal symptoms and prevents osteoporosis. It also plays a role in protecting the heart. A goal of this treatment also is managing weight, stress reduction, vagina lubrication, etc. Steroids, moisturizers, and oral contraceptives may be used to treat menopause.[15,22]

No specific diet is advised other than avoiding those that have been mentioned above for other conditions.

32.7 Scientific Basis of Ayurvedic Therapies

Our literature search found very few scientific studies and clinical trials on Ayurvedic therapies. These studies are reviewed and summarized here.

32.7.1 Clinical Studies on Compound Formulas

In one study[24] on leucorrhea (n = 52), the resin of *Shorea robusta* was given at a dose of 1 g/day in divided doses for 30 days. Externally, a *Terminalia chebula* decoction was administered for vaginal douche. At the end of 30 days of treatment, there was 100% improvement in the symptoms of leucorrhea. Of the 12 cases infected with trichomonas infection at the baseline, 10 cases showed a negative smear test for trichomonas infection at the end of treatment. Similarly, 5 cases of erosion of cervix showed complete healing of erosion at the end of the treatment. The authors of the study reported that there were no adverse reactions observed during the full length of the study.

In the second study (n = 32) on leucorrhea, Masilamani et al.[25] reported that the combination of oxidized alum ash (*padigara barpam*) in the dosage of 300 mg three times/day with milk, along with a vaginal douche and a decoction of *T. chebula,* showed promising results. The duration of the study was 30 days. Of the 32 patients, 26 (81%) were clinically cured and 6 (19%) were clinically relieved of their symptoms of leucorrhea. There are no follow-up data or any adverse event information given in the article.

Ashokarishta, a very popular formulation for gynecological disorders, was studied for its efficacy in 22 subjects suffering from menorrhagia (dysfunctional uterine bleeding) for 3 months. A dose of 25 ml three times/day was given until the onset of the next menstruation. It was continued for another 2 months from the fourth day of the menstrual cycle with another break during the next cycle. The trial drug was continued for three consecutive cycles. Results of the study indicate that *ashokarishta* gave relief from excessive bleeding and pain in all the cases. Subjects who had *vata-* and *kapha*-predominant symptoms showed relief within 3 days after starting the formulation. One patient with a follicular cyst and one patient with an ovarian cyst had to undergo a hysterectomy after 3 months of the study. An interesting finding of this study was that the hemoglobin automatically increased as soon as the bleeding was stopped. With the help of this study, we can infer that the properties of *Saraca indica* — oxytocic, hemostatic, and analgesic — have been investigated.[26]

32.7.2 Pharmacological Studies on Single Herbs and Bhasmas

32.7.2.1 Saraca indica

Research has found that *Saraca indica* (saracin) is a good uterine tonic, which is effective in normalizing menstruation and reducing associated symptoms.[27,28] In another study,[29] saracin seems to be an interesting immunomodulator for the mammalian immune system. It has been found to be mitogenic for human lymphocytes, and this mitogenic activity could be inhibited in presence of fetuin. It also revealed that treatment with saracin could induce secretion of interleukin-2 (IL-2) in a culture of resting human peripheral blood mononuclear cells after 48 h. The study found that saracin has a higher affinity for the CD8(+) than the CD4(+) T-cells.

32.7.2.2 Aloe vera

In an interesting study,[30] the aqueous extract of *Aloe barbadensis* Miller in an *in vitro* culture of *Trichomonas vaginalis* revealed that within 24 h, percentages of inhibition greater than 50% were obtained from concentrations of 20.8 μg/ml. The researchers studied three strains of this parasite. The aqueous extracts were used as an initial concentration of 400 mg/ml of the extract and double serial dilutions were performed; final concentrations based on the dried weight of the extract were 10.4, 20.8, 41, 83, and 160 mg/ml. The inhibition of growth was greater than 50% even when tried with lower concentrations of the extract but it took 48 to 72 h for such an action.

In another study,[31] CARN 750 (injectable acemannan), a polydispersed beta-(1,4), linked acetylated mannan isolated from the *A. barbadensis* plant, was evaluated for its multiple therapeutic properties. It was found helpful in wound repair and acts as a biological agent for the treatment of neoplasia in animals; it was also noted for its ability to activate macrophages.

It was also found that CARN 750 directly or indirectly has significant hematoaugmenting properties. Subcutaneous administration of CARN 750 significantly increased splenic and peripheral blood cellularity, as well as hematopoietic progenitors in the spleen and bone marrow as determined by the IL-3-responsive colony-forming unit culture assay and the high-proliferative-potential colony-forming cell assay (a measure of primitive hematopoietic precursors) in myelosuppressed (7 Gy) C57BL/6 mice. It was observed that the greatest hematopoietic effect was obtained after sublethal irradiation in mice receiving 1 mg of CARN 750/animal, with less activity observed at higher or lower doses. Results showed activity equal to or greater than the injection of an optimal dose of granulocyte-colony-stimulating factor in myelosuppressed mice when CARN was injected daily.

In another study,[32] lyophilized *A. barbadensis* at concentrations of 7.5 and 10% proved to be spermicidal when used along with zinc acetate. The action was attributed to the multiple microelements boron, barium, calcium, chromium, copper, iron, potassium, magnesium, manganese, phosphorus, and zinc; these elements were toxic to the tail and caused instant immobilization. The two compounds did not show any signs of irritation or cause ulceration of rabbit vaginal epithelium. These results suggest the possibility of using zinc acetate and lyophilized *A. barbadensis* as a new, effective, and safe vaginal contraceptive.

The effects of another species of aloe on some physiological and biochemical parameters of reproduction in immature female rats based on the history of their use by the folklore medicine in Cameroon was studied.[33] *Aloe buettneri, Justicia insularis, Hibiscus macranthus,* and *Dicliptera verticillata* were given in different doses daily to 22-day-old rats for 5, 10, 15, 20, and 25 days by gastric intubation. The weights of ovaries and uteri, levels of uterine and ovarian proteins, ovarian cholesterol, and serum estradiol were evaluated at the end of each experimental period. The results of the study showed a decrease in growth rate of animals treated with 94 mg/kg/day at the end of the experimental period. Interestingly enough, the ovarian and uterine weights increased in all treated groups, especially within the pubertal period (36 to 41 days old), when compared with the respective controls. During the same period, other parameters that were also observed showed significant differences in treated rats when compared with the controls. Ovarian and uterine protein levels, as well as serum estradiol, also increased in the groups given 49 or 94 mg/kg/day of the plant extracts. The investigators concluded that these results suggest a possible presence of estrogenic compounds in the plant extracts.[33]

The study was repeated with the aqueous extract of the leaf mixtures of *A. buettneri, Dicliptera verticillata, Hibiscus macranthus,* and *Justicia insularis* at doses of 13, 49, and 94 mg/kg/day for 15 days given by oral route to immature female rats. Results showed that the extracts induced a significant increase in ovarian and uteri weight as well as serum and ovarian estradiol.[34]

Aloe vera was also studied for its anti-inflammatory property. In this study, the effects of aqueous, chloroform, and ethanol extracts of *A. vera* gel on carrageenan-induced edema in the rat paw and neutrophil migration into the peritoneal cavity stimulated by carrageenan were studied. The results showed that the aqueous and chloroform extracts decreased the edema induced in the hind-paw and the number of neutrophils migrating into the peritoneal cavity; the ethanol extract decreased only the number of neutrophils. The mechanism of action of the aqueous extract was due to the inhibited prostaglandin-E2 production from [^{14}C]arachidonic acid. The investigators conducted an assay of the extracts and found that the aqueous extract contained anthraglycosides, reductor sugars, and cardiotonic glycosides; in the ethanol extract, the chemical tests performed for saponins, carbohydrates naftoquinones, sterols, triterpenoids, and anthraquinones turned out positive. The chemical tests performed in the chloroform extract showed positive reaction for sterols type delta 5 and anthraquinones. On the basis of these findings, it was concluded that the extracts of *A. vera* gel have anti-inflammatory activity and suggested its inhibitory action on the arachidonic acid pathway via cyclooxygenase.[35]

32.7.2.3 Muktashukti Bhasma

Muktashukti bhasma, a compound formulation consisting of pearl, *A. vera,* and vinegar, inhibited acute and subacute inflammation in albino rats as induced by subplanter injection of carrageenan, histamine, serotonin (5-HT), nystatin, and subcutaneous implant of cotton pellets. The anti-inflammatory response of 1000 mg/kg MSB was comparable with the response observed with 300 mg/kg acetylsalicylic acid (ASA) in all the test procedures. According to the investigators, the anti-inflammatory activity of the compound was attributed to its ability to cause inhibition of prostaglandins, histamine, and 5-HT and stabilization of the lysosomal membranes. The anti-inflammatory activity of MSB seems to be only one third to half as potent as ASA.[36]

32.7.2.4 Glycerrhiza glabra

Glycyrrhyzin, a constituent of *Glycerrhiza glabra,* inhibits inflammation and prostaglandin synthesis. It blocks estrogen effects binding to estrogen receptors. In other studies for treating menopausal syndrome, licorice was found an effective source of estrogen.

Glycyrrhizae radix is found to suppress estradiol-17 beta (E2)-induced expression of c-fos/jun in uterine corpus and inhibited *N*-methyl-*N*-nitrosourea and E2-induced endometrial carcinogenesis in mice. The probable mode of action could be through suppression of estrogen-induced c-fos/jun expression and could be promising in preventing agents for endometrial cancers.[37,38]

Tamir et al.[16] reported that the stimulatory effects of 2.5 to 25 μg/animal glabridin were similar to those of 5 μg/animal estradiol. Glabridin, the major isoflavon in licorice root, was tested for the estrogenic properties, in view of the resemblance of its structure and lipophilicity to those of estradiol. The results indicate that glabridin is a phytoestrogen, binding to the human estrogen receptor and stimulating creatine kinase activity in rat uterus, epiphyseal cartilage, diaphyseal bone, aorta, and left ventricle of the heart. During the course of the study, the researchers found that the position of the hydroxyl groups has a significant role in binding to the human estrogen receptor and in proliferation-inducing activity. There was a biphasic effect of increasing concentrations of glabridin on the growth of breast-tumor cells. It showed an estrogen-receptor–dependent, growth-promoting effect at low concentrations (10 n*M* to 10 μ*M*) and estrogen-receptor–independent antiproliferative activity at concentrations of >15 μ*M*. The investigators concluded that glabridin and its derivatives exhibited varying degrees of estrogen-receptor agonism in different tests and demonstrated growth-inhibitory actions on breast cancer cells.

32.7.2.5 Curcuma longa

It has been proven that this herb has antibacterial, anticancerous, antihemorrhagic, and anti-inflammatory properties and hence can be effective in menstrual difficulties like menorrhagia or abnormal uterine bleeding, vaginitis, and leukorrhea. Laboratory research has shown that it may modulate estrogen and progesteron activity.[39]

32.7.2.6 Nardostachys jatamansi (Jatamansi)

The clinical trials showed reduced restlessness, insomnia, and aggressiveness. These properties are very useful in menopause as well as in PMS.

A study was proposed to evaluate the protective effect of *Nardostachys jatamansi* on neurobehavioral activities, thiobarbituric acid reactive substance, reduced glutathione, thiol group, and catalase and sodium-potassium adenosine triphosphatase activities in the middle cerebral artery (MCA) occlusion model of acute cerebral ischemia in rats. Findings showed that the changes induced by ischemia were significantly attenuated by a 15-day pretreatment of *N. jatamansi* (250 mg/kg orally) and correlated well with histopathology by decreasing the neuronal cell death after MCA occlusion and reperfusion. The study provided first evidence of effectiveness of *N. jatamansi* in focal ischemia probably by virtue of its antioxidant property.[40]

32.7.2.7 Zingiber officinale (Ginger)

Ginger was found effective in the symptoms such as nausea and vomiting in pregnant women. In a randomized, placebo-controlled, double-blind trial (n = 70),[41] women received either oral ginger 1 g/day or an identical placebo for 4 days. At a follow-up visit 7 days later, all participants except three in the placebo group remained in the study. After the therapy, nausea decreased significantly in the ginger group (2.1 ± 1.9) compared with the placebo group (0.9 ± 2.2, p = .014). The number of vomiting episodes also decreased significantly in the ginger group (1.4 ± 1.3) compared with the placebo group (0.3 ± 1.1, $p < 0.001$). No adverse effect of ginger on pregnancy outcome was detected. It can also be used in PMS symptoms such as nausea and vomiting.

32.7.2.8 *Commiphora mukul (Myrrh)*

In laboratory research, *Commiphora mukul* showed antibacterial and antifungal properties, especially in *Candida albicans*. Therefore, it can be used in vaginitis and related leukorrhea.[42]

In a study on the species *Commiphora guidotti*, known as scented myrrh, all sesquiterpenes were isolated and characeterized. Seven compounds, with cadinane, guaiane, oplopane, and eudesmane skeletons, were obtained. Two of seven are new and two are reported from a natural source for the first time. The present study was planned to compare the effects of the minor sesquiterpenes with those of the previously isolated major component, T-cadinol, which has shown to possess smooth muscle-relaxing properties. The results showed that the minor sesquiterpenes are more efficient in reducing K(+)-induced contractions than those induced by the alpha-adrenoceptor agonist phenylephrine. However, they were all less potent than T-cadinol in their action.[43]

In another study, Kimura et al.[44] reported that myrrhanol A, a new triterpene isolated from *Balsamodendron* or *C. mukul* Hook-gum resin, showed a potent anti-inflammatory effect on exudative pouch fluid, angiogenesis, and granuloma weights in the adjuvant-induced air-pouch granuloma of mice. The interesting finding of this study is that its effects were more marked than those of hydrocortisone and the 50% aqueous methanolic extract of the crude drug.

32.7.2.9 *Withania somnifera*

Withania somnifera is found effective in combination with other rejuvenating drugs like licorice in menopausal syndrome in studies conducted by National Institute of Ayurveda, Jaipur, India. It increases levels of estrogen and helps reduce the symptoms like hot flashes, fatigue, and depression because of its antioxidant.[45,46] It also has immunomodulatory,[47] antidepressant,[48] anti-inflammatory, and adaptogenic effects.[49,50] Information on the studies on these effects are available in other chapters.

32.7.2.10 *Tinospora cordifolia*

The active principles of *Tinospora cordifolia*, cordioside (TC-2), cordiofolioside A (TC-5), and cordiol (TC-7) are found to possess the macrophage activation. Syringin (TC-4) and TC-7 inhibited the *in vitro* immunohaemolysis of antibody-coated sheep erythrocytes by guinea pig serum. The anticomplementary and immunomodulatory activities were found to be caused by inhibition of the C3-convertase of the classical complement pathway. Higher concentrations showed constant inhibitory effects. The authors reported that the compounds also gave rise to significant increases in immunoglobin-G (IgG) antibodies in serum. Humoral and cell-mediated immunity were also enhanced but were dose dependant.[51]

In another study,[52] *T. cordifolia* extract (100 mg/kg body weight for 15 days) given to CCl4 intoxicated rats was found to protect the liver, as indicated by enzyme level in serum. A significant reduction in serum levels of serum glutamic oxaloacetic transaminase (SGOT), serum glutamate pyruvate transaminase (SGPT), alkaline phosphatase (ALP), and bilirubin were observed after *T. cordifolia* treatment during CCl4 intoxication. The extract also deleted the immunosuppressive effect of CCl4.

32.7.2.11 *Asparagus recemosus*

Asparagus recemosus was tried in menopausal syndrome for relieving symptoms like hot flashes, excessive sweating, tiredness, and sleep disturbances in a study conducted by

Government Ayurveda College, Trivandrum, India. The report reads that the treatment was effective. No further details were available about the author, dosage, and or duration.

In another study,[50, 53–55] *A. recemosus, T. cordifolia, W. somnifera,* and *Picrorhiza kurrooa* were tested on the functions of macrophages obtained from mice treated with the carcinogen ochratoxin A (OTA). At the end of 17 weeks of treatment, the chemotactic activity of murine macrophages was significantly decreased with OTA compared with controls. Production of interleukin-1 (IL-1) and tumor necrosis factor (TNF) was also markedly reduced. OTA-induced suppression of chemotactic activity and production of IL-1 and TNF-alpha by macrophages was significantly inhibited with the treatment with *A. racemosus, T. cordifolia, W. somnifera,* and *P. kurroa.* It was also noted that *W. somnifera* treated macrophage chemotaxis and *A. recemosus*-induced excess production of TNF-alpha when compared with controls.

Mandal et al.[56] studied the antibacterial activity of *A. racemosus* and compared it with chloramphenicol. The methanol extract of the roots of *A. recemosus* were given in concentrations of 50, 100, and 150 μg/ml. Results showed considerable *in vitro* antibacterial efficacy against *Escherichia coli, Shigella dysenteriae, Shigella sonnei, Shigella flexneri, Vibrio cholerae, Salmonella typhi, Salmonella typhimurium, Pseudomonas putida, Bacillus subtilis,* and *Staphylococcus aureus.*

Antioxytocic action of saponin isolated from *A. recemosus* on uterine muscle was further studied.[57] The details of this study could not be accessed. Similar studies[58,59] on the lactogoggue effect of *Asparagus recemosus* showed positive effects, but details were not available.

References

1. Carlson, K.J. and Ziporyn Terra, E.S., *Harvard Guide to Women's Health,* Harvard University Press, Cambridge, 1996.
2. Kjerulff, K.H., Erickson, B.A., et al. Chronic gynecological conditions reported by US women: findings from the National Health Interview Survey, 1984 to 1992, *Am. J. Public Health,* 86(2), 195-199, 1996.
3. Nayak, B., Ed., *Menarche to Menopause,* Ayurmedline, Banglore, India, 2002.
4. Martin, M.C., Infertility, in *Current Obstetrics & Gynecologic Diagnosis & Treatment,* 8th ed., Decherney, A.H. and Permoll, M.L., Eds., Appleton & Lange, Norwalk, CT, 1994, pp. 996–1006.
5. Rannestad, T., Eikeland, O.J., Helland, H., and Qvarnstrom, U., Quality of life, pain, and psychological well-being in women suffering from gynecological disorders, *J. Womens Health Gender-Based Med.,* 9(8), 897–903, 2000.
6. Agadjanian, V., Women's choice between indigenous and Western contraception in urban Mozambique, *Women Health,* 28(2), 1–17, 1998.
7. Bhishagratna, K.L., Ed., *Sushrut Samhita,* Chaukhambha Orientalia, Varanasi, India, 1981.
8. Sharma, P., Ed., *Charaka Samhita,* 1st ed., Vol. 2., Chaukhambha Orientalia, Varanasi, India, 1983.
9. Neldner, K.H., Complementary and alternative medicine, *Dermatol. Clin.,* 1, 189–193, 2000.
10. Mishra, S.S., Management of gynecological problems, in *Menarche to Menopause,* Nayak, B., Ed., Ayurmedline, Banglore, India, 2002.
11. Vartak, D., *Dosha-Dhatu-Mala Vignyan,* The Pragnya Press, Maharashtra, India, 1962.
12. Frawley, D., *Ayurvedic Healing a Comprehensive Guide,* Motilal Banarasidas Publishers Pvt. Ltd., Delhi, India, 1992.
13. Tripathi, A., Ed., Uttara vasti: uterine and utero-vesicle enema, in *Menarche to Menopause,* Nayak, B., Ed., Ayurmedline, Banglore, India, 2002.
14. Bhavamishra, A., *Bhavaprakash Nighantu,* Chaukhambha Bharati Academy, Varanasi, India, 1984.

15. Decherney, A.H. and Permoll, M.L., *Current Obstetrics & Gynecologic Diagnosis & Treatment*, 8th ed., Appleton & Lange, Norwalk, CT, 1994.
16. Tamir, S., Eizenberg, M., Somjen, D., et al., Estrogenic and antiproliferative properties of glabridin from licorice in human breast cancer cells, *Cancer Res.*, 60(20), 5704–5709, 2000.
17. Anon., Effect of Takradhara in Menorrhagia, *Ayurveda Update,* 1, 6–8, 1998.
18. Syamalakumari, S. et al., Effect of Kashmarya kutaja ghrita in Menorrhagia, thesis, Government Ayurveda College, Trivandrum, India, 1992.
19. Anon., Effect of Ashokarishta and Musalikhadiradi Kwatha in Menorrhagia, M.D. thesis, Government Ayurveda College, Trivandrum, India, 2002.
20. Anon., Effect of Kutajashtaka lehyam in DUB and Menorrhagia, M.D. thesis, Government Ayurveda College, Trivandrum, India, 2002.
21. Venugopal, S., Role of *Saraca indica, Aloe vera* and Cyperus rotundus in oligomenorrhea, *Antiseptic,* 95, 329–330, 1998.
22. Kulkarni, K.S., Menopause and its management modalities, in *Menarche to Menopause,* Nayak, B., Ed., Ayurmedline, Banglore, India, 2002.
23. Novaes, C., Almeida, O.P., et al., Mental health among perimenopausal women attending a menopause clinic: possible association with premenstrual syndrome?, *Climacteric,* 1(4), 264–270, 1998.
24. Rajalakshmi, S.V.G., Clinical evaluation of Kungila Barpam and Kadukkai decoction in the management of Vellai Noi (leukorrhea), *J. Res. Ayurveda Siddha,* 17, 157–161, 1996.
25. Masilamani, G. and Subbulakshmi, A.A., Clinical study of vellainoi (leukorrhea). V, *J. Res. Ayurveda Siddha,* 16, 125–133, 1996.
26. Geeta, A. and Nalini, A.M., Treatment of pradara with ashokarishta. VI, *J. Res. Ayurveda Siddha,* 16, 177–180, 1996.
27. Satyavati, G.V., Prasad, D.N., Sen, S.P., and Das, P.K., Oxytocic activity of a pure phenolic glycoside (P2) from *Saraca indica* Linn (ashoka): a short communication, *Indian J. Med. Res.,* 58(5), 660–663, 1970.
28. Satyavati, G.V., Prasad, D.N., Sen, S.P., and Das, P.K., Further studies on the uterine activity of *Saraca indica* Linn., *Indian J. Med. Res.,* 58(7), 947–960, 1970.
29. Ghosh, S., Majumder, M., Majumder, S., Ganguly, N.K., and Chatterjee, B.P., Saracin: a lectin from *Saraca indica* seed integument induces apoptosis in human T-lymphocytes, *Arch. Biochem. Biophys.,* 371(2), 163–168, 15 1999.
30. Rojas, L., Matamoros, M., Garrido, N., and Finlay, C., The action of an aqueous extract of Aloe barbadensis Miller in an in-vitro culture of Trichomonas vaginalis, *Rev. Cubana Med. Trop.,* 47(3), 181–184, 1995.
31. Egger, S.F., Brown, G.S., Kelsey, L.S., Yates, K.M., Rosenberg, L.J., and Talmadge, J.E., Hematopoietic augmentation by a beta-(1,4)-linked mannan, *Cancer Immunol. Immunother.,* 43(4), 195–205, 1996.
32. Fahim, M.S. and Wang, M., Zinc acetate and lyophilized aloe barbadensis as vaginal contraceptive. *Contraception,* 53(4), 231–236, 1996.
33. Telefo, P.B., Moundipa, P.F., Tchana, A.N., Tchouanguep Dzickotze, C., and Mbiapo, F.T., Effects of an aqueous extract of Aloe buettneri, Justicia insularis, Hibiscus macranthus, Dicliptera verticillata on some physiological and biochemical parameters of reproduction in immature female rats, *J. Ethnopharmacol.,* 63(3), 193–200, 1998.
34. Telefo, P.B., Moundipa, P.F., and Tchouanguep, F.M., Oestrogenicity and effect on hepatic metabolism of the aqueous extract of the leaf mixture of Aloe buettneri, Dicliptera verticillata, Hibiscus macranthus and Justicia insularis, *Fitoterapia,* 73(6), 472–478, 2002.
35. Vazquez, B., Avila, G., Segura, D., and Escalante, B., Antiinflammatory activity of extracts from *Aloe vera* gel, *J. Ethnopharmacol.,* 55(1), 69–75, 1996.
36. Chauhan, O., Godhwani, J.L., Khanna, N.K., and Pendse, V.K., Antiinflammatory activity of *muktashukti bhasma, Indian J. Exp. Biol.,* 36(10), 985-989, 1998.
37. Mori, H., Niwa, K., Zheng, Q., Yamada, Y., Sakata, K., and Yoshimi, N., Cell proliferation in cancer prevention; effects of preventive agents on estrogen-related endometrial carcinogenesis model and on an *in vitro* model in human colorectal cells, *Mutat. Res.,* 480–481, 201–207, 2001.

38. Niwa, K., Hashimoto, M., Morishita, S., Yokoyama, Y., Mori, H., and Tamaya, T., Preventive effects of Glycyrrhizae radix extract on estrogen-related endometrial carcinogenesis in mice, *Jpn. J. Cancer Res.*, 90(7), 726–732, 1999.
39. Garg, S.K., Effect of *Curcuma longa* (rhizomes) on fertility in experimental animals, *Planta Med.*, 26(3), 225–227, 1974.
40. Salim, S., Ahmad, M., Zafar, K.S., Ahmad, A.S., and Islam, F., Protective effect of *Nardostachys jatamansi* in rat cerebral ischemia, *Pharmacol. Biochem. Behav.*, 74(2), 481–486, 2003.
41. Vutyavanich, T., Kraisarin, T., and Ruangsri, R., Ginger for nausea and vomiting in pregnancy: randomized, double-masked, placebo-controlled trial, *Obstet. Gynecol.*, 97(4), 577–582, 2001.
42. Dolara, P., Corte, B., Ghelardini, C., et al., Local anaesthetic, antibacterial and antifungal properties of sesquiterpenes from myrrh, *Planta Med.*, 66(4), 356–358, 2000.
43. Andersson, M., Bergendorff, O., Shan, R., Zygmunt, P., and Sterner, O., Minor components with smooth muscle relaxing properties from scented myrrh (Commiphora guidotti), *Planta Med.*, 63(3), 251–254, 1997.
44. Kimura, I., Yoshikawa, M., Kobayashi, S., et al., New triterpenes, myrrhanol A and myrrhanone A, from guggul-gum resins, and their potent anti-inflammatory effect on adjuvant-induced air-pouch granuloma of mice, *Bioorg. Med. Chem. Lett.*, 11(8), 985–989, 2001.
45. Archana, R. and Namasivayam, A., Antistressor effect of *Withania somnifera*, *J. Ethnopharmacol.*, 64(1), 91–93, 1999.
46. Scartezzini, P. and Speroni, E., Review on some plants of Indian traditional medicine with antioxidant activity, *J. Ethnopharmacol.*, 71(1–2), 23-43, 2000.
47. Davis, L. and Kuttan, G., Immunomodulatory activity of *Withania somnifera*, *J. Ethnopharmacol.*, 71(1–2), 193–200, 2000.
48. Battacharya, S.K., Attacharya, B.A., Sairam, K., and Ghosal, S., Anxiolytic-antidepressant activity of *Withania somnifera* glycowithanolides: an experimental study, *Phytomedicine*, No. 7, 463–469, 2000.
49. Mishra, L.C., Singh, B.B., and Dagenais, S., Scientific basis for the therapeutic use of *Withania somnifera* (ashwagandha): a review, *Altern. Med. Rev.*, 5(4), 334–346, 2000.
50. Dhuley, J.N., Adaptogenic and cardioprotective action of ashwagandha in rats and frogs, *J. Ethnopharmacol.*, 70(1), 57–63, 2000.
51. Kapil, A. and Sharma, S., Immunopotentiating compounds from *Tinospora cordifolia*, *J. Ethnopharmacol.*, 58(2), 89–95, 1997.
52. Bishayi, B., Roychowdhury, S., Ghosh, S., and Sengupta, M., Hepatoprotective and immunomodulatory proprties of *Tinospora cordifolia* in CCl4 intoxicated mature albino rats, *J. Toxicol. Sci.*, 27(3), 139–146, 2002.
53. Dhuley, J.N., Effect of some Indian herbs on macrophage functions in ochratoxin A treated mice, *J. Ethnopharmacol.*, 58(1), 15–20, 1997.
54. Dhuley, J.N., Effect of ashwagandha on lipid peroxidation in stress-induced animals, *J. Ethnopharmacol.*, 60(2), 173–178, 1998.
55. Dhuley, J.N., Nootropic-like effect of ashwagandha (*Withania somnifera* L.) in mice, *Phytotherapy Res.*, 15(6), 524–528, 2001.
56. Mandal, S.C., Nandy, A., Pal, M., and Saha, B.P., Evaluation of antibacterial activity of Asparagus racemosus willd. root, *Phytotherapy Res.*, 14(2), 118–119, 2000.
57. Gaitonde, B.B. and Jetmalani, M.H., Antioxytocic action of saponin isolated from Asparagus racemosus Willd (Shatavari) on uterine muscle, *Arch. Int. Pharmacodyn. Ther.*, 179(1), 121–129, 1969.
58. Joglekar, G.V., Ahuja, R.H., and Balwani, J.H., Galactogogue effect of Asparagus racemosus, Preliminary communication, *Indian Med. J.*, 61(7), 165, 1967.
59. Sharma, S., Ramji, S., Kumari, S., and Bapna, J.S., Randomized controlled trial of Asparagus racemosus (shatavari) as a lactogogue in lactational inadequacy, *Indian Pediatr.*, 33(8), 675–677, 1996.

Appendix 1:

Ayurvedic Words and Their English Meanings

Abhyanga oil massage
Adhimamsa fleshy growth
Adhimamsarma pterygium
Adhimantha glaucoma
Adhisthana site
Adhoga Amlapitta regurgitation through the rectum
Adhyarbuda recurrence of tumor
Adhyasana frequent eating
Agantuka exogenous factors
Agni fire, digestive juice, hormones
Agnikarma heat therapy
Ahara diet
Ahara rasa absorbed digested nutrients
Ahara Rasayana herbal dietary supplement
Ahara sakti digestive power
Aheerata eagerness, anxiety
Ahigata injury
Ahishyanda conjunctivitis
Ahita incompatible
Ajakajat prolapse of the iris
Ajasrik Rasayana dietary supplement to keep the process of new tissue formation
Ajirna indigestion
Akrti general appearance
Akshepaka spasm/convulsion
Akshipakatyaya panophthalmitis
Alochaka pitta pitta located in the retina responsible for eyesight
Ama-Atisara enterotoxic diarrhea
Ama dosa undigested food and other materials
Amaja anaha a variety of constipation due to undigested materials
Amasaya stomach
Amavata rheumatoid arthritis
Amla sour
Amladhyashita subacute glaucoma
Amlapitta hyperacidity
Amritikarana the process of heating the product in presence of some herbal drugs
Amruthaprasa rasayanam a preparation of herbal drugs in concentrated jaggary syrup
Anaha bloated abdomen due to the accumulation of stool
Anguli fingers

Anjan ophthlmic preparation to be applied or rubbed gently on the conjunctiva
Anna food
Antarvyavartana entropion
Antuja unmada psychosis due to exterior origin
Anubandh binding
Anubandhya principal
Anuvanshaja hereditary
Anuvasan a kind of enema
Anuvasan vasti enema with medicated oils
Anuvsana basti oil enema
Anyasthaniyakshaya body-weight loss
Anyatovata supraorbit neuralgaia
Apachi glandular swelling
Apana vata responsible for the excretion of urine and feces
Aparipakvasana eating improperly cooked food
Apasmaara epilepsy
Apatarparna fat reducing
Apathya harmful food
Apathyaja acquired due to unhealthy lifestyle
Apaya loss, going away, destruction of
Arbud carcinomas
Arbuda neoplasm; fibroid
Arista preparation obtained by fermentation
Arjun subconjunctival hemorrhage
Arshas hemorrhoids
Artava ovum/menses
Artavajanana ovulation inducing
Aruchi anorexia
Aruhyakam general well-being
Asadhya incurable
Asadhya vrana incurable ulcers
Asathmya bhojana hypersensitive or incompatible food items
Ashchyotana eyedrop
Ashmari urolithiasis, urinary calculi
Astavidha pariksa eight-point examination
Asthapana basti herbal decoction enema
Asthayi transient lipids
Asthi bones
Asthipatal/drishtipatal retina
Ati sthulya obesity and morbid obesity
Atisara diarrhea
Atma spirit
Aushadhi medicine
Avagalana or utplavana subluxation of lens
Avapeedna instillation of nasal drops
Avara weak
Avipaka acid indigestion
Avrana Shukla corneal opacities
Awaleha sugar-based semisolid preparation
Ayana path/channel
Ayu-kshaya decrease in life span

Ayurveda knowledge of life; Vedic health science
Bala strength
Bala thailam medicine prepared in oil for improving strength
Baluka sveda sand fomentation
Basti medicated enema
Beejadosha genetic disorder
Beeja poshana treatise to better the quality and quantity of semen
Bhaishajya kalpana formulation of a dosage form
Bhasma literally ash; incinerated metal or minerals
Bhauma earth
Bhavana drava trifala decoction
Bheda histopathological differentiation
Bhedan and lekhan incise and drainage
Bhedana penetrating
Bhutavidya science of evil spirit
Bhutonmada *grahavesa* (sychosis)
Brimhan repletion of the body tissue
Buddhi intellect
Buddhimandya mentally retarded
Cetana consciousness
Chakrikas small cakes
Chikitsa therapy
Chinabandha bandage of eye
Churna powder
Daiva spiritual
Daivavyapasraya cikitsa spiritual treatment
Darun vicar serious diseases
Dashavidha pariksha ten methods of examination
Dashmool roots of ten herbs
Deergham ayu long life
Deva vyapashraya chikitsa devine therapy
Dhamani nerve supply to artieries
Dhamapana insufflation
Dhara steady flow of liquids
Dhasamoola Rishtam hot-water extract of roots of the ten herbal medicines that is fermented
Dhatu tissues
Dhatukshaya degeneration of essential constituents
Dhatupak janya vikriti a disease caused by a defective metabolism leading to derangement in body-tissue (seven dhatus) transformation process
Dhatus tissues; there are seven *dhathus*: *rasa* (ingested food), *raktha* (blood), *mamsa* (muscles), *medas* (fat), *asthi* (bone), *majja* (bone marrow), and *shuklam* (semen); *rasa* is converted to *raktha* and so on until it is finally converted into *shuklam*
Dhatuvahasrotas place of conversion of tissues
Dhatu-vriddhi tissue growth
Dhatwagni deranged metabolism
Dhatwagni chikitsa correction of metabolic defects
Dhoomra medicated smoking
Dhuma nasya smoke inhalation
Dhumapana medicated smoking
Dhwaja bhangam erectile dysfunction

Dipana materials that stimulate digestive juices
Divavyapashraya spiritual interventions
Divyausadhi divine medicinal plants
Dola yantra, khalva yantra, musha yantra instruments used in preparation of *bhasmas*
Dooshti vitiation
Dooshyas tissues that are the site of a disease
Dosa biomaterials, bioenergy, bodily humor
Dosasushti vitiation of *dosa*
Dravaka liquefacients
Dravya Rasayana therapy with dietary supplements
Drishtimani lens
Dushtavrana infected ulcer
Dushya that which can get vitiated like tissues
Dushyas culpable
Dwirarbuda metastasis of tumor
Ekadesavriddhi enlargement of particular tissue
Gairika red chalk
Gala throat
Galaganda goiter
Garbhini pregnant women
Ghee, Ghrita, or Ghruta dehydrated butter
Ghritika buttermilk
Gomutra cow urine
Grahani irritable colon
Grahan restrained movement
Grahas planets
Grahavesa influence of planets
Granthi minor neoplasm
Gridhra eagle
Gridhrasi sciatica
Gudabhramsa rectal prolapse
Gulma intra-abdominal swellings
Guna attribute or respect
Gunas-sattva, raja, tama three qualities of mind, mental constitution
Halimaka fulminant hepatic failure
Haridra meha yellowish urine (like turmeric)
Hasti meha urine similar to an elephant in rut
Hima cold infusion
Hingula cinnabar
Hrdaya heart
Hritkantha Daha burning sensation rising up from the stomach or lower chest toward the neck
Iksu meha urine similar to sugarcane juice and very sweet
Indriyartha sensorial
Ingalekam cinnabar
Jangama ausadhis prepared from animal products
Jangha thigh
Janu knee
Jara-janya manasa vikara psychiatric problems of the aged
Jatharagni digestive fire
Jeevaneya ganam group of herbs to increase the vigor and vitality

Jeevaneya ghrutham ghee-based medicine used to prolong life
Jihva tongue
Jvara-Atisara infective diarrhea
Kajjali amalgum of sulfur and mercury
Kala time, rhythm
Kalaka choroid
Kala meha black urine
Kalka crushed plant material
Kalyanakam ghrutham a preparation in liquefied butter used for treating oligospermia
Kalyanakam kashayam water extract of certain herbs indicated for oligospermia
Kamala hepatitis
Kamsya bell, metal
Kamya Rasayana rasayana given with certain special aim
Kandaras tendons
Kandu itching
Kanji rice gruel
Kapha biological material, water humor, mucus, *dosa*
Kapha and raktavaha srotasa lymphatic and circulatory system
Kaphadhara Kala mucous lining of the stomach
Kapha dosa mucus and mucoid, interlinking functions and constituents of the body
Kapha Grahani dysentery predominant
Kaphahara/Kaphashamaka measures or drugs that pacify *kapha*
Kaphaja granthi or arbuda adenoma
Kaphaja Linganasha mature cataract
Kaphaj linganash mature cataract
Karma action
Karna ear
Karnika cornea
Karshan the depletion of body tissues
Kasa cough
Kashay rasa astringent
Kashaya/kwatha decoction
Kastha ausadhi herbal preparation
Kati low back
Katu pungent
Katu vipak bitter
Kavalika dressing
Kaya chikitsa medicine
Khalva stone mortar
Khanja monoplegia
Khara hard
Klaibyam impotence
Klama fatigue
Kleda waste products of adipose tissues
Kledaka one of the five types of *kapha dosa*
Klinnavartma blephritis
Kosta intestine
Kostashakhasrita kamala hemolytic jaundice
Kotham necrosis
Kricchravitka, alpavitka passing small quantity of stool
Krimi helminthiasis including microbial infection

Krimijanya due to worms
Krishnapatal iris
Krura koshtha extremely harsh bowel
Ksara meha the urine is like a solution of alkali in smell, color, and taste
Kshara alkali
Ksharakarma application of caustics
Kshaudrameha excessive urine with sweet taste like honey
Kshayaja due to emaciation
Ksheernartava amenorrhea
Ksudraka svasa asthma
Kukunder oscoccygis bone
Kumba kamala hepatic failure
Kupipakwa vidhi procedure used for preparing mercury *bhasma*
Kushta bhasma-like preparation of *Unani-tibb*
Kutipraveshika patient/concerned specialized living in a hut
Kwatha decoction
Laala meha the urine is slimy and contains threads like that of saliva
Lagan chalazion
Laghu lightweight, small
Lakshanika chikitsa symptomatic treatment
Langhana depletion or reducing therapy, no food intake
Lavan salty
Leen lens falling back into vitreous chamber
Lehyam medicinal preparation in jaggary syrup
Lekhan scraping
Lekhana scraping
Lepa ointment
Lepana application of medicated paste
Linga symbol of male organ
Linganasha dosha liquified lenticular material
Lingarsha genital growths, genital wart
Lingavridhikara yoga drugs used for enlargement of penis
Loha iron
Loka-purusa samya balance with universe
Maans muscle
Maans lolup greedy to flesh
Madhumeha diabetes
Madhur sweet
Madhyama middle path or medium
Madhyama koshtha moderate bowel
Mahamarma very important vital organ
Maharasa main metals, also used for mercury
Mahasrotas gastrointestinal tract
Majja bone marrow
Majja meha the urine looks like marrow
Mala excretion, stool
Mamsa muscle, soft tissue
Mamsarbuda neoplasm of soft tissue
Mamsashrit Patal fleshy part or choroid
Manas mind
Manasika psychological factors

Manas Rasayana rasayana for the improvement of intellect
Manassila arsenic
Manayah gems
Mandal orbits
Mandbudhi low intelligence
Manjistha meha foul-smelling urine that is slightly red
Manodaihika vyadhis psychosomatic diseases
Manovaha srtoas psychological channels
Mansa dhatwagni digestive power in the muscle tissues
Marana the process of burning or calcination
Margavaran obstruction of passage
Marma vital part
Marma ghat vital's trauma
Matruj avayava maternal organ ovum
Meda fat
Medadhatu adipose tissue
Medaja originated from fatty tissue
Medas patal choroid
Medhaja granthi or arbuda lipoma lipid tumor or lipoma
Medhya intellect
Medhya Rasayana brain tonics
Medodhatwagni fat-specific energy
Medomay steostasis
Medoposhakansh nutritive food, fatty food
Medoroga disease of the fat tissue
Meha immunity
Mithyaaharavihara unwholesome diet and regimen
Mool root
Mrudu koshtha extremely weak bowel
Mukha oral cavity
Mula sthana center of origin
Mulika root
Murccha, Moha, Tamaka loss of consciousness, fainting
Mutra urine
Nadi pulse
Nadi svedan steam fomentation by tube
Nadipariksa pulse examination
Naimittic Rasayana rasayana is given only for partial period for certain number of days
Naishthiki chikitsa spiritual therapy
Nakulandhyatva retinoblastoma
Nanatmaj vadhis many kinds of *vataj* diseases
Napumsaka eunuch
Narasimha rasayanam a formula to delay the aging process
Nasa nose
Nash destruction
Nashtartava menopause
Nasya nasal drops
Nasya karma errhines therapy
Nasya karma nasal infiltration
Navana nasya inunction errhine
Netra eyes

Nidan diagnosis
Nidana pancake five methods of diagnosis
Nidana purvarupa immediate signs, premonitory symptoms
Nija endogenous factors
Nila meha bluish urine
Nirama stool without enterotoxin
Niruha vasti medicated enema with decoction
Nirutthalvarttara end product of *nirutthikarana*
Nirutthikarana filtration/separation
Ojakashaya immunity
Ojas the final product of all seven *dhathus*
Ojas meha urine that looks like honey
Onychomycosis ringworm of the nails
Pachaka Pitta digestive enzymes
Pachana digestant
Pakshma heat therapy
Pakshmakopa trichiasis, blephritis
Pakvasaya lower part of gastrointestinal tract
Palashmakopa entropion
Panaki hepatorenal syndrome
Pancamahabhuta five basic elements
Pancendriya pariksa examination of the five sense organs
Panchakarma five cleansing procedures (*vaman, virechan, siro-virechan, anuvasan,* and *nirooha vastis*)
Pandu anemia
Pangu paraplegia
Parada, rasa, suta, maharasa, rasendra various names for mercury
Paratantra kamala obstructive jaundice
Parinama Sula ulcerative dyspepsia, duodenal ulcer
Parooshakadi ganam group of herbs starting with *Phoenix pusilla*
Parpams term for *bhasmas* used in Siddha medicine system
Parpati, rasayoga mercury preparations
Parthive substances derived from earth
Pashchat karma postoperative procedures
Patal coats
Patana yantra a pot pertaing to an apparatus used for sublimation or distillation for preparing *bhasma*
Patra pind sveda poultice
Phalasarpis preparation in liquefied butter, mainly used for women to increase fertility
Phalavarti, snehavarti anal suppositories
Phanita hot infusion
Pichu cotton plug
Pipali *Piper longum*
Pishti triturated drug with specified liquids prepared by exposing to sun or moon
Pista meha urine that is white and thick; similar to a solution of corn flour
Pitta biological fire, metabolic catabolic enzymes
Pitta dosa the functions of tissue interchange and conversion
Pittaja originated from *pitta*
Pittala brass
Pittashaya gall bladder
Pittaviridhi serum bilirubin

Poorvakarma preoperative procedures
Pooyastrava panopthalmitis, hypopion ulcer
Pothaki trachoma
Prabhava unique action
Pradhana dhatu primary metal
Pradhana karma main cleansing procedures
Prakopa transformation of growth into metastatic tumors
Prakriti constitution
Prakritisthapani chikitsa restorative treatment
Pralepa application of thin medicament paste in the affected part
Pramana build, size
Pramana vijnana anthropometry
Pramehas urinary disorders
Pramoha impairment in functioning of mind
Prana respiration
Pranavaha srotas respiration
Pranyama breathing exercises
Prasara metastasis
Prasna pariksa interrogation
Prasrutha measure/equivalent of one handful
Prastari Arma pterygium
Prasuti delivery
Pratimarsha topical application
Pravahika dysentery
Pravala shells
Pravara type of body constitution
Prayoga experiment
Purishaja anaha variety of constipation due to stool accumulation
Purishasanga, purishanaha accumulation of feces
Purva karma preparatory procedures
Purvarupa prodromal signs/symptoms
Pushta overweight
Putapaka heating with cow dung cakes
Puttam cow dung cake or made pits with cow dung cakes
Puyalasak dacryocystitis
Raja menstrual blood
Rajas prakriti authoritarian mental constitution
Rajata silver
Rajayakshma tuberculosis
Rajonivritti menopause
Rakta blood
Raktaarbudanasna anticancer drug
Rakta-Atisara hemorrhagic diarrhea
Rakta meha blood red
Raktamokshana bloodletting
Rakta-pradara menorrhagia
Raktarbuda tumors that exudate blood
Raktashodhaka blood purifier
Raktasrava profuse hemorrhage
Raktavaha srotas circulatory system
Rakthasthambhaka styptics

Ranjaka pitta type of biliary fluid
Ras blood
Rasa absorbed food nutrients, mercury preparations
Rasa ausadhi metallic preparation
Rasa dhatu plasma tissue
Rasa karpur mercuric subchloride
Rasalinga symbol of power
Rasashala laboratory of an alchemist
Rasashastra Ayurvedic pharmacy of mercury preparations, metallurgy
Rasavadins alchemists
Rasayana Ayurvedic drug preparation to increase the life span
Rasvidya Indian alchemy
Ratna gems
Rihti pupil
Roga disease
Roganashani chikitsa curative therapy
Rogibala ability to defend against diseases
Rog pariksha clinical examination
Rog viakhya clinical description
Rohini sixth layer of skin, similar to epithelium
Ropana healing
Ruk pain
Ruksha dry
Rupa clinical manifestation
Sabda voice
Sadanga pariksa six-point examination
Sadhya curable
Sadhyasadhyata prognosis
Sahaja genetic
Sahaya dhatu secondary metal
Sama stool with enterotoxin
Samana balanced
Samana vata vata that stimulates the digestive enzymes
Saman vikruti decreased hepatic conjugation
Samanya shodhana general purification
Samasanhanan nara proportionate body
Samhanana body structure
Samhita text
Samprapti pathogenesis
Samshodhana purification procedures
Samshodhana chikitsa detoxification therapy
Samskara process
Samudra-sauviram mercuric perchloride
Samyak vedhan proper pricking
Sanair meha urine passes very slowly
Sanchaya localization of growth
Sandhi junctions
Sandhigat vata osteoarthritis and rheumatoid arthritis
Sandrajala vetrious humor
Sandra meha urine kept overnight
Sang biliary stasis

Santarpan restorative treatment
Sara quality of tissues
Sastra chikitsa surgical treatment
Sathavari gulam preparation of herbs made with jaggary used for female infertility
Sathavaryadi ghrutham medicine prepared in liquefied butter for female infertility
Sathya Yuga time period in history when the rule of justice prevailed and all people were happy
Satmya adaptability
Sattva pharmaceutical process, consciousness, intelligence
Sattvavajaya counseling therapy
Sattvika prakrti examination of the psyche
Satva liquid containing active ingredient
Satvavajaya chikitsa psychotherapy
Sauvarcala, saindhava, vida, audbhida types of salt
Savrana Shukla corncal ulcers with perforations
Seka fomentation
Sesa *Sesamum indicum* oil
Shakhasrita kamala intra- and extra-hepatic jaundice
Shalya tantra surgery
Shamana pacifying, palliative
Sharava mud tray
Sharira human body
Shashkakshipaka ophthalmoplegaia
Shatadhoutha Ghrita medicated ghee
Sheeta cold
Shefa penis
Shilajit asphaltum
Shiro head
Shiro vasti flow of liquid on the head
Shleshak kapha type of *kapha dosa*
Shleshma another name for kapha or phlegm
Shodana chikitsa therapy by elimination of vitiated pathogens
Shodhana detoxification
Shodhana karma measures of internal purification
Shonitarma pterygium
Shotha localized swelling/edema
Shothahara anti-inflammatory
Shrunga horn of a cow
Shuddha, sishra, pooti loha quality of iron *bhasma*
Shukadosha diseases of external genitalia caused by the use of irritants
Shuklam semen
Shuklarma pterygium
Shukra semen
Shuktika bitot's spots/xeophthalmia
Shwetapatal sclera-white of eye
Shweta-pradara mucous in the urine
Siddha dugdha medicated milk
Siddha ghruta smedicated ghee
Siddh Makardhwaja preparation containing oxide form of mercury
Sikata meha urine contains sandlike particles
Sindoora drug prepared by the process of sublimation

Sira different channels
Siraharsha scleritis
Sirajal acute orbital cellulites
Siravedha bloodletting
Sirobasti treatment of head and neck with oils
Sirotpat episcleritities
Sirstalvantargatam manah skull
Sisa, naga lead
Sita meha urine is sweet and very cold
Smriti memory
Smruti memory
Smrutim Medha good intellect, good recalling ability
Snana bath
Snayu ligament
Snehana oleation
Snehana chikitsa oleation therapy
Snehapan intake of medicated fats
Sodhana chikitsa purification therapy
Sokatisara diarrhea due to sorrow
Somana chikitsa curative therapy
Sopham swelling
Soul spirit
Spandan muscle spasm
Sparsahsnutwam tenderness
Sparsa skin/touch
Sphik gluteous
Srotamsi channels, microscopic pores
Srotas channels, pores
Srotas pariksa examination of channel
Srotorodh channel blockage
Stambha numbness
Sthana samsraya secondary growth
Sthayi stored form
Sthoulyam hugeness
Sthula obese
Streeroga gynecological disorders
Streeshareer anatomy of the female reproductive system
Stree stanya breast milk
Sukra dhatu reproductive tissue, semen
Sukra meha urine mixed with semen
Sukravahasrotas path through which semen passes
Sukshma minute, delicate
Sukumaram ghrutham a preparation of herbals in liquefied butter for the treatment of male and female infertility
Sukumaram kashayam water extract of certain herbs, used for male and female infertility
Sukumaram lehyam a preparation of herbs in concentrated jaggary syrup used to treat male and female infertility
Sura meha urine resembles wine (sura) with a clear top and cloudy at the bottom
Surya-namaskar sun-yoga-asana (body positions)
Suwarna gold
Svasa increased or difficult breathing, dyspnea

Svedana fomentation
Svedana karma sudation therapy
Swaras fresh juices
Swarna bhasma gold bhasma
Swasthavritta and ritucharya daily and seasonal health regimens
Swatantra kamala hepatocellular jaundice
Taila oil
Takra buttermilk
Talaka arsenic trisulphide
Talu palate
Tamaka svasa bronchial asthma
Tamas inertia
Tamra copper
Tandra lassitude
Tantriks practitioners of black magic
Tantu threads
Tara pupil
Taraka iris
Tarunam vayah ability to remain young
Teekshna pointed
Teevravastha acute phase
Tejojalashrit Patal outermost layer in which there exists aqueous humor
Tikshna guna severe taste
Tiksna sharp
Tikta bitter
Tikta-Amlodgara bitter and acid regurgitation
Tilapista nibha clay-colored stool
Timira refractive errors, premature cataract, or other serious causes of blindness
Toda paresthesia
Trapa tin
Tridosa three *dosas* (*vatta, pitta, and kapha*)
Trikatu three bitter herbs
Triphala group of three herbs (*Embelica officinalis, Terminalia belerica,* and *Terminalia chebula*)
Tritiya patalgat dushti disorders of the third coat
Trivanga bhasma bhasma containing lead, tin, and zinc
Twak bark
Udaka water
Udaka meha urine is clear; is in large amounts; and is white, cold, and odorless
Udara abdomen
Udaram, jalodhar, or asadhya ascites
Unmada roga psychosis
Uparasa there are eight *uparasa*: *gandhaka* (sulphur), *gairic* (ochre), *kasis* (ferrous sulphate), *sphatica* (potash alum), *hartal* (orpiment), *manashila* (realgar), *anjana* (lead), *kankustha* (rhubarb)
Upasaya-anupasay exacerbating and relieving factors
Upataraka cilliary body
Urdhvaga Amlapitta regurgitation through the mouth
Urdhwajatrugat of the upper level of the clavicle
Uru thigh
Ushna veerya dry

Ushnavata cystitis/urethritis
Uthara sthanam last volume
Utklesha hypersalivation
Utsangini chalation
Utsangini lagan chalazion
Vadanasthapana analgesics
Vaikrintaka tourmaline
Vajikarana aphrodisiac therapy
Vaman therapeutic emesis
Vamathu vomiting
Vapavahan visceral and omental fat
Vardhanana Rasayana rasayana dose is increased slowly to the highest level, maintained at that level, and then decreased slowly to the base line
Vartka a mixture of five metals
Vartma eyelids
Vasa fatty substance
Vasa meha urine looks like liquid muscle fat and may be passed frequently
Vasti Ayurvedic enema therapy; karma-enema
Vata biological humor related to nervous system
Vatadoshas represents functions of movements or propulsions
Vata grahani constipation predominant
Vataja caused by vitiated *vata*
Vataparyay supraorbital neuralgia
Vata rakta gouty arthritis
Vatatapika rasayana treatment that can be given to outdoor patients
Vata vyadhi nervous disorders
Vati, gutika, or guggulu preparations in pill form
Vaya age and aging
Vayu air, wind; another name of *vata*
Veda knowledge
Vedana severe pain
Veerya potency
Vega Dhara a controlling natural urges
Viadhi heitu etiology
Vibandha constipation
Vidaryadi kashayam water extract of some herbs to enhance body tissues repair
Vidaryadi lehyam preparation of herbs in jaggary syrup for body tissue repair
Vikriti imbalance of *dosas*
Vilekhan scraping
Vipaka postdigestive effect
Virecana karma purgation therapy
Virek purgation
Viruddha Ahara incompatible food
Viruddh asana incompatible exercise
Viryalpata impotence
Visa poison
Vishaghna detoxifier
Vishesha shodhana special purification
Vishtambha obstruction
Vismriti amnesia
Vitiated dosas toxic materials

Vrana ulcer
Vriddhipatra shastra scalpal
Vrisya aphrodisiac
Vrukkas fat around the body organs
Vyadhi disease
Vyadhi hetu etiology
Vyakti expression of symptoms
Vyayama sakti physical strength
Yakrut liver
Yakruta dhatwagni manya decreased hepatic uptake
Yakruta shotha hepatocellular damage
Yakrutodara hepatomegaly
Yakrutshosh cirrhosis
Yapya difficult to treat
Yavakshara salt of potassium and sodium
Yonidhavana vaginal douche
Yoniroga/yonivyapat vaginal diseases
Yuktivyapashraya nondrug and drug modalities
Yukti vyapashraya chikitsa rational therapy

Appendix 2:

Ayurvedic Herbs and Botanical Names

Botantical Name	Ayurvedic Name	Parts Used
Abroma angusta Linn.	*Bharadwaji*	Root
Abies pindrow Royale	*Talispatra*	Leaves
Abrus precatorius Linn.	*Gunja*	Leaf, root, seed
Abutilon indicum G. Don	*Atibala*	Entire plant
Acaia arabica Willd.	*Babbula*	Entire plant, resin
Acacia catechu Willd.	*Khadirasara*	Sara
Acacia concinna DC.	*Phenika*	Fruit
Acacia farnesiana Willd.	*Irimeda*	Bark
Acacia latiosum	*Kinkirat*	Stem, bark, fruit
Acalypha indica Linn.	*Akakiya*	Sara
Achyranthes aspera	*Apamarga*	Enitre plant
Aconitum chasmanthum	*Sringivisa*	Root
Aconitum heterphyllum Wall.	*Ativisa*	Root
Aconitum napellus Linn.	*Vatsanabha*	Root
Acorus calamus Linn.	*Vaca*	Root
Actiniopteris dichotoma	*Mayurasikha*	Entire plant
Adansonia digitatat Linn.	*Gorakha cinca*	Fruit, leaf, bark
Adenanthera pavonia Linn.		*Ravan amlika*
Adhatoda vasica Nees	*Vasa*	Complete plant
Adiantum lunulatum Burm.	*Hansaraja*	Complete plant
Aegle marmelos Corr.	*Bilwa*	Leaves, fruit, root
Agaricus campestris Linn.	*Chatraka*	Complete plant
Ailanthus excelsa Roxb.	*Aralu*	Bark, seed
Alangium salvifolium	*Ankola*	Root, bark, oil
Albizzia lebbeck Benth.	*Sirisa*	Bark, seed
Alhagi pseudalhagi	*Yavasakam*	Complete plant
Allium cepa	*Palandu*	Root (*kanda*)
Allium sativum	*Lasuna*	Root
Alocasia indica	*Manakanda*	*Kanda*
Aloe barbadensis	*Kumari*	Exudation
Alpinia galanga	*Kulinjana*	Root
Alstonia scholaris	*Saptaparna*	Bark
Alternanthera sessilis	*Matsyaksi*	Complete plant
Amomurn sublatum Roxb.	*Sthulaila, Badi Ilaichi*	Seeds
Amorphophallus campanulatus Blume.	*Surana*	*Kanda*
Amorphophallus sylvaticus	*Banya surana*	*Kanda*
Amranthus blitum	*Tanuliyaka*	Leaf, root
Amranthus spinosus Linn.	*Tanuliyaka*	Complete plant
Anacardius occidentale	*Kaju*	Seed
Anacyclus pyrethrum DC.	*Akarakarabha*	Root
Anamirta cocculus	*Kakamari*	Fruit
Andrographis paniculata Nees.	*Yavatikta, kalamegha*	Complete plant

Andropogon iwaraneusa jones	*Lamajjaka*	Root
Andropogon schoenanthus	*Rohisa trina*	Root
Anethum sowa Kurz.	*Satapuspa*	Seed, oil, arka
Annona atemoya	*Sitaphala*	Fruits
Anogeissus latifolia	*Dhava*	Bark, gum
Anisomeles malabarica	*Sprikka*	Whole plant
Anthocephalus cadamba Mig.	*Kadamba*	Bark, leaf, flower
Anthocephalus chinensis	*Kadamba*	Fruits, leaves, bark
Aquilaria agallocha	*Agar*	Wood
Aquilaria agallocha Roxb.	*Aguru*	Wood, oil
Areca catechu Linn.	*Pugaphala*	Fruit
Argemone mexicana	*Swarnaksiri*	Complete plant
Argyreia speciosa	*Briddhadaru*	Root, leaf, seed
Aristolochia bracteata	*Kitamari*	Complete plant
Aristolochia indica Linn.	*Ishwarimula*	Root
Artemisia siversiana	*Damanaka*	Complete plant
Artemisia vulgaris Linn.	*Saraparna*	Flower
Artocarpus lakoocha Roxb.	*Lakuca*	Fruit
Arundo donax	*Nala*	Whole plant
Asparagus adscendens Roxb.	*Krisna Musali*	Root
Asparagus racemosus Willd.	*Satavari*	Root
Asparagus sarmentosa Linn.	*Maha satawari*	Root
Asteracantha longifolia Nees.	*Kokilaksa, Iksuraka*	Seeds, complete plant
Averrhoa carambola	*Karmaranga*	Fruit
Azadirachta indica A. Juss	*Nimba*	Seeds, oil, resin
Balanites aegyptiaca	*Ingudi*	Fruit, oil
Balanites arundinacea Willd.	*Vamsalocana*	Whole plant
Balospermum mantanum	*Danti*	Seed, oil, root
Balsamodendron myrrha	*Bola, gandharasa*	Exudate
Bambusa arundinacea Willd.	*Vamsalocana*	
Barleria prionitis	*Saireyaka, sahacara*	Complete plant
Barringtonia acutangula	*Samudraphala*	Fruit
Bassia latifolia	*Madhuka*	Flower, seed, oil, bark
Bauhinia racemosa	*Asmantaka*	Leaf, bark
Bauhinia variegata Linn.	*Kancanar*	Bark, leaf, root
Benincasa hispida Thunb.	*Kusmanda*	Fruit, seed
Berberis aristata	*Rasanjana*	Whole plant
Bergenia ligulata	*Pashna bheda*	
Betula utilis D. Don.	*Bhojapatra*	Leaf, bark
Bixa orellana	*Sinduri*	Seeds
Blepharis edulis Pers.	*Ucata*	Seeds
Boerhaavia diffusa	*Punarnava*	Complete plant
Boerhaavia verticillata	*Vrushiva*	Complete plant
Borassus flabellifer Linn.	*Tada*	Fruit, root, seed
Boswellia serrata Roxb.	*Sallaki*	Exudate
Brassica juncea	*Rajika*	Seed, oil
Brassica nigra Koch.	*Sarsapa*	Seed, leaf, oil
Bryonopsis laciniosa	*Sivalingi*	Seed
Buchanania lanzan	*Badam*, almond	Faruit, seed
Buchanania lanzan Spr.	*Priyal*	Oil
Butea frondosa	*Palasha, dhaka*	Seed, root, leaf, flower
Butea monosperma	*Palasha, dhaka*	Seed, root, leaf, flower
C. angustifolia roxb.	*Tavaksiri*	*Kanda curna*
C. cetilissineus	*Karkatika*	Fruit, seed
C. long Linn.	*Rajani*	Rhizome
C. zedoaria rose	*Kachur*	Rhizome

Caesalpinia bonducella	*Kuberaksa*	Complete plant, seed
Caesalpinia digyna Rottler.	*Ghrita karanji*	Root
Caesalpinia sappan Linn.	*Patrang*	Wood
Cajanus indicus	*Adhaki*	Leaf, seed
Calamus rotang	*Vetra*	*Prakanda*
Calophyllum inophyllum Linn.	*Punnag*	Oil
Calotropis gigantean	*Arka*	Complete plant, *ksira*
Calotropis procera	*Arka*	Complete plant, *ksira*
Cannabis sativa Linn.	*Bhanga*	Leaves, *manjari, kandastha*
Canscora decussata	*Sankh holi*	Whole plant
Capparis aphylla	*Karira*	Fruit, flower, root
Capparis horrida	*Kinkini*	Fruit
Capparis sepiaria	*Himsra*	Fruits, flowers, root
Capparis zeylanica	*Vyaghranakhi*	Root
Capsicum annum	*Katuvira*	Fruit, seeds
Capsicum frutescens	*Toksna*	Fruits, seed
Careya arborea	*Kumbhi*	Fruit, bark
Carica papaya Linn.	*Madhu karkati*	Fruit, seed, leaf
Carissa carandas	*Karamarda*	Fruit
Carum ajamoda	*Ajamoda*	Seed, fruit
Carum carvi	*Krishn jiraka*	Seeds
Carum copticum	*Yavani, ajowan*	Fruits, leaves, root
Carum opticum	*Yavani*	Seed, oil
Carum roxburghianum	*Yavani*	Seeds
Carthamus tinctorius	*Kusumbha*	Complete plant, oil
Caryophyllus aromaticus	*Lavanga*	Flower, oil
Caseria asculenta	*Satacakra*	Flower, oil
Cassia absus	*Caksusya*, Indian almond tree	Seed
Cassia angustifolia	*Markandi*	Leaf, fruit
Cassia auriculata	*Avartaki*	Leaf, bark, fruit
Cassia deodara Roxb.	*Devadaru*	Stem, oil
Cassia fistula	*Aragwadha*	Complete plant, pulp of the fruit
Cassia occidentalis	*Kasamarda*	Seed, root, leaf
Cassia tora Linn.	*Cakramarda*	Leaf, seed
Cayratia trifolia	*Amlata*	Leaves, root
Cedrus deodaru	*Devdaru*	Leaves, bark
Ceiba pentandra	*Salmali*	Complete plant, fruit, root
Celastrus paniculata Willd.	*Jyotismati*	Seed, oil
Celosia argentea	*Siri balika*	Root, leaf, seed
Centella asiatica	*Mandukparni*	Whole plant, leaves
Celosia cristata	*Murva*	Seeds, flowers
Centipeda minima Linn.	*Chikkika*	Complete plant
Chichorium intybus	*Kasani*	Leaves
Cicer arietinum	*Chanakamla*	Leaf
Cinchona sps.	*Kunayan*	Bark, extract
Cinnamomum camphora	*Bhimasenikarpura*	Extract
Cinnamomum cassia	*Twakpatra*	Bark
Cinnamomum tamala	*Tamala*	Leaf
Cinnamomum zeylancium	*Twak*	Bark, oil
Cissampelos pareira Linn.	*Patha*	Root, complete plant
Cissus quadrangularis Linn.	*Asthisrinkhla*	Complete plant, *kanda*
Citrullus lanatus	*Indravaruni*	Whole plant
Citrus acida	*Nimbuka*	Fruit, seed, oil, leaves
Citrus limetta	*Madhu jambira*	Fruit
Citrus limon Linn.	*Jambira*	Fruit
Citrus sp.	*Amla vetas*	Root, fruit
Cleome viscosa	*Karna sphota*	Leaf, seed

Clerodendrum infortunatum	*Bhandir*	Root
Clerodendrum multiflorum	*Agnimantha*	Leaves, roots
Clerodendrum phlomidis	*Agnimantha*	Complete plant, root
Clerodendrum serratum Linn.	*Bharangi*	Root
Clitorea ternatea	*Aparajita*	Complete plant, root, seed
Coccinia indica W & A	*Bimbi*	Complete plant, root
Cocculus hirsutus Linn.	*Patala garudi*	Complete plant, leaf
Cocculus villosus Linn.	*Patala garudi*	Complete plant
Cocos nucifera	*Sriphala*	Fruit, oil
Coleus vettiveroides	*Hribera*	Leaves
Commiphora mukul	*Guggulu*	Resin
Convolvulus pluricaulis	*Sankhapuspi*	Complete plant
Coptis teeta Wall.	*Pikta mula*	Root
Corallocarpus epigaeus	*Nahi kanda*	*Kanda*
Corchorus fascicularis	*Bahuphali*	Complete plant
Cordia latifolia	*Slesmatak*	Leaf, bark, fruit
Coriandrum sativum	*Dhanyak*	Seed, leaf, oil
Coscinium fenestratum	*Kaliyaka*	Leaves
Cotoneaster racemiflora	*Yavasasarkara*	*Suskasara*
Crataeva nurvala	*Varuna*	Root, bark, leaf
Cressa cretica	*Rudanti*	Complete plant
Crinum latifolium	*Sudarsan*	*Kanda*, leaf
Crocus sativus Linn.	*Kumkum*	Pollen grains
Crotalaria juncea	*Shana*	Seed, fruit, leaf
Crotalaria verrucosa	*Shanapuspi*	Leaf, seed
Croton oblongifolius	*Asti danti*	Root
Croton tiglium Linn.	*Jayapala*	Seed
Cryptolepis buchanan	*Krisna sariva*	Bark
Cucumis melo	*Kharbuja*	Fruit, seed
Cucumis utilissimus	*Eravaru*	
Cuminum cyminum	*Jirak*	Seed, fruit
Curculigo orchioides	*Bhutala*	Leaves, root
Curculigo orchioides Gaertn.	*Swetamusali*	*Kanda*, root
Curcuma amada Roxb.	*Amragandhi hridra*	Rhizome
Cyamopsis tetragonoloba	*Guwar*	Fruit, seed, leaf
Cydonia vulgaris	*Vrihi*	Seed, fruit
Cymbopogon citratus	*Jambira truna*	Leaves, oil
Cynodon dactylon	*Durva*	Complete plant
Cynomorium coccineum	*Malta fungus*	Whole plant
Cyperus rotundus	*Musta*	Leaves, flower, root
D. stramonium	*Krisa dhattura*	Complete plant, seeds, leaves, flowers
D. zalil	*Trayamana*	Complete plant, flower
Dacus carota	*Gajar*	Seed, root, *kanda*
Daemia extensa	*Yugma kantaka*	Leaf
Dalbergia sissoo Roxb.	*Shimsapa*	Bark, stems
Datura alba	*Dhattura*	Complete plant
Datura metal	*Dhattura*	Complete plant
Delphinium denudatum	*Nirvisi, jadwar shireen*	Root, *kanda*, seed
Dendropthoe falicata	*Vriksadani*	Complete plant
Desmodium gangeticum	*Salaparni*	Complete plant
Desmostachya bipinnata	*Darba, kusa*	Root
Dichrostachys cinerea	*Virataru*	Complete plant
Digitalis purpura	*Tilapuspi*	Leaf
Dillenia indica	*Bhavya*	Fruit, leaf
Dioscorea bulbifera	*Varahi kanda*	*Kanda*
Dioscorea opposita	*Vidari bheda*, common yam	Tuber

Diospyros peregrina	*Tinduka*	Bark, fruit, oil
Digitalis purpura	*Tilapuspi*	Leaf
Dolichos biflorus	*Kulattha*	Seed
Dracaena cinnabari	*Rakta niryas*	Resin
E. glandulifera	*Dravanti*	Seed, oil, fruit
E. nerifolia	*Snuhi*	Root, stem, milk
Echinops schinatus	*Urkantaka*	Root, seed
Eclipta alba Hassk.	*Bringaraja*	Complete plant
Eichhorinia crassipes	*Jalakumbhi*	Complete plant
Elaeocarpus ganitrus Roxb.	*Rudraksa*	Seed
Elettaria cardomum	*Suksma ela*	Seed, bark
Embelia ribes Burm.	*Vidanga*	Seed
Emblica officinalis Gaertn.	*Amalaki*	Fruit, complete plant
Enicostemma littorale Blume.	*Mamajjak*	Complete plant
Ephedra vulgaris	*Soma*	Complete plant
Erythrina indica	*Paribhadra*	Leaf, bark
Eugenia caryophyllus	*Long*	Dried flower buds
Eulophia campestris	*Munjataka*	Root, *kanda*
Eulophia nuda	*Malakanda*	*Kand* (root)
Eupatorium ayapana	*Vishalyukarni ajaparna*	Leaf
Euphorbia antiquorum	*Snuhi (tridhara)*	Root
Exogonium purga	*Revakandam*	Root
F. lacor Buch-Ham.	*Plaksa*	Bark, fruit
F. religiosa Linn.	*Aswattha*	Complete plant
F. retusa	*Nandi vriksha*	Complete plant
Fagonia arabica	*Duralabha*	Complete plant
Feronia limonia	*Kapittha*	Fruit, leaf
Ferula alliacea (narthex)	*Hingu*	Resin
Ficus bengalensis Linn.	*Vata*	Prop roots, complete plant
Ficus glomerata Roxb.	*Udumbara*	Fruit, root, complete plant, milk
Ficus hispida Linn.	*Kakodumbara*	Complete plant
Foeniculum vulgare	*Misi*	Seed, root, flower
Fritillaria roylei	*Fritillary*	Whole plant
Fumaria parviflora	*Ksetra parpata*	Complete plant
G. herbaceum Linn.	*Karpasa*	Complete plant, oil, leaf
G. morella Desr.	*Kankustha*	Resin
G. tiliaefolia	*Dhanvana*	*Antastwak*
Garcinia indica Chois.	*Vriksamla*	Fruit, oil
Garcinia pedunculata	*Amlavetas*	Fruit
Gardenia gummifera	*Nadihingu*	Resin
Gloriosa superba Linn.	*Langali*	Root, *kanda*
Glycyrrhiza glabra	*Madhu yasti*	*Praknad*
Gmelina arborea Linn.	*Gambhari*	Root, bark, leaf
Gossypium arboreum	*Aranya karpasa*	Complete plant
Grewia asiatica	*Parusaka*	Fruit, bark
Grewia populifolia	*Nagabala*	Complete plant, root, bark
Gymnema sylvestre R. Br.	*Madhu nasini*	Leaf
Gymnosporia montana	*Vikankat*	Complete plant, leaf
Gynandropsis pentaphylla	*Tilaparni*	Leaf, seed
Hedychium spicatum	*Sati*	*Kanda*
Helianthus annus	*Suryapuspi*	Seed
Helicteria isora	*Avarta phala*	Fruit, root
Hemidesmus indicus R. Br.	*Anantamul*	Root
Hibiscus abelmoschus	*Latakasturi*	Seed, leaf, root
Hibiscusrosa-sinensis	*Japa*	Flower, root
Hiptage benghalensis	*Madhavi*	Root
Holarrhena antidysenterica	*Indrayava*	Seed, bark

Hordeum vulgare	*Yava, yavaksara*	Seed, *ksara*
Hydnocarpus laurifolia	*Katukapitha*	Seed, fruit, oil, pulp
Hydrocotyl asiatica	*Brahmamanduki*	Complete plant
Hyocyamus niger Linn.	*Parasik yavani*	Seed, leaf
Indigofera tinctoria	*Nili*	Flower, leaf, root, seed
Inula racemosa Hook.	*Puskaramula*	Root
Ipomoea arvensis	*Prasarinee*	Complete plant
Ipomoea digitata Linn.	*Ksiravidari*	*Kanda*
Ipomoea paniculata	*Vidar Kund*	Whole plant, root
Ipomoea reniformis	*Akhuparni*	Complete plant
Iris germanica Linn.	*Haimavati*	Root
Jasminum grandifolium Linn.	*Jati*	Flower, leaf, oil
Jasminum officinale	*Jati*	Fruits
Jasminum pubescens	*Kund*	Fruit
Jasminum sambac Linn.	*Mallika*	Flower, leaf, root
Juglans regia	*Aksota*	Fruit
Juniperus communis	*Hapusa*	Fruit
Kalanchoe pinnata	*Parnabija*	Leaf
Lagenaria siceraria	*Ikswaku*	Complete plant
Lagenaria vulgaris	*Ikswaku*	Complete plant
Lannea grandis	*Jingini*	Bark, resin
Lawsonia alba	*Madayantika*	Flower, leaf, seed
Lawsonia inermis	*Mehndi*	Leaves, flower, seeds, bark
Leonotis nepetifolia	*Dipamala*	Flower, leaf
Lepidium sativum	*Chandrasura*	Seed
Leptadenia reticulata	*Jivanti*	Whole plant, leaf
Letaria stalica	*Kangu*	Seed
Leucas cephalotes	*Dronapuspi*	Complete plant
Linum usitatissimum	*Atasi,* flaxseed husk	Seed, oil
Lippia nodiflora	*Jalapippali*	Whole plant
Liquidambar orientalis	*Silhaka*	Resin
Loranthus longiflorus	*Vandaka*	Whole plant
Luffa acutangula Linn.	*Kosataki*	Fruit, root
Madhuca longiflora	*South Indian Mahua*	Flower, fruits
Maerua arenaria	*Marata*	Whole plant
Malaxis acuminata	*Jeevak*	Whole plant
Malaxis muscifera	*Rishabak*	Whole plant
Mallotus philippinensis	*Kampillaka*	Fruits
Mammea suriga	*Nagkesar*	Flowers
Mangifera indica	*Amra*	Complete plant, resin
Mannaobambusa arundnacium	*Vasmalochana*	Whole plant
Marsdenia roylei	*Murva*	Complete plant
Melia azadirachta	*Mahanimba*	Fruit, pulp
Mentha piperita	*Podina,* peppermint	Leaves
Mentha sylvestris	*Putiha*	Complete plant
Merium odorum	*Karavira*	Root, flower, leaf
Mesua ferrea	*Nagakesara*	Stamen
Michelia champaca	*Survarna champak*	Flower, bark
Mimosa pudica	*Lajjalu*	Complete plant, seed
Mimusops elengi	*Bakula*	Fruit, flower, bark
Mimusops hexandra	*Ksirini*	Fruit, bark
Mirabilis jalapa	*Nakata*	Flower, root, *kanda*
Momordica charantia Linn.	*Karavellaka*	Fruit, leaf
Momordica cymbalaria	*Ksudrakaravellaka*	Leaf, root, fruit
Momordica dioica	*Karkotak*	Fruit, *kanda* (root)
Moringa oleifera	*Sigru*	Complete plant, fruit
Morus alba	*Tooda*	Fruit
Mucuna prurita Hook.	*Kapikachu*	Seed, fruit
Murraya koenigii	*Kaidarya*	Leaf
Musa paradisiacal	*Kadali,* plantain banana	Complete plant, root

Myrica esculenta	*Katphala*	Fruits, bark
Myrica nagi	*Katphala*	Stembark
Myristica fragrans	*Jayaphal*	Flower, seed, *kosa*
Nardostachys jatamansi DC	*Jatamansi*	Root, complete plant
Nelumbium speciosum	*Padmabija*	Seed, flower, leaf
Nelumbo nucifera	*Indian lotus*	Seeds, flowers, leaves, rhizomes
Nicotiana tabacum Linn.	*Tamakhu*	Leaf
Nigella sativa Linn.	*Prithvika*	Seed
Nyctanthes arbortristis Linn.	*Parijata*	Leaf, flower
Nymphaea alba	*Swetakamal*	Flower, leaf, root, pulp
Nymphaea rubra	*Raktakamal*	Flower, leaf, root, pulp
Nymphaea stellata	*Nilakamal, Indivari*	Flower, leaf, seed, pulp
Ochrocarpus longifolius	*Surapunnagaa*	Stamen, style, stigma
Ocimum basilum	*Tulsi*	Complete plant, leaves
Ocmum gratissimum	*Ajagandha*	Complete plant, seed
Ocimum sanctum	*Tulsi*	Leaf, seed, root
Operculina turpethum	*Trivrita, nishoth*	Root, bark, leaves
Orchis latifolia	*Munjataka*	Root, *kanda*
Origanum majorana	*Maruvaka*	Seed
Oroxylum indicum	*Syonaka*	Root, bark, seed
Oryza sativa	*Shalimula*	Root
Ougeinia dalbergioides	*Tinisa*	Seed
Oxalis corniculata	*Cangeri*	Leaf
Paederia foetida	*Gandhaprasarini*	Complete plant
Paeonia emodi	*Uood saleeb*	Seeds, flowers, roots
Pandanus odoratissimus	*Keora*	Whole plant
Pandanus tectorius	*Ketaki*	Flower, root, oil, pollen grain
Papaver somniferum	*Ahifena*	Fruit extract
Parmelia perforata	*Saileya*	*Sarvanga*
Paspalum scrobiculatum	*Kodrava*	Seed
Pavonia odorata	*Balaka*	Leaves, root
Pedalium murex Linn.	*Brihad goksura*	Fruit, complete plant
Pentapetes phoenicea	*Bandhuk*	Flower
Peristrophe bicaliculata	*Kakajangha*	Complete plant
Phaseolus mungo	*Mung Bean*	Seeds, root
Phaseolus trilobus	*Mudgaparni*	Complete plant, seed
Phoenix dactylifera	*Kharjura*	Fruit, seed
Phragmites maxima	*Nal*	Complete plant
Phyllanthus urinaria	*Bhumyamalaki*	Complete plant
Picrorhiza kurroa	*Kutaki*	Root
Pimpinella anisum	*Saunf*	Seeds
Pinus roxburghii Sargent.	*Gandhabiroja*	*Ral*, resin
Pinus succinifera	*Trinakant*	*Niryasa*
Piper aurantiacum	*Renuka*	Seeds, root
Piper betel Linn.	*Cavika*	Complete plant
Piper chaba	*Cavya*	Leaves
Piper cubeba	*Kankola*	Seed, oil
Piper longum Linn.	*Pippali*	*Kanda*, root, fruit
Piper nigrum Linn.	*Marica*	Fruit, grain
Pistacia integerrima Stewart	*Pista*	Fruit
Plantago ovata	*Snigdhajirika*, psyllium husk	Seeds
Pluchea lanceolata BC Clarke	*Rasna*	Leaf, complete plant
Plumbago indica	*Rakta Citraka*	Root
Plumbago zeylanica Linn.	*Citraka*	Root, leaf
Plumeria acutifolia	*Campak*	Flower, leaf
Polyalthia longifolia	*Devdaru*	Bark
Polygonum aviculare	*Granthi truna*	Complete plant
Pongamia glabra	*Karanja*	Bark
Pongamia pinnata	*Karnaja*	Flowers, seed, leaves, bark, root
Portulaca oleracea	*Lonika*	Leaf, seed

Prosopis spicigera	*Sami*	Leaf, bark, flower, buds, *kanda*
Prunus alochia	*Alukam*	Fruit
Prunus amygdalus	*Badam*	Fruit, seeds, bark, oil
Prunus cerasus	*Ela waluka*	Fruit
Prunus domestica	*Arkam*	Fruit
Prunus mahaleb	*Gandhapriyangu*	Fruit
Prunus persica	*Aluka, peach*	*Kanda*, fruit
Prunus puddum	*Padmakh*	Stem
Psidium guajava	*Amritaphal, Paruka*	Fruit, leaf
Psoralea corylifolia Linn.	*Bakuchi*	Seed, oil
Pterocarpus marsupium Roxb.	*Bijak*	Bark, extract, stern, resin
Pterocarpus santalinus Linn.	*Raktacandan*	*Kastha*
Ptychotis ajowan	*Yavani*	Seeds
Pueraria tuberosa	*Vidarikanda*	*Kanda*
Punica granatum Linn.	*Dadima*	Complete plant
Putranjiva roxburghii Wall.	*Putrajivak*	Fruit, root
Quercus infectoria	*Mayaphal*	Fruit
Randia dumetorum	*Madanaphala*	Fruit
Randia uliginosa	*Pinditaka*	Root, fruit
Raphanus sativa	*Mulaka, Muli*	Complete plant
Rauwolfia serpentina	*Sarpagandha*	Root
Rheum emodi Wall.	*Cuka*	Root, leaf, branch
Rhinecanthus communis	*Yudhikaparni*	Complete plant
Rhus parviflora	*Tntidaka*	Fruit
Ricinus communis Linn.	*Ernada*	Leaf, root, seed, oil
Rosa damascena	*Satapatri*, rose	Flower
Rubia cordifolia	*Manjistha*	Root, stem
Rumex vesicarius	*Cuka*	Leaf, seed
Saccharum arundinaceum	*Sara*	Root, *kandu*
Saccharum officinarum Linn.	*Iksu*	Root, stem
Saccharum spontaneum Linn.	*Kasa*	Rot
Salix alba	*Vetasa*	Stem
Salix caprea	*Vatasa*	Stem
Salmalia malabarica	*Salmali*	*Niryasa*
Salvadora oleoides	*Brihat pilu*	Leaf, fruit, oil
Salvadora persica Linn.	*Sweta candan*	*Kastasana*, oil
Santalum album	*Chandan*	Wood, oil
Sapindus trifoliatus	*Aristaka*	Fruit
Saraca indica	*Asoka*	Bark
Saussurea lappa	*Kustha*	Root
Saxifraga ligulata	*Pasanabheda*	Root
Schleichera oleosa	*Kusumbha*	Flower, seed, oil
Schrebera swieteniodes	*Muskaka*	*Ksara*
Scindapsus officinalis	*Gajapippali*	Fruit
Scirpus kysoor	*Kaseruka*	*Kanda*
Semecarpus anacardium	*Bhallatak*	Seed, fruit, pulp, bark, oil
Sesamum indicum Linn.	*Tila*	Seed, oil, root
Sesbania grandiflora	*Agastya*	Complete plant
Shorea robusta Gaertn.	*Rala, sala*	*Niryasa*
Sida cordifolia Linn.	*Bala*	Root, leaf, seed
Sida humilis	*Nagabala*	Complete plant, root
Silkworm cocoon	*Kosa*	*Kosa*
Sloanum indicum Linn.	*Brihati*	Complete plant
Smilax china	*Dwipantara vaca*	Root, rhizome
Smilax zeylanica	*Badara valli*	Root
Solanum nigrum Linn.	*Kakamaci*	Complete plant, fruit
Solanum torvum	*Kakamaci*	Whole plant, fruits, leaves, root
Solanum xanthocarpum	*Kantakari*	Complete plant
Soymida febrifuga	*Rohini*	Bark
Spathodea falcate	*Mesasringi*	Root, bark, leaf
Sphaeranthus indicus	*Sravani/mundi, Mundika*	Complete plant

Spilanthes acmella	*Maharastri*	Flower
Spinacia oleracea	*Palakya*	Leaf, seed
Spirogyra (rhizome)	*Saivala*	Complete plant
Spondias mangifera	*Amrataka*	Fruit
Stephania japonica	*Patha*	Leaves, bark, root
Stereospermum suaveolens	*Patola*	Root, fruit
Streblus asper	*Sakhotak*	Bark, *ksira*
Strychnos nux-vomica Linn.	*Visatinduka*	Seed
Strychnos potatorum Linn.	*Katak*	Seed
Styrax benzoin	*Lohabana*	Resin
Swertia chirata	*Kiratatikta*	Complete plant
Symplocos racemosa	*Lodhra*	Bark
Syzygiu m aromaticum	*Longa*	Dried flower buds
Syzygium cumini	*Jambu*	Fruit, seed, leaves, bark
Syzygium jambos	*Jambu*	Bark
Tamarindus indica	*Chinca*	Fruit, complete plant
Tamarix aphylla	*Phabuka*	Bark, *niryasa*
Taraxacum officinale	*Dugdhapheni*	Root
Taxus baccata	*Talisapatra*	Leaf
Tecoma undulata	*Raktarohitaka*	Bark
Tectona grandis	*Saka*	Flower, seed, root
Tephrosia purpurea	*Sarapunkha*	Complete plant
Terminalia arjuna	*Arjuna*	Bark
Terminalia belerica	*Bibhitaki*	*Kashta*, bark, fruit
Terminalia chebula Retz.	*Haritaki*	Fruit, bark
Terminalia tomentosa	*Sadada*	Bark
Thespesia populnea Willd.	*Parishapippali*	Leaf, flower, seed
Tinospora cordifolia Willd.	*Amrita*	Complete plant
Tragia involucrata	*Vriscikali*	Root, leaf
Trianthema monogyna Linn.	*Varsabhu*	Complete plant
Tribulus terrestris Linn.	*Goksura*	Fruit, complete plant
Trachyspermum ammi	*Yavani*	Fruits, seeds, leaves, root
Trichosanthes dioica	*Patola*	Fruits, leaves, root
Trichosanthes indica	*Patola*	Fruits, leaves, root
Trichosanthes palmata	*Mahakal*	Fruit
Trigonella foenum-graecum	*Methika*	Seed, leaf
Triticum aestivum	*Godhuma*	Whole plant
Typha elephantina	*Eraka*	Flower, root
Uraria picta	*Prisniparni*	Complete plant
Urginea indica	*Vanapalandu*	*Kanda*
Valeriana officinalis	*Tagara*	Rhizomes
Valeriana wallichii	*Tagar*	*Kasta*, root
Vanda tessellata	*Ichneumon* plant	Whole plant
Vernonia anthelmintica	*Krsnajiraka*	Seed, fruit
Vernonia cinerea	*Sahadevi*	Complete plant
Vetiveira zizanioides	*Usira*	Leaves, root
Vigna mungo	*Masha*, black gram	Seeds, root
Vitex agnus-castus	*Renuka bija*	Seed
Vitex negundo	*Nirgundi*	Seed, fruit
Vitis vinifera	*Draksa*	Fruit
Withania somnifera	*Aswagandha*	Root
Woodfordia fruticosa	*Dhataki*	Flower, root
Xanthoxylum alatum	*Tumbaru*	Seed, fruit
Zingiber officinale	*Sunthi*	Dry root
Zingiber officinale	*Ardraka*	*Kanda*
Zizyphus jujuba	*Badari*	Fruit, seed, leaf, root
Zizyphus vulgaris	*Sauvira*	Fruit pulp

Appendix 3:

List of Ayurvedic Scientific Journals

1. *Journal of Research in Ayurveda and Siddha*
   Publisher: Central Council for Research in Ayurveda and Siddha (CCRAS)
   Director: CCRAS
   Jawahar Lal Nehru Bhartiya Chikitsa Avum Homeopathy Anusandhan Bhavan
   No. 61-65
   Institutional Area
   Opp. 'D' Block
   Janakpuri, New Delhi, 110 058, India
   Tel.: 91-011-5614970/71/72
   Fax: 91-011-5528748
   E-mail: ccras@ndf.vsnl.net.in or ccras@del6.vsnl.net.in
2. *Bulletin of Medico-Ethno-Botanical Research*
   Publisher: CCRAS
3. *Bulletin of Indian Institute of History of Medicine*
   Publisher: CCRAS
4. *Ancient Science of Life*
   Publisher: AVR Educational Foundation of Ayurveda
   1382 Trichy Rd.
   Coimbatore, 641 018, India
5. *Arya Vaidyan*
   Publisher: Publication Division, Arya Vaidya Sala
   Kottakkal, 676 503, Kerala State, India
6. *Ayu*
   Publisher: Gujarat Ayurved University
   Jamnagar, Gujarat, India

For combined general and scientific articles:

1. *Heritage Healing*
   Publisher: Healthcare Communications Pvt. Ltd.
   #8, 5th Cross Extension
   Bakthavachalam Nagar, Adyar
   Chennai, 600 020, India

Tel.: 91-44-4422780
E-mail: heritagehealing@usa.net

2. *Holistic Healing*
Publisher: Indian Express Newspapers Pvt. Ltd.
Business Publication Division
1st Floor, Manandi Plaza, Express Towers
Nariman Point, Mumbai, 400 021, India
Tel.: 2301020
E-mail: bpdhqbom4.vsnl.net.in
3. *Ayur Medline*
Publisher: Seetharam Prasad
124/2, near Ganesh Temple
7th B- main road iv the Block Jaynagar
Bangalore, 560 011, India
Tel.: 91-080/6349314
E-mail: ayurmedline@mailcity.com

For publishing matters related to any aspect of medicinal plant research, the following journals can be considered:

1. *Indian Journal of Medical Research* (ICMR)
2. *Indian Journal of Experimental Biology*
3. *Indian Journal of Pharmacology*
4. *Indian Journal of Physiology and Pharmacology*
5. *Current Science*
6. *Journal of Phytotaxonomy*
7. *Indian Drugs*
8. *Indian Journal of Pharmaceutical Sciences*
9. *Indian Journal of Medical Sciences*
10. *Journal of Natural Remedies*

Appendix 4:

Ayurvedic Product Manufacturers

Manufacturers of Ayurvedic products were identified by the chapter contributors and are listed in alphabetic order. Sequoia Inc. USA may be contacted for further information.

AIMIL Pharmaceuticals Pvt. Ltd.
2994/4, Street No. 17
New Delhi, 110 008
India

Almasaguda Village
Badangpet P.O. Hyderabad, 500 058
India
Tel.: 040-24652472(O), 24751490 (R)
Fax: 040-4759109
Web site: www.amritayaurveda.com

Anglo-French Drugs and Industries Ltd.
41, 3rd cross, 5th Block
Rajaji Nagar, Bangalore, 560 010
India

Anjali Pharma, 48-B.Sector
'C' Mandi-Deep, Pin: 462 046
India
Tel.: 07480-33905, 52050
Fax: 07480-33634

Arya Aushadhi Pharmaceutical Works
Indore, 452 008
India
E-mail: kuki@bom4.vsnl.net.in

Arya Vaidya Pharmacy (Coimbatore) Ltd.
326, Perumal Koli St.
Ramanathapuram, Coimbatore, 641 045
India

Arya Vaidya Sala
Kottakal, 676 503
Kerala, India
Tel.: 742216-19,744261-64
Fax: 0493-742210/742572
E-mail: kottakal@vsnl.com
Web site: kottakal@md3.vsnl.net.in

Ayucare Pharma
Near Income Tax Office
Ashram Road
Ahmedabad, India
Tel.: 079-7541814

Ayudrugs
Shop No. 4, Fancy Bazar
Guwahati, 781 001
Assam, India

Ayurvedeeya Arkashala Ltd.
1915/4, Mannar's Market, Shivrampet
Mysore, 570 001
India

Bajaj Consumer Care Ltd.
17-1-204-8, Saidabad
Hyderabad, 500 059
India

Ban Labs Ltd.
Ban House, Gondal Rd.
Rajkot, 360 004
India
E-mail: banlabs@bigfool.com
Web site: www.banlab.com

Capro Labs Exports India Ltd.
1109, S.H. Layout
Kaval Byrasandra
P.B. No. 3240
Bangalore, 560 032
India

Charak Pharmaceuticals
Evergreen Ind. Estate
Mumbai, 400 011
India

Dabur Ayurvedic Specialities Ltd.
Koushambi, Sahibabad, 201010
Gaziabad (UP), India

Dey's Medical Stores Pvt. Ltd.
41 Chowringhee Rd.
Calcutta, India

Dindayal Aushadhalaya
Daulataganja
Gwalior, 474 001
India

Dubagunta Nivas
Kari Marx Rd .
Vijayawada, Hydarabad, 520 002
India
Fax: 0866-571666
E-mail: imispharma@etn.net

Fraco-Indian Pharmaceuticals Ltd.
No. 20, Dr. E. Moses Rd.
Mumbai, 400 011
India

Garry and Son
550E Plum Lane, Suite 301/306
Reno, Nevada 89502
U.S.A.

Herbal Doctor Remedies
499 Cumber St.
Monterey Park, California
U.S.A.

Herbicure Pvt. Ltd.
Herbochem Remedies, India (P) Ltd.
Regd. Office & Works at Narendrapur
743508 Sales Office: 45
Pratap Aditya Palace
Calcutta, Bengal, 700 026
India

Himalaya Drug House
Makali, Bangalore, 562 123
India

Himalayan Drug Company
Lowrence Rd.
New Delhi, India
Web site: www.thehimalayadrugco.com

Imis Pharmaceuticals Pvt. Ltd.
Dubagunta Nivas, Karl Marx Rd.
Vijayawada, Hyderabad, 520 002
India

Indian Medical Practitioner's
Co-operative Pharmacy & Stores —
(IMPCOPS) Ltd.
X-185, 34-37, Kalki Krishnamurthy
Salai, Thiruvan miyur
Chennai, 600 041
India
Tel.: 11029, 4911189, 4917344
Fax: 4913313. GRAMS. DASAMULA, P.B.
No. 8602
E-mail: impcops@vsnl.net

Indian Medicines Pharmaceutical Corporation
Ltd. (IMPCL)
Mohan, Almora
Ramnagar 244 715
Uttranchal, India

J & J Dechane Lab. Pvt. Ltd.
4-1-324, Residency Rd.
Hyderabad, 500 001
India

Jamana Pharma
48.B. Sector ‘C’, Mandi Deep
Bhopal, Madhya Pradesh, 462 046
India
Web site: www.jamanapharma.com
Tel.: 33905, 52050

Jark Pharma Pvt. Ltd.
13/12, M.P.Shah, Municipal Industrial Estate
Sarusecation Rd.
Jamnagar, 361 002
Gujarat, India
Tel.: (0)0288-664200
Fax: 91-288-540267
Web site: www.globalremediesindia.com

Kerala Ayurveda Pharmacy Ltd.
Athani Post Office, 683 585
Aluva, Kerala, India

KV Health Care Pdts. Pvt. Ltd.
304, Lokhandwala Complex
Mumbai, 400 058
Maharashtra, India

Maharshi Ayurveda Corp. Ltd.
A14 Mohan Estate, Mathura Rd. N.
Delhi, 110 044
India
E-mail: mprl@blr.vsnl.net.in

Merind Pharmaceuticals Ltd. (MPL)
G.P. Box 10081
Mulund Goregaon Link Rd. Bhandup
Mumbai, 400 067
India

Millenium Herbal Care Ltd.
Film Centre, Ground Floor
68 Tardeo Rd.
Mumbai, 400 034
India

Multani Pharmaceuticals Ltd.
New Delhi, India
E-mail: multaniayurveda@hotmail.com
Web site: www.multaniayurveda.com

Nagarjuna Herbal Concentrates Ltd.
Kalayanthani
Thodupuzha, 685 588
Idukki Dt.
Kerala, India

Nagarjuna Pharmaceuticals
c-1/1114 -B, Phase-IV, g.i.d.c. aroda
Ahemadabad, 382 330
Gujarat, India

Nupal Remedies Pvt. Ltd.
Nupal Rd.
Kadavanthra P.O., P.B. No. 2051
Kochi, 682 020
India
E-mail: inquiry@nupalremedies.com
Web site: www.nupalremedies.com

Penn Herb Company
Philadelphia, Pennsylvania 19154
U.S.A.
Tel.: 022-4307021/4304517-18
Fax: 022-4375491

Phyto Pharma Pvt. Ltd.
Plot No. 3, "E", Torna Nagar, Sagarmal
Kolhapur, 416 008
Maharashtra, India

Rajashree Ayurvedic Pharmacy
Rajashree Main Rd.
Ambalpady
Udupi, 576 103
Kerala, India

Rucha Pharma, Opp.
Daria Purgat, Ahmedabad
Gujrat, India
Tel.: 079-2123495

Sandu Brothers Pvt. Ltd.
Sandu Nagar
D.K. Sandu Marg
Chembur, Mumbai, 400 071
Maharashtra, India

Sequoia Inc., Division of
Ayurvedic Dietary Supplements and
Text Formulations
13505 Cleveland Dr.
Rockville, Maryland 20850
U.S.A.
Tel.: 301-762-8262
Web site: www.Lcmishra.com

Shree Baidyanath Ayurved Bhawan Ltd.
1 Gupta Lane
Calcutta, 700 006
Bengal, India
Web site: www.baidyanathayurved.com

Shree Bhuvaneshwari Aushadhashram
Gondal, 360 311
Gujarat, India
Tel.: 02825-22445/22446/22447
Fax: 02825-21195/20599
E-mail: bhuvaneshwaripith@usa.net

Shree Dhanwantari Ayurvedic Pharmacy
277 East Mohan Nagar
Amritasar, Punjab, India

Shree Dhoothpapaeshwar Ltd.
135, Nanubhai Desai Rd.
Khetwadi, Mumbai
Maharashtra, 400 004
India
Tel.: 022-3825888
Fax: 022-3881308
E-mail: sdiho@sdindia.com;
sales@sdindia.com

Sri Dhanwantari Matam Ayurvedics Pvt. Ltd.
Ambujavilasam Rd.
Pulimoodu, Trivandrum 695 001
India

Swastik Formulations Pvt. Ltd.
Gangotri II, B-27/35-8, Ravindrapuri Extn.
Varanasi, 221 005
U.P., India
Tel.: +91 222 4307021
Fax: +91 222 4375491

Unjha Ayurvedic Pharmacy
Station Road, Unjha, 384 170
Gujarat, India
Tel.: (02767)53583
Fax: (02767) 54836

UNJHA, UAP Pharma Pvt. Ltd.
Mahagujarath Industrial Estate
Plot No.423/98, A-B Sarkhej Bawala Rd.
Moraiya, 382 213
Tq. Sanand Dist., Ahmedabad
India

Vaidyaratnam Oushadhasala,
Ollur, Thaikkattussery
Thrissur, 680 322
India
E-mail: vaidyaratnam@yahoo.com
Web site: www.vaidyaratnam-moss.com

Vasu Pharmaceuticals Ltd.
967/4, GIDC, Makarpura
Vadodara, 390 010
India

Venkateswara Ayurveda Nilayam Pvt. Ltd.
Chintaluru, 533 232
A.P., India

Viable Herbal Solutions Comp.
Morrisville, Pennsylvania
U.S.A.

Vyas Pharmaceuticals
98-C, Sanwar Road, Sector-E,
Behind Choutha Sansar,
Indore, 452 015
Madhya Pradesh, India
Web site: www.aryavaidyasala.com

Zandu Pharmaceutical Works Ltd.
70, Gokhale Road South
Mumbai 400 025
Maharqashtra, India
Tel.: (022) 4307021, 4304517, 4304518
Telegram: "Zandu" Mumbai
Fax: (91) (22) 4375491
E-mail: zanduho@giasbm01.vsnl.net.in

Index

E

F

G

I

N

Q

R

U

V

W

Y

Z